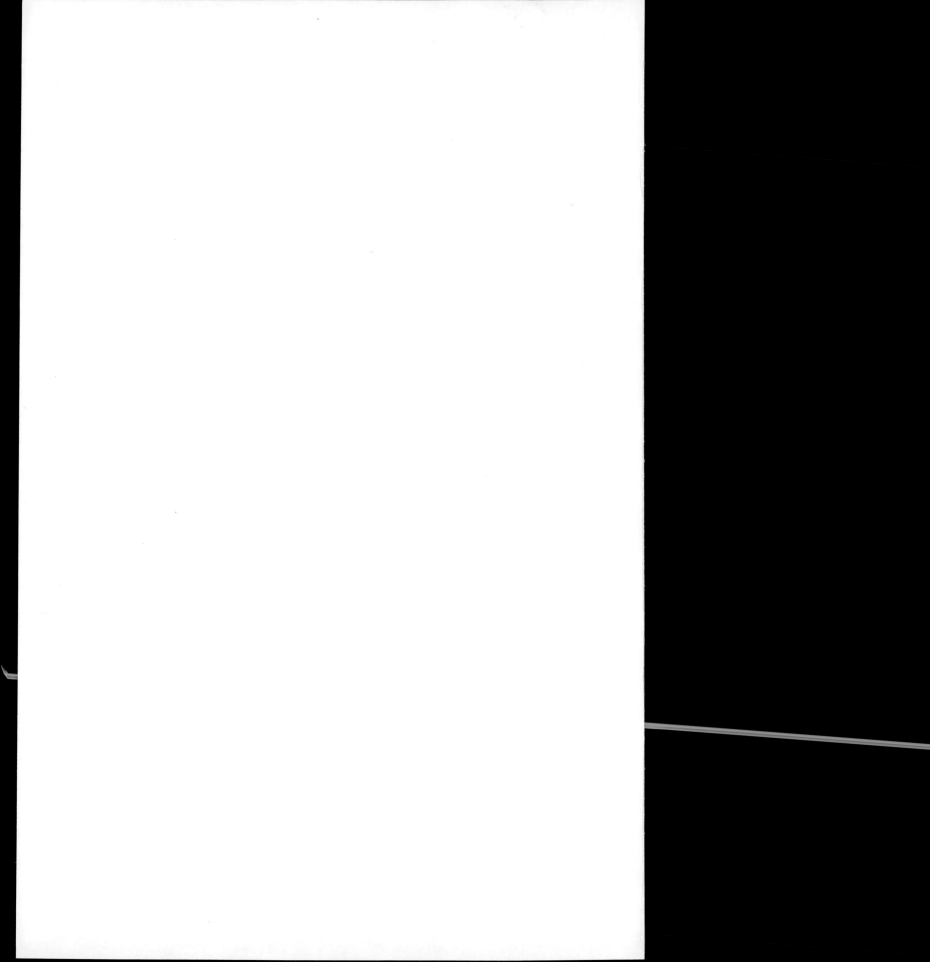

Streptococcal Infections

Streptococcal Infections

Clinical Aspects, Microbiology, and Molecular Pathogenesis

Edited by

DENNIS L. STEVENS, M.D., Ph.D.

Chief, Infectious Diseases
Veterans Affairs Medical Center
Boise, Idaho
Professor of Medicine
University of Washington School of Medicine
Seattle, Washington

and

EDWARD L. KAPLAN, M.D.

Professor of Pediatrics
University of Minnesota Medical School
Minneapolis, Minnesota

New York   Oxford
OXFORD UNIVERSITY PRESS
2000

Oxford University Press

Oxford   New York
Athens   Auckland   Bangkok   Bogotá   Buenos Aires   Calcutta
Cape Town   Chennai   Dar es Salaam   Delhi   Florence   Hong Kong   Istanbul
Karachi   Kuala Lumpur   Madrid   Melbourne   Mexico City   Mumbai
Nairobi   Paris   São Paulo   Singapore   Taipei   Tokyo   Toronto   Warsaw

and associated companies in
Berlin   Ibadan

Library of Congress Cataloging-in-Publication Data
Streptococcal infections : clinical aspects, microbiology, and molecular pathogenesis /
edited by Dennis L. Stevens and Edward L. Kaplan.
p.   cm.   Includes bibliographical references and index.
ISBN 0-19-509921-4
1. Streptococcal infections.
I. Stevens, Dennis L.   II. Kaplan, Edward L.
[DNLM: 1. Streptococcal Infections—physiopathology.   2. Streptococcal Infections—microbiology.
3. Streptococcal Infections—prevention & control.
WC 210 S9156 1999]   RC116.S84S775   1999   616.9'2—dc21
DNLM/DLC   for Library of Congress   98-55466

The science of medicine is a rapidly changing field. As new research and clinical experience broaden our knowledge, changes in treatment and drug therapy do occur. The author and the publisher of this work have checked with sources believed to be reliable in their efforts to provide information that is accurate and complete, and in accordance with the standards accepted at the time of publication. However, in light of the possibility of human error or changes in the practice of medicine, neither the author, nor the publisher, nor any other party who has been involved in the preparation or publication of this work warrants that the information contained herein is in every respect accurate or complete. Readers are encouraged to confirm the information contained herein with other reliable sources, and are strongly advised to check the product information sheet provided by the pharmaceutical company for each drug they plan to administer.

1 2 3 4 5 6 7 8 9

Printed in the United States of America
on acid-free paper

This book is dedicated to the millions of children and adults who have experienced one of the many types of streptococcal infections and their sequelae. The impact, whether from a comparatively simple infection such as pharyngitis, impetigo, and otitis media, or from a more serious and life-threatening consequence of infection such as rheumatic heart disease, toxic shock syndrome, pneumonia, meningitis, or neonatal sepsis is always significant. It is perhaps ironic that through the resulting pain and suffering of these patients, unique and innovative epidemiologic, clinical, and basic science observations have provided insight into the pathogenesis of these infections. The significance and the impact of streptococcal infections have been evident in the large and still recurring epidemics that have affected enormous numbers of people during the last centuries. Though much of our understanding of the epidemiology of all streptococcal infections is based upon studies from industrialized countries, the magnitude of these infections appears to continue to be much greater in developing countries. It is our responsibility as clinicians and scientists to assure that this suffering can be transcribed into faster and more accurate diagnosis, new and more efficient treatments, and—equally important—cost-effective preventive measures.

This volume is also dedicated to the clinicians, epidemiologists, individuals with expertise in public health issues, and basic scientists who have made prodigious contributions to our still admittedly incomplete understanding of the pathogenetic mechanisms and epidemiology of streptococcal infections and their sequelae. Although this book describes, acknowledges the importance of, and references their work, we would specifically like to acknowledge posthumously their dedication and contributions. It is impossible to cite everyone, but special mention should be made of O.T. Avery, Burtis Breese, Edwin Beachey, Alvin Coburn, George and Gladys Dick, Hugh C. Dillon, Alphonse R. Dochez, F. Griffith, Rebecca Lancefield, Charles W. Rammelkamp, Jr., Jiri Rotta, and Lewis W. Wannamaker.

We all—patients, clinicians, and laboratory scientists alike—also must acknowledge another group of individuals who have made major contributions to the understanding of streptococcal infections and who continue to serve as mentors, colleagues, and sometimes even as knowledgeable critics. It is their work, guidance, and ideas that provide direction for contemporary and future research efforts: Joseph Alouf, Robert Austrian, Paul Beeson, Geoffrey Coleman, Richard Facklam, Issac Ginsberg, Richard Krause, Benedict Massell, W.R. Maxted, Macylyn McCarty, Tom Parker, Robert Petersdorf, Gene Stollerman, Angelo Taranta, Werner Köhler, R.E.O. Williams, and many others who are too numerous to acknowledge here.

Preface

For centuries the streptococci and the resulting infections have continued as enigmas, whether for the practicing medical professional, the epidemiologist, the public health expert, or the basic scientist. The infections caused by these organisms have never been completely understood. Thus, the control and prevention of these infections and their sequelae, either for benefit of the individual patient or for the public's health, have remained problematic. The late 20th century resurgence of group A streptococcal infections and their complications confirms this.

Having been responsible for major outbreaks associated with significant morbidity and mortality in the past, the group A streptococcus has remained a major pathogen in all geographic and socioeconomic settings. Group A streptococcal infections continue to be very common in children; yet, in the industrialized world, acute rheumatic fever has become extraordinarily uncommon. This is in marked contrast to the industrializing countries of the world, countries that constitute almost two-thirds of the world's population, where streptococcal problems in general and rheumatic fever in particular remain very significant health problems.

But the group A streptococcus is not alone in its capability to baffle practitioners and scientists alike. The lethality of group B streptococci for otherwise normal newborns has had a significant impact on the practice of both pediatrics and of obstetrics. The mysterious and relatively sudden appearance of strains of *Streptococcus pneumoniae* with resistance to multiple antibiotics (including penicillin) has resulted in important modifications in the management of patients with pneumococcal infection, whether otitis media or meningitis. The role of the oral streptococci, whether as a cause of dental caries and gingivitis or as the etiologic agents in infective endocarditis, has not been completely defined. Finally, the enterococci have emerged as major nosocomial pathogens, not because of increased virulence but because of absolute antibiotic resistance.

As one examines the epidemiologic history of the streptococcal species, it appears that from the end of the first half of the 20th century to the beginning of the 1980s, many of these organisms were essentially ignored and were almost considered nuisance infections. This changed rapidly, with the result that suddenly practitioners and public health authorities were confronted with organisms that no longer could be taken for granted and were no longer necessarily easily controlled. Despite a virtual explosion in the knowledge and understanding about the streptococci resulting in significant progress in the ability to understand their physiology in the laboratory and to further define their epidemiology in the field, numerous important questions remain unanswered as the next millennium begins.

Upon reflection, we realized that no comprehensive volume specifically addressing the problems created by these streptococci had been published in many years. With this in mind, we have attempted to bring together the assessment of recognized authorities in order to define the current understanding of epidemiology, physiology, and pathophysiology of these microorganisms. Thanks to the unselfish contributions made by our many colleagues who have contributed, we hope this volume will assist readers in understanding more about these organisms and perhaps encourage further advances in the understanding of the epidemiology and pathogenesis of streptococcal infections and their resulting complications. The book is not meant for any single group of scientists or practitioners. We hope that an encompassing approach will prove beneficial to those in all of these involved disciplines, and ultimately to the care of patients.

Boise, Idaho   D.L.S.
Minneapolis, Minn.   E.L.K.
September 1999

Contents

Contributors

BASCOM F. ANTHONY, M.D.
Biologics Consulting Group, LLC
Alexandria, VA

ARIS P. ASSIMACOPOULOS, M.D.
Department of Microbiology
University of Minnesota Medical School
Minneapolis, MN

ELIA M. AYOUB, M.D.
Department of Pediatrics
University of Florida College of Medicine
Gainesville, FL

CAROL J. BAKER, M.D.
Departments of Pediatrics, Microbiology, and
    Immunology
Baylor College of Medicine
Houston, TX

ALAN BISNO, M.D.
Department of Medicine
Veteran's Affairs Medical Center
University of Miami School of Medicine
Miami, FL

DAVID BRILES, PH.D.
Department of Microbiology
University of Alabama at Birmingham
Birmingham, AL

PATRICK CLEARY, PH.D.
Department of Microbiology
University of Minnesota Medical School
Minneapolis, MN

MADELAINE W. CUNNINGHAM, PH.D.
Departments of Microbiology and Immunology
University of Oklahoma Health Sciences Center
Oklahoma City, OK

JAMES B. DALE, M.D.
Department of Medicine
Veteran's Affairs Medical Center
University of Tennessee, Memphis
Memphis, TN

JUDY A. DALY, PH.D.
Department of Pathology
Primary Children's Medical Center
University of Utah Medical School
Salt Lake City, UT

FLOYD W. DENNY, JR., M.D.
Department of Pediatrics
University of North Carolina School of Medicine
Chapel Hill, NC

KATHRYN EDWARDS, M.D.
Department of Pediatrics
Vanderbilt University School of Medicine
Nashville, TN

JOSEPH FERRETTI, PH.D.
Department of Microbiology and Immunology
University of Oklahoma Health Sciences Center
Oklahoma City, OK

PATRICIA FERRIERI, M.D.
Departments of Pediatrics, Laboratory Medicine
    and Pathology
University of Minnesota Medical School
Minneapolis, MN

VINCENT A. FISCHETTI, PH.D.
Laboratory of Bacterial Pathogenesis and
    Immunology
The Rockefeller University
New York, NY

J. MILTON GAVIRIA, M.D.
Department of Medicine
University of Washington School of Medicine
Seattle, WA

MICHAEL A. GERBER, M.D.
National Institute of Allergy and Infectious
    Diseases
National Institutes of Health
Bethesda, MD

MICHAEL S. GILMORE, PH.D.
Departments of Microbiology and Immunology, and
    Ophthalmology
University of Oklahoma Health Sciences Center
Oklahoma City, OK

BARRY GRAY, M.D.
Departments of Pediatrics, Microbiology and
    Immunology
Medical University of South Carolina
Spartanburg Regional Medical Center
Spartanburg, SC

MARK HERZBERG, D.D.S., PH.D.
Department of Preventive Sciences
University of Minnesota School of Dentistry
Minneapolis, MN

STIG HOLM, M.D.
Department of Clinical Bacteriology
University of Umea
Umea, SWEDEN

EDWARD L. KAPLAN, M.D.
Department of Pediatrics
University of Minnesota Medical School
Minneapolis, MN

DENNIS L. KASPER, M.D.
Channing Laboratory
Department of Medicine
Brigham and Women's Hospital
Harvard Medical School
Boston, MA

MALAK KOTB, PH.D.
Departments of Surgery, Microbiology and
    Immunology

Veteran's Affairs Medical Center
University of Tennessee, Memphis
Memphis, TN

MILTON MARKOWITZ, M.D.
Department of Pediatrics
University of Connecticut Medical School
Farmington, CT

DIANA R. MARTIN, PH.D.
New Zealand Communicable Disease Center
Institute of Environmental Science and Research
Porirua, NEW ZEALAND

WILLIAM MICHAEL MCSHAN, M.D.
Departments of Microbiology and Immunology
University of Oklahoma Health Sciences Center
Oklahoma City, OK

VICTOR NIZET, M.D.
Department of Pediatrics
University of California San Diego School of
    Medicine
San Diego, CA

ANNIKA NORDSTRAND, PH.D.
Department of Clinical Bacteriology
University of Umea
Umea, SWEDEN

MARI NORGREN, PH.D.
Department of Clinical Bacteriology
University of Umea
Umea, SWEDEN

KRISTEN HOIKKA PRITCHARD, M.D.
Department of Microbiology
University of Minnesota Medical School
Minneapolis, MN

MANUELA ROGGIANI, M.D.
Department of Microbiology
University of Minnesota Medical School
Minneapolis, MN

CRAIG RUBENS, M.D., PH.D.
Department of Pediatrics
Children's Hospital and Regional Medical Center
University of Washington School of Medicine
Seattle, WA

PATRICK SCHLIEVERT, PH.D.
Department of Microbiology
University of Minnesota Medical School
Minneapolis, MN

STANFORD T. SHULMAN, M.D.
Department of Pediatrics
Children's Memorial Hospital
Northwestern University Medical School
Chicago, IL

DENNIS L. STEVENS, M.D., PH.D.
Department of Medicine
Veteran's Affairs Medical Center
Boise, ID
University of Washington School of Medicine
Seattle, WA

LARRY J. STRAUSBAUGH, M.D.
Department of Medicine
Veteran's Affairs Medical Center
Oregon Health Sciences University
Portland, OR

EDWIN SWIATLO, M.D.
Department of Microbiology
University of Alabama at Birmingham
Birmingham, AL

ROBERT R. TANZ, M.D.
Department of Pediatrics
Children's Memorial Hospital
Northwestern University Medical School
Chicago, IL

MICHAEL R. WESSELS, M.D.
Channing Laboratory
Department of Medicine
Brigham & Women's Hospital
Harvard Medical School
Boston, MA

History of Hemolytic Streptococci and Associated Diseases

FLOYD W. DENNY, JR.

The history of hemolytic streptococci and the diseases associated with this remarkable organism is exceedingly complex. Streptococci cause a wide array of suppurative infections in most organs of the body and, and in addition, cause the nonsuppurative sequelae rheumatic fever and glomerulonephritis. The diseases caused by the streptococcus were described many years before the streptococcus was recognized and the relationship between group A streptococci and the nonsuppurative sequelae was not recognized until well into the 20th century. This history will attempt to paint a picture of this remarkable bacterium in all of its many roles in this saga.

THE STREPTOCOCCUS

Globular organisms growing in chains were recognized by many investigators in the last part of the 19th century [1]. Billroth is credited with using the term streptococcus (from two Greek words: *streptos*, meaning twisted or chain, and *kokhos*, meaning a berry or seed) in 1874 [2]. Classification of these bacteria proved to be a large problem. Because specific diseases, such as scarlet fever, erysipelas, and puerperal fever, had been recognized for many years, streptococci were frequently classified according to the source from which they were recovered—*Strep-*

tococcus erysipelatis, Streptococcus scarlatinae, Streptococcus puerperalis and *Streptococcus pyogenes* [1]. Classification began to show some order when Schotmüller, in 1903, determined that streptococci produced various kinds of hemolysis on blood agar plates [1]. In 1919 Brown, in an extensive treatise, described the hemolysis produced by streptococci on blood agar as we know it today: alpha, partial, or green hemolysis; beta, clear hemolysis; and gamma, no hemolysis [3]. It was left to the grand lady of the streptococcus, Rebecca Lancefield (Fig. 1.1) to develop the system for classifying the streptococcus serologically; she first classified the organism according to the group-specific polysaccharide and then categorized group A strains into specific types according to the M protein in the cell wall [4]. M protein is especially important; in addition to allowing classification, it is also a virulence factor and antibodies developed to it are protective. At about the same time of Lancefield's observations Griffith differentiated group A strains into types with a slide agglutination test based on T rather than M antigens [5].

There are several other highlights in the history of the streptococcus that deserve mention. In 1932 Todd developed a test for measuring antibodies to streptolysin O, thus allowing demonstration of the host's response to the organism

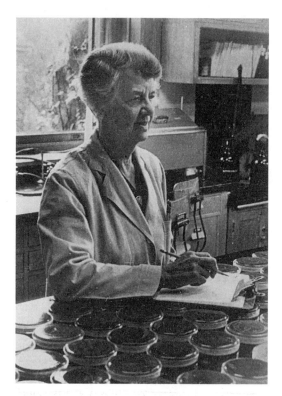

Figure 1.1 Rebecca C. Lancefield. (From Denny [21], with permission.)

[6]. Methods were developed later to measure antibodies to other extracellular antigens such as hyaluronidase and deoxyribonuclease B. The erythrogenic toxins (now termed pyrogenic exotoxins) were described by the Dicks in 1924 [7,8]. Also noteworthy was the finding that sheep red blood cells incorporated into agar plates simplified the isolation and identification of hemolytic streptococci, especially group A organisms [9]. This has become the standard for use in streptococcal laboratories throughout the world. Finally, the development of rapid methods for identifying group A carbohydrates in swabs of the throat, the so-called rapid strep test, facilitated management of patients with pharyngitis [10].

At least 13 serological groups of streptococci have been identified. The group A streptococcus, *Streptococcus pyogenes*, is the most important of these and is the streptococcus that is most intimately associated with the history of hemolytic streptococci. Non–group A streptococci can also cause occasional infections in humans.

The group B streptococcus is a common cause of serious infections in the newborn period and since the 1960s has been the most frequent cause of neonatal meningitis [11]. Groups C and G can also cause pharyngitis but do not cause rheumatic fever and only group C has been associated rarely with acute glomerulonephritis [12,13]. Several of the non–group A organisms are the cause of infections in animals. The remainder of this history will be restricted to the history of the group A streptococcus and associated human diseases.

DISEASES ASSOCIATED WITH GROUP A STREPTOCOCCUS

The diseases associated with the group A streptococcus are listed in Table 1.1. Several of these—scarlet fever, erysipelas, puerperal fever and pharyngitis—were recognized long before streptococci were described and have histories that are peculiar to each. They will be addressed separately below. The remainder of the chapter will be devoted to the relationship of the group A streptococcus to rheumatic fever and acute glomerulonephritis.

Scarlet Fever

Scarlet fever has been recognized as a clinical entity for centuries, but it was not until Syden-

Table 1.1 Diseases Associated with the Group A Streptococcus

Suppurative Infections	Nonsuppurative Sequelae
Arthritis	Acute rheumatic fever
Cellulitis	Acute glomerulonephritis
Erysipelas	
Fasciitis	
Impetigo	
Lymphadenitis	
Mastoiditis	
Meningitis	
Osteomyelitis	
Otitis media	
Pericarditis	
Peritonitis	
Pharyngitis	
Pneumonia/empyema	
Puerperal fever	
Scarlet fever	
Sinusitis	
Vaginitis	

ham, in the latter part of the 17th century, gave it its present name and separated it clinically from measles [1]. Shortly after the recognition of the streptococcus several investigators associated these organisms with typical cases of scarlet fever. For some time it was not clear whether the streptococcus was the cause of scarlet fever or a secondary infection. About the turn of the century typical streptococci were identified from the throats of most scarlet fever cases. This observation, plus the isolation of the streptococcus from the blood of a surprisingly high proportion of severe infections, established the streptococcus as the cause of scarlet fever. Extensive efforts were made to classify these organisms, first called *Streptococcus scarlatinae*, but they were not adequately classified until much later. Another hotly debated issue was whether the streptococcus produced scarlet fever by a direct action of the organism itself or a toxin produced by the streptococcus. This issue was at least partly resolved in 1918 when Schultz and Charlton showed that serum from a convalescent scarlet fever patient caused blanching of the rash when injected intradermally into the skin of a patient with active disease (Schultz-Charlton test) [1,2]. This was confirmed further by the Dicks who showed that a toxin separated from the organism produced localized erythematous reactions when injected into the skin of susceptible patients. Conversely, the failure to produce a reaction indicated an immune subject (Dick test) [7,8]. The erythrogenic toxins of the streptococcus (now called streptococcal pyrogenic exotoxins) have received a lot of attention; at least 3 have been identified (A, B, and C), the last as recently as 1960 [14]. It is being postulated that these exotoxins are associated with presently occurring severe infections, but at this time their precise role in disease is not clear.

In recent years scarlet fever has been a mild disease, frequently described as a usual case of streptococcal pharyngitis with a rash. This is in sharp contrast to the devastating infections seen in the 19th century [15]. Precise epidemiological, clinical, and laboratory data are not available to make an adequate comparison between the two eras, but the recent reappearance of severe streptococcal infections, including rheumatic fever, in the 20th century suggests a cyclic phenomenon and that we again may be faced with scarlet fever as a killing disease.

Erysipelas

Erysipelas (from two Greek words meaning red skin), freqently called St. Anthony's fire, has been recognized as long as there have been written records of disease [1]. Until the streptococcus was recognized as its cause, it is probable, however, that other clinical diseases were included in these early descriptions. Fehleisen in 1882–1883 was the first to accurately associate the streptococcus with erysipelas [1]. Subsequently, for many years the streptococci isolated from typical cases were called *Streptococcus erysipelatis* because of the possibility that all cases of erysipelas were caused by a single strain of bacteria. It was not until the modern classification of streptococci by Lancefield was developed that this issue was clarified. The great frequency of erysipelas in the last half of the 19th century is in sharp contrast to its infrequency today. The reason for this is unknown but possibly is related to the great decrease in all severe streptococcal infections at the same time.

Puerperal Fever

Historically, puerperal fever ("childbed fever" was also used at one time) was clearly one of the most deadly of all diseases; outbreaks with a mortality rate of 50% or more were not unusual [16]. Its history can be divided conveniently into two eras, before and after the middle of the 19th century. The first era was characterized by its recognition as a contagious disease and its control by aseptic techniques. In 1795, Alexander Gordon, determined that puerperal fever was a communicable disease. This was confirmed in the mid-1800s by Thomas Watson in England and Oliver Wendell Homes in the United States who proposed that infections were spread from infected patients and autopsies by the hands of physicians and medical students. These observations were hotly opposed by the obstetric community until Semmelweis, in 1846, presented unequivocal proof that puerperal fever can be caused by lack of hand washing of attending physicians and medical students. When Semmelweis' techniques were practiced the mortality of puerpual fever was reduced. This era occurred before the streptococcus was recognized as its most frequent cause.

The second era extended from the time of discovery of the streptococcus until the present time. At first strains isolated from patients were classified as *Streptococcus puerperalis* because it was thought that, as with other streptococcal entities, a single strain of bacteria was the cause [1]. At one time puerperal fever was associated so frequently with erysipelas it was postulated that they were caused by the same streptococcus. Subsequently, *Streptococcus pyogenes* was proposed as the hemolytic streptococcus that caused both entities, as well as other septic conditions.

The relative role of the streptococcus as a cause of puerperal fever is not clear. While it is universally accepted as the major cause, other streptococci, as well as other types of bacteria, have been shown to cause puerpual fever. As with all other streptococcal infections, a clearer role for this organism was possible only after Lancefield's classification.

Puerperal fever due to the group A streptococcus is now a rare event. How much of this great decrease is caused by aseptic techniques, the use of antimicrobials, or a natural decrease in "virulence" of the streptococcus is not clear.

Pharyngitis

The story of the role of the streptococcus as a cause of pharyngitis is an exceedingly interesting one. Although pharyngitis is the most common group A streptococcal infection, it has been the last to be defined. For many years sore throat was known to accompany scarlet fever, erysipelas, and puerpual fever, but little emphasis was placed on this aspect of these infections. Shortly after the streptococcus was described, they were associated with milk-borne epidemics, but it was not until the turn of the century that the association of streptococci with these milk-borne epidemics was generally accepted. In these epidemics, the term "septic sore throat" was applied to the throat infections, which were a common finding. The importance of these milk-borne epidemics is emphasized by Williams who recorded 83 published accounts of these between 1867 and 1929 [1]. The importance of the

streptococcus in these epidemics was recognized by classifying isolated streptococci as *Streptococcus epidemicus*. Little progress was made in defining the role of streptococci in pharyngitis as a clinical entity until after World War II when throat cultures became readily available to clinicians. Breese, Stillerman, and Markowitz, among others, led the way in establishing a more precise role of the streptococcus [17–19] in pharyngitis. Unfortunately, the diagnosis of streptococcal pharyngitis is still an incompletely resolved issue. As recently as 1983, Wannamaker concluded his presentation at the conference on the Management of Pharyngitis in an Era of Declining Rheumatic Fever as follows: "At best, the differential diagnosis of streptococcal infection of the upper respiratory tract is an inexact science, one requiring the use and careful evaluation of all available clues and pieces of evidence" [20]. The importance of streptococcal pharyngitis in relationship to acute rheumatic fever and acute glomerulonephritis will be addressed in more detail in the next section.

Rheumatic Fever[1]

Rheumatic fever as we know it today is a syndrome encompassing three separate but intimately related clinical entities: arthritis, carditis, and chorea (Fig. 1.2) [22]. The concept of this syndrome evolved from the potpourri of manifestations known in the seventeenth century as "rheumatism" and described first by Guillaume Du Baillou in France and by Thomas Syndenham in England. Deformities of heart valves were described by Morgagni in Italy in 1761, but the clinical description of rheumatic heart disease had to await the invention of the stethoscope by Laennec in 1819. In the Harvean Lecture of 1898, Walter Butler Cheadle (Fig. 1.3) offered a full description of the rheumatic fever syndrome as we know it today: carditis, polyarthritis, and chorea, as well as subcutaneous

---

[1]This section was adapted from A 45-Year Perspective in the Streptococcus and Rheumatic Fever: The Edward H. Kass Lecture in Infectiuos Disease History, presented at the meeting of the Infectious Diseases Society of America on October 16, 1993 and published in Clin Infect Dis 1994; 1110–1122 [21].

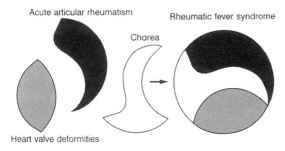

Figure 1.2 Historical development of the concept of the rheumatic fever syndrome, consisting of disease manifestations previously described independently of each other. (From Denny [21], with permission.)

nodules and erythema marginatum [23,24]. Thus, rheumatic fever was first described about 100 years ago. It is interesting to speculate on what rheumatic fever might have been like before the 19th century. English, and Taranta and Markowitz have speculated that before the crowding produced by urbanization, it might have been infrequent [22,25].

The streptococcus entered the picture at about the same time that rheumatic fever was being described, but it was not until the early 1930s that the association of the group A streptococcus with rheumatic fever was demonstrated convincingly by Coburn in the United States (Fig. 1.4) and by Collis in England [26,27]. Despite the evidence obtained by these researchers, it was still not agreed in all quarters for some time that the group A streptococcus was the only cause of rheumatic fever. As late as 1941, no lesser authority than Dr. John Paul, the well-known epidemiologist from Yale, accepted that "hemolytic streptococcal infections have something to do with rheumatic fever" but questioned whether the hemolytic streptococcus was the only infectious agent responsible [28]. In addition, there was little appreciation in civilian or military medicine of the role that the group A streptococcus played in upper respiratory infections. The story in the U.S. military is an astounding one. Lowell Rantz, in his history of streptococcal infection in World War II, states that "for a number of reasons disease caused by

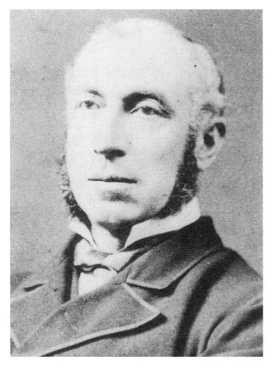

Figure 1.3 Walter Butler Cheadle. (From Denny [21], with permission.)

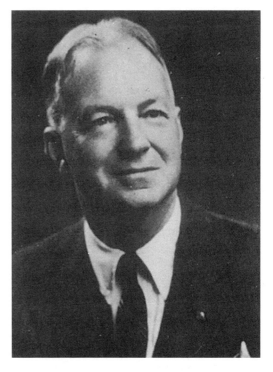

Figure 1.4 Alvin F. Coburn. (From Denny [21], with permission.)

these organisms was not recognized as an important military problem before World War II" [29]. He goes on to point out that during the Civil War 145,000 cases of "acute rheumatism"—most of which were presumably cases of acute rheumatic fever—were documented in 5.2 years, for an annual incidence of 65 cases/1000. Moreover, during World War I there were 24,750 admissions for acute articular rheumatism, but rheumatic fever was not mentioned as a problem.

Streptococcal infections and rheumatic fever posed a huge problem in World War II. Table 1.2 lists data from Rantz's report on the occurrence of rheumatic fever at selected U.S. Army installations [29]. The highest incidence rate was at Fort Francis E. Warren in Wyoming: 49.9/1000 personnel for the year 1943 alone. Rantz further reports that there were 29,512 cases of rheumatic fever in the U.S. Army between 1942 and 1945. During this same interval there were 21,000 cases of rheumatic fever in the U.S. Navy [30]. Unfortunately, the intimate relationship between streptococcal infections and rheumatic fever was not appreciated in the military. In addition, physicians, both military and civilian, were not trained to distinguish between streptococcal and nonbacterial respiratory infections, and bacteriologic diagnostic methods were not readily available. Consequently, little could be done to ameliorate this situation.

During World War II another important event occurred: the publication in 1944 of the classic paper by T. Duckett Jones (Fig. 1.5) entitled "The Diagnosis of Rheumatic Fever" [31]. Dr. Jones described major and minor manifestations of rheumatic fever whose use as diagnostic criteria could prevent under- and overdiagnosis. These criteria, subsequently termed "Jones criteria," standardized and revolutionized

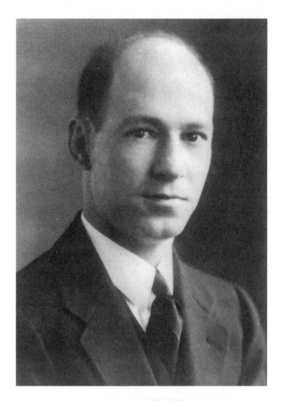

Figure 1.5 T. Duckett Jones. (From Denny [21], with permission.)

the diagnosis of rheumatic fever and have been used successfully by generations of physicians. Jones criteria have been modified and revised several times, since their original delineation, but these changes have been relatively minor and have mostly emphasized the importance of the previous streptococcal infection.

In spite of our lack of knowledge, the picture with regard to streptococcal infections was not as gloomy during this period as it may sound, as demonstrated by the following examples. For whatever reason, scarlet fever as a fatal disease had largely disappeared from England and Wales before the discovery of sulfonamides or penicillin (Fig. 1.6). Likewise, the incidence of rheumatic fever in Denmark declined steadily after 1900 (Fig. 1.7) [32]. The severity of rheumatic fever also decreased in the United States (Fig. 1.8); mortality from rheumatic fever declined sharply well before sulfonamides became available [33]. In the face of these positive trends, however, rheumatic fever continued to be an enormous problem all over the world.

Table 1.2 Incidence of Rheumatic Fever at Selected U.S. Army Installations in 1943

Station	Cases	Rate per 1000
Fort Francis E. Warren, Wyoming	806	49.9
Lowry Field, Colorado	620	30.0
Camp Crowder, Missouri	420	12.2
Buckley Field, Colorado	343	26.4
Kearns Field, Utah	250	14.4

Adapted from Rantz [29], with permission.

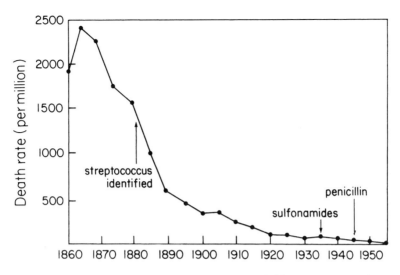

Figure 1.6 Mean annual death rate from scarlet fever among children <15 years of age in England and Wales, 1860–1950. (From Denny [21], with permission.)

The story of the streptococcus and rheumatic fever after World War II can be divided into three parts: the prevention of recurrences of rheumatic fever in subjects who had had one or more acute attacks through continuous prophylaxis of streptococcal infections; the prevention of acute rheumatic fever in nonrheumatic subjects through the treatment of streptococcal infections; and the prevention of streptococcal infections in large populations through the administration of antimicrobial prophylaxis to selected individuals at high risk. The first intervention was implemented in civilian populations, while the second and third were carried out in the military.

Secondary prevention—the prevention of recurrences in "rheumatic" subjects—was first demonstrated in 1939 by Coburn and Moore

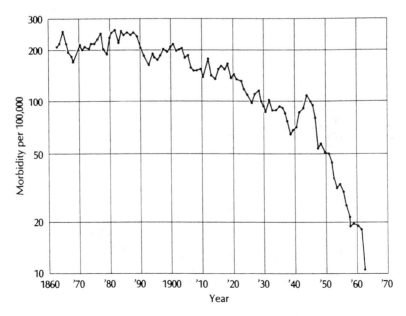

Figure 1.7 Steady decline in the incidence of rheumatic fever in Copenhagen, beginning about 1900. (From Denny [21], with permission.)

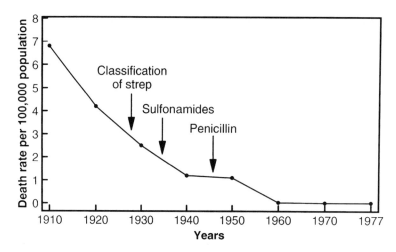

Figure 1.8 Crude death rates from rheumatic fever in the United States, 1910–1977. (From Denny [21], with permission.)

[34] and by Thomas and France [35] and involved the use of sulfanilamide. Thereafter, numerous reports confirmed the success of continuous prophylactic doses of the sulfonamides, primarily sulfadiazine. Antimicrobial resistance, which posed a substantial problem when drugs were used to prevent streptococcal infections in military populations, was not a problem in rheumatic subjects. In 1947 several investigators reported the successful use of oral penicillin in prophylaxis [36]. Then in 1952, Stollerman and Rusoff reported the use of injectable benzathine penicillin [37]. Recent figures on the comparative effectiveness of three prophylactic regimens are shown in Fig. 1.9 [22]. Injectable benzathine penicillin remains the gold standard. Through the use of these regimens, rheumatic recurrences can be virtually eliminated.

The prevention of initial attacks of rheumatic fever in nonrheumatic subjects and the prevention of streptococcal infections in large populations were entirely different matters. Studies to elucidate these problems were carried out in the military, primarily at the Streptococcal Disease

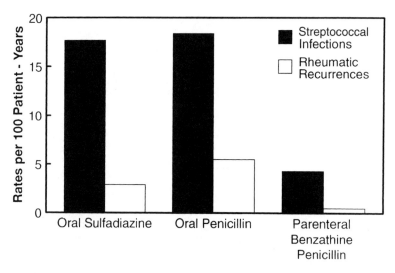

Figure 1.9 Rates of streptococcal infection and rheumatic fever among persons receiving one of three prophylactic regimens. (From Denny [21], with permission.)

Table 1.3 Hospital Admissions for Streptococcal Infections and Rheumatic Fever at Warren Air Force Base, Wyoming, 1949–1953

| Year | Hospitalizations | |
	Streptococcal Infection	Rheumatic Fever
1949	2206	117
1950	1853	54
1951	3586	144
1952	2835	125
1953	2204	136
Total	12,684	576

Laboratory at Warren Air Force Base, Wyoming. This laboratory, established in 1948, was under the aegis of the Commission on Acute Respiratory Diseases and the Commission on Streptococcal Diseases of the Armed Forces Epidemiological Board (AFEB) [38].

The AFEB is an arm of the military made up of civilian scientists whose duty is to advise the military services on matters epidemiological and on infectious disease. The Commission on Acute Respiratory Diseases, operating under the aegis of the AFEB and directed by John Dingle, at Case Western Reserve University School of Medicine, was responsible for administration of the Laboratory. The Commission on Streptococcal Diseases, under the leadership of Dr. William Tillett, shared with the Commission on Acute Respiratory Diseases the scientific oversight of the Laboratory. Charles H. Rammelkamp, Jr., of Case Western University, was the director of the Laboratory.

The picture of streptococcal infections and rheumatic fever at Warren Air Force Base in 1949 was a remarkable one. The figures on hospitalization for respiratory infections in 1949–1953 are shown in Table 1.3 (unpublished data, Commission on Streptococcal Diseases). During this interval there were 20,958 admissions for acute respiratory infections, of which 12,684 were due to streptococci. During the same time period there were 576 admissions for acute rheumatic fever. The types of group A streptococci associated with these cases are shown in Table 1.4 (unpublished data, Commission on Streptococcal Diseases). These types are listed so that they can be compared with the types implicated in virulent disease and rheumatic fever in the late 1980s and

early 1990s. The enormity of the task faced by the Laboratory is indicated by Figures 1.10 and 1.11. Figure 1.10 shows the attack rate for rheumatic fever during the first 3 years of study [39]. Note that the vertical axis depicts the number of cases per 1000 troops per month. Thus, at times of peak incidence on the base, with a population of about 10,000, there would be 30–40 admissions for rheumatic fever in a month's time. Figure 1.11 shows typical figures for admissions for streptococcal pharyngitis. During intervals of peak incidence, 100–300 cases per week would be seen (unpublished data, Commission on Streptococcal Diseases). Streptococcal infections and rheumatic fever abounded at this Air Force base in Wyoming, and methods to control these conditions were urgently needed.

Over the next 5 years a basis was established for the control of streptococcal infections and rheumatic fever. The greatest accomplishment of the laboratory was the demonstration that acute rheumatic fever could be prevented by adequate treatment of group A streptococcal infections. Table 1.5 shows the results of studies with depot penicillin G that were reported in 1950 and 1951 [40,41]. The effectiveness of other antimicrobial agents in the prevention of rheumatic fever was also studied [42–45]. It was shown subsequently that prevention was predicated on eradication of the streptococcus [46], that rheumatic fever was prevented if the streptococcal infection was treated within 9 days of its onset [47], and that a 10-day course of penicillin treatment was more effective than a 5-day course [48]. In 1954 the Streptococcal Disease Laboratory received the Lasker Award for demonstrating that rheumatic fever could be prevented by the treatment of streptococcal infections.

Table 1.4 Streptococcal M Types Isolated from Patients at Warren Air Force Base, Wyoming, 1949–1953

Year	Predominant Type	Common Types
1949	14	24, 5
1950	14	5
1951	14	5, 1, 6
1952	30	14, 3, 18
1953	30	19, 3, 14

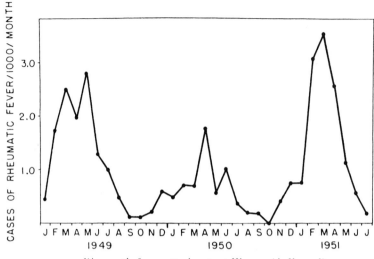

Rheumatic fever attack rate at Warren Air Force Base.

Figure 1.10 Attack rate for rheumatic fever at Warren Air Force Base, Wyoming, 1949–1951. (From Denny [21], with permission.)

Other major contributions of the laboratory included the following: *(1)* Several antimicrobial agents, including penicillin G, were shown to shorten the clinical course of streptococcal pharyngitis [49,50]. *(2)* The effect of cortisone and other anti-inflammatory drugs on the course of acute rheumatic fever in young adults was demonstrated [51–53]. *(3)* Studies showed that the environment was important in the epidemiology of streptococcal infections, but only because of close contact; fomites were not important [54–57]. *(4)* The protection provided by type-specific, or anti-M protein, immunity was demonstrated in humans [54]. *(5)* Certain "epidemic" strains of group A streptococci were more infectious than "nonepidemic" strains [54]. *(6)* The effectiveness of oral and injectable benzathine penicillin in preventing streptococcal infections was demonstrated in large military populations [58–60].

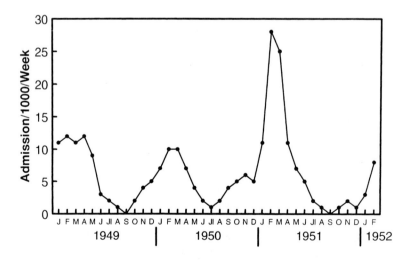

Figure 1.11 Attack rate for streptococcal respiratory disease at Warren Air Force Base, Wyoming, 1949–1952.

Table 1.5 Effects of Pencillin Therapy for Streptococcal Infections on Occurrence of Rheumatic Fever

Treatment	Streptococcal Infections	No. (%) Cases with Rheumatic Fever Developing
None	996	28 (2.8)
Penicillin	978	2 (0.2)

Adapted from Wannamaker et al. [41], with permission.

By the mid-1950s the tools were available for the control of streptococcal infections and rheumatic fever in both military and civilian populations. It had been well established that the continuous administration of prophylactic sulfonamides or penicillin to rheumatic patients would prevent the vast majority of streptococcal infections and hence recurrent rheumatic fever. Injectable benzathine penicillin proved to be an almost perfect form of prophylaxis, eliminating the problems involved in compliance with a daily oral regimen. Rheumatic fever could be prevented in nonrheumatic individuals through the adequate treatment of streptococcal pharyngitis. Continuous penicillin prophylaxius in healthy military personnel showed that streptococcal infections could be prevented in large populations as well.

The story then became rather dramatic. In programs coordinated through the Commission on Streptococcal and Staphylococcal Infections, the military initiated prophylactic penicillin administration to recruit populations. Within a short period streptococcal infections and rheumatic fever virtually disappeared from the military [30,61]. Among civilians the story was almost as dramatic. If patients with rheumatic fever were identified and given adequate prophylaxis, recurrences were infrequent. In nonrheumatic populations the frequency of rheumatic fever decreased rapidly so that by the 1970s cases were rare. This situation led to the organization in February 1983 of a conference sponsored by the American Heart Association and Ross Laboratories, entitled "Management of Pharyngitis in an Era of Declining Rheumatic Fever" [62]. Dr. Milton Markowitz opened the conference with "Thirty Years' War Against the Streptococcus: A Historic Perspective" [63]. His approach was so imaginative that

I have taken the liberty of using it here, with a few additions.

Dr. Markowitz categorized the decades from 1950 through 1980 as follows:

From 1950 to 1960 was the decade of discovery. First attacks of rheumatic fever could be prevented by treating patients with streptococcal pharyngitis. It was learned that the clinical diagnosis of streptococcal pharyngitis was uncertain. Finally, the throat culture was developed as a diagnostic tool.

From 1960 to 1970 was the decade of dissemination. The principles of management of pharyngitis were widely accepted, the throat culture was in wide use, and there was a high level of satisfaction among doctors and patients regarding prevention of rheumatic fever.

From 1970 to 1980 was the decade of dissonance; things began to come loose at the seams. It was found that the throat culture could not distinguish the acutely ill patient from the carrier. We became aware of treatment failures and the difficulty in their management. Most important of all, rheumatic fever virtually disappeared.

This was the situation in 1983 at the time of the Ross Conference. As a result of this conference, some of the recommendations regarding the management of pharyngitis were changed. In general, there was relaxation of the vigorous approach that had characterized the previous search for and treatment of patients with streptococcal pharyngitis. It was recommended that patients be cultured only if they had symptoms, that follow-up cultures as tests of cure be done only if the patient developed symptoms, and that family contacts be cultured only if they had symptoms. At the time these changes seemed rather dramatic but justified in view of the very small risk of developing rheumatic fever. Then, much to our surprise, the decade between 1980 and 1990—called here the decade of dismay—brought the return of rheumatic fever and very severe streptococcal infections.

The story of the disappearance of rheumatic fever is an interesting one. This was summarized beautifully by Leon Gordis in the T. Duckett Jones Memorial Lecture in 1984 [33]. Gordis reported that rheumatic fever had disappeared in

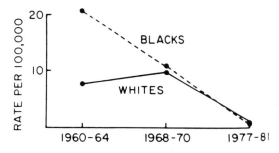

Figure 1.12 Average annual incidence of first attacks of rheumatic fever among persons 5–19 years of age, by race, in Baltimore, 1960–1981. (From Denny [21], with permission.)

Baltimore by the late 1970s (Fig. 1.12), and he attributed this phenomenon, at least in part, to the recognition and treatment of streptococcal pharyngitis. Milton Markowitz, in the Lewis W. Wannamaker Memorial Lecture in 1984, came to the same conclusion [64]. Rheumatic fever had all but disappeared by the late 1970s in Chicago (Fig. 1.13) [32]. As already shown, figures for Denmark and for the United States

as a whole showed that the severity and incidence of rheumatic fever decreased long before antimicrobial agents became available. Massell et al. attributed the marked decrease in morbidity and mortality from rheumatic fever to the introduction of penicillin in the 1940s [65]. However, the complete explanation for the decline in rheumatic fever remains unclear.

In 1987 our complacency was shattered by the report from Utah by Veasy and co-workers of a sharp increase in the number of hospital admissions of children with acute rheumatic fever [66]. This report was followed quickly by descriptions of similar increases in incidence from widely separated sites in the Unites States, although this reappearance of rheumatic fever did not appear to be uniform in all areas of the country. Concurrent with its resurgence in civilian populations, rheumatic fever also reappeared in military populations, in which prophylaxis had been discontinued [30,61].

Almost simultaneous with the reappearance of rheumatic fever were reports of very severe, sometimes life-threatening, group A streptococc-

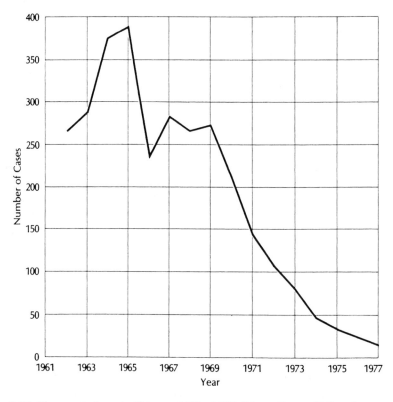

Figure 1.13 Rheumatic fever in Chicago, 1961–1977. (From Denny [21], with permission.)

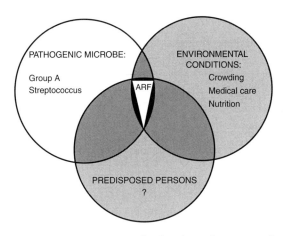

Figure 1.14 Factors involved in the pathogenesis of acute rheumatic fever (ARF). (From Denny [21], with permission.)

cal infections. The first reports came from the Rocky Mountain area, where a toxic shock–like syndrome was documented at about the same time as the increase in rheumatic fever [67–71]. These infections occurred mostly in adults and were often associated with skin and soft-tissue infections (frequently described as fasciitis) and hypotension. This so-called toxic strep syndrome differed from staphylococcal toxic shock in that most patients exhibited sepsis. Mortality was high—30% in the largest reported series. Severe and invasive group A streptococcal infections did not always take the form of toxic shock syndrome; there were also widespread reports of severe invasive infections that did not meet the criteria for this syndrome. This increase has not been restricted to the United States; similar infections have been reported from other countries, including several European nations and Australia [72].

The reasons for the return of rheumatic fever and the occurrence of severe streptococcal infections are entirely speculative at this time. The possible explanations, as discussed by Ayoub (Fig. 1.14), are changes in the host, the environment, and/or the streptococcus [73]. Changes in the host seem improbable. Changes in the environment, including the treatment and prevention of streptococcal infections, have already been mentioned. Attention has been directed mainly toward the streptococcus itself as the most logical focus of change. Several things have been learned about the strains isolated from patients

with severe infections and/or from their contacts. A large proportion of colonies of freshly isolated strains have a highly mucoid appearance. This appearance is characteristic of heavily encapsulated strains that are also rich in M protein. Both heavy encapsulation and high M protein content are associated with increased virulence. Strains isolated recently from patients have been classified as M types 1, 3, 5, 6, 14, 18, 19, and 24—all of which were associated with rheumatic fever in years past and were documented in Wyoming, but were isolated infrequently during the years when the incidence of rheumatic fever was low [74,75]. In the last few years, M types 3 and 18 have been most frequently associated with rheumatic fever and M types 1, 3, and 18 with severe infections. Stollerman and others have presented a substantial body of evidence that these M protein types (or strains of these types) have increased rheumatogenic potential [76,77].

Other factors have been implicated in the increased severity of group A streptococcal infections. Foremost among these factors is the production of pyrogenic exotoxins, although relevant data are inconsistent. Some investigators analyzing recent isolates have found exotoxin A, which had not been detected in streptococcal strains for many years, while others have documented the production of exotoxin B or of exotoxins B and C [72].

The present status of rheumatic fever and severe group A streptococcal infections is pertinent. In 1994 Veasy et al. reported on the continued occurrence of rheumatic fever in their hospital (Fig. 1.15) [78]. The incidence peaked in 1985. There was a slow decline in rheumatic fever admissions to a level similar to that seen in the 1960s and early 1970s. Thus, although there appear to be fewer cases now than in the 1980s, more cases are being seen than in the years from 1975 to 1985. A communication with Dr. Edward L. Kaplan, director of the World Health Organization's Collaborating Center for Reference and Research on Streptococci at the University of Minnesota, confirmed the impression that rheumatic fever is continuing to occur but not at the peak level seen in the late 1980s. Dr. Kaplan also confirmed the continuing occurrence of severe and invasive streptococcal infections.

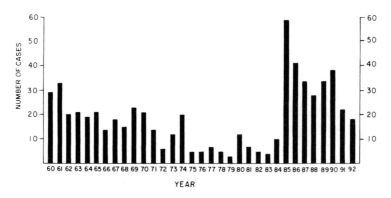

Figure 1.15 Acute rheumatic fever at Primary Children's Medical Center in Salt Lake City, Utah, 1960–1992. (From Denny [21], with permission.)

The final point to be emphasized is the occurrence of rheumatic fever in developing countries. Precise data are hard to obtain for these countries, as they are for the United States. It has been suggested that rheumatic fever is decreasing in some developing countries, but data to support this idea are lacking. In contrast, data do exist to support the continued occurrence of rheumatic fever cases in large numbers in many developing nations. The data in Table 1.6 [79], for example, show an incidence of rheumatic fever 60–200 times higher in developing countries (or in disadvantaged populations in developed countries) than in Baltimore. A recent report from the Top End of Australia's Northern Territory showed an annual incidence of rheumatic fever in Aboriginal populations of 651 per 100,000 [80].

It is difficult to know how to interpret recent events relating to group A streptococcus and rheumatic fever. The history of medicine is replete with examples of the waxing and waning of infectious diseases. Thus the saga of the streptococcus and rheumatic fever is not a new story but merely the repetition of an old one. Whether the present resurgence of disease will continue, get worse, or recede, we can only speculate.

Acute Glomerulonephritis

The relationship between nephritis and some of the diseases now known to be caused by the group A streptococcus has been recognized for several centuries [1,77,81]. This association apparently was made with scarlet fever in the 1600s and subsequently with erysipelas. Over the years nephritis was recognized in patients with scarlet fever who had severe "angina" and then in patients with "angina" alone. Richard Bright (1789–1858) clearly differentiated cardiac from renal dropsy and also noted the association between acute disease, particularly scarlet fever, and acute nephritis [82]. When the streptococcus was recognized in the last half of the 19th century, the situation was gradually clarified. The problem at that time was determining if the nephritis was caused by direct invasion of the kidney by the streptococcus or by some "toxin" produced at the site of infection and in some way affecting the kidneys. About the turn of the century it was recognized that a latent period frequently occurred between the infection and the renal disease. Schick attributed this to sensitiv-

Table 1.6 Incidence of Rheumatic Fever in Various Locales

Locale	Year	No. cases/ 100,000 population
Kuwait	1985	31
Iran	1972	58–100
Sri Lanka	1978	140
New Zealand	1972	
Maori		88
Non-Maori		9
United States		
Hawaii	1976–1980	
Chinese		4
Samoan		96
Baltimore, Maryland	1978–1980	0.5

Adapted from Markowitz [79] with permission.

ity to a product of the streptococcus, similar to other reactions he described at about the same time [77]. Although considerable understanding had been gained regarding the streptococcus and glomerulonephritis, many questions still remained. As late as 1928 Longcope wrote, "Though the facts collected suggest that the streptococcus producing the infection in these cases is also the cause of the nephritis, it is not possible to obtain proof for this contention" [83]. Lancefield's classification of the streptococcus at about the same time allowed clarification of the streptococcus involved. A large puzzle continued to puzzle investigators, however: the proportion of patients with streptococcal infections in different epidemics who developed nephritis was vastly different. It approached zero in some but was as high as 15%–20% in others. The answer to this was provided by Rammelkamp who demonstrated that certain serological types of streptococci (or even different strains of the same type) were the causes of the nephritis—so-called nephritogenic types and strains [84]. Another highlight in the history of the streptococcus and acute glomerulonephritis is the recognition that, in contrast to rheumatic fever, infections not involving the throat, as well as those involving the throat, are capable of causing nephritis. The most frequent of these is streptococcal pyoderma or impetigo [85]. Comprehensive studies of the epidemiology, bacteriology, immunology, and natural history of pyoderma-associated nephritis by Wannamaker in Minnesota, Potter et al. in Trinidad, and Dillon et al. in Alabama have greatly increased our understanding of this disease [85–87]. The M protein streptococcal types most frequently associated with pharyngitis-associated nephritis are 1, 4, 12, and 25; those associated with pyoderma-associated nephritis include type 1 but also the higher types 49, 55, 57, 59, 60, and 61 [77].

At this time the whole story regarding the pathogenesis of poststreptococcal acute glomerulonephritis is incompletely understood. While there is rather general consensus that the group A streptococcus causes most cases of acute glomerulonephritis, there is some evidence that there may be other causes as well, albeit infrequently occurring ones.

REFERENCES

1. Williams AW. In: Streptococci in Relation to Man in Health and Disease. Baltimore: Williams and Wilkins, 1932.
2. McCarty M. Streptococci. In: Davis BD, Dulbecco R, Eisen HN, Ginsberg HS (eds). Microbiology, Including Immunology and Molecular Genetics. Philadelphia: Harper and Row, 1980; 607–622.
3. Brown JH. The Use of Blood Agar for the Study of Streptococci. Monogr No 9. New York: Rockefeller Institute of Medical Research, 1919.
4. Lancefield RC. A serological differentiation of human and other groups of hemolytic streptococci. J Exp Med 1933; 57:571–595.
5. Griffith F. The serological classification of *Streptococcus pyogenes*. J Hyg 1934; 34:542–584.
6. Todd EW. Antigenic streptococcal hemolysis. J Exp Med 1932; 55:267–280.
7. Dick GF, Dick CH. Skin test for susceptibility to scarlet fever. JAMA 1924; 82:265–266.
8. Dick GF, Dick CH. Scarlet Fever. Chicago: Yearbook Publishers, 1938.
9. Feller AE, Stevens DA. Sheep blood agar for the isolation of Lancefield groups of beta-hemolytic streptococci. J Lab Clin Med 1952; 39:484–491.
10. Kaplan EL. The rapid identification of group A beta-hemolytic streptococci in the upper respiratory tract. Pediatr North Am 1988; 35:535–542.
11. Anthony BF. Group B streptococcal infections. In: Feigin RD, Cherry JD (eds). Pediatric Infectious Diseases, 3rd ed. Philadelphia: W.B. Saunders, 1992; 1305–1316.
12. Barnham M, Thornton TV, Lange K. Nephritis caused by *Streptococcus zooepidemicus* (Lancefield group C). Lancet 1983; 1:945–948.
13. Duca E, Teodorovici GR, Radu C, Vita A, Talasman-Niculescue P, Bernescu E, Feldi C, Rosca V. A new nephritogenic streptococcus. J Hyg 1969; 67:691–698.
14. Watson DW. Host-parasite factors in group A streptococcal infections. Pyrogenic and other effects of immunologic distinct exotoxins related to scarlet fever toxins. J Exp Med 1960; 111:255–283.
15. Katz AR, Morens DM. Severe streptococcal infections in historical perspectives. Clin Infect Dis 1992; 14:298–307.
16. Charles J, Charles D. Postpartum infection. In: Charles D (ed). Obstetric and Perinatal Infections. St. Louis: C.V. Mosby, 1993; 60–84.
17. Breese BB, Disney FA. The accuracy of the diagnosis of beta hemolytic streptococcal infections on clinical grounds. J Pediatr 1954; 44:670–673.
18. Stillerman M, Bernstein SH. Streptococcal pharyngitis: Evaluation of clinical syndromes in diagnosis. Am J Dis Child 1961; 101:476–489.
19. Markowitz M. Cultures of the respiratory tract in pediatric practice. Am J Dis Child 1963; 105:12–18.

20. Wannamaber LW. Diagnosis of pharyngitis: clinical and epidemiologic features. In: Shulman ST (ed). Management of Pharyngitis in an Era of Declining Rheumatic Fever. Report of the Eighty-Sixth Ross Conference on Pediatric Research. Columbus, OH: Ross Laboratories, 1984; 25–42.

21. Denny FW Jr. A 45-year perspective on the streptococcus and rheumatic fever: the Edward Kass Lecture in Infectious Disease History. Clin Infect Dis 1994; 19:1110–1122.

22. Taranta A, Markowitz M. Rheumatic Fever, 2nd ed. Boston: Kluwer Academic, 1989.

23. Cheadle WB. The Various Manifestations of the Rheumatic State as Exemplified in Childhood and Early Life. London: Smith, Elder, 1889.

24. Stollerman GH. Rheumatic Fever and Streptococcal Infection. New York: Grune and Stratton, 1975; 1–19.

25. English PC. Emergence of rheumatic fever in the nineteenth century. Milbank Q 1989; 67(Suppl 1):33–49.

26. Coburn AF. The Factor of Infection in the Rheumatic State. Baltimore: Williams and Wilkins, 1931.

27. Collis WRF. Acute rheumatism and haemolytic streptococci. Lancet 1931; 1:1341–1345.

28. Paul JR (ed). The Epidemiology of Rheumatic Fever and Some of Its Public Health Aspects, 2nd ed. New York: Metropolitan Life Insurance Co. Press, 1943.

29. Rantz LA. Hemolytic streptococcal infections. In: Coates JB Jr (ed). Preventive Medicine in World War II, Vol 4. Communicable Diseases Transmitted Chiefly Through Respiratory and Alimentary Tracts. Washington, DC: Office of the Surgeon General, 1958; 229–257.

30. Gray GC, Escamilla J, Hyams KC, Struewing JP, Kaplan El, Tupponce AK. Hyperendemic *Streptococcus pyogenes* infection despite prophylaxis with penicillin G benzathine. N Engl J Med 1991; 325:92–97.

31. Jones TD. The diagnosis of rheumatic fever. JAMA 1944; 126:481–484.

32. Stollerman GH. The return of rheumatic fever. Hosp Pract (Off Ed) 1988; 23(11):100–106, 109–113.

33. Gordis L. The virtual disappearance of rheumatic fever in the United States: lessons in the rise and fall of disease. T. Duckett Jones Memorial Lecture. Circulation 1985; 72:1155–1162.

34. Coburn AF, Moore LV. The prophylactic use of sulfanilamide in streptococcal respiratory infections with special reference to rheumatic fever. J Clin Invest 1939; 18:147–155.

35. Thomas CB, France R. A preliminary report of the prophylactic use of sulfanilamide in patients susceptible to rheumatic fever. Bull Johns Hopkins Hosp 1939; 64:67–77.

36. Denny FW Jr. The prophylaxis of streptococcal infections. In: McCarty M (ed). Streptococcal In-

fections. New York: Columbia University Press, 1954; 176–196.

37. Stollerman GH, Rusoff JH. Prophylaxis against group A streptococcal infections in rheumatic fever patients: use of new repository penicillin preparation. JAMA 1952; 150:1571–1575.

38. Woodward TE. The Armed Forces Epidemiological Board. Its First Fifty Years. Falls Church, VA: Office of the Surgeon General, 1990.

39. Rammelkamp CH Jr, Denny FW, Wannamaker LW. Studies on the epidemiology of rheumatic fever in the armed services. In: Thomas L (ed). Rheumatic Fever, a Symposium. Minneapolis: University of Minnesota Press, 1952; 72–89.

40. Denny FW, Wannamaker LW, Brink WR, Rammelkamp CH Jr, Custer EA. Prevention of rheumatic fever: treatment of the preceding streptococcic infection. JAMA 1950; 143:151–153.

41. Wannamaker LW, Rammelkamp CH Jr, Denny FW, Brink WR, Houser HB, Hahn EO, Dingle JH. Prophylaxis of acute rheumatic fever by treatment of the preceding streptococcal infection with various amounts of depot penicillin. Am J Med 1951; 10:673–695.

42. Houser HB, Eckhardt GC, Hahn EO, Denny FW, Wannamaker LW, Rammelkamp CH Jr. Effect of aureomycin treatment of streptococcal sore throat on the streptococcal carrier state, the immunologic response of the host, and the incidence of acute rheumatic fever. Pediatrics 1953; 12:593–606.

43. Chamovitz R, Catanzaro FJ, Stetson CA, Rammelkamp CH Jr. Prevention of rheumatic fever by treatment of previous streptococcal infections. I. Evaluation of benzathine penicillin G. N Engl J Med 1954; 251:466–471.

44. Catanzaro FJ, Brock L, Chamovitz R, Perry WD, Siegel AC, Stetson CA, Rammelkamp CH Jr, Houser HB, Stolzer BL, Wannamaker LW, Hahn EO. Effect of oxytetracycline therapy of streptococcal sore throat on the incidence of acute rheumatic fever. Ann Intern Med 1955; 42:345–357.

45. Morris AJ, Chamovitz R, Catanzaro FJ, Rammelkamp CH Jr. Prevention of rheumatic fever by treatment of previous streptococcic infections: effect of sulfadiazine. JAMA 1956; 160:114–116.

46. Catanzaro FJ, Rammelkamp CH Jr, Chamovitz R. Prevention of rheumatic fever by treatment of streptococcal infections. II. Factors responsible for failures. N Engl J Med 1958; 259:51–57.

47. Catanzaro FJ, Stetson CA, Morris AJ, Chamovitz R, Rammelkamp CH Jr, Stolzer BL, Perry WD. The role of the streptococcus in the pathogenesis of rheumatic fever. Am J Med 1954; 17:749–756.

48. Wannamaker LW, Denny FW, Perry WD, Rammelkamp CH Jr, Eckhardt GC, Houser HB, Hahn EO. The effect of penicillin prophylaxis on

streptococcal disease rates and the carrier state. N Engl J Med 1953; 249:1–7.

49. Brink WR, Rammelkamp CH Jr, Denny FW, Wannamaker LW. Effect of penicillin and aureomycin on the natural course of streptococcal tonsillitis and pharyngitis. Am J Med 1951; 10:300–308.

50. Denny FW, Wannamaker LW, Hahn EO. Comparative effects of penicillin, aureomycin and terramycin on streptococcal tonsillitis and pharyngitis. Pediatrics 1953; 11:7–14.

51. Clark EJ, Houser HB. Comparative effects of 3-hydroxy-2-phenylcinchoninic acid (HPC) and aspirin on the acute course of rheumatic fever and the occurrence of rheumatic valvular disease. Am Heart J 1953; 45:576–588.

52. Houser HB, Clark EJ, Stolzer BL. Comparative effects of aspirin, ACTH and cortisone on the acute course of rheumatic fever in young adult males. Am J Med 1954; 16:168–180.

53. Stolzer BL, Houser HB, Clark EJ. Therapeutic agents in rheumatic carditis: comparative effects of acetylsalicylic acid, corticotropin and cortisone. Arch Intern Med 1955; 95:677–688.

54. Wannamaker LW. The epidemiology of streptococcal infections. In: McCarty M (ed). Streptococcal Infections. New York: Columbia University Press, 1954; 157–175.

55. Perry WD, Siegel AC, Rammelkamp CH Jr, Wannamaker LW, Marple EC. Transmission of group A streptococci. I. The role of contaminated bedding. Am J Hyg 1957; 66:85–95.

56. Perry WD, Seigel AC, Rammelkamp CH Jr. Transmission of group A streptococci. II. The role of contaminated dust. Am J Hyg 1957; 66:96–101.

57. Rammelkamp CH Jr, Morris AJ, Catanzaro FJ, Wannamaker LW, Chamovitz R, Marple EC. Transmission of group A streptococci. III. The effect of drying on the infectivity of the organism for man. J Hyg 1958; 56:280–287.

58. Chancey RL, Morris AJ, Conner RH, Catanzaro FJ, Chamovitz R, Rammelkamp CH Jr. Studies of streptococcal prophylaxis: comparison of oral penicillin and benzathine penicillin. Am J Med Sci 1955; 229:165–171.

59. Davis J, Schmidt WC. Benzathine penicillin G: its effectiveness in the prevention of streptococcal infections in a heavily exposed population. N Engl J Med 1957; 256:339–342.

60. Morris AJ, Rammelkamp CH Jr. Benzathine penicillin G in the prevention of streptococcic infections. JAMA 1957; 165:664–667.

61. Wallace MR, Garst PD, Papadimos TJ, Oldfield EC III. The return of acute rheumatic fever in young adults. JAMA 1989; 262:2557–2561.

62. Shulman ST (ed). Management of Pharyngitis in an Era of Declining Rheumatic Fever. Report of the Eighty-Sixth Ross Conference on Pediatric Research. Columbus, OH: Ross Laboratories, 1984.

63. Markowitz M. Thirty years' war against the streptococcus: a historic perspective. In: Shulman ST (ed). Management of Pharyngitis in an Era of Declining Rheumatic Fever. Report of the Eighty-Sixth Ross Conference on Pediatric Research. Columbus, OH: Ross Laboratories, 1984; 2–7.

64. Markowitz M. The decline of rheumatic fever: role of medical intervention. Lewis W. Wannamaker Memorial Lecture. J Pediatr 1985; 106:545–550.

65. Massell BF, Chute CG, Walker AM, Kurland GS. Penicillin and the marked decrease in morbidity and mortality from rheumatic fever in the United States. N Engl J Med 1988; 318:280–286.

66. Veasy LG, Wiedmeier SE, Orsmond GS, Ruttenberg HD, Boucek MM, Roth SJ, Tait VF, Thompson JA, Daly JA, Kaplan EL, Hill HR. Resurgence of acute rheumatic fever in the intermountain area of the United States. N Engl J Med 1987; 316:421–427.

67. Cone LA, Woodard DR, Schlievert PM, Tomory GS. Clinical and bacteriologic observations of a toxic shock-like syndrome due to *Streptococcus pyogenes*. N Engl J Med 1987; 317:146–149.

68. Bartter T, Dascal A, Carroll K, Curley FJ. "Toxic strep syndrome": a manifestation of group A streptococcal infection. Arch Intern Med 1988; 148:1421–1424.

69. Stevens DL, Tanner MH, Winship J, Swarts R, Ries KM, Schlievert PM, Kaplan EL. Severe group A streptococcal infections associated with a toxic shock-like syndrome and scarlet fever toxin A. N Engl J Med 1989; 321:1–7.

70. Givner LB, Abramson JS, Wasilauskas B. Apparent increase in the incidence of invasive group A beta-hemolytic streptococcal disease in children. J Pediatr 1991; 118:341–346.

71. Stollerman GH. Changing group A streptococci: the reappearance of streptococcal "toxic shock" [editorial]. Arch Intern Med 1988; 148:1268–1270.

72. Bisno AL. Group A streptococcal infections and acute rheumatic fever. N Engl J Med 1991; 325:783–793.

73. Ayoub EM. The search for host determinants of susceptibility to rheumatic fever: the missing link. T. Duckett Jones Memorial Lecture. Circulation 1984; 69:197–201.

74. Johnson DR, Stevens DL, Kaplan EL. Epidemiologic analysis of group A streptococcal serotypes associated with severe systemic infections, rheumatic fever, or uncomplicated pharyngitis. J Infect Dis 1992; 166:374–382.

75. Kaplan EL, Johnson DR, Cleary PP. Group A streptococcal serotypes isolated from patients and sibling contacts during the resurgence of rheumatic fever in the United States in the mid-1980's. J Infect Dis 1989; 159:101–103.

76. Stollerman GH. Rheumatogenic streptococci and

autoimmunity. Clin Immunol Immunopathol 1991; 61:131–142.

77. Bisno AL. Nonsuppurative poststreptococcal sequelae: rheumatic fever and glomerulonephritis. In Mandell GL, Bennett JE, Dolin R (eds). Principles and Practice of Infectious Diseases, 4th ed. New York: Churchill Livingstone, 1995; 1799–1810.

78. Veasy LG, Tani LY, Hill HR. Persistence of acute rheumatic fever in the intermountain area of the United States. J Pediatr 1994; 124:9–16.

79. Markowitz M. Streptococcal disease in developing countries. Pediatr Infec Dis J 1991; 10(10)(Suppl):S11–S14.

80. Carapetis JR, Wolff DR, Currie BJ. Acute rheumatic fever and rheumatic heart disease in the Top End of Australia's Northern Territory. Med J Aust 1996; 164:146–149.

81. Peters JH. Pathogenesis of glomerulonephritis. In: Strauss MB, Welt LG (eds). Diseases of the Kidney. Boston: Little, Brown, 1963; 233–254.

82. Bright R. Cases and observations, illustrative of renal disease accompanied with the secretion of albuminous urine. Guys Hosp Rep 1836; 1:338–379.

83. Longcope WT, O'Brien DP, McGuire J, Hansen OC, Denny ER. Relationship of acute infections to glomerular nephritis. J Clin Invest 1928; 5:7–30.

84. Rammelkamp CH Jr, Weaver RS. Acute glomerulonephritis: the significance of the variations in the incidence of the disease. J Clin Invest 1953; 32:345–358.

85. Wannamaker LW. Differences between streptococcal infections of the throat and of the skin. N Engl J Med 1970; 282:23–31.

86. Potter EV, Ortiz JS, Sharrett R. Changing types of nephritogenic streptococci in Trinidad. J Clin Invest 1971; 50:1197–1205.

87. Dillon HC, Derrick CW, Dillon MS. M-antigens common to pyoderma and acute glomerulonephritis. J Infect Dis 1974; 130:257–267.

2

Group A Beta-Hemolytic Streptococci: Virulence Factors, Pathogenesis, and Spectrum of Clinical Infections

DENNIS L. STEVENS

Group A streptococcal (GAS) infections have been described since the time of Hippocrates. In the 16th century, severe forms of pharyngitis occurring in Spain were referred to as "garitillo," and in England in the 18th century were known as "Fothergill's sore throat." Complications of pharyngitis such as mastoiditis, and thrombosis of the cavernous sinus, tonsillar vein, and lateral sinus were still reported as complications of GAS infections in the 1930s and carried a mortality of 55% [1]. Perhaps the earliest clinical evidence of mastoiditis was found in pre-Columbian skulls (8000–6500 B.C.) recovered from an archeological excavation in the Americas [2]. Throughout history there have been numerous epidemics of other forms of GAS infections such as scarlet fever, rheumatic fever, impetigo, and erysipelas, demonstrating that (1) group A streptococcus causes a variety of clinical illnesses, (2) the severity of each type of infection can independently wax and wane, and (3) an epidemic of only one type of GAS infection may materialize in a specific period of time. In contrast, the annual prevalence of GAS pharyngitis has remained quite constant over decades. Thus, these historical perspectives provide solid clues that many different strains of group A streptococci may be present in a given geographical site at a specific point in time. Over a 10-year period, one strain may emerge as a dominant strain, only to be replaced by one or more different strains [3]. That this dynamic process affects the expression of disease with a regular periodicity is suggested by the work of Kohler, who demonstrated that the severity of scarlet fever varied in 6- to 7-year cycles and correlated with the appearance of M-1 strains producing streptococcal pyrogenic exotoxin A [4].

Over the last 40 years in the Western world, streptococcal pharyngitis, erysipelas, and scarlet fever have become milder diseases and the prevalence of acute rheumatic fever and post-streptococcal glomerulonephritis have reached all-time lows. Since 1985, several epidemics of rheumatic fever [5] and severe invasive GAS infections (reviewed in ref. [6]) have been described from many sites around the world. In addition, the prevalence of streptococcal infections of all types remains high in undeveloped countries. Despite the abundance of epidemiologic examples of disease variation, a clear understanding of the interaction between host and pathogen has been lacking. Thus, at the present time it seems prudent to aggressively diagnose and treat GAS infections of the throat to prevent not only rheumatic fever but also extension of infection into the vital structures of the head and neck and to prevent life-threatening invasive infections such as bacteremia, necrotizing fasciitis, and streptococcal toxic shock syndrome (streptococcal TSS).

THE PATHOGEN

General Characteristics of the Pathogen

Streptococcus pyogenes, or group A streptococcus (GAS), is a facultative, gram-positive coccus that grows in chains and causes numerous infections in humans, including pharyngitis, tonsillitis, scarlet fever, cellulitis, erysipelas, rheumatic fever, poststreptococcal glomerulonephritis, necrotizing fasciitis, myonecrosis, and lymphangitis. The only known reservoirs for GAS in nature are the skin and mucous membranes of the human host. The clinical diseases produced by group A streptococci have been well described; however, the pathogenic mechanisms underlying them are poorly understood, largely because each is the culmination of highly complex interactions between the human host defense mechanisms and specific virulence factors of the streptococcus.

Microbiological Characteristics

Group A streptococci require complex media containing blood products, grow best in an environment of 10% carbon dioxide, and on blood agar plates produce pinpoint colonies that are surrounded by a zone of complete (beta) hemolysis (Plate 1). The exhaustive work of Rebecca Lancefield established the classification of streptococci into types A through O based upon acid-extractable carbohydrate antigens of cell wall material [7]. In addition, group A streptococci have also been subdivided according to the surface expression of M and T antigens (see also Chapters 15, 19, and 20). Subtyping of strains of group A streptococcus has proven invaluable for epidemiological studies, in much the same way that phage typing has been useful for defining the epidemiology of *Staphylococcus aureus.* High-resolution genotyping provides a more specific determination of relatedness among

strains isolated from outbreaks of GAS infections [8]. Finally, rapid sequencing of the gene encoding M protein is providing a definitive way of comparing M-typeable and M-nontypeable strains (see Chapter 15).

Virulence Factors

Capsule Streptococcus

Some strains of S. *pyogenes* possess thick capsules of hyaluronic acid resulting in large mucoid colonies on blood agar (Plate 2). Luxuriant production of M protein may also impart a mucoid colony morphology, a trait that has been associated most commonly with M-18 strains [9]. Using an isogenic mutant of an M-18 strain, Wessels et al. showed that the strains producing hyaluronic acid capsule were resistant to phagocytosis and were virulent in mice, whereas the hyaluronic acid–deficient strain was nonvirulent and readily killed by phagocytes [10]. Interestingly, the non–hyaluronic acid–producing strain adhered to macrophages with greater avidity than the mucoid strain [10]. This suggests that hyaluronic acid capsule, like M protein, confers resistance to phagocytosis but that these capsules also interfere with adherence to eukaryotic cells. Streptococci possessing hyaluronic acid capsule adhere to keratinocytes through specific (CD44) receptors [11].

Cell Wall

The cell wall consists of a peptidoglycan backbone with integral lipoteichoic acid components (Figure 2.1). The main function of these components is structural stability of the microbe, although the exact function of lipoteichoic acid is unknown. Lipoteichoic acid may play a role in pathogenesis by facilitating the adherence of group A streptococci to pharyngeal epithelial cells [12]. Peptidoglycan, like endotoxin from gram-negative bacteria, is capable of activating the alternative complement pathway [13–15].

M Proteins

Over 80 different M protein types of GAS are currently described. The protein is a coiled-coil consisting of four regions of repeating amino

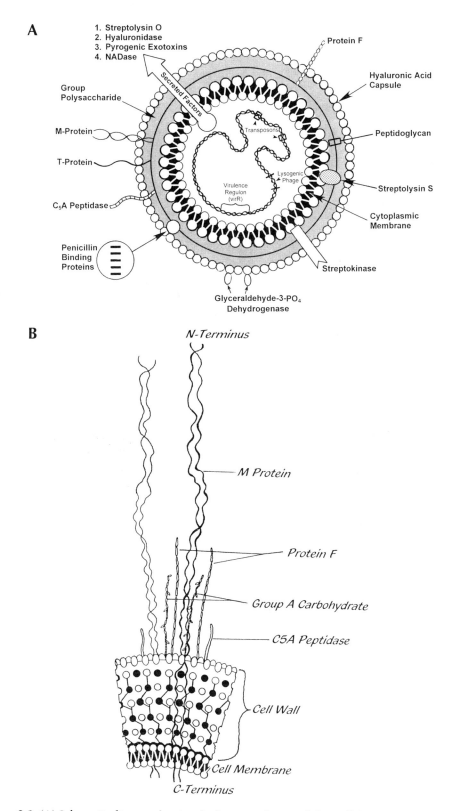

A

1. Streptolysin O
2. Hyaluronidase
3. Pyrogenic Exotoxins
4. NADase

Protein F

Hyaluronic Acid Capsule

Secreted Factors

Group Polysaccharide

M-Protein

T-Protein

Transposons

Peptidoglycan

C$_5$A Peptidase

Lysogenic Phage

Streptolysin S

Virulence Regulon (virR)

Cytoplasmic Membrane

Penicillin Binding Proteins

Streptokinase

Glyceraldehyde-3-PO$_4$ Dehydrogenase

B

N-Terminus

M Protein

Protein F

Group A Carbohydrate

C5A Peptidase

Cell Wall

Cell Membrane

C-Terminus

Figure 2.1 *(A)* Schematic diagram showing the location of intracellular, cellular, and extracellular virulence factors and genetic regulators of their expression. *(B)* Expanded view of the cell wall and its components.

21

acids (A–D), a proline/glycine–rich region that serves to intercalate the protein into the bacterial cell wall, and a hydrophobic region that acts as a membrane anchor [16]. Region A near the N-terminus is highly variable, and antibodies to this region confer type-specific protection. Within the more conserved B–D regions lies an area that binds one of the complement regulatory proteins (factor H), stearically inhibiting antibody binding and complement-derived opsonin deposition, and effectively camouflaging the organism against humoral immune surveillance [17] (Fig. 2.1). M protein also protects the organism against phagocytosis by polymorphonuclear leukocytes [18], although this property can be overcome by type-specific antisera [7,16,19]. Observations by Lancefield suggest that the quantity of M protein produced decreases with passage on artificial media but increases rapidly with passage through mice [7]. In humans, the quantity of M protein produced by an infecting strain progressively decreases during convalescence and with prolonged carriage [7]. Nontypeable strains of group A streptococcus may express minute amounts of M protein, may lack M protein altogether, or may be of a totally new M type. Recently, 60 nontypeable strains that had been isolated from upper respiratory sources in Southeast Asia were found to be resistant to phagocytosis in normal serum or plasma, suggesting that these strains do in fact produce M protein [20]. These data are compatible with the view that new M types are constantly emerging. This could result from mutational events within the *emm* gene, producing novel M proteins that no longer cross-react with standard polyvalent typing sera. Evidence that heterogeneity within this gene locus does in fact occur has recently been demonstrated among strains typed as M-1 [21]. In subsequent studies by these investigators, roughly 50% of randomly collected human sera opsonized seven strains of M-1 GAS [22]. In contrast, the remaining 50% of serum samples opsonized only some of these strains, prompting the authors to conclude that opsonic antibody may not be type-specific, but rather strain-specific [22]. See Chapters 19 and 20 for additional information about M proteins and two different strategies for vaccine development.

Immunoglobulin-Binding Proteins (M-like proteins)

Group A streptococcus produces a family of proteins that share structural similarities to M proteins and also bind immunoglobulins, including IgG, IgM, and IgA. Unlike M protein, these molecules do not inhibit phagocytosis in the absence of type-specific antibody. Nonetheless, these molecules, like M protein, may play a role in pathogenesis by interfering with complement activation. This was nicely shown by Thern et al. [23] who demonstrated that IgG-binding protein from GAS selectively bound C4b-binding protein (C4BP), a protein that is intimately involved in the regulation of the complement system. The authors concluded that this protein might interfere with opsonization by down-regulating complement activation, but acknowledged that it could also serve as a ligand between GAS and host cells [23] and thus may actually facilitate nonimmune phagocytosis.

Fibronectin-Binding Protein (protein F)

Binding of GAS to fibronectin appears to enhance the adherence of GAS to epithelial surfaces. Hanski and Capron [24] described protein F, a 659 amino acid protein with two fibronectin-binding domains [24] (Fig. 2.1). It was suggested that protein F might be found in abundance in isolates from patients with invasive GAS infections [25]. Yet studies that defined the distribution of protein F among various M types indicated that M types 1 and 3, the two most common strains isolated from patients with invasive GAS infections, did not produce protein F [25]. These authors were able to demonstrate that high carbon dioxide concentrations increase the expression of protein F. Thus, protein F or perhaps other fibronectin binding proteins might play an important role in the adhesion of GAS to mucosal or skin surfaces.

Protein Streptococcal Complement Inhibitory Protein

Akesson et al. have described a novel, extracellular protein of 305 amino acid residues that inactivates the membrane attack complex of complement [26]. Streptococcal complement inhibitory protein (SIC) was found only in M types

1 and 57. In addition, the *sic* gene is located in the mga regulon of M type 1 GAS, directly adjacent to the *emm* gene [26]. Clearly, through this mechanism the organism could evade destruction by the membrane attack complex (C5–C9) generated by either the alternative or classical complement pathway.

Opacity Factor

The opacity factor (OF) has been found largely in group A streptococci but has recently also been detected in group G and C streptococci, *Streptococcus dysgalactiae*, and *Streptococcus equisimilis* [27]. The OF is a type-specific lipoprotein lipase whose role in pathogenesis is unknown. Recent evidence suggests a relationship with the presence of OF and arrangement of specific *emm* genes. Specifically, OF is associated with M types that are largely skin strains [28].

Streptolysin O

Streptolysin O belongs to a family of oxygen-labile, thiol-activated cytolysins, and causes the broad zone of beta hemolysis surrounding colonies of *Streptococcus pyogenes* on blood agar plates [29] (Plate 1). Thiol-activated cytolysins bind to cholesterol on eukaryotic cell membranes, creating toxin–cholesterol aggregates that contribute to cell lysis via a colloid-osmotic mechanism. Cholesterol inhibits both toxicity in isolated myocytes and hemolysis of red blood cells in vitro. In situations where serum cholesterol is high (i.e., nephrotic syndrome), falsely elevated ASO titers may occur because both cholesterol and anti-ASO antibody will neutralize streptolysin O. Striking amino acid homology exists between streptolysin O and thiol-activated cytolysins from other gram-positive bacteria [30].

Streptolysin S

Streptolysin S is a cell-associated hemolysin that does not diffuse into the agar media. Purification and characterization of this protein have been difficult and its only role in pathogenesis may be through direct, contact-dependent cytotoxicity.

Deoxyribonucleases A, B, C, and D

Expression of deoxyribonucleases (DNases) in vivo, especially DNase B, elicits production of anti-DNase antibody following either pharyngeal or skin infection.

Hyaluronidase

This extracellular enzyme hydrolyzes hyaluronic acid in deeper tissues and may facilitate the spread of infection along fascial planes. Anti-hyaluronidase titers rise following *Streptococcus pyogenes* infections, especially those infections involving the skin.

Nicotine-Adenine-Dinucleotidase (NADase)

This extracellular enzyme, also called NAD glycohydrolase, is produced by many strains of GAS [31]. It is not known what function this enzyme has for the organism per se and it is also unclear what role NADase may play in the pathogenesis of any GAS infection. Recently it was shown that NADase is expressed in M-1 and M-3 strains of GAS, but not in noninvasive strains [32]. Interestingly, in a survey done 20 years ago, NADase was not found in M-1 strains [31].

Streptokinase

Streptokinase is produced by all strains of GAS and is located in the extracellular milieu. In contrast, a plasminogen binding site is found on the surface of strains of GAS [33]. Once plasminogen is bound, streptokinase proteolytically converts bound plasminogen to active plasmin [33]. Plasmin then cleaves fibrin into fragments known as fibrin degradation products. Interestingly, bound plasmin can not be inhibited by endogenous antiproteases such as alpha-l anti-trypsin [33]. The role of streptokinase in GAS infections is unclear, although it may play a role in post-streptococcal glomerulonephritis. (see Chapter 9 for current concepts in the pathogenesis of poststreptococcal glomerulonephritis.)

Pyrogenic Exotoxins

Streptococcal pyrogenic exotoxins (SPE) type A, B, and C, also called scarlatina or erythrogenic toxins, induce lymphocyte blastogenesis, potentiate endotoxin-induced shock, induce fever, suppress antibody synthesis, and act as superantigens [34]. The identification of these three different types of pyrogenic exotoxins may explain in part why some individuals may have multiple attacks of scarlet fever. The gene for pyrogenic exotoxin A (*Spe*A) is transmitted by bacteriophage, and stable production depends upon lysogenic conversion in a manner analogous to toxin production by *Corynebacterium diphtheriae* [35]. Although control of SPEA production is not yet understood, this is likely an important mechanism since it is well established that the quantity of SPEA produced by strains varies dramatically from decade to decade (see also Chapter 3). In addition, point mutations in the *Spe*A gene result in dramatic changes in the potency of SPEA toxin [36]. Historically, SPEA- and B-producing strains have been associated with severe cases of scarlet fever and more recently, with streptococcal toxic shock syndrome (TSS) [37,38].

Although all strains of group A streptococci are endowed with the gene for SPEB (*spe*B), not all strains produce SPEB, and even among those strains which produce SPEB, the quantity of toxin produced varies greatly from strain to strain [4,35,37,39].

Pyrogenic exotoxin C, like SPEA, is bacteriophage mediated and expression is likewise highly variable. Recently, mild cases of scarlet fever in England and the United States have been associated with SPEC–positive strains [39]. Two new superantigens, mitogenic factor [40,41] and streptococcal superantigen [42], have been described; however, their roles in pathogenesis have not been fully investigated. Additional information about the pyrogenic exotoxins can be found in Chapter 3, Group A Streptococcal Genetics and Virulence, and Chapter 4, Exotoxins of *Streptococcus pyogenes*.

EPIDEMIOLOGY

Natural Reservoir

Group A streptococcus is purely a human pathogen. This statement is based upon the observations that (*1*) natural GAS infection in animals is rare; (*2*) laboratory animals do not develop spontaneous postinfectious sequelae such as rheumatic fever or poststreptococcal glomerulonephritis; (*3*) the inoculum needed to cause infection in laboratory animals is orders of magnitude greater than that estimated to cause infection in humans; and (*4*) group A streptococci have developed highly sophisticated defensive molecules that bind, inactivate, or destroy human immune response molecules, such as immunoglobulin [16] and complement [43] (see also Chapters 19 and 20).

Relationship to Humans

The highest incidence of most GAS infections is in children younger than age 10 years [9]. The asymptomatic prevalence is also higher (15% to 20%) in children compared to adults (<5%). Age is not the only factor since crowded conditions in temperate climates during the winter months are associated with epidemics of pharyngitis in military recruits as well as in school children (see Chapter 5). Impetigo is most common in children from ages 2 to 5, and may occur throughout the year in tropical areas or largely in the summer in temperate climates (see Chapter 8). Similarly, 90% of cases of scarlet fever occur in children 2 to 8 years old, and like pharyngitis, it is most common in temperate regions during the winter months.

In contrast to pharyngitis, impetigo, and scarlet fever, the age-specific attack rate of bacteremia is highest in the elderly and in neonates [44]. Between 1986 and 1988, however, the prevalence of bacteremia increased 800% to 1000% in adolescents and adults in Western countries [45]. Although some of this increase is attributable to intravenous drug abuse and puerperal sepsis, most cases involve streptococcal TSS [44]. This recent clinical manifestation of streptococcal infection may be in part related to the emergence of more virulent strains [37,46–48] (see also Chapter 10).

Colonization and Transmission

Human skin and mucous membranes serve as the natural reservoirs of *Streptococcus pyogenes*. Pharyngeal or cutaneous acquisition is by person-to-person spread via aerosolized microdroplets or direct contact, respectively. Epidemics of pharyngitis and scarlet fever have also occurred following ingestion of contaminated nonpasteurized milk or food. Epidemics of impetigo have been reported particularly in tropical areas, day care centers, and among underprivileged children. Group A streptococcal infections in hospitalized patients occur during child delivery (puerperal sepsis), times of war (epidemic gangrene), surgical convalescence (surgical wound infection, surgical scarlet fever), or as a result of burns (burn wound sepsis). Thus, in most clinical streptococcal infections, the mode of transmission and the portal of entry are easily ascertained. In contrast, among patients with streptococcal TSS, the portal of entry is obvious in only 50% of cases [48].

PATHOGENESIS

Adherence

Adherence of cocci to the pharyngeal mucosal epithelium is necessary but not sufficient to cause disease in all cases, since prolonged asymptomatic carriage is well documented. Complex interactions between host epithelium and streptococcal factors such as M protein, lipoteichoic acid, peptidoglycan, and fimbriae are necessary for adherence [12,49]. Fibronectin-binding protein (protein F) also contributes to adherence since protein F–deficient mutants are less capable of binding to epithelial cells than protein F–rich strains [24]. In addition, there appear to be additional, as-yet uncharacterized proteins produced by GAS that bind fibronectin [25]. Direct interaction of GAS with eukaryotic membrane proteins can also result in adhesion. For example, Frick et al. demonstrated that protein H, a member of the M protein family, binds specific neural-cell adhesion molecules (N-CAM) [50]. Similarly, Okada et al. have demonstrated a highly specific ligand interaction between the C-repeat region of M protein and the membrane cofactor protein (MCP) or CD46 on the surface of normal human skin keratinocytes [51]. The presence of a hyaluronic acid capsule appears to inhibit adherence to some eukaryotic cells [10] but may facilitate binding to keratinocytes [11].

Phagocytosis

On the surface of respiratory epithelial cells or within the tissues, streptococci may evade opsonophagocytosis by destroying or inactivating complement-derived chemoattractants and opsonins (C5a peptidase) [52] and by binding immunoglobulins. Expression of M protein, in the absence of type-specific antibody, also protects the organism from phagocytosis by polymorphonuclear leukocytes and monocytes. This is related in part to the inhibition of complement activation via the alternative pathway [15]. Interestingly, in some mucoid strains resistance to phagocytosis appears to be related more to the presence of a hyaluronic acid capsule than to expression of M protein [10]. For example, Dale et al. demonstrated that despite the observation that C3b was deposited on both an encapsulated (hyaluronic acid capsule) and unencapsulated strain of M-18, only the encapsulated strain was completely resistant to phagocytosis [53]. Thus, the hyaluronic acid capsule physically attenuated the interaction between complement-opsonized strains and the phagocyte [53].

Zabriske et al. demonstrated that antibody against the group A polysaccharide was a complement-fixing antibody that enhanced opsonophagocytosis by phagocytes [54]. Interestingly, the authors suggested that previous studies demonstrating a dominant role for type-specific anti-M protein antibody had generally been performed in heparinized blood that had potent anti-complement effects. When these investigators used EDTA (ethylenediaminetetraacetic acid), complement fixation was not affected and potent phagocytosis and killing of GAS was observed. The role of complement in immunity to GAS is made more complex by the observation that SIC, a novel extracellular protein produced by GAS, inhibits the function of the membrane attack complex (MAC) of complement [26]. In addition, certain IgG-binding proteins of GAS bind the human complement regulatory protein, C4b-binding protein, effectively interfering with the classical pathway of complement activation [23]. The C-repeat region of M protein also binds factor H, a fluid phase complement regulatory serum protein [17]. Once factor H is bound to the M protein molecule, inhibition or reversal of the formation of C3b complexes ensues with conversion of C3b to the inactive form (iC3b), thus preventing complement-dependent phagocytosis [17].

M protein may also shroud itself by binding to fibrinogen in plasma, effectively reducing opsonization by type-specific antibody against the M protein [55]. This phenomenon appears to be M-type-specific since unencapsulated M-24 strains but not M-18 strains were resistant to phagocytosis in plasma or whole blood but not serum [53]. This appeared to be related to the observation that M-18 protein contained only one B-repeat region, whereas M-24 protein contained five B-repeats [53]. The M-24 strain bound 10 times more fibrinogen than the M-18, presumably via the B-repeat segments of M protein [53]. Paradoxically, fibrinogen could serve as a ligand between the streptococcus and phagocyte since the iC3b receptor of phagocytes, CD11b/CD18, binds fibrinogen [56]. Although this may not be an important mechanism for resting phagocytes, activated or primed phagocytes dramatically increase the level of expression of these cell surface receptors. That this might be an important mechanism was suggested by German investigators [57] who demonstrated that M protein resistance to phagocytosis could be overcome by first activating the phagocyte. Finally, there is some evidence that SPEB may cleave the amino-terminal portion of M proteins, rendering the bacteria more susceptible to phagocytosis [58].

Inflammation, Cytokines, and Shock

In tissues, streptolysin O secreted in high concentrations may destroy approaching phagocytes. Distal to the focus of infection, lower concentrations of streptolysin O stimulate polymorphonuclear leukocyte adhesion to endothelial cells, effectively preventing continued granulocyte migration and promoting vascular damage [59]. In the nonimmune host, streptolysin O, streptococcal pyrogenic exotoxin A, and other streptococcal components stimulate host cells to produce tumor necrosis factor (TNF) and interleukin-1 (IL-1), cytokines that mediate hypotension and stimulate leukostasis, resulting in shock, microvascular injury, multi-organ failure, and if excessive, death [44]. A unique feature of the pyrogenic exotoxins [60] and of some M protein

fragments [61] is their ability to interact with certain $V\beta$ regions of the T cell receptor in the absence of classical antigen processing. Such antigens are called *superantigens* and they induce massive clonal proliferation of T lymphocytes and production of the lymphokines TNF-β, interferon gamma (IFN-γ), and IL-2 [62] (see Chapter 4, Exotoxins of *Streptococcus pyogenes*, and Chapter 10, Life-Threatening Streptococcal Infections). Streptococcal pyrogenic exotoxin B is related to the proteinase precursor and may play a role in the pathogenesis of necrotizing fasciitis and myositis. It may also contribute to shock in streptococcal TSS through its ability to cleave pre-IL-β into active IL-1β [63] or kininogen into kinins [64]. Thus, in streptococcal TSS, toxins, lymphokines, monokines, and bradykinin may all contribute to shock and microvascular injury [44,65].

Immunological responses of the host to GAS infections are also responsible for the pathology observed in the postinfectious sequelae, acute rheumatic fever and post-streptococcal glomerulonephritis (see Chapters 6 and 9 for definitive discussion of these diseases).

CLINICAL TYPES OF INFECTION

Pharyngitis and the Asymptomatic Carrier

Group A streptococcus may be isolated from the throats of 1%–70% of the population, many of whom are asymptomatic. The lowest carriage rates are in adults, whereas children living in crowded conditions in temperate climates during the winter months are highly affected. Patients with pharyngitis have abrupt onset of sore throat, submandibular adenopathy, fever, and chilliness, but usually not frank rigors. Cough and hoarseness are rare but pain on swallowing is characteristic. The uvula is edematous, tonsils are hypertrophied, the pharynx is erythematous with exudates that may be punctate or confluent (Plate 3). Uncomplicated pharyngitis is usually self-limited, and pain, swelling, and fever resolve spontaneously in 3 to 4 days even without treatment. In recent times the main reason to treat streptococcal pharyngitis was to prevent rheumatic fever. However, depending upon the nature of the infecting strain and on the immunologic state of the host, pharyngitis may progress to scarlet fever, bacteremia, suppurative head and neck infections, rheumatic fever, poststreptococcal glomerulonephritis, or streptococcal TSS. Definitive diagnosis of streptococcal pharyngitis is difficult when based solely upon clinical parameters, especially in infants where rhinorrhea may be the dominant manifestation. Even in older children having all of the above physical findings, the correct clinical diagnosis is made in only 75% of patients. Absence of any one of the classic signs greatly reduces the diagnostic specificity (see also Chapter 5).

Scarlet Fever

During the last 30 to 40 years, scarlet fever in the Western world has been infrequent and of such a mild nature that some have referred to it as pharyngitis with a rash or benign scarlet fever. In contrast, in the latter half of the 19th century, mortalities of 25% to 35% were reported in the United States, Western Europe, and Scandinavia [66]. The fatal or malignant forms of scarlet fever have been described as either septic or toxic. Children with septic scarlet fever had prolonged courses and succumbed 2 to 4 weeks after the onset of pharyngitis, frequently due to complications such as upper-airway obstruction, otitis media with perforation, meningitis, mastoiditis, invasion of the jugular vein or carotid artery, and bronchopneumonia. The second form of severe or malignant scarlet fever was referred to as toxic scarlet fever and, though rare, was associated with profound hyperpyrexia (temperatures of 107°–113°F), delirium, convulsions, and death. All these suppurative complications of streptococcal pharyngitis as well as the malignant forms of scarlet fever have been markedly less common since the advent of antibiotics. Currently, scarlet fever in the Western world has been mild, caused by strains of GAS producing pyrogenic exotoxin type C.

Erysipelas

Erysipelas is usually caused by *Streptococcus pyogenes*, although recently groups C, G, and B have also been isolated from patients with this illness [67]. Distinctive features include an abrupt onset, fiery red, salmon, or scarlet rash with well-defined margins—particularly along the nasolabial fold—rapid progression, and intense pain (Plate 4). Flaccid bullae may develop during the second to third day of illness, yet extension to deeper soft tissues is rare. Surgical debridement is rarely necessary and treatment with penicillin has been very effective. Swelling may progress despite treatment, though fever, pain, and the intense redness diminish. Desquamation of the involved skin occurs 5 to 10 days into the illness. In contrast to acute streptococcal tonsillitis, which is more common among children and young people under the age of 30, erysipelas affects mostly elderly people, who may suffer recurrent episodes of this infection [68]. Historically, erysipelas, like scarlet fever, was more severe prior to the turn of the century. Although erysipelas is most common on the face, it may occur anywhere in the body. The portal of entry is usually the skin when it occurs on an extremity, although even here no portal of entry can be found in 26% of cases. The oropharynx likely serves as the source of bacteria and portal of entry when erysipelas occurs on the face. Norrby et al. have demonstrated that many different M types of GAS were associated with erysipelas infections in Sweden [68]. Although M types 1 and 8 were most common, they accounted for <50% of the infections. These strains produced low quantities of SPEA; larger quantities of SPEB and SPEC and 26 of the 38 strains were OF positive [68].

Streptococcal Pyoderma (Impetigo Contagiosa)

Impetigo is most common in patients with poor hygiene or malnutrition. It may occur on the face, but is more common on the extremities. Colonization of the unbroken skin occurs first, then intradermal inoculation is initiated by minor abrasions, insect bites, etc. Single or multiple thick-crusted, golden-yellow lesions develop within 10 to 14 days (Plate 5). Penicillin orally or parenterally, and bacitracin or mupuricin topically are effective treatments for impetigo and also reduce transmission of streptococci to susceptible individuals. None of these treatments including penicillin, prevents poststreptococcal glomerulonephritis. (See Chapter 8 for details of the epidemiology and clinical characteristics of impetigo and Chapter 9 for the clinical characteristics and pathogenesis of post-streptococcal glomerulonephritis).

Cellulitis

Group A streptococcus is the most common cause of cellulitis; however, alternative diagnoses may be obvious when associated with a primary focus such as an abscess or boil (*Staphylococcus aureus*), dog bite (*Capnocytophaga canimorsus*), cat bite (*Pasteurella multocida*), fresh-water injury (*Aeromonas hydrophila*), or sea-water injury (*Vibrio vulnifica*) [69]. Clinical clues to diagnosis are important because aspiration of the leading edge or punch biopsy yields a causative organism in only 15% and 20% of cases, respectively [70]. Predisposing factors for GAS cellulitis include lymphedema of any cause such as lymphoma, filariasis or postsurgical regional lymph node dissection (mastectomy, carcinoma of the prostate, etc.), and chronic venous stasis. Recently, recurrent saphenous vein donor site cellulitis has also been attributed to group A, C, or G streptococci (see Chapter 13). Cellulitis without a portal of entry such as those described above is most likely to be caused by streptococcus. Nonetheless, careful examination may reveal cracks between the toes or eczema. Group A streptococci may invade the epidermis and subcutaneous tissues, resulting in local swelling, erythema, and pain. The skin becomes indurated and, unlike the brilliant redness of erysipelas, is a pinkish color. Streptococcal cellulitis responds quickly to penicillin, but in some cases where staphylococcus is of concern, nafcillin or oxacillin may be a better choice.

Epidemics of GAS cellulitis in surgical wards or burn centers were well described before antibiotics but are currently uncommon. Little is known about the pathogenesis of streptococcal cellulitis; however, it is likely that endogenous mediators such as TNF and IL-1 as well as extracellular bacterial toxins play an important role in the clinical manifestations. This is supported by the observation that cultures of skin biopsy yield bacteria in <20% of cases, thus much of the erythema likely represents diffusion of bacterial toxins or endogenous mediators away from the site of actual infection.

Lymphangitis

Cutaneous infection such as cellulitis or erysipelas, with bright red streaks ascending proximally, is commonly due to group A streptococcus. Bacteremia and systemic toxicity develop rapidly once streptococci reach the bloodstream via the thoracic duct. Lymphangitis is a serious infection and patients should be admitted to the hospital and treated with parenteral antibiotics initially to prevent systemic complications.

Necrotizing Fasciitis

Necrotizing fasciitis, originally called streptococcal gangrene, is a deep-seated infection of the subcutaneous tissue that results in progressive destruction of fascia and fat but may spare the skin itself. Subsequently, "necrotizing fasciitis" has become the preferred term, since *Clostridium perfringens*, *C. septicum*, *Staphylococcus aureus*, and mixed aerobic/anaerobic flora of the mouth or gastrointestinal tract can produce a similar pathologic process. Infection may begin at the site of trivial or inapparent trauma. Within the first 24 h, swelling, heat, erythema, and tenderness develop and rapidly spread proximally and distally from the original focus. During the next 24 to 48 h, the erythema darkens, changing from red to purple and then to blue, and blisters and bullae form that contain clear yellow fluid (Plate 6). On the fourth or fifth day, the purple areas become frankly gangrenous (see also Chapter 10).

Myositis

Historically, streptococcal myositis has been an extremely uncommon infection, with only 21 cases being documented from 1900 to 1985. Recently, the prevalence of streptococcal myositis has increased in the United States, Norway, and Sweden. Although bacteria may be delivered to muscle by penetrating trauma, translocation of streptococci from the pharynx to the site of deep (nonpenetrating) trauma (muscle) also occurs hematogenously. Severe pain may be the only presenting symptom, and swelling and erythema may be the only signs of infection. In most cases, a single muscle group is involved; however, because patients are frequently bacteremic, multiple sites of myositis or abscess can occur. Distinguishing streptococcal myositis from spontaneous gas gangrene due to *C. perfringens* or *C. septicum* may be difficult, although the presence of crepitus or gas in the tissue would favor clostridial infection. Myositis is easily distinguished from necrotizing fasciitis anatomically by surgical exploration or incisional biopsy, however, clinical features of both conditions overlap (Plate 7). In published reports, the case–fatality rate of necrotizing fasciitis is between 20% and 50%, whereas that of streptococcal myositis is between 80% and 100%. Aggressive surgical debridement is extremely important because of the poor efficacy of penicillin described in human cases as well as in experimental models of streptococcal myositis (see In Vivo Efficacy of Antibiotics, below).

Pneumonia

Pneumonia caused by GAS is most common in women in the second and third decades of life, and is associated with the rapid appearance of large pleural effusions and empyema in 40% of patients. Chest tube drainage is mandatory, however, management is complicated by thick fibrinous pleural effusions forming loculations. In the past, this has required multiple chest tube placements and prolonged hospitalization despite penicillin treatment. Early thoracoscopy and decortication of the pleura may prevent these complications and, perhaps more importantly, may prevent the development of restrictive lung disease. Recently, pneumonia caused by GAS has also been associated with streptococcal TSS.

Streptococcal Toxic Shock Syndrome

In the late 1980s, invasive GAS infections associated with bacteremia, deep soft-tissue infection, shock, multiorgan failure, and death in 30%–70% of cases were reported from North America and Europe (reviewed in ref. [6]). Such cases have been defined as the streptococcal toxic shock syndrome [71]. Though all age-groups may be affected, most cases have occurred sporadically in previously healthy individuals who are between 20 and 50 years of age. Over 50% of patients have experienced a viral-like prodrome, minor trauma, recent surgery, or varicella infection. In cases that progress to necrotizing fasciitis, the infection may begin at the site of a break in the skin and extend deep in the soft tissue, or alternatively, infections may begin deep at the site of blunt trauma such as a hematoma or muscle strain and extend through muscle and fascia to the superficial skin layers. Although preceding symptomatic pharyngitis is rare, the pharyngeal mucosa is the likely bacterial source. Presumably a transient bacteremia from pharyngeal colonization seeds the site of trauma.

The abrupt onset of severe pain is a common initial symptom of streptococcal TSS. The pain most commonly involves an extremity, but may also mimic peritonitis, pelvic inflammatory disease, acute myocardial infarction, Herpes zoster infection, headache, toothache, meningitis, or sinus infection. Treatment with nonsteroidal anti-inflammatory agents may mask the presenting symptoms or predispose to more severe complications such as shock.

Fever is the most common presenting sign, although some patients present with profound hypothermia secondary to shock. Confusion is present in over half of patients, and may progress to coma or combativeness. On admission, 80% of patients have tachycardia and over half will have a systolic blood pressure of <110 mm Hg. Of those with normal blood pressure on admission, most become hypotensive within 4 h. Soft-tissue infection evolves to necrotizing fasciitis or myositis in 50% to 70% of patients and these require emergent surgical debridement, fasciotomy, or amputation. An ominous sign is progression of soft-tissue swelling to violaceous or bluish vesicles or bullae. Invariably this indicates necrotizing fasciitis or myonecrosis and demands immediate surgical exploration. Many other clinical presentations may be associated with streptococcal TSS, including endophthalmitis, myositis, perihepatitis, peritonitis, myocarditis, meningitis, septic arthritis, and overwhelming sepsis. Patients with shock and multiorgan failure without signs or symptoms of local infections have a worse prognosis since definitive diagnosis and surgical debridement may be delayed. In addition, infection involving the soft tissues of the head and neck are problematic because surgical debridement may be disfiguring or impossible (see also Chapter 10).

Puerperal Sepsis

Puerperal sepsis occurs during pregnancy or abortion when group A streptococcus, colonizing the patient, invades the endometrium and surrounding structures as well as the lymphatics and bloodstream. The result is acute endometritis and bacteremia complicated by pelvic thrombophlebitis and peritonitis. This disease reached epidemic proportions in Europe [72] and the United States [73] during the mid-1800s, largely as the result of contamination of women by attending physicians. Currently, in the United States there has been a re-emergence of these types of infection associated with streptococcal TSS; these cases appear, however, to be sporadic, isolated events, and not nosocomial as in the last century. Unless there is a high index of suspicion, puerperal sepsis may not be recognized largely because abdominal pain, the hallmark of this infection is not uncommon after a normal delivery. Increasingly severe pain associated with unexplained fever and leukocytosis should prompt a careful examination of the patient by the physician. Computed tomography (CT) scans and magnetic resonance images (MRIs) may only show swelling of the uterus and an increase in peritoneal fluid. Prompt surgical exploration and hysterectomy may be lifesaving.

Vulvovaginitis

Group A streptococcus is a common cause of vulvovaginitis in the prepubertal female. Symptoms include a serous vaginal discharge, erythema of the vulvar area, and intense pruritis. Oral antibiotics such as Pen V K are usually curative.

Funisitis and Omphalitis

Omphalitis is an infection of the umbilical cord and surrounding tissues. Etiologic organisms include GAS, *Staphylococcus aureus*, group B streptococcus, and gram-negative enteric organisms. Appropriate Gram stain and cultures should guide therapy, although oxacillin and/or gentamicin is reasonable empiric treatment.

Endocarditis

Endocarditis due to streptococci is generally caused by viridans streptococci and enterococci. Group A streptococcus has been a very rare cause of endocarditis in the antibiotic era. Interestingly, the Infectious Disease Society of America Hotline Network on Emerging Pathogens has recently documented 32 cases of endocarditis caused by beta hemolytic streptococci, including several due to GAS (D.L. Stevens, unpublished data). The epidemiology of such infections has not yet been defined. Fortunately, most antibiotic treatments for acute or subacute endocarditis would cover these strains, although it is likely that the course of endocarditis caused by these strains could be much more fulminant than those caused by viridans streptococci.

Postinfectious Sequelae (Rheumatic Fever and Poststreptococcal Glomerulonephritis)

See Chapter 6, Pathogenesis of Rheumatic Fever, Chapter 7, Rheumatic Fever, and Chapter 9, Acute Poststreptococcal Glomerulonephritis for discussion of postinfectious sequelae.

LABORATORY DIAGNOSIS

Rapid antigen detection tests in the office setting have a sensitivity and specificity of 40% to 90% (see Chapter 5). A popular approach in clinical practice is to obtain two throat swab samples from the posterior pharynx or tonsillar surface. A rapid strep test is performed on the first sample and if positive, the patient is treated with antibiotics and the second swab discarded. If the rapid strep test is negative, the second sample is sent for culture and treatment is withheld pending a positive culture. Bacitracin susceptibility remains an excellent presumptive test for GAS. Alternatively, rapid Lancefield group typing can be performed using latex agglutination tests. Acute pharyngitis results in sufficient antigenic stimulation to induce antibody production directed against M protein, streptolysin O, DNase and hyaluronidase, and, if present, pyrogenic exotoxins. An increase in titer of any of these is indicative of a recent streptococcal infection. The anti-hyaluronidase test is the best test for infections involving the skin. (See Chapter 5, Streptococcal Pharyngitis, and Chapter 15, Laboratory Evaluation of Streptococci, for more definitive information on laboratory aids to diagnosis).

TREATMENT

Antibiotic Resistance

The group A streptococcus remains exquisitely sensitive to penicillin and other beta lactam antibiotics, but resistance to sulfonamides and tetracyclines has been recognized since World War II [74]. Erythromycin resistance has been found in as high as 70% of GAS isolates in Japan [75] and nearly 50% of pharyngeal isolates in Finland [76]. Currently, in the United States erythromycin resistance is found in only about 5% of clinical isolates (D.L. Stevens, unpublished data). Resistance to clindamycin and lincomycin has also been reported sporadically over the last 20 years [77,78]. Although cross-resistance to macrolide and lincosamide antibiotics has been observed among a variety of gram-positive bacteria, this multiple-resistance phenomenon does not commonly occur among strains of group A streptococci [79]. For example, in a recent investigation, 28 erythromycin-resistant strains of GAS were found to be susceptible to clindamycin [79]. Erythromycin resistance appears to be due a macrolide efflux mechanism [79].

In Vivo Efficacy of Antibiotics

Numerous studies have demonstrated the clinical efficacy of penicillin, cephalosporins, erythromycin, and clindamycin in the treatment of streptococcal pharyngitis, erysipelas, impetigo, and cellulitis. In addition, Wannamaker et al. [80] demonstrated that penicillin therapy prevented the development of rheumatic fever following streptococcal pharyngitis if therapy was begun within 8 to 10 days of the onset of sore throat. Nonetheless, some clinical failures of penicillin treatment of streptococcal infection do occur. One problem with penicillin treatment of *Strep-*

tococcus pyogenes has been the inability of the drug to eradicate bacteria from the pharynx in 5% to 20% of patients with documented streptococcal pharyngitis [81–83]. In addition, more aggressive GAS infections (such as necrotizing fasciitis, empyema, burn wound sepsis, subcutaneous gangrene, and myositis) respond less well to penicillin and continue to be associated with high mortality and extensive morbidity [38,44,84]. For example, a recent study of 25 cases of streptococcal myositis reported an overall mortality of 85% despite penicillin therapy [84]. Finally, several studies using experimental models suggest that penicillin fails when large numbers of organisms are present [85,86]. For example, experimental studies of GAS myositis demonstrate that penicillin was ineffective when treatment was delayed ≥2 h after initiation of infection [86]. Interestingly, erythromycin and clindamycin had significantly greater efficacy [86,87]. Eagle suggested that penicillin failed in this type of infection because of the "physiologic state of the organism" [85]. This phenomenon has recently been attributed to both in vitro and in vivo inoculum effects [88,89].

Penicillin and other β-lactam antibodies are most efficacious against rapidly growing bacteria. We hypothesized that large inocula reach the stationary phase of growth sooner than smaller inocula both in vitro and in vivo. The finding that high concentrations of *Streptococcus pyogenes* accumulate in deep-seated infection is supported by data from Eagle [85]. We compared the penicillin-binding protein (PBP) patterns from membrane proteins of group A streptococci isolated from different stages of growth, i.e., mid-log phase and stationary phase. Binding of radiolabeled penicillin by all PBPs was decreased in stationary cells and remarkably, PBPs 1 and 4 were undetectable in late stationary phase [88]. Thus, the loss of certain PBPs during stationary-phase growth in vitro may be responsible for the inoculum effect observed in vivo and may account for the failure of penicillin in both experimental and human cases of severe streptococcal infection.

The greater efficacy of clindamycin is likely multifactorial. First, its efficacy is not affected by inoculum size or stage of growth [88,90]. Second, clindamycin is a potent suppressor of bacterial toxin synthesis [91,92]. Third, clindamycin facilitates phagocytosis of *Streptococcus pyogenes* by inhibiting M protein synthesis [92]. Fourth, clindamycin suppresses synthesis of PBP, which, in addition to being targets for penicillin, are also enzymes involved in cell wall synthesis and degradation [90]. Fifth, clindamycin has a longer postantibiotic effect than β-lactams such as penicillin. Lastly, we have shown that clindamycin causes suppression of lipopolysaccharide-induced monocyte synthesis of TNF-α [93]. Thus, clindamycin's efficacy may also be related to its ability to modulate the immune response. In summary, a combination of penicillin and clindamycin seems warranted because resistance to clindamycin has been described, albeit rarely. In addition, there are no antagonistic effects between these two antibiotics and at very low concentrations there is modest synergy [94].

Although antibiotic selection is critically important, other measures such as prompt and aggressive exploration and debridement of suspected deep-seated *Streptococcus pyogenes* infection are mandatory and provide material for Gram stain and culture. Thus, it is critically important that our surgical colleagues be involved early in such cases; later in the course of treatment, surgical intervention may be impossible because of toxicity or because infection has extended to vital areas that are impossible to debride.

Anecdotal reports suggest that hyperbaric oxygen has been used in a handful of patients with necrotizing fasciitis, but no controlled studies are underway, nor is it clear if this treatment is useful.

Because of intractable hypotension and diffuse capillary leak in streptococcal TSS, massive amounts of intravenous fluids (10–20 liters/day) in adults are often necessary. Pressors such as dopamine are used frequently, however, no controlled trials of streptococcal TSS have been performed. In patients with intractable hypotension, vasoconstrictors such as epinephrine have been used, but symmetrical gangrene of digits seems to result frequently (D.L. Stevens, unpublished observations), often with loss of limb. In these cases it is difficult to determine if symmetrical gangrene is due to pressors or infection or both.

Neutralization of circulating toxins would be a desirable therapeutic modality in scarlet fever and streptococcal TSS, yet appropriate antitoxins are not commercially available in the United States or Europe. Several small, nonrandomized studies describe successful use of intravenous gamma globulin (IVIG) in the treatment of streptococcal TSS [95–97]. Several studies have demonstrated that some batches of IVIG contain neutralizing antibodies against streptococcal pyrogenic exotoxins [98,99]. Thus, the rationale for IVIG is sound [101], and although double-blind control studies have not yet been performed, comparative observational studies are encouraging [102].

REFERENCES

1. Keefer CS, Ingelfinger FJ, Spink WW. Significance of hemolytic streptococcic bacteremia; a study of two hundred and forty-six patients. Arch Intern Med 1937; 60:1084–1097.
2. Brothwell D, Sandison AT. Antiquity of diseases caused by bacteria and viruses. In: Brothwell D, Sandison AT (eds). Diseases in Antiquity: A Survey of the Diseases, Injuries and Surgery of Early Populations. Springfield: Charles C. Thomas, 1967; 122–124.
3. Gaworzewska E, Colman G. Changes in the patterns of infection caused by *Streptococcus pyogenes*. Epidemiol Infect 1988; 100:257–269.
4. Kohler W, Gerlach D, Knoll H. Streptococcal outbreaks and erythrogenic toxin type A. Zentralbl Bakteriol Mikrobiol Hyg 1987; 266:104–15.
5. Veasy LG, Wiedmeier SE, Orsmond GS. Resurgence of acute rheumatic fever in the intermountain area of the United States. N Engl J Med 1986; 316:421–427.
6. Stevens DL. Streptococcal toxic shock syndrome: spectrum of disease, pathogenesis and new concepts in treatment. Emerg Infect Dis 1995; 1:69–78.
7. Lancefield RC. Current knowledge of type specific M antigens of group A streptococci. J Immunol 1962; 89:307–313.
8. Stanley J, Desai M, Xerry J, Tanna A, Efstratiou A, George R. High-resolution genotyping elucidates the epidemiology of group A streptococcus outbreaks. J Infect Dis 1996; 174:500–506.
9. Stevens DL. *Streptococcus pyogenes* infections. In: Stein JH (ed). Internal Medicine, 4th ed. St. Louis: C.V. Mosby, 1994; 2078–2086.
10. Wessels MR, Moses AE, Goldberg JB, DiCesare TJ. Hyaluronic acid capsule is a virulence factor

for mucoid group A streptococci. Proc Natl Acad Sci USA 1991; 88:8317–8321.

11. Schrager HM, Albertis S, Cywes C, Dougherty GJ, Wessels MR. Hyaluorinic acid capsule modulates M protein–mediated adherence and acts as a ligand for attachment of group A streptococcus to CD44 on human keratinocytes. J Clin Invest 1998; 101:1708–1716.

12. Hasty DL, Itzhak O, Courtney HS, Doyle RJ. Minireview: multiple adhesions of streptococci. Infect Immun 1992; 60:2147–2152.

13. Greenblatt J, Boackle RJ, Schwab JH. Activation of the alternate complement pathway by peptidoglycan from streptococcal cell wall. Infect Immun 1978; 19:296–303.

14. Verhoef J, Kalter E. Bacterial Endotoxins: Structure, Biomedical Significance and Detection with the Limulus Amebocyte Lysate Test. Alan R. Liss, 1985.

15. Bisno AL. Alternate complement pathway activation by group A streptococci: role of M-protein. Infect Immun 1979; 26:1172–1176.

16. Fischetti VA. Streptococcal M protein. Sci Am 1991; 264(6):58–65.

17. Fischetti VA, Horstmann RD, Pancholi V. Location of the complement factor H binding site on streptococcal M6 protein. Infect Immun 1995; 63:149–153.

18. Peterson PK, Schmeling D, Cleary PP, Wilkinson BJ, Kim Y, Quie PG. Inhibition of alternative complement pathway opsonization by group A streptococcal M protein. J Infect Dis 1979; 139:575–585.

19. Dale J, Chiang E. Intranasal immunization with recombinant group A streptococcal M protein fragment fused to the B subunit of Escherichia coli labile toxin protects mice against systemic challenge infections. J Infect Dis 1995; 171:1038–1041.

20. Tran PT, Johnson DR, Kaplan EL. The presence of M protein in nontypeable group a streptococcal upper respiratory tract isolates from southeast Asia. J Infect Dis 1994; 169:658–661.

21. Single LA, Martin DR. Clonal differences within M-types of the group A streptococcus revealed by pulsed field gel electrophoresis. FEMS Microbiol Lett 1992; 91:85–90.

22. de Malmanche SA, Martin DR. Protective immunity to the group A streptococcus may be only strain specific. Med Microbiol Immunol 1994; 183:299–306.

23. Thern A, Stenberg L, Dahlback B, Lindahl G. Ig-binding surface proteins of Streptococcus pyogenes also bind human C4b-binding protein (C4BP), a regulatory component of the complement system. J Immunol 1995; 154:375–386.

24. Hanski E, Caparon M. Protein F, a fibronectin-binding protein, is an adhesin of the group A streptococcus Streptococcus pyogenes. Proc Natl Acad Sci USA 1992; 89:6172–6176.

25. Natanson S, Sela S, Moses A, Musser J, Caparon M, Hanski E. Distribution of fibronectin-binding proteins among group A streptococci of different M types. J Infect Dis 1995; 171:871–878.

26. Akesson P, Sjoholm AG, Bjorck L. Protein SIC, a novel extracellular protein of Streptococcus pyogenes interfering with complement function. J Biol Chem 1996; 271:1081–1088.

27. Katerof V, Lindgren P, Totolain A, Schalen C. Serum opacity factor activity among group C and group G streptococci. In: Program and Abstracts of the ASM Conference on Streptococcal Genetics, Washington, D.C.: American Society for Microbiology, 1998.

28. Bessen DE, Sotir CM, Readdy T, Hollingshead SK. Genetic correlates of throat and skin isolates of group A streptococci. J Infect Dis 1996; 173:896–900.

29. Alouf JE, Geoffroy C. Structure activity relationships in sulfhydryl-activated toxins. In: Freer JH, Jeljaszewicz J (eds). Bacterial Protein Toxins. London: Academic Press, 1984; 165–171.

30. Tweten RK. Nucleotide sequence of the gene for perfringolysin O (theta-toxin) from Clostridium perfringens: significant homology with the genes for streptolysin O and pneumolysin. Infect Immun 1988; 56:3235–3240.

31. Lutticken R, Lutticken D, Johnson DR, Wannamaker LW. Application of a new method for detecting streptococcal nicotinamide adenine dinucleotide glycohydrolase to various M types of Streptococcus pyogenes. J Clin Microbiol 1976; 3:533–536.

32. Stevens DL, McIndoo E, Bryant AE, Zuckerman D. Production of NADase in clinical isolates of Streptococcus pyogenes [abstract]. In: Interscience Conference on Antimicrobial Agents and Chemotherapy, Toronto. Washington, D.C.: American Society for Microbiology, Abstract # K-158, p. 356.

33. Lottenberg R, Broder CC, Boyle MDP. Identification of a specific receptor for plasmin on a group A streptococcus. Infect Immun 1987; 55:1914–1928.

34. Barsumian EL, Schlievert PM, Watson DW. Non-specific and specific immunological mitogenicity by group A streptococcal pyrogenic exotoxins. Infect Immun 1978; 22:681–688.

35. Nida SK, Ferretti JJ. Phage influence on the synthesis of extracellular toxins in group A streptococci. Infect Immun 1982; 36:745–750.

36. Kline JB, Collins CM. Analysis of the superantigenic activity of mutant and allelic forms of streptococcal pyrogenic exotoxin A. Infect Immun 1996; 64:861–869.

37. Hauser AR, Stevens DL, Kaplan EL, Schlievert PM. Molecular analysis of pyrogenic exotoxins from Streptococcus pyogenes isolates associated with toxic shock-like syndrome. J Clin Microbiol 1991; 29:1562–1567.

38. Stevens DL, Tanner MH, Winship J, Swarts R, Reis KM, Schlievert PM, Kaplan E. Reappearance of scarlet fever toxin A among streptococci in the Rocky Mountain West: severe group A streptococcal infections associated with a toxic shock-like syndrome. N Engl J Med 1989; 321:1–7.

39. Hallas G. The production of pyrogenic exotoxins by group A streptococci. J Hyg (Camb) 1985; 95:47–57.

40. Iwasaki M, Igarashi H, Hinuma Y, Yutsudo T. Cloning, characterization and overexpression of a *Streptococcus pyogenes* gene encoding a new type of mitogenic factor. FEBS Lett 1993; 331:187–192.

41. Norrby-Teglund A, Newton D, Kotb M, Holm SE, Norgren M. Superantigenic properties of the group A streptococcal exotoxin SpeF (MF). Infect Immun 1994; 62:5227–5233.

42. Mollick JA, Miller GG, Musser JM, Cook RG, Grossman D, Rich RR. A novel superantigen isolated from pathogenic strains of *Streptococcus pyogenes* with aminoterminal homology to staphylococcal enterotoxins B and C. J Clin Invest 1993; 92:710–719.

43. Cleary PP, Peterson J, Chen C, Nelson C. Virulent human strains of group G streptococci express a C5a peptidase enzyme similar to that produced by group A streptococci. Infect Immun 1991; 59:2305–2310.

44. Stevens DL. Invasive group A streptococcus infections. Clin Infect Dis 1992; 14:2–13.

45. Martin PR, Hoiby EA. Streptococcal serogroup A epidemic in Norway 1987–1988. Scand J Infect Dis 1990; 22:421–429.

46. Cleary PP, Kaplan EL, Handley JP, Wlazlo A, Kim MH, Hauser AR, Schlievert PM. Clonal basis for resurgence of serious *Streptococcus pyogenes* disease in the 1980s. Lancet 1992; 339:518–521.

47. Musser JM, Hauser AR, Kim MH, Schlievert PM, Nelson K, Selander RK. *Streptococcus pyogenes* causing toxic-shock-like syndrome and other invasive diseases: clonal diversity and pyrogenic exotoxin expression. Proc Natl Acad Sci USA 1991; 88:2668–2672.

48. Stevens DL, Tanner MH, Winship J, Swartz R, Ries KM, Schlievert PM, Kaplan E. Group A streptococcal infections and a toxic shock–like syndrome. N Engl J Med 1989; 321:2545–2546.

49. Caparon MG, Stephens DS, Olsen A, Scott JR. Role of M protein in adherence of group A streptococci. Infect Immun 1991; 59:1811–1817.

50. Frick I-M, Crossin KL, Edelman GM, Bjorck L. Protein H—a bacterial surface protein with affinity for both immunoglobulin and fibronectin type III domains. EMBO J 1995; 14:1674–1679.

51. Okada N, Liszewski MK, Atkinson JP, Caparon M. Membrane cofactor protein (CD46) is a keratinocyte receptor for the M protein of the group A streptococcus. Proc Natl Acad Sci USA 1995; 92:2489–2493.

52. Simpson WJ, Lapenta D, Chen C, Cleary PP. Coregulation of type 12 M protein and streptococcal C5a peptidase genes in group A streptococci: evidence for a virulence regulon controlled by the *virR* locus. J Bacteriol 1990; 172:696–700.

53. Dale JB, Washburn RG, Marques MB, Wessels MR. Hyaluronate capsule and surface M protein in resistance to opsonization of group A streptococci. Infect Immun 1996; 64:1495–1501.

54. Salvadori IG, Blake MS, McCarty M, Tai JY, Zabriskie JB. Group A streptococcus–liposome ELISA antibody titres to group A polysaccharide and opsonophagocytic capabilities of the antibodies. J Infect Dis 1995; 171:593–600.

55. Whitnack E, Beachey EH. Anti-opsonic activity of fibrinogen bound to M protein on the surface of group A streptococci. J Clin Invest 1992; 69:1042–1045.

56. Wright SD, Weitz JI, Huang AJ, Levin SM, Silverstein SC, Loike JD. Complement receptor type three (CD11b/CD18) of human polymorphonuclear leukocytes recognizes fibrinogen. Proc Natl Acad Sci USA 1988; 85:7734–7738.

57. Schnitzler N, Schweizer K, Podbielski A, Haase G, Spellerberg B, Holland R, Lutticken R. Activation of granulocytes by phorbol-12-myristate (PMA) enhances phagocytosis of *Streptococcus pyogenes*. Adv Exp Med Biol 1997; 418:897–902.

58. Raeder RH, Woischnik M, Podbielski A, Boyle MDP. A secreted streptococcal cysteine protease can cleave a surface expressed M1 protein and alters its immunoglobulin-binding properties. Res Microbiol 1998; 149:539–548.

59. Bryant AE, Kehoe MA, Stevens DL. Streptococcal pyrogenic exotoxin A and streptolysin O enhance PMNL binding to protein matrixes. J Infect Dis 1992; 166:165–169.

60. Marrack P, Kappler JW. The staphylococcal enterotoxins and their relatives. Science 1990; 248:705–711.

61. Kotb M, Ohnishi H, Majumdar G, Hackett S, Bryant A, Higgins G, Stevens D. Temporal relationship of cytokine release by peripheral blood mononuclear cells stimulated by the streptococcal superantigen pep M5. Infect Immun 1993; 61:1194–1201.

62. Hackett SP, Stevens DL. Superantigens associated with staphylococcal and streptococcal toxic shock syndromes are potent inducers of tumor necrosis factor beta synthesis. J Infect Dis 1993; 168:232–235.

63. Kappur V, Majesky MW, Li LL, Black RA, Musser JM. Cleavage of Interleukin 1β (IL-1β) precursor to produce active IL-1β by a conserved extracellular cysteine protease from *Streptococcus pyogenes*. Proc Natl Acad Sci USA 1993; 90:7676–7680.

64. Herwald H, Collin M, Muller-Esterl W, Bjorck L. Streptococcal cysteine proteinase releases kinins: a novel virulence mechanism. J Exp Med 1996; 184:1–9.

65. Shanley TP, Schrier D, Kapur V, Kehoe M, Musser JM, Ward PA. Streptococcal cysteine protease augments lung injury induced by products of group A streptococci. Infect Immun 1996; 64:870–877.

66. Rotch TM. Pediatrics: The Hygienic and Medical Treatment of Children. Philadelphia: J.B. Lippincott, 1896.

67. Bernard P, Bedane C, Mounier M, Denis F, Catanzano G, Bonnetblanc JM. Streptococococcal cause of erysipelas and cellulitis in adults. Arch Dermatol 1989; 125:779–782.

68. Norrby A, Eriksson B, Norgren M, Ronstrom CJ, Sjöblom AC, Karkkonen K, Holm SE. Virulence properties of erysipelas-associated group A streptococci. Eur J Clin Microbiol Infec Dis 1992; 11:1136–1143.

69. Stevens DL. Soft tissue infections. In: Isselbacher KJ, Braunwald E, Wilson JD, Martin JB, Fauci AS, Kasper DL (eds). Harrison's Textbook of Medicine, 13th ed. New York: McGraw-Hill, 1994; 561–563.

70. Duvanel T, Auckenthaler R, Rohner P, Harms M, Saurat JH. Quantitative cultures of biopsy specimens from cutaneous cellulitis. Arch Intern Med 1989; 149:293–296.

71. The Working Group on Severe Streptococcal Infections. Defining the group A streptococcal toxic shock syndrome: rationale and consensus definition. JAMA 1993; 269:390–391.

72. Carter KC, Carter BR. Childbed Fever: A Scientific Biography of Ignaz Semmelweis. Westport, CT: Greenwood Press, 1994.

73. Holmes OW. In: Holmes OW (ed). Medical Essays 1842–1882: The writings of Oliver Wendell Holmes. Boston: Houghton, Mifflin, 1891.

74. Eickhoff TC, Finland M. In vitro susceptibility of group A beta hemolytic streptococci to 18 antibiotics. Am J Med Sci 1965; 249:261–268.

75. Mitsuhashi S, Inoue M, Fuse A. Drug resistance in Streptococcus pyogenes. Jpn J Microbiol 1974; 18:98–99.

76. Seppala H, Nissenen A, Jarvinen H, Huovinen S, Henriksson T, Herva E, et al. Resistance to erythromycin in group A streptococci. N Engl J Med 1992; 326:292–297.

77. Drapkin MS, Karchmer AW, Moellering RC. Bacteremic infections due to clindamycin-resistant streptococci. JAMA 1976; 236:263–265.

78. Kohn J, Hewitt JH, Fraser CAM. Group A streptococci resistant to clindamycin. BMJ 1968; 1:1.

79. Sutcliffe J, Tait-Kamradt A, Wondrack L. Streptococcus pneumoniae and Streptococcus pyogenes resistant to macrolides but sensitive to clindamycin: a common resistance pattern mediated by an efflux system. Antimicrob Agents Chemother 1996; 40:1817–1824.

80. Wannamaker LW, Rammelkamp CH Jr, Denny FW, Brink WR, Houser HB, Hahn EO, Dingle JH. Prophylaxis of acute rheumatic fever by treatment of the preceding streptococcal infection with various amounts of depot penicillin. Am J Med 1951; 10:673–695.

81. Kim KS, Kaplan EL. Association of penicillin tolerance with failure to eradicate group A streptococci from patients with pharyngitis. J Pediatr 1985; 107:681–684.

82. Gatanaduy AS, Kaplan EL, Huwe BB, McKay C, Wannamaker LW. Failure of penicillin to eradicate group A streptococci during an outbreak of pharyngitis. Lancet 1980; 2: 498–502.

83. Brook I. Role of beta-lactamase-producing bacteria in the failure of penicillin to eradicate group A streptococci. Pediatr Infect Dis 1985; 4:491–495.

84. Adams EM, Gudmundsson S, Yocum DE, Haselby RC, Craig WA, Sundstrom WR. Streptococcal myositis. Arch Intern Med 1985; 145:1020–1023.

85. Eagle H. Experimental approach to the problem of treatment failure with penicillin. I. Group A streptococcal infection in mice. Am J Med 1952; 13:389–399.

86. Stevens DL, Bryant-Gibbons AE, Bergstrom R, Winn V. The Eagle effect revisited: efficacy of clindamycin, erythromycin, and penicillin in the treatment of streptococcal myositis. J Infect Dis 1988; 158:23–28.

87. Stevens DL, Bryant AE, Yan S. Invasive group A streptococcal infection: new concepts in antibiotic treatment. Int J Antimicrob Agents 1994; 4:297–301.

88. Stevens DL, Yan S, Bryant AE. Penicillin binding protein expression at different growth stages determines penicillin efficacy in vitro and in vivo: an explanation for the inoculum effect. J Infect Dis 1993; 167:1401–1405.

89. Yan S, Mendelman PM, Stevens DL. The in vitro antibacterial activity of ceftriaxone against Streptococcus pyogenes is unrelated to penicillin-binding protein 4. FEMS Microbiol Lett 1993; 110:313–318.

90. Yan S, Bohach GA, Stevens DL. Persistent acylation of high-molecular weight penicillin binding proteins by penicillin induces the post antibiotic effect in Streptococcus pyogenes. J Infect Dis 1994; 170:609–614.

91. Stevens DL, Maier KA, Mitten JE. Effect of antibiotics on toxin production and viability of Clostridium perfringens. Antimicrob Agents Chemother 1987; 31:213–218.

92. Gemmell CG, Peterson PK, Schmeling D, Kim Y, Mathews J, Wannamaker L, Quie PG. Potentiation of opsonization and phagocytosis of Streptococcus pyogenes following growth in the

presence of clindamycin. J Clin Invest 1981; 67: 1249–1256.

93. Stevens DL, Bryant AE, Hackett SP. Antibiotic effects on bacterial viability, toxin production, and host response. Clin Infect Dis 1995; 20:S154–S157.

94. Stevens DL, Madaras-Kelly KJ, Richards DM. In vitro antimicrobial effects of various combinations of penicillin and clindaymcin against four strains of *Streptococcus pyogenes*. Antimicrob Agents Chemother 1998; 42:1266–1268.

95. Barry W, Hudgins L, Donta S, Pesanti E. Intravenous immunoglobulin therapy for toxic shock syndrome. JAMA 1992; 267:3315–3316.

96. Yong JM. Letter. Lancet 1994; 343:1427.

97. Kaul R, McGeer A, Norrby-Teglund A, Kotb M, Low DE. Intravenous immunoglobulin (IVIG) therapy in streptococcal toxic shock syndrome (STSS): results of a matched case–control study. Am J Med 1997; 103:18–24.

98. Norrby-Teglund A, Kaul R, Low DE, McGeer A, Andersson J, Andersson U, Kotb M. Evidence for the presence of streptococcal-superantigen-neutralizing antibodies in normal polyspecific immunoglobulin G. Infect Immun 1996; 64:5395–5398.

99. Norrby-Teglund A, Basma H, Andersson J, McGeer A, Low DE, Kotb M. Varying titres of neutralizing antibodies to streptococcal super-antigens in different preparations of normal polyspecific immunoglobulin G (IVIG): implications for therapeutic efficacy. Clin Infect Dis 1998; 26:631–638.

100. Stevens DL. Editorial response: rationale for the use of intravenous gamma globulin in the treatment of streptococcal toxic shock syndrome. Clin Infect Dis 1998; 26:639–641.

101. Norrby-Teglund A, Stevens DL. Novel therapies in streptococcal toxic shock syndrome attenuation of virulence factor expression and modulation of the immune response. Curr Opin Infect Dis 1998; 11:285–291.

102. Kaul R, McGeer A, Norrby-Teglund A, Kotb M, Schwartz B, O'Rourke K, Talbot J, Low DE, and The Canadian Streptococcal Study Group. Intravenous immunoglobulin therapy for streptococcal toxic shock syndrome—a comparative observational study. Clin Infect Dis 1999; 28(4): 800–807.

3

Group A Streptococcal Genetics and Virulence

P. PATRICK CLEARY
KRISTEN H. PRITCHARD
W. MICHAEL McSHAN
JOSEPH J. FERRETTI

The discovery by Avery, MacLeod, and McCarty that DNA was the genetic material represents one of the most important discoveries of modern biology. DNA obtained from an encapsulated (smooth) strain of *Streptococcus pneumoniae* was used to transform a capsule-deficient (rough) strain to produce capsule, thus establishing a molecular basis for the study of genetics [1]. Although these experiments also signaled the beginning of streptococcal genetics as a field of study, the difficulty in working with these organisms led researchers to pursue other microorganisms that were less fastidious in growth requirements as well as less pathogenic.

EXTRACHROMOSOMAL ELEMENTS

Recombinant DNA technology and the techniques of modern molecular biology provided new approaches to the study of streptococcal genetics. Gene cloning and sequencing, and the ability to employ natural (transduction and conjugal transfer of plasmids) and artificial (electrotransformation) methods of gene transfer, have allowed great progress to be made in further understanding the biology, epidemiology,

and virulence factors associated with streptococcal diseases. This chapter will focus on the genetics of group A streptococci.

Bacteriophages

Bacteriophages of both the virulent and temperate forms are known to infect *Streptococcus pyogenes*. These phages are morphologically similar to *Escherichia coli* phage lambda, with a head containing double-stranded DNA and a long, flexible tail. Historically, streptococcal phages have been known since the 1930s, however, the body of information available about them is limited compared to what is known about phages of other organisms. A significant problem in their study has been the low plating efficiency of many of these phages, which is probably because many have a low burst size and some have difficulty penetrating the hyaluronic acid capsule of the host. Gene-transfer experiments via transduction in the group A streptococci were first accomplished with the virulent phage A25 [2].

Bacteriophages are common among streptococci with estimates as high as 98% of all strains being lysogenized and containing at least one phage genome in its chromosome. Streptococcal phages are of considerable medical significance since they are known to carry the *spe*A and *spe*C genes, specifying erythrogenic toxin A and C, respectively [3,4]. Streptococcal erythrogenic toxin A (SPE A), also known as pyrogenic exotoxin A, increases the virulence of strains and is frequently found in strains associated with severe invasive infections. Epidemiological studies have shown that the *spe*A gene is found with a high frequency in serotype M1, M3, and M49 strains and rarely in serotype M2, M4, M6, and M12 strains. In contrast, *spe*C is found primarily in serotype M2, M4, M6, and M12 strains and rarely in M1, M3, and M49 strains [5].

The best-studied temperate phage is T12, a phage carrying the *spe*A gene encoding erythrogenic toxin A. Phage T12 is a member of a family of *spe*A-containing phages, three of which have been shown to have distinct physical maps and genomes that range in size from 32 kb to 40 kb [6]. The 35 kb chromosome of T12 has been sequenced and contains all of the information for establishing and maintaining lysogeny, including an attachment region that is located adjacent to the *spe*A gene (W.M. McShan and J.J. Ferretti, unpublished results; see Fig. 3.1). The attachment region is homologous to a 96 bp prophage attachment region in the *Streptococcus pyogenes* chromosome and following entry into the bacterial cell, the phage genome becomes inserted into the bacterial chromosome in a Campbell-like fashion characteristic of other lysogen-forming phages. Insertion of the phage at the homologous attachment site results in a duplication of that region without loss of genetic continuity in that particular region of bacterial DNA. In the case of phage T12, the bacterial attachment region is in the gene for a serine-tRNA [7]. Other streptococcal temperate phages appear to have their own characteristic insertion site. The location of *spe*A next to the phage attachment site suggests that this gene was incorporated into the phage genome during an abnormal excision event from an unknown organism. Additionally, the presence of a signal peptide coding region in *spe*A indicates that SPE A is a secreted protein, and its gene is most likely of bacterial origin. The identity of the source of the *spe*A gene remains unknown and its progenitor organism may have been lost during evolution. It is speculated that this organism is also the evolutionary source of the *Staphylococcus aureus* enterotoxin B protein, a secreted protein that has a high degree of amino acid identity with SPE A as well as similar biological properties. The *spe*A gene is not an essential bacteriophage gene since specific *spe*A inactivation does not alter phage function. Finally, bacteriophages have been isolated that share the same attachment site as T12 and possess an identical integrase gene but do not contain *spe*A, as well as bacteriophages that have *spe*A but use an integrase and attachment site that is distinct from T12 [8]. This information suggests that recombination plays an important role in the generation of

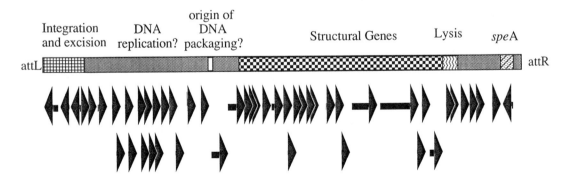

Figure 3.1 Genomic organization of bacteriophage T12. The genome is shown in the integrated prophage arrangement. The function of several regions of the genome has been identified by biological activity (*spe*A and the integrase) or by homology to previously identified phage genes from other bacteriophages (other regions indicated). Beneath the genome are arrows indicating the potential open reading frames in the genome and direction of transcription (W.M. McShan and J.J. Ferretti, unpublished results).

phage diversity and the spread of these phage-associated toxin genes.

Lysogeny is predicted to be maintained by the presence of a repressor, which controls in a negative fashion all phage functions except *spe*A. SPE A, on the other hand, is synthesized continuously during lysogen growth. Induction of the prophage from the lysogenic state occurs by interruption of DNA synthesis following exposure to ultraviolet light or mitomycin C, presumably since the RecA protease activity cleaves the repressor and allows lytic function to proceed.

Phage T12 contains all of the information essential for excision from the host as well as for synthesis of all of the proteins of the lytic phase of phage growth. One of the enzymes formed during the lytic phase of many streptococcal phages is a hyaluronidase, capable of cleaving the hyaluronic acid capsule found on the *Streptococcus pyogenes.* surface. The identification of multiple variants of phage hyaluronidases confirms the presence of a variety of different phages, some of which may be defective phages.

Plasmids

Plasmids or extrachromosomal genetic elements capable of autonomous replication and which are not necessary for cell function are found in low frequency in the group A streptococci. Most plasmids identified to date confer an antibiotic resistance phenotype to the cell, predominantly resistance to erythromycin, kanamycin, streptomycin, gentamicin, tetracycline, or chloramphenicol. Erythromycin and chloramphenicol-resistance determinants have been found as parts of conjugative plasmids capable of being transferred to other organisms [9]. Chromosomal conjugative transposons or composite elements have been identified in streptococci and are discussed below.

Plasmids have served as vectors for recombinant DNA experiments and plasmids from virtually all streptococci have been found to replicate efficiently in the group A streptococci [10,11]. Use of shuttle vectors containing a replicon each from *E. coli* and streptococci have proven useful for performing manipulations first in *E. coli* and then transferring the plasmid to

streptococci. Possible problems of methylation of streptococcal DNA sequences while in *E. coli* have not proven to be a problem in further molecular biology analyses or manipulations. Another group of plasmids that has gained widespread use are integration or suicide vectors [12,13]. These plasmids replicate only in *E. coli* and if they contain streptococcal DNA and an antibiotic resistance marker, the only possible fate is integration of the streptococcal DNA into the genome via a recombination event. Recently, novel vectors have been designed that incorporate the integrase and phage attachment site from phage T12, allowing site-specific recombination of the plasmid at the unique bacterial attachment site [14]. Such a phage-derived vector has been used to replace a nephritis-associated with a non–nephritis-associated allele of streptokinase [15].

Transposons and Insertion Sequence Elements

Conjugative transposons are widespread in gram-positive bacteria and have an important role in the spread of antibiotic resistance. Conjugative transposons differ from the well-studied transposons of *E. coli* and other gram-negative bacteria in several ways, particularly in the process of replication and spread to new hosts. Transposition in conjugative transposons occurs by an integration–excision process reminiscent of lambdoid bacteriophages and proceeds through a nonreplicative circular intermediate capable of conjugation-like transfer between donor and recipient cells. Additionally, these transposons have a wide host range; Tn*916*, for example, has been found in at least 47 species in 23 genera encompassing both gram-positive and gram-negative organisms [16]. Genes conferring antibiotic resistance to the host are a usual feature of conjugative transposons, and often multiple drug resistance markers are associated with a single transposon. Antibiotic resistance to tetracycline, erythromycin, chloramphenicol, kanamycin, and the macrolide (MLS) group is specified by various members of these genetic elements. Transposons appear to be the major vectors for dissemination of these resistance markers in gram-positive bacteria; plasmid-associated resistance genes are uncommon in contrast to the situation in *E. coli* and other gram-negative organisms. The review by Clewell [17] discusses the biology of conjugative transposons in depth.

Two well-studied conjugative transposons are found in *Streptococcus pyogenes*, Tn*916* and Tn*3701*. Tn*916*, first isolated from *Enterococcus faecalis*, is an 18 kb transposon specifying tetracycline resistance (*tet*M). The closely related transposon Tn*1545* is a 25.3 kb element that also carries *erm* and *aph*A-3 genes. Tn*916* has coding regions on one end of the transposon with similarity to the *int* and *xis* genes of temperate bacteriophages, and the products of both of these genes appear to play key roles in the integration/excision of Tn*916* by a Campbell-like process. Integration occurs at AT-rich target sites, and some degree of specificity appears to be involved since integration preferentially occurs in sequences with some degree of homology to the ends of Tn*916*. Multiple insertions of Tn*916* into the donor chromosome after mating are not uncommon. Tn*3701*, originally isolated from *Streptococcus pyogenes*, is a larger, composite transposon that contains a region homologous to Tn*916* [18]. Inserted into the right end of the Tn*916*-like region is an erythromycin resistance marker (*erm*). This subelement is named Tn*3703* and is occasionally found as an independent element and separate from the rest of the transposon. Tn*3703* can undergo transposition from a plasmid to the chromosome but apparently cannot undergo independent conjugative transfer as Tn*3701* can. The *erm* element is sometimes deleted from the transposon and may represent an additional subelement acquired in the evolution of this transposon.

Few insertion sequence (IS) elements have been observed in group A streptococci; however, the number will probably increase as genomic analysis proceeds. Kapur et al. [19] found a 1,110 bp element, IS*1239*, that was harbored by 33% of the *Streptococcus pyogenes* strains examined. IS*1239* has the capacity to encode a 326 amino acid peptide with homology to the *E. coli* IS*30* transposase. This element can exist in multiple copies in the host chromosome, and one serotype of DLS M15 strains was found to contain at least 12 copies. Whether this IS element ever forms a portion of a larger, composite transposon is yet unknown.

Gene Transfer

Transduction, the bacteriophage-mediated transfer of genetic material, was the first type of gene exchange described in the group A streptococci [2]. Use was made of virulent phages such as A25 to transfer primarily laboratory-induced antibiotic resistance genes to other group A strains. These genes conferred a phenotype that could be readily selected in the presence of the respective antibiotic in the growth medium. Although several linkage groups of resistance genes were identified, transduction has been limited in its ability to further define the genetics of the organism [20]. The main reasons for this limitations are the complex growth requirements of the organism and the inability to select directly for a phenotype since the group A streptococci lack many of the genes essential for the synthesis of amino acids, nucleotides, cofactors, etc.

Although conjugation has been observed in the group A streptococci, the transfer of genes has been primarily limited to naturally occurring antibiotic resistance genes. Conjugative plasmids carrying a number of antibiotic resistance genes have been shown to transfer between group A, B, D, and H streptococci [21]. Additionally, conjugation has been used to transfer an *emm* gene in group A streptococci [22].

Transformation has been the historical method of choice for introduction of DNA into microorganisms and initial studies with this method of gene transfer focused on those organisms that possessed a competence stage that naturally took up DNA into the cell, providing the opportunity for a recombination event to take place between homologous regions. The group A streptococci are not known to be naturally competent, thus introduction of DNA into the cell had to occur by artificial means. Transformation of streptococci by artificial means is most efficiently achieved by exposing the organism to high-voltage pulses, which apparently changes cell wall and membrane permeability, allowing DNA to enter the cell [23]. This process is known as electrotransformation and can be used to introduce either plasmid or linear DNA into the cell. It should be noted that transformation of plasmid DNA into the group A streptococci results in an approximately 1000-fold greater efficiency than introduction of linear

DNA. Whereas many strains of streptococci are easily transformed via electrotransformation, some strains remain refractory to this technique. The reason for the inability to transform is not clear, although capsule presence and cell wall characteristics of some strains may represent barriers to the uptake process.

The ability to transform group A streptococci has been most important for genetic engineering experiments directed at understanding the role of various factors involved in its virulence and pathogenicity. For example, individual genes can be insertionally inactivated via linear DNA [24] or integration or suicide vectors to produce strains containing a defective or mutant gene [12]. Genes inactivated in individual strains include streptolysin O, streptokinase, proteinase (erythrogenic toxin B), M protein, C5a peptidase, and immunoglobulin-binding protein genes.

Chromosome Organization

The construction of a physical map of *Streptococcus pyogenes* was made possible by the use of restriction enzymes with specificity for rare sequences that cut the genome only several times and the ability to separate large fragments

of DNA (>50 kb) from each other by pulsed-field gel electrophoresis (PFGE). Once a physical map was constructed, the approximate location of individual genes was determined by Southern hybridization. A physical and genetic map of an M1 strain of *Streptococcus pyogenes* is shown in Figure 3.2 [25]. The genome size of this strain was estimated to be 1920 kb, less than half the size of the genome of *E. coli* (4700 kb) or *Bacillus subtilis* (5700 kb). Several genes thought to be important for the expression of a virulence phenotype (e.g., *emm*, *ska*, *slo*, *plr*, *spe*B, *scp*A, and *tee*) were found to be located in a region spanning approximately 320 kb. Whether other virulence-associated genes will be found in this region is yet to be determined. The streptokinase gene is the only virulence gene in a 9.8 kb region consisting of a total of six genes [26]. The exact location of all of these genes with respect to each other will be confirmed in the near future when the entire nucleotide sequence of the genome is completed.

Although the location of individual genes on the map can be expected to be quite similar or even identical among the different M type strains, there is considerable heterogeneity of physical maps. For example, analysis of restriction fragment length polymorphism (RFLP) pat-

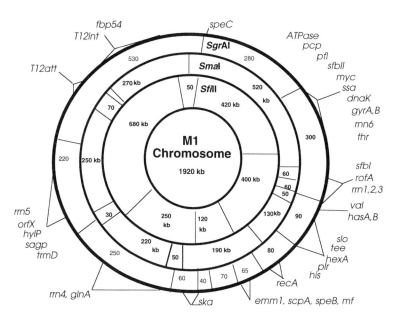

Figure 3.2 Physical and genetic map of the chromosome of an M type 1 strain of *Streptococcus pyogenes*. (From Suvorov and Ferretti [25], with permission.)

terns by PFGE of 90 different M1 strains isolated in New Zealand showed at least six different RFLP patterns [27]. Similarly, an analysis of 54 different M1 strains from nine countries showed seven different RFLP patterns. RFLP analysis will be an important tool for epidemiological surveillance, particularly in outbreaks and epidemics of streptococcal disease. Individual M-type strains also differ in RFLP patterns from each other and may also exhibit heterogeneity of RFLP patterns within the same M type (Fig. 3.3). Evolutionary changes involving chromosomal rearrangements, deletions, insertions, point mutations, and introduction of mobile genetic elements account for this heterogeneity and suggest that our once-simplified view of only 80 types of *Streptococcus pyogenes* strains based on M-type serological analysis is much more complex and continuing to change.

GENETIC DETERMINANTS OF *STREPTOCOCCUS PYOGENES* VIRULENCE

The group A streptococci elicit barriers to both innate and adaptive components of the immune response. Virulence depends on a cadre of extracellular and surface macromolecules. The application of molecular biology techniques to a genetic analysis of these organisms has provided a wealth of new information concerning virulence properties and dramatically advanced our understanding of their role in pathogenesis. The reader is referred to the proceedings of several conferences on streptococcal genetics [10,11,28,29], Lancefield international symposia on streptococcal diseases and review articles [31] and other sources [32] which provide detailed information on individual studies and techniques.

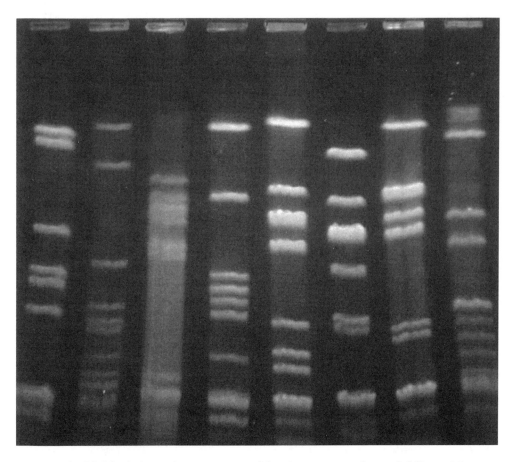

Figure 3.3 Pulsed field gel electrophoresis pattern of the chromosomes of several different M type strains of *Streptococcus pyogenes* which exhibit restriction fragment length polymorphisms.

Extracellular Products

The group A streptococci are reported to secrete more than 20 different extracellular proteins into the extracellular milieu, many of which are thought to be involved in the initiation of tissue damage and have a variety of pharmacologic and toxic activities. Genes producing extracellular proteins are generally thought to be accessory genes since their products are not essential for survival of the organism or in vitro growth. Nevertheless, their potent activities towards tissue and the ability to elicit responses from the immune system suggest an important role in the disease process.

Streptolysin O is the hallmark of group A streptococcal extracellular products and is the oxygen-labile hemolysin responsible for the characteristic beta-hemolytic pattern surrounding colony growth on blood agar plates. Streptolysin O is a membrane-damaging protein toxin that has been shown to have cardiotoxic properties. The *slo* gene has been cloned and is present in a highly conserved form in all strains of streptococci [33,33a]. The N-terminal region of streptolysin O is quite sensitive to proteolytic cleavage and the secreted protein product of the *slo* gene can be found in several sizes, most of which retain hemolytic activity. Little is known about the regulation of *slo*, but recent studies have shown that in some strains a site-specific rearrangement takes place in the *slo* region of the chromosome, resulting in a new genetic context and level of expression (D. Savic, personal communication).

Streptokinase is a protein secreted by group A, C, and G streptococci and is thought to be a virulence factor by virtue of its ability to facilitate the spread of these organisms by promoting the lysis of blood clots. Streptokinase binds stoichiometrically to mammalian plasminogen, and this complex can convert other plasminogen molecules to the serine protease plasmin. Once formed, plasmin can act on a variety of proteins, including the fibrin found in the matrix of blood clots. The discovery that the streptococci possess specific surface receptors capable of binding plasminogen, which is converted to plasmin in the presence of streptokinase, offers the organism the ability to have associated with it a proteolytic enzyme capable of causing tissue destruction. Streptokinase genes from a number of different streptococci have been cloned [34] and sequence analysis has shown the presence of two regions of high variability [35,36]. There have been suggestions that specific changes in amino acid sequence encoded in these regions may confer a specificity of binding of streptokinase–plasminogen complexes to glomerular structures. A streptokinase-deficient strain has been employed in preliminary animal studies to test the hypothesis that streptokinases from nephritogenic strains of streptococci may play a role in the pathogenesis of poststreptococcal glomerulonephritis [37].

Extensive sequence analysis of genes surrounding the group C streptococci streptokinase gene (*skc*) have identified a gene upstream encoding a leucine-rich protein and two downstream genes identified as *orf*1 and *rel*. The *orf*1 gene is of unknown function and the *rel* gene is homologous to two *E. coli* genes, *spo*A and *rel*A, which function in the metabolism of guanosine $5',3'$-guanosine polyphosphates [(p)ppGpp] [38]. A similar arrangement of genes is found in the group A streptococci [26].

Streptococcal erythrogenic toxins, also known as pyrogenic exotoxins, are found in several forms designated A, B, and C toxins. The *spe*A and *spe*C genes are carried by bacteriophages and are present with varying frequencies among group A strains. The *spe*A gene is found in about 15% of general group A strains, and in a higher frequency (~50%) in strains associated with more severe diseases—e.g., scarlet fever, toxic shock syndrome, necrotizing fasciitis, and rheumatic fever [39]. Streptococcal erythrogenic toxin A (SPE A) is a superantigen which activates and expands T cells to release cytokines such as tumor necrosis factor alpha (TNF-α), interleukin-2 (IL-2), and interferon gamma (IFN-γ) [40,41]. These cytokines are known to produce many of the symptoms consistent with the development of toxic shock syndrome. The *spe*A gene is carried by a family of phages related to the prototype phage T12, three of which have been identified [6]. Sequence analysis of a number of *spe*A genes from a variety of strains shows the presence of three alleles that encode toxins differing by a single amino acid change, and another allele encoding a toxin with 26 amino acid changes [42].

The erythrogenic toxin B gene (speB) encodes a protein shown to be identical to the precursor form of streptococcal proteinase, a cysteine proteinase [43]. The speB gene is a chromosomal gene found in all strains of *Streptococcus pyogenes* [5], although all strains may not produce the protein in vitro [44]. Production of the SPE B protein in vitro occurs only in the late logarithmic and stationary phases of growth, suggesting the presence of a regulatory element not effective on other extracellular products. Sequence analysis of speB from a variety of strains indicates that the gene is highly conserved [45]. Streptococcal proteinase may act on a number of targets, thus contributing to the organism's virulence and pathogenicity. For example, proteinase action can release as M protein, C5a peptidase, and certain IgG-binding proteins from the cell surface in biologically active forms [46]. Additionally, proteinase can act on host proteins such as the precursor of IL-1β to produce an active IL-1β, as well as fibronectin and vitronectin [45].

The speC gene is found in about half of all group A strains and like speA, also encodes a protein that has been shown to be a superantigen. The speC gene has been sequenced from a number of strains and two alleles have been found, although there were no changes in amino acids of the toxin encoded by these genes [47]. Little is known about the phage carrying speC, but many similarities with speA carrying phages are expected. Several other recently identified genes that have superantigen activity are mitogenic factor (mf), streptococcal superantigen (ssa), and streptococcal mitogenic exotoxin Z (smeZ). The gene encoding mitogenic factor is also known as speF and is a chromosomal gene found in all strains of streptococci. MF protein has no sequence identity with other streptococcal exotoxins such as SPE A or SPE C. The ssa gene is found in about 50% of all strains examined, suggesting that it is part of a mobile genetic element. The protein encoding ssa has sequence identity with other superantigens, with a higher identity to staphylococcal enterotoxin B and C than to SPE A. The smeZ gene product (SME Z) was originally thought to be a variant of SPE A, but amino acid and DNA sequencing revealed that this protein was distinct from any previously identified exotoxin [48]. SME Z, a 28 kDa peptide with an acidic isoelectric point, is a potent mitogen and superantigen.

Hyaluronidase has long been identified as one of the spreading factors of the group A streptococci because of its ability to cleave the hyaluronic acid found in the ground substance of human tissues. A gene responsible for extracellular production of hyaluronidase has not been discovered, although two genes from bacteriophages which lack signal peptides essential for secretion have been described [49]. One of these phage genes (hylP) contains an internal sequence of 10 Gly-X-Y amino acid triplets that closely resembles the characteristics repeating sequences found in collagen. The 90 bp sequence encoding the collagen-like sequence in hylP is widely disseminated in strains, but its origin remains unknown. Speculation that this collagen-like sequence might be responsible for the induction of antibodies that cross-react with human connective tissue and account for the polyarthritis associated with rheumatic fever has not been tested. The phage-encoded hyaluronidases described to date have no sequence identity with the extracellular hyaluronidases recently sequenced from the group B streptococci or *Streptococcus pneumoniae*.

Neuraminidase (sialidase) was thought to be an extracellular product of group A streptococci, but it is now clear that assays done in early studies with extracts of these organisms employed a mucin substrate contaminated with hyaluronic acid. These early assays were really measuring a hyaluronidase activity and recent highly specific assays for neuraminidase show that the group A streptococci do not produce a neuraminidase [50]. Other extracellular products are known to be produced by the group A streptococci, such as streptolysin S (SLS), NADase, and four DNases. The chromosomal region for the production of SLS has been identified independently by two laboratories [51] (B. Beall, personal communication); however, the genes encoding the other activities have not been identified to date. Another novel protein, a CAMP factor homologous to the protein produced by group B streptococci, has been also added to the growing list of extracellular products [52]. CAMP factor is a ceramide-binding protein that can participate in the synergistic lysis of erythrocytes in combination with a sphingomyelinase such as the beta-toxin of *Staphylococcus aureus* [53]. The biological role of CAMP factor in either group A or group B streptococci remains undiscovered.

Bacteriocins

Bacteriocins are protein antibiotics that are bactericidal to the same or related species as the producing bacterium. The best-studied bacteriocins are the colicins of *E. coli* that are defined by a narrow species spectrum of activity, a protein moiety responsible for the bactericidal activity, attachment to a specific surface receptor on the sensitive cell, plasmid-borne genes for bacteriocin production and host cell immunity, and induced (SOS) release of the bacteriocin upon cell death of the producing strain. The bacteriocins of gram-positive bacteria, including *Streptococcus pyogenes*, share some of these characteristics but differ in others (for an extensive recent review, see ref. [54]). In general, the bacteriocins from gram-positive bacteria have a much wider spectrum of action, killing not only closely and distantly related gram-positive species but sometimes killing gram-negative organisms as well. Bacteriocins of gram-positive bacteria may be carried on plasmids, as are the colicins, or may exist as part of a transposon. Klaenhammer [55] has proposed a classification scheme for the gram-positive bacteriocins based upon molecular weight, post-translational modifications, and complexity.

The gram-positive bacteriocins are characteristically synthesized as prepeptides that undergo post-translational modification and cleavage. One class of these bacteriocins, the lantibiotics (Klaenhammer's class I), contain unusual amino acid residues such as lanthionine, B-methyl lanthionine, didehydroalanine, and didehydrobutyrine after modification. These atypical residues may stabilize the conformation of the peptide or provide reactive groupings to increase the biological activity. Lantibiotics are formed as prepeptides with a leader sequence that is cleaved to release the mature bacteriocin; however, post-translational modifications occur before cleavage of the leader peptide, and the leader is required for the introduction of lanthionine and the other modified amino acids into the mature protein. The antimicrobial activity of lantibiotics appears to result from the interaction of the protein with the cell membrane of the target bacterium. Barrel-stave poration complexes have been proposed to form between one or more of the proteins, resulting in ion leakage, loss of membrane potential, and ultimately, cell death.

Although many strains of *Streptococcus pyogenes* have been observed to have bacteriocin or antibacterial activity, only streptococcin A-FF22 (SA-FF22) has been characterized in any detail. This bacteriocin was first identified by Tagg et al. [56], and is a member of the class of lantibiotics. The primary amino acid sequence of SA-FF22 has been determined by direct analysis as well as deduced from the gene structure; the prepeptide consists of a 25 amino acid leader peptide followed by 26 amino acids that comprise the mature propeptide sequence. The mature protein contains one lanthionine and two 3-methyllanthionine residues [57]. The structural gene, *scn*A, appears to be part of a nisin-like operon located on a transposon. Upstream of *scn*A and oriented in the opposite direction is *scn*R, a gene encoding a 232 amino acid peptide with high homology to response regulators found in two component regulatory systems [58].

The gene for salivaricin A (*sal*A), a bacteriocin from *Streptococcus salivarius* with bactericidal activity against most strains of *Streptococcus pyogenes*, has been cloned and sequenced [59]. Many *Streptococcus pyogenes* strains carry a closely related gene with over 95% homology to *sal*A [60]. The function of this gene in group A streptococci remains unknown since the carrier strains produce no detectable salivaricin activity. Whether this gene specifies a salivaricin homologue with antimicrobial activity against an unknown target species or some other biological activity remains to be determined.

Surface Associated Virulence Factors

Group A streptococci elicit barriers to both innate and adaptive components of the immune response. Virulence depends on a cadre of surface and extracellular macromolecules. The application of molecular biology and genetics to streptococcal research has dramatically advanced our understanding of their pathogenesis. The fibrillar surface of this organism is a mosaic of protein and polysaccharide that determines its fate once it contacts host tissue. The proteins that compose this fibrous layer vary among the more than 80 M serotypes of group A streptococci and sometimes vary within a serotype. The genetic basis for this variation has been and will continue to be the subject of intense investigation. A major surface protein is the M protein [61]. Rebecca Lancefield originally defined the M proteins as antiphagocytic proteins that determine the serotype of a strain and showed that serotype-specific antibody promotes phagocytosis by neutrophils in fresh human blood. Until recently, surface fibrils of virulent strains were thought to be composed entirely of the α-helical rod-like M protein. It is now clear that this layer also contains a variety of proteins, including enzymes. Two enzymes that have been studied more extensively are the apolipoproteinase (SOF), which is used as an epidemiological marker and also binds fibronectin [62], and the C5a peptidase (SCPA), which destroys the C5a complement protein that is the chemotactic signal that initially attracts neutrophils to sites of infection [63]. Immunoglobulin-binding proteins may also protrude into the aqueous phase, ready to nonspecifically capture IgG and IgA immunoglobulins [64,70]. Surprisingly, genetic studies have revealed that M proteins and immunoglobulin binding proteins are similar in primary sequence and architecture. They represent a family of proteins generally termed M-like proteins. A single strain can express as many as four M-like proteins, each with the capacity to bind different human plasma proteins [64].

Subclassification of group A streptococci by serotype has historically depended on the antigenic specificity of the M antigen and T antigen. The T antigen or antigens are a variable repertoire of cell-surface, trypsin-resistant antigens that are identified by a battery of agglutinating antisera. The pattern of agglutination reactions predictably limits the number of potential M antigens associated with a given strain. The *tee*6 antigen gene was cloned and sequenced [65]. From sequence the T6 antigen was deduced to contain the conserved cell wall anchor motif, LPSTGE, but was otherwise unrelated to other proteins of known sequence. It is very likely that T antigens are unrelated to each other and merely represent trypsin-resistant epitopes associated with a variety of unrelated cell wall proteins.

The *vir* Regulon

The infectious process is anticipated to be a multistep pathway, proceeding from initial adherence of bacteria to mucosal tissue, to invasion of deeper tissue, and occasional penetration of the bloodstream. Therefore, out of necessity, group A streptococci have evolved mechanisms to coordinate expression of the proteins that are bound to the surface and critically interact with components of the host's inflammatory and adaptive immune responses. Genes that encode M-like proteins are linked in a cluster immediately adjacent to the C5a peptidase gene (*scp*A) (Fig. 3.4); [66,67]. Sequence comparisons suggest that M-like genes have descended from one another as products of gene duplication and unequal intergenic recombination [66]. The number and nature of tandem genes vary with serotype. Although only three common arrays are shown here, several others are known to exist [67]. Transcription of each gene in the cluster is initiated from its own promoter and is dependent on the multiple gene activator (Mga), formerly termed VirR [68] and Mry [69]. All serotypes can be divided into two major phylogenetic groups by their capacity to produce SOF. The simplest cluster contains only an *emm* gene (M protein gene) and an *scp*A gene. These strains usually lack SOF activity. SOF$^+$ strains, such as serotype M49, may have three M-like genes [66,67]. In this and related serotypes, the most 5' gene is *mrp* (originally termed *fcr*A) [70], which encodes type II immunoglobulin-binding proteins. Interspersed between the *emm* and *scp*A genes is the *enn* gene. *enn* genes code for IgA-binding proteins. Both *mrp* and *enn* genes are more conserved than *emm* genes, suggesting that they are under less intense selective pressure by the human immune response or that change is restricted by their need to retain immunoglobulin-binding activity. The prevalence of *mrp* and *enn* genes among many serotypes suggests that they play key roles in virulence, but the importance of immunoglobulin binding to pathogenesis or the biology of the organism is, however, still not understood [71].

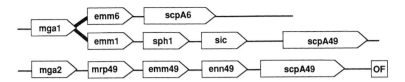

Figure 3.4 Diversity in M gene clusters.

A highly virulent clone of serotype M1 emerged in the late 1980s to become responsible for a major increase in systemic infections in Europe and North America [72–74]. Thus, serotype M1 strains have become the focus of molecular studies. *mrp* and *enn* genes are not present in the *vir* regulon of this serotype. Instead, *sph* and *sic* genes reside between *emm* and *scp*A [75]. *sph* encodes protein H, an IgG-binding protein that is unrelated to the immunoglobulin-binding proteins coded by *mrp* genes. In addition to binding IgG, protein H also binds fibrinogen and factor H, both of which are properties of M protein. Whether M1 protein, protein H, or both impart resistance to phago-cytosis is unknown. The protein product of the *sic* gene is an extracellular protein that is completely unrelated to M-like proteins. The SIC protein binds two plasma proteins, clustering and the histidine-rich protein (HRG), both of which are regulators of the complement membrane attack complex (C5b–C9). Interaction of SIC with these plasma proteins inhibits complement-mediated lysis of sensitized erythrocytes [75]. Gram-positive bacteria lack an outer membrane and are generally resistant to the membrane attack complex; therefore, it is unclear how this activity of SIC impacts on virulence. Another 2.2 kb of sequence between *sic* and *scp*A has not been defined. Serotype M1 clinical isolates are not entirely homogeneous; some lack an *sph* gene (P.P. Cleary, unpublished data). Clinical isolates representing the M1 clone that is responsible for worldwide disseminated disease are internalized by epithelial cells at an unusually high frequency [76]. The relationship of intracellular invasion to the frequent isolation of M1 strains from blood is of interest. Not surprisingly, insertional inactivation of *mga* in a serotype M1 strain greatly diminished its capacity to invade human lung epithelial cells. This finding suggests that some gene in the *vir* regulon is required for high-efficiency uptake by human epithelial cells [77].

The *emm* Gene Family

The dogma that type specificity and resistance to phagocytosis are solely dependent on M proteins is beginning to crumble as more serotypes are investigated at the molecular level. The first 150 or more base pairs of more than 80 *emm* genes are sequenced. Most were identified and sequenced from polymerase chain reaction (PCR) products using *emm*-specific primers [78]. On the basis of primer specificity and position in the regulon, investigators assumed that the sequenced genes encode serotype-specific, antiphagocytic M proteins. This assumption proved to be incorrect in both respects. Among 79 different M serotypes, nine pairs of strains of different M type were found to have the same *emm* nucleotide sequence [78]. Therefore, in these cases the *emm* gene does not determine serotype specificity, and the determinant of type specificity is unknown. Only *emm*1 [79], *emm*2 [80], *emm*5 [81], *emm*6 [82], *emm*12 [83], *emm*24 [84], *emm*49 [66], and *emm*57 [85] were shown to code for the type-specific antigen. Moreover, inactivation of the *emm* gene by plasmid insertion into *emm*49 had little or no impact on resistance to phagocytosis [86]. Podbielski's data suggest that both *mrp*49 [87] and *emm*49 are required for full resistance to phagocytosis, but they do not rule out the possibility that Mga controls expression of another unidentified macromolecule that imbues streptococci with the capacity to resist phagocytosis. Furthermore, the capacity of serotype M18 strains to resist phagocytosis is entirely dependent on expression of a hyaluronic acid capsule [88].

The potential of M proteins to undergo antigenic change has seriously retarded efforts to develop a protective vaccine. Although antisera are able to distinguish at least 80 M serotypes, the number of serotypes is potentially much greater. Classification is further complicated due to strong selective pressure for individual M proteins to undergo antigenic change. Comparison of an M1 protein sequence to a cross-reactive M1 variant protein showed that the N-termini of M proteins are prone to accumulate nonsynonymous mutations and small nucleotide insertions [79]. Moreover, intragenic recombination between the A repeats within the emm6 gene is a second mechanism by which the M protein can vary antigenically [82]. Several studies suggest that hybrid M proteins also arise from intergenic recombination between different M-like genes on the same chromosome [89,90] or between M-like genes introduced from another strain by some unknown mechanism. Although sequence comparisons and hybridization studies suggest that emm genes are horizontally transferred between different strains of group A streptococci [67,90,91] as well as to other groups of streptococci [92], this has not yet been reproducibly demonstrated in the laboratory.

Hyaluronic Acid Capsule

Many clinical isolates produce large hyaluronic acid (HA) capsules when grown on agar plates, prompting investigators to speculate that capsule plays an important role in streptococcal virulence. The HA biosynthetic genes, hasA, hasB, and hasC were found by transposon mutagenesis to be clustered on the chromosome in an operon [88,93,94]. These genes code for hyaluronate synthetase, UDP-glucose dehydrogenase and UDP-glucose pyrophosphorylase, respectively. The degree of encapsulation is highly variable and genetically unstable when the organism is cultivated on laboratory media. Molecular events responsible for this instability and variability between strains are poorly understood. An analysis of the has operon showed that promoters of a highly encapsulated M18 strain and a poorly encapsulated M3 strain differed in sequence by a few nucleotides. These cis-acting difference were determined to affect the expression of hyaluronic acid synthesis three-

fold [95]. The simultaneous expression of hyaluronidases by streptococci, and similar activities in human body fluid question the relevance of HA capsules in vivo. For some serotypes capsule is required for resistance to phagocytosis in vitro and for colonization of the nasopharynx [88].

Regulation of Virulence

Group A streptococcal virulence is clearly dependent on several cell-bound proteins. The need for these proteins more than likely depends on the bodily fluid or tissue in which the organism finds itself. Surface proteins required for persistence and growth in blood may be very different from those required for colonization of the skin. Experiments to date suggest that regulatory circuits that control expression of these proteins are complex. Transcription of individual genes in the vir gene cluster is dependent on the multiple gene activator protein, Mga. Since Mga was first found to be required for emm12 expression [68,83], it has been shown to act in trans to activate transcription of the emm12 [96,97], the emm6 [69], the emm49 [86,98] and the emm1 gene clusters [99]. Transcription of Mga is autoactivated and is initiated from two promoters [100,101]. Although the mga genes of SOF$^+$ and SOF$^-$ strains share significant sequence similarity, they have clearly diverged from each other [86]. The mga49 (SOF$^+$) gene showed 76% overall homology to the mga12 (SOF$^-$) gene. The 3' end of mga49 is highly conserved when compared to 20 other SOF$^+$ serotypes, but is completely unrelated to the 3' end of mga genes of SOF$^-$ strains [86]. In SOF$^+$ strains, Mga also controls expression of SOF even though this gene is not closely linked to the vir gene cluster [98]. In a serotype M1 strain, Mga is required for expression of HA capsule [77]. Preliminary experiments suggest that Mga either directly or indirectly downregulates the expression of Streptolysin S. Mga$^-$ mutants produce larger amounts of Streptolysin S and are more cytotoxic for human lymphocytes [99].

Mga contains domains that are common to two-component response regulators of signal transduction systems. In the simplest form, such regulatory systems contain a sensor component that detects changes in the external environment and a DNA-binding component that activates transcription of genes under its control. The DNA-binding function of Mga was confirmed by McIver et al. [102], whose experiments showed that Mga binds to a 45 bp consensus sequence, which overlaps the promoters of the *emm* and *scp*A genes and was previously predicted by sequence comparisons [69,90]. It is also predicted to bind to the promoter regions of several other M-like genes. The sensor that interacts with Mga is unknown. Superimposed on Mga-mediated control of virulence is a metastable phase-switching mechanism. Expression of the *vir* regulon fluctuates between "on-off" states at frequencies between 1×10^{-3} and 1×10^{-4} per colony-forming unit [103]. Some M$^-$ variants are products of mutation, but most result from phase variation and readily revert back to the virulent M$^+$ form. Cultures can become M$^-$ and avirulent following multiple transfers in laboratory media. Virulence can be regained by passing cultures in mice or rotating them in phagocytic human blood. This instability of *vir* regulon expression, although intriguing to geneticists, is problematic for students of streptococcal virulence and epidemiology. It is not possible to control day-to-day variation in experiments due to phase switching. Earlier investigators assumed that M protein was the primary determinant of virulence, because when they isolated spontaneous M$^-$ variants, they found that these variants had also lost the capacity to resist phagocytosis and to kill mice following intraperitoneal injection. However, it is now known that most spontaneous M$^-$ variants lack the entire set of proteins encoded by the *vir* regulon. *emm*, *mrp*, and *scp*A co-vary simultaneously between "on-off" states [96,104]. More recent experiments show that *mga* expression itself phase-varies [101]. Recent data suggest the existence of a regulatory circuit linking HA and SpeA toxin expression. The *has* operon and *spe*A gene expression also phase-vary in concert with Mga-controlled genes. SpeA expression, however, was found to be independent of Mga. A common, variable genetic switch that controls surface protein expression and toxin synthesis has been suggested [77], but the nature of that switch has not been determined.

Differential Expression of Virulence Factors

As an organism attempts to establish itself within a host, it is faced with determining when to express various components of its virulence arsenal. Throughout the infectious process, the organism must adapt to survive in various microenvironments including blood, tissues, and the interior of cells. For many pathogens it has been determined that control of virulence gene expression involves complex networks that connect the sensing of environmental signals to gene expression. These signals may include temperature, osmolarity, pH, iron availability, and O_2/CO_2 levels [105]. Group A streptococci encounter many different environments as they colonize the skin or nasopharynx and then invade to deeper tissues. Regulation of gene expression in these streptococci throughout this process is just beginning to be understood.

Although Mga is required for high-level expression of the genes in the *vir* regulon, members of the regulon are activated at different levels. In a serotype M49 strain, transcripts from the *enn* 49 gene were much less abundant than transcripts from the other *vir* regulon genes [66,86]. Similarly in a serotype M2 strain, Bessen and Fischetti [80] reported that the *enn* homologue *emm*L2.2 is transcribed at a level 32-fold less than the *emm*L2.1 transcript. The genetic basis for differences in the level of expression of these Mga-activated genes is unknown. It is possible that minor sequence variations in the Mga-binding sequence [102] reduce Mga-mediated transcription initiation. There may also be other unidentified regulatory factors involved. In a serotype M12 strain, the genetic basis for differential expression between the *emm*12 gene and the *scp*A12 gene was determined. In this strain, the *scp*A12 gene is expressed at a level three- to fourfold lower than the *emm*12 gene because of a novel mechanism for downregulation of gene expression in *Streptococcus pyogenes*. The leader mRNA of *scp*A12 contains an inverted repeat sequence that acts as a transcription terminator. As shown in Figure 3.5, the inverted repeat sequence forms a transcription-terminating hairpin structure, resulting in truncated *scp*A12 transcripts that do not extend into the structural gene [106]. The presence of this

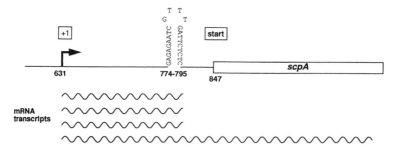

Figure 3.5 Transcription termination and differential gene expression in the *vir* regulon.

inverted repeat down-regulates *scp*A12 gene expression by 70%–80% relative to expression of the *scp*A12 gene with the inverted repeat removed. It is unknown whether the formation of the transcription terminator is regulated or if the level of *scp*A12 mRNA transcription is constitutively low. Nearly identical inverted repeat sequences are located at the 3′ ends of at least 15 group A streptococcal genes from 12 different M serotypes; however, their functions have not been studied.

In addition to Mga, the only other known transcriptional regulator of putative virulence genes in *Streptococcus pyogenes* is RofA. RofA influences expression of one of the several fibronectin-binding proteins, protein F [107]. In addition to protein F, other streptococcal fibronectin-binding proteins include SfbI (which is closely related to protein F), the 28 kDa antigen, glyceraldehyde-3-phosphate dehydrogenase, M3 protein, FBP54, and SfbII and Sof22 [62,108,109,111,112,113]. The *rof*A gene is located immediately upstream of the *prt*F gene (encoding protein F), and the two genes are divergently transcribed [114]. RofA functions in *trans* to activate transcription of the *prt*F gene. In one extensively passaged laboratory strain, the *rof*A gene appears to be truncated, and its protein product causes high-level constitutive expression of *prt*F. It is believed that this strain contains a mutant form of the *rof*A gene. Other strains in which *prt*F is not constitutively expressed contain a larger *rof*A gene. In these strains, the regulatory mechanisms of RofA have not been determined. RofA is now known to regulate other genes.

Differential regulation of gene expression is necessary to enable the organism to display the appropriate amounts of each protein in the various microenvironments within the host. For an organism to change its surface in response to its surroundings, it must be able to sense the local environment. Although environmental regulation of virulence is a common theme in many pathogens, it is not well understood in *Streptococcus pyogenes*. The transcriptional activators Mga [68,69] and RofA [114] both have homology to the activator component of two-component regulatory systems, but no complementary sensory proteins have been identified. Despite this lack of knowledge, it has been demonstrated that the expression of RofA- and Mga-activated genes are influenced by the environment. In some strains, transcription of *prtF* is up-regulated by increased levels of O_2 [115], resulting in increased fibronectin binding and increased adherence to respiratory epithelial cells. These observations suggest that protein F is required for streptococcal infection at locations where the concentration of O_2 is high, such as skin surfaces and mucous membranes. In fact, it was demonstrated that protein F also mediates adherence of streptococci to Langerhans cells in the skin [107]. This is consistent with a role in attachment during the early stages of infection. Conversely, transcription of *mga* and consequently of *emm* and *scpA* is increased by increased levels of CO_2 [107] and anaerobiosis [97]. M protein–mediated binding to human skin sections was increased when the bacteria were cultured in high CO_2 concentrations [107]. This suggests a possible role for M protein in deeper tissues where the CO_2 concentration would presumably be higher. Although expression of these proteins under in vivo conditions has not been examined, the in vitro assays demonstrate that the gaseous environment significantly influences the adhesive capacity of group A streptococci and may therefore have an impact on the tissue specificity of infection.

Other physical and metabolic conditions also alter expression of the *vir* regulon. Recently, expression of *emm*6 was shown to decrease under conditions of low temperature, high salt, iron limitation, and vigorous aeration [116]. These conditions are known to regulate virulence in other pathogens, but their roles in the virulence of group A streptococci infection have not been investigated. Growth phase is also an important influence on the infective capabilities of bacterial pathogens, and many virulence genes are induced as the bacteria enter stationary phase. In *Streptococcus pyogenes* the *emm* gene is expressed at higher levels when the cells enter late-log growth phase [97,106,117]; (K.H. Pritchard and P.P. Cleary, unpublished observation). The late-log increase in *emm* expression may have an impact on the capacity of streptococci to invade epithelial tissue. LaPenta et al. [76] showed that stationary-phase group A streptococci invade a human epithelial cell line more efficiently than mid-log-phase bacteria. M protein can also act as an adhesin in a tissue-dependent manner. Okada et al. [107] showed that M protein can serve as an adhesin for keratinocytes, and Courtney et al. [118] demonstrated the capacity of M protein to mediate adhesion to HEp-2 cells and mouse oral epithelial cells. Preliminary evidence from our laboratory shows that mutations in *mga*, which knock out expression of M protein and other Mga-activated genes, reduce the ability of group A streptococci to invade epithelial cells [117,118a].

In contrast to the late-log-phase induction of *emm*, the amount of *scp*A12 expression remains constant throughout the growth cycle. The potential role of the C5a-inactivating SCPA protein in group A streptococcal infection has been examined using a mouse air sac model. Within 4 h of infection into a connective tissue air sac, SCPA$^-$ bacteria were cleared more efficiently than wild-type SCPA$^+$ bacteria [119]. This finding suggests that SCPA acts early in the infectious process to delay recruitment of immune cells to the infection site, allowing group A streptococci to colonize and spread before the onslaught of an immune response.

The current data suggest a complex presentation of several proteins that allow for attachment, colonization, and dissemination of *Streptococcus pyogenes*. Although several virulence genes are coordinately regulated by the Mga protein, maximal expression of each may be required at different stages of infection. As the bacteria first encounter the host on the surface of the skin or pharynx, protein F and SCPA may be important virulence determinants. With the relatively high O_2 concentration of these locations, protein F would be expressed and could mediate attachment to epithelial cells and fibronectin. The expression of SCPA at this time would delay the influx of polymorphonuclear cells to the site of infection and allow the bacteria to multiply. Constant, low-level production of SCPA may be more important than a burst of activity as the organism enters stationary phase. Then as the organism becomes established and penetrates deeper into tissues and into the blood, the role of M protein and the many immunoglobulin-binding proteins may become much more important. In deeper tissues, the CO_2 concentration may be higher, inducing high-level M protein expression. The antiphagocytic M protein plays a major protective role wherever phagocytic cells are present. The role of the immunoglobulin-binding proteins is less clear. Since the organism is capable of binding several blood proteins via many of its own proteins, these interactions are likely to be very important. The bacteria may coat themselves with host proteins to camouflage themselves, or the blood proteins may serve as signalling molecules. This intriguing property of group A streptococci is the subject of much current research.

Over the past 15 years significant progress has been made toward defining the genes that encode and regulate the multitude of virulence factors produced by group A streptococci. We are beginning to understand the complex and dynamic processes that occur when these bacteria interact with the host. These insights may lead us to better methods for combatting infections. Antibiotics are becoming less effective due to bacterial resistance, and the standard models and assays for new antibiotic discovery have become less useful. Although old antibiotics are "rediscovered," new ones are increasingly more difficult to identify. A therapeutic that globally shuts down expression of several virulence factors at once could disarm the microbe so that it can be readily cleared by a host's defenses. This problem acts as further impetus to continue to investigate genetic regulatory circuits and their environmental signals in pathogenic streptococci. New targets on which to focus antibiotic discovery and vaccine development may be revealed.

REFERENCES

1. McCarty M. The Transforming Principle: Discovering That Genes Are Made of DNA. New York: W.W. Norton, 1985.
2. Malke H. In: Wannamaker LW, Matsen JM (eds). Streptococci and Streptococcal Diseases: Recognition, Understanding and Management. New York: Academic Press, 1972; 120–131.
3. Weeks CR, Ferretti JJ. Nucleotide sequence of the type A streptococcal exotoxin (erythrogenic toxin) gene from Streptococcus pyogenes bacteriophage T12. Infect Immun 1986; 52:144–150.
4. Goshorn SC, Schlievert PM. Nucleotide sequence of streptococcal pyrogenic exotoxin C. Infect Immun 1988; 56:2518–2520.
5. Yu CE, Ferretti JJ. Frequency of the erythrogenic toxin genes (speB and speC) among clinical isolates of group A streptococci. Infect Immun 1991;91:211–215.
6. Yu CE, Ferretti JJ. Molecular characterization of new group A streptococcal bacteriophages containing the gene for streptococcal erythrogenic toxin A (speA). Mol Gen Genet 1991; 231:161–168.
7. McShan WW, Tang Y-F, Ferretti JJ. Bacteriophage T12 of Streptococcus pyogenes integrates into the gene encoding a serine tRNA. Mol Microbiol 1997; 23:719–728.
8. McShan WM, Ferretti JJ. Genetic diversity in temperate bacteriophages of Streptococcus pyogenes: identification of a second attachment site for phages carrying the erythrogenic toxin A gene. J Bacteriol 1997; 179:6509–6511.
9. Clewell DB, Gawron-Burke C. Conjugative transposon and the dissemination of antibiotic resistance in streptococci. Annu Rev Microbiol 1986; 40:635–659.
10. Ferretti JJ, Curtiss R III. (eds). Streptococcal Genetics. Washington, DC: American Society for Microbiology, 1987.
11. Dunny G, Cleary P, McKay L. Genetics and Molecular Biology of Streptococci, Enterococci, and Lactococci. Washington, DC: American Society for Microbiology, 1991.
12. Macrina FL, Evans RP, Tobian JA, Hartley DL, Clewell DB, Jones KR. Novel shuttle plasmid vehicles for Escherichia-Streptococcus transgeneric cloning. Gene. 1983; 25:145–150.
13. Tao L, LeBlanc DJ, Ferretti JJ. Novel streptococcal-integration shuttle vectors for gene cloning and inactivation. Gene 1992; 120:105–110.
14. McShan WM, McLaughlin RE, Nordstrand A, Ferretti JJ. Vectors containing streptococcal bacteriophage integrases for site-specific gene insertion. Meth Cell Sci 1999; (in press).
15. Nordstrand A, McShan WM, Ferretti JJ, Holm SE, Norgren M. Allele substitution of the streptokinase gene and its effect on nephritogenic capacity of group A streptococcal strain NZ131. Infect Immun 1999; (in press).
16. Clewell DB, Flannagan SE, in Clewell DB, Bacterial Conjugation. New York: Plenum Press, 1993; 369–393.
17. Clewell DB. Movable genetic elements and antibiotic resistance in enterococci. Eur Clin Microbiol Infect Dis 1990; 9:90–102.
18. LeBouguenec CL, Cespedes GD, Horaud T. Molecular analysis of a composite chromosomal conjugative element (Tn3701) of Streptococcus pyogenes. J Bacteriol 1988; 170:3930–3936.
19. Kapur V, Reda KB, Li L-L, Ho L-J, Rich RR, Musser JM. Characterization and distribution of insertion sequence IS1239 in Streptococcus pyogenes. Gene 1994; 150:135–140.
20. Wannamaker LW. In: Schlessinger D (ed). Microbiology 1982. Washington, DC: American Society for Microbiology, 1982; 112–116.
21. Malke H. Conjugal transfer of plasmids determining resistance to macrolides, lincosamides and streptogrami-B type antibiotics among group A, B, D and H streptococci. FEMS Microbiol Lett 1979; 5:335–338.
22. Scott JR, Guehthner PC, Malone LM, Fischetti, VA. Conversion of an M⁻ group A streptococcus to M⁺ by transfer of a plasmid containing an M6 gene. J Exp Med 1986; 164:1641–1651.
23. McLaughlin RE, Ferretti JJ. Electrotransformation of Streptococci. In: Nickoloff JA (ed). Electroporation and Electrofusion of Microorganisms. Methods Mol Biol 1995; 47:185–193.
24. Simon D, Ferretti JJ. Electrotransformation of Streptococcus pyogenes with plasmid and linear DNA. FEMS Microbiol Lett 1991; 82:219–224.
25. Suvorov AN, Ferretti JJ. Physical and genetic chromosomal map of an M type 1 strain of Streptococcus pyogenes. J Bacteriol 1996; 178:5546–5549.
26. Frank C, Steiner K, Malke H. Conservation of the organization of the streptokinase gene region among pathogenic streptococci. Med Microbiol Immunol 1995; 184:139–146.
27. Single LA, Martin DR. Cloncal differences within M-types of the group A streptococcus revealed by pulsed field gel electrophoresis. FEMS Microbiol Lett 1992; 91:85–90.
28. Schlessinger D. Microbiology—1982. Washington, DC: American Society for Microbiology 1982.

29. Ferretti JJ, Gilmore MS, Klaenhammer T (eds). Genetics of Streptococci, Enterococci, and Lactococci. Dev Biol Stand 1995; 85.

30. Orefici G. New Perspectives on Streptococci and Streptococcal Infections. Zentralbl. Bakteriol Mikrobiol Hyg 1992; 22.

31. Totolian A (ed). Pathogenic Streptococci: Present and Future. St. Petersburg, Russia: Lancer Publication, 1994.

32. Caparon MG, Scott JR. Genetic manipulation of pathogenic streptococci. Methods Enzymol 1991; 204:556–586.

33. Kehoe MA, Timmis KN. Cloning and expression in *Escherichia coli* of the streptolysin O determinant from *Streptococcus pyogenes*: characterization of the cloned streptolysin O determinant and demonstration of the absence of substantial homology with determinants of other thiol-activated toxins. Infect Immun 1987; 43:804–810.

33a. Kehoe MA, Miller ML, Walker JA, Boulnois GJ. Nucleotide sequence of the streptolysin O (*slo*) gene: structural homologies between SLO and other membrane damaging thiol-activated toxins. Infect Immun 1987; 55:3228–3232.

34. Malke H, Ferretti JJ. Streptokinase: cloning, expression, and excretion in *E. coli*. Proc Natl Acad Sci USA 1984; 81:3557–3561.

35. Huang T-T, Malke H, Ferretti JJ. The streptokinase gene of group A streptococci: cloning, expression in *Escherichia coli*, and sequence analysis. Mol Microbiol 1989; 3:197–205.

36. Malke H. Polymorphism of the streptokinase gene: implications for the pathogenesis of post-streptococcal glomerulonephritis. Zentralbl Bakteriol Mikrobiol Hyg 1993; 278:246–257.

37. Holm SE, Ferretti JJ, Simon D, Johnston KH. In: Orefici G (ed). New Perspectives on Streptococci and Streptococcal Infections. Zentralbl Bakteriol Mikrobiol Hyg 1992; Suppl 22:261–263.

38. Mechold U, Cashel ML, Steiner K, Gentry D, Malke H. Functional analysis of *relA/spoT* gene homolog from *Streptococcus equisimilis*. J Bacteriol 1996; 178:1401–1411.

39. Yu CE, Ferretti JJ. 1989. A molecular epidemiologic analysis of the type A streptococcal exotoxin (erythrogenic toxin) gene (*speA*) among clinical *Streptococcus pyogenes* strains. Infect Immun 57:3715–3719.

40. Braun MA, Gerlach D, Hartwig UF, Ozegowski JH, Romagne F, Carrel S, Kohler W, Fleischer B. Stimulation of human T cells by streptococcal "superantigen" erythrogenic toxins (scarlet fever toxins). J Immunol 1993; 150:2457–2466.

41. Schlievert PM. Role of superantigens in disease. J Infect Dis 1993; 167:997–1002.

42. Nelson K, Schlievert PM, Selander RK, Musser JM. Characterization and clonal distribution of four alleles of the *speA* gene encoding pyrogenic exotoxin A (scarlet fever toxin) in *Streptococcus pyogenes* J Exp Med 1991; 174:1271–1274.

43. Chaussee M, Gerlach D, Yu CE, Ferretti JJ. Inactivation of the streptococcal erythrogenic toxin B (*speB*) gene in *Streptococcus pyogenes*. Infect Immun 1993; 61:3719–3723.

44. Chaussee MS, Liu J, Stevens DL, Ferretti JJ. Genetic and phenotypic diversity among isolates of *Streptococcus pyogenes* from invasive infections. J Infect Dis 1996; 173:901–908.

45. Kapur V, Topouzis S, Majesky MW, Li LL, Hamrick MR, Hamill RJ, Patti JM, Musser JM. A conserved *Streptococcus pyogenes* extracellular cysteine protease cleaves human fibronectin and degrades vitronectin. Microb Pathog 1993; 15:327–346.

46. Berge A, Bjorck L. Streptococcal cysteine proteinase releases biologically active fragments of streptococcal surface proteins. J Biol Chem 1995; 270:9862–9867.

47. Kapur V, Nelson K, Schlievert PM, Selander RK, Musser JM. Molecular population genetic evidence of horizontal spread of two alleles of the pyrogenic exotoxin C gene (*speC*) among pathogenic clones of *Streptococcus pyogenes*. Infect Immun 1992; 60:3513–3517.

48. Kamezawa Y, Nakahara T, Nakano S, Abe Y, Nozaki-Renard J, Isono T. Streptococcal mitogenic exotoxin Z, a novel acidic superantigenic toxin produced by a T1 strain of *Streptococcus pyogenes*. Infect Immun 1997; 65:3828–3833.

49. Hynes WL, Hancock L, Ferretti JJ. Analysis of a second bacteriophage hyaluronidase gene from *Streptococcus pyogenes*: evidence for a third hyaluronidase involved in extracellular enzyme activity. Infect Immun 1995; 63:3015–3020.

50. Savic D, Ferretti JJ. Group A streptococci do not produce neuraminidase (sialidase). Med Microbiol Lett 1994; 3:358–362.

51. Borgia SM, Betschel S, Low DE, de Azavedo JC. Cloning of a chromosomal region responsible for streptolysin S production in *Streptococcus pyogenes*. Adv Exp Med Biol 1997; 418:733–736.

52. Gase K, McShan WM, Ferretti JJ. The CAMP-factor of group A streptococci: strain characterization and gene cloning. Infect Immun 1999; (in press).

53. Sterzik B, Fehrenbach FJ. Reaction components influencing CAMP factor induced lysis. J Gen Microbiol 1985; 131:817–820.

54. Jack RW, Tagg JR, Ray B. Bacteriocins of gram-positive bacteria. Microbiol Rev 1995; 59:171–200.

55. Klaenhammer TR. Genetics of bacteriocins produced by lactic acid bacteria. FEMS Microbiol Rev 1993; 12:39–86.

56. Tagg JR, Wannamaker LW. Streptococci A-FF22: nisin-like antibiotic substance produced by a group A streptococcus. Antimicrob Agents Chemother 1978; 14:36–39.

57. Hynes WL, Ferretti JJ, Tagg JR. Cloning of the gene encoding streptococcin A-FF22, a novel

lantibiotic produced by *Streptococcus pyogenes*, and determination of its nucleotide structure. Appl Environ Microbiol 1993; 59:1969–1971.

58. Hynes WL, Ferretti JJ. A response regulator gene controls production of the lantibiotic streptococcin A-FF22. In: Ferretti JJ, Gilmore MS, Klaenhammer TR, Brown F (eds). Genetics of Streptococci, Enterococci and Lactococci. Dev Biol Stand 1995; 85:635–637.

59. Ross KF, Ronson CW, Tagg JR. Isolation and characterization of the lantibiotic salivaricin A and its structural gene *sal*A from *Streptococcus salivarius* 20P3. Appl Environ Microbiol 1993; 59:2014–2021.

60. Simpson WJ, Ragland NL, Ronson CW, Tagg JR. A lantibiotic gene family widely distributed in *Streptococcus salivarius* and *Streptococcus pyogenes*. In: Ferretti JJ, Gilmore MS, Klaenhammer TR, Brown F (eds). Genetics of Streptococci, Enterococci and Lactococci. Dev Biol Stand 1995; 85:639–643.

61. Fischetti VA. Streptococcal M protein: molecular design and biological behavior. Clin Microbiol Rev 1989; 2:285–314.

62. Rakonjac JV, Robbins JC, Fischetti VA. DNA sequence of the serum opacity factor of group A streptococci: identification of a fibronectin-binding repeat domain. Infect Immun 1995; 63:622–631.

63. Wexler DE, Nelson RD, Cleary PP. Human neutrophil chemotactic response to group A streptococci: bacteria-mediated interference with complement-derived factors. Infect Immun 1983; 39:239–246.

64. Boyle MDP, Raeder R, Flosdorff A, Podbielski A. Role of *emm* and *mrp* genes in the virulence of group A streptococcal isolate 64/14 in a mouse model of skin infection. J Infect Dis 1998; 177:991–997.

65. Schneewind O, Jones KF, Fischetti VA. Sequence and structural characteristics of the trypsin-resistant T6 surface protein of group A streptococci. J Bacteriol 1990; 172:3310–3317.

66. Haanes ED, Cleary PP. Identification of a divergent M protein gene and an M protein–related gene family in *Streptococcus pyogenes* serotype 49. J Bacteriol 1989; 171:6397–6408.

67. Hollingshead SK, Readdy TL, Yung DL, Bessen D. Structural heterogeneity of the *emm* gene cluster in group A streptococci. Mol Microbiol 1993; 8:707–717.

68. Chen C, Bormann N, Cleary PP. VirR and Mry are homologous *trans*-acting regulators of M protein and C5a peptidase expression in group A streptococci. Mol Gen Genet 1993; 241:685–693.

69. Perez-Casal J, Caparon MG, Scott JR. Mry, a trans-acting positive regulator of the M protein gene of *Streptococcus pyogenes* with similarity to the receptor proteins of two-component regulatory systems. J Bacteriol 1991; 173:2617–2624.

70. Heath DG, Cleary PP. Fc receptor and M protein genes of group A streptococci are products of gene duplication. Proc Natl Acad Sci USA 1989; 86:4741–4745.

71. Cleary PP, Retnoningrum D. Group A streptococcal immunoglobulin-binding proteins: adhesins, molecular mimicry or sensory proteins. Trends Microbiol 1994; 2:131–136.

72. Cleary PP, Kaplan EL, Handley JP, Wlazlo A, Kim MH, Hauser AR, Schlievert PM. Clonal basis for resurgence of serious streptococcal disease in the 1980's. Lancet 1992; 321:518–521.

73. Schlievert PM, Assimacopoulos AP, Cleary PP. Severe invasive group A streptococcal disease: clinical description and mechanisms of pathogenesis. J Lab Clin Med 1996; 127:13–22.

74. Musser JM, Kapur V, Szeto J, Pan X, Swanson DS, Martin DR. Genetic diversity and relationships among *Streptococcus pyogenes* strains expressing serotype M1 protein: recent Intercontinental spread of a subclone causing episodes of invasive disease. Infect Immun 1995; 63:994–1003.

75. Akesson P, Sjoholm AG, Bjorck L. Protein SIC, a novel extracellular protein of *Streptococcus pyogenes* interfering with complement function. J Biol Chem 1996; 271:1081–1088.

76. LaPenta D, Rubens C, Chi E, Cleary PP. Group A streptococci efficiently invade human respiratory epithelial cells. Proc Natl Acad Sci USA 1994; 91:12115–12119.

77. Cleary PP, McLandsborough L, Ikeda L, Cue D, Krawczak J, Lam H. High-frequency intracellular infection and erythrogenic toxin A expression undergo phase variation in M1 group A streptococci. Mol Microbiol 1998; 28:157–167.

78. Whatmore A, Kapur V, Sullivan DJ, Musser JM, Kehoe MA. Non-congruent relationships between variation in emm gene sequences and the population genetic structures of group A streptococci. Mol Microbiol 1994; 14:619–631.

79. Harbaugh MP, Podbielski A, Hugl S, Cleary PP. Nucleotide substitutions and small-scale insertion produce size and antigenic variation in group A streptococcal M1 protein. Mol Microbiol 1993; 8:981–991.

80. Bessen DE, Fischetti VA. Nucleotide sequence of two adjacent M or M-like protein genes of group A streptococci: different RNA transcript levels and identification of a unique immunoglobulin A binding protein. Infect Immun 1992; 60:124–35.

81. Kehoe MA, Poirer TP, Beachey EH, Timmis KN. Cloning and genetic analysis of serotype 5 M protein determinant of group A streptococci: evidence for multiple copies of the M5 determinant in the *Streptococcus pyogenes* genome. Infect Immun 1985; 48:190–197.

82. Hollingshead SK, Fischetti VA, Scott JR. Size variation in group A streptococcal M protein is

generated by homologous recombination between intragenic repeats. Mol Gen Genet 1987; 207:196–203.

83. Robbins J, Spanier JG, Jones SJ, Simpson WJ, Cleary P. *Streptococcus pyogenes* type 12 M protein gene regulation by upstream sequences. J Bacteriol 1987; 169:5633–5640.

84. Mouw A, Beachey EH, Burdett V. Molecular evolution of streptococcal M protein: cloning and nucleotide sequence of the type 24M protein gene and relation to other genes of *Streptococcus pyogenes*. J Bacteriol 1988; 170:676–684.

85. Manjula BN, Khandke KM, Fairwell T, Relf WA, Sriprakash KS. Heptad motifs within the distal subdomain of the coiled-coil rod region of M protein from rheumatic fever and nephritis associated serotypes of gruop A streptococci are distinct from each other: nucleotide sequence of the M57 gene and relation of the deduced amino acid sequence to other M proteins. J Prot Chem 1991; 10:369–384.

86. Podbielski A, Flosdorff A, Weber-Heynemann J. The group A streptococcal *vir49* gene controls expression of four structural *vir* regulon genes. Infect Immun 1995; 63:9–20.

87. Podbielski A, Schnitzler N, Beyhs P, Boyle MD. M-related protein (Mrp) contributes to group A streptococcal resistance to phagocytosis by human granulocytes. Mol Microbiol 1996; 19:429–441.

88. Wessels MR, Bronze MS. Critical role of the group A streptococcal capsule in pharyngeal colonization and infection in mice. Proc Natl Acad Sci USA 1994; 91:12238–12242.

89. Heden L, Lindahl G. Conserved and variable regions in protein Arp, the IgA receptor of *Streptococcus pyogenes*. J Gen Microbiol 1993; 139:2067–2074.

90. Podbielski A, Hawlitzky J, Pack TD, Flosdorff A. A group A streptococcal Enn protein potentially resulting from intergenomic recombination exhibits atypical immunoglobulin-binding characteristics. Mol Microbiol 1994; 12:725–736.

91. Whatmore AM, Kehoe MA. Horizontal gene transfer in the evolution of group A streptococcal *emm*-like genes: gene mosaics and variation in *vir* regulons. Mol Microbiol 1994; 11:363–374.

92. Simpson WJ, Musser JM, Cleary PP. Evidence consistent with horizontal transfer of the gene (*emm*12) encoding serotype M12 protein between group A and group G pathogenic streptococci. Infect Immun 1992; 60:1890–1893.

93. DiAngelis PL, Papaconstantinou J, Weigle PH. Isolation of a *Streptococcus pyogenes* gene locus that directs hyaluronan biosynthesis in acapsular mutants and in heterologous bacteria. J Biochem 1993; 268:14568–14571.

94. Crater DL, Dougherty BA, van de Rjin I. Molecular Characterization of *has*C from an operon required for hyaluronate synthesis in group A streptococcus. J Biol Chem 1995; 270:28676–28680.

95. Alberti S, Ashbaugh CD, Wessels MR. Structure of the *has* operon promoter and regulation of hyaluronic acid capsule expression in group A streptococcus. Mol Microbiol 1998; 28:343–353.

96. Simpson WJ, LaPenta D, Chen C, Cleary PP: Coregulation of type 12 M protein and streptococcal C5a peptidase genes in group A streptococci: evidence for a virulence regulon controlled by the virR lcous. J Bacteriol 1990; 172:696–700.

97. Podbielski A, Peterson JA, Cleary PP. Surface protein-CAT reporter fusions demonstrate differential gene expression in the *vir* regulon of *Streptococcus pyogenes*. Mol Microbiol 1992; 6:2253–2265.

98. McLandsborough L, Cleary PP. Insertional inactivation of virR´ in *Streptococcus pyogenes* M49 demonstrates that VirR functions as a positive regulator of ScpA, FcRA, OF, and M protein. FEMS Microbiol. Lett 1995; 128:45–52.

99. Kihlberg B, Cooney J, Caparon MG, Olsen A, Bjorck L. Biological properties of a *Streptococcus pyogenes* mutant generated by Tn*916* insertion in mga. Microbiol Pathol 1995; 19:299–315.

100. Okada N, Geist RT, Caparon MG. Positive transcriptional control of *mry* regulates virulence in the group A streptococcus. Mol Microbiol 1993; 7:893–903.

101. Bormann NE, Cleary PP. Transcriptional analysis of *mga*, a regulatory gene in *Streptococcus pyogenes*: identification of monocistronic and bicistronic transcripts that phase vary. Gene 1997; 200:125–134.

102. McIver KS, Heath AS, Green BD, Scott JR. Specific binding of the activator Mga to promoter sequences of the *emm* and *scp*A genes in the group A streptococcus. J Bacteriol 1995; 177: 6619–6624.

103. Simpson W, Cleary PP. Expression of M-type 12 protein by a group A streptococcus exhibits phase-like variation: evidence for coregulation of colony opacity determinants and M protein. Infect Immun 1987; 55:2448–2455.

104. LaPenta D, Zhang XP, Cleary PP. *Streptococcus pyogenes* type IIa IgG Fc receptor expression is co-ordinately regulated with M protein and streptococcal C5a peptidase. Mol Microbiol 1994; 12:873–879.

105. Mekalanos JJ. Environmental signals controlling expression of virulence determinants in bacteria. J Bacteriol 1992; 174:1–7.

106. Pritchard KH, Cleary PP. Differential expression of genes in the *vir* regulon of *Streptococcus pyogenes* is controlled by transcription termination. Mol Gen Genet 1996; 250:207–213.

107. Okada N, Pentland AP, Falk P, Caparon MG. M protein and protein F act as important de-

terminants of cell-specific tropism of *Streptococcus pyogenes* in skin tissue. J Clin Invest 1994; 94:965–977.

108. Talay SR, Ehrenfeld E, Chhatwal GS, Timmis KN. Expression of the fibronectin-binding components of *Streptococcus pyogenes* in *Escherichia coli* demonstrates that they are proteins. Mol Microbiol 1991; 5:1727–1734.

109. Courtney HS, Hasty DL, Dale JB, Poirier TP. A 28-kilodalton fibronectin-binding protein of group A streptococci. Curr Microbiol 1992; 25:245–250.

110. Pancholi V, Fischetti VA. A major surface protein on group A streptococci is a glyceraldehyde-3-phosphate dehydrogenase with multiple binding activities. J Exp Med 1992; 176:415–426.

111. Schmidt KH, Mann K, Cooney J, Kohler W. Multiple binding of type 3 streptococcal M protein to human fibrinogen, albumin and fibronectin. FEMS Immun Med Microbiol 1993; 7:135–144.

112. Courtney HS, Li Y, Dale JB, Hasty DL. Cloning, sequencing, and expression of a fibronectin/fibrinogen-binding protein from group A streptococci. Infect Immun 1994; 62:3937–3946.

113. Kreikemeyer B, Talay SR, Chhatwal GS. Characterization of a novel fibronectin-binding surface protein in group A streptococci. Mol Microbiol 1995; 17:137–145.

114. Fogg GC, Gibson CM, Caparon MG. The identification of *rof*A, a positive-acting regulatory component of *prt*F expression: use of an mgd-based shuttle mutagenesis strategy in *Streptococcus pyogenes*: Mol Microbiol 1994; 11:671–684.

115. VanHeyningen T, Fogg G, Yates D, Hanski E, Caparon M. Adherence and fibronectin binding are environmentally regulated in the group A streptococci. Mol Microbiol 1993; 9:1213–1222.

116. McIver KS, Heath AS, Scott JR. Regulation of virulence by environmental signals in group A streptococci: influence of osmolarity, temperature, gas exchange, and iron limitation on *emm* transcription. Infect Immun 1995; 63:4540–4542.

117. McIver KS, Scott JR. Role of *mga* in growth phase regulation of virulence genes of group A streptococcus. J Bacteriol 1997; 179:5178–5187.

118. Courtney HS, Bronze MS, Dale JB, Hasty DL. Analysis of the role of M24 protein in group A streptococcal adhesion and colonization by use of W-interposon mutagenesis. Infect Immun 1994; 62:4868–4873.

118a. Dombek P, Cue D, Sedgewick J, Lam H, Ruschkowski S, Finlay B, Cleary P. High-frequency intracellular invasion of epithelial cells by serotype M1 group A Streptococci: M1 protein-mediated invasion and cytoskeletal rearrangements. Mol Microbiol 1999; 859–870.

119. Ji YL, McLandsborough L, Kondagunta A, Cleary PP. C5a peptidase alters clearance and trafficking of group A streptococci by infected mice. Infect Immun 1996; 64:503–510.

4

Exotoxins of
Streptococcus pyogenes

MANUELA ROGGIANI
ARIS P. ASSIMACOPOULOS
PATRICK M. SCHLIEVERT

Group A streptococci, which are pathogens of humans only, produce a wide variety of illnesses, ranging from relatively mild pharyngitis and impetigo to life-threatening septicemia and toxic shock syndrome (TSS). In addition, certain strains of the organism are associated with production of apparently autoimmune delayed sequelae, including rheumatic fever, acute glomerulonephritis, erythema nodosum, and occasionally guttate psoriasis.

Streptococci elaborate a variety of extracellular factors that facilitate their ability to cause human disease. Among these factors are the streptococcal pyrogenic exotoxins (SPEs, scarlet fever toxins, erythrogenic toxin [type A]) and related toxins, the hemolysins streptolysin O and S, a variety of nucleases and proteases, and the hyaluronic acid capsule.

There is considerable evidence to suggest that SPEs and hemolysins contribute significantly to human diseases. Most notably, the recognition of SPEs as members of a large family of pyrogenic toxin superantigens, including also TSS toxin-1 and staphylococcal enterotoxins, has led to a large body of information regarding their role in severe streptococcal diseases. This chapter reviews current studies of SPE and hemolysin structure and function. The readers are referred to previous reviews for extensive discussions of older literature [1–9].

STREPTOCOCCAL PYROGENIC EXOTOXINS AND RELATED TOXINS

General Properties

Pyrogenic exotoxins secreted by streptococci (SPEs) were first identified in supernates of cultures from scarlet fever strains; initially their biological activity was thought to be limited to the induction of the erythematous rash typical of scarlet fever [10]. Later, Watson provided evidence that the toxins are pyrogenic [11]. Today the SPEs, designated serotypes A, B, and C, are recognized to be part of a large family of exotoxins that include also SPE F, streptococcal superantigen, staphylococcal TSST-1 and enterotoxins A, B, Cn, D, E, G, and H, and non–group A streptococcal pyrogenic exotoxins. Recently, several investigators have isolated, from streptococcal supernates, other secreted products that share at least some of the properties of this group of toxins.

The members of this large family of toxins are generically called pyrogenic toxins because of their ability to induce fever [11], but they share several other immunobiological properties. The best characterized among these properties is superantigenicity. Superantigens are a group of molecules of both bacterial and viral origin that induce proliferation of a large number of host T lymphocytes, independent of their antigenic specificity, but dependent on the composition of the variable part of the β chain (Vβ) of the T cell receptor (TCR). It is estimated that superantigens can stimulate up to 20% of the T cell repertoire, and in TSS patients the T cell population expanded by a superantigen can constitute up to 70% of the total peripheral blood T lymphocytes [12]. T cell activation by superantigens requires binding to class II major histocompatibility complex (MHC) molecules, which occurs outside the typical antigenic peptide binding groove, does not involve antigen processing, and is not or only minimally influenced by the antigenic peptide presented in the MHC groove [3,13]. Superantigenic activation is not MHC restricted, although each superantigen has greater affinity for some HLA alleles than for others [3,13].

At least in part a consequence of superantigenicity is the toxin's ability to induce host cell release of massive amounts of cytokines of the inflammatory (interleukin [IL]-1α, IL-1β, IL-6, tumor necrosis factor [TNF]-α, TNF-β) and antinflammatory (sIL-1ra,) groups, of the TH1 (IL-2, IL-12, interferon [IFN]-γ) and TH2 (IL-4, IL-5, IL-10, IL-13) T cell subsets, and hematopoietic cells (IL-3, granulocyte-macrophage colony-stimulating factor [GM-CSF]) [14–23]. It is generally accepted that capillary leak is the prime factor that leads to hypotension and shock [24–28], the most severe manifestations of streptococcal TSS. Circulating cytokines released by the direct action of the pyrogenic toxins on immune cells is thought to provide a very important contribution to capillary leak [27,28].

Another property of the pyrogenic toxins that may contribute significantly to capillary leak and shock is the ability to amplify host susceptibility to endotoxin by a factor of $>10^5$ [29,30]. This effect may occur through impairment of the liver's ability to clear endotoxin derived from the endogenous gram-negative flora [31], with subsequent elevation of endotoxin levels in the blood circulation, binding of endotoxin with

lipopolysaccharide-binding protein, and release of TNF-α from macrophages. The significance of this property in the pathogenesis of TSS is supported by the observation that shock can be prevented in animal models in part by administration of polymyxin B [32], or in studies performed on pathogen-free animals [30]. Lastly, a final contributor to the onset of hypotension and shock may be direct damage to endothelial cells, shown to occur in vitro with TSST-1 [33].

Additional immunobiologic properties of the pyrogenic toxins are T cell–dependent B cell immunosuppression [34]; inhibition of inflammatory responses caused by the exceedingly high level of circulating TNF-α (antichemotactic for polymorphonuclear leukocytes [PMNs]) [15,16,35]; and enhancement of delayed type hypersensitivity, proposed to cause the rash of scarlet fever [36].

In addition to properties shared with the other members of the larger pyrogenic toxin family, the SPEs also enhance host susceptibility to myocardial damage induced by either endotoxin or streptolysin O [37]. This cardiotoxic property, the association of SPEs with rheumatic fever isolates [38], and their superantigenicity may implicate the SPEs in the early events leading to this autoimmune disease. SPEs have also been shown to cross the blood-brain barrier [39], and thus are thought to induce fever also by acting on macrophage-like cells in the hypothalamic area.

Structural and Biological Properties

The toxins of the larger pyrogenic family share variable degrees of primary amino acid sequence similarity, ranging between 70% and 20% (Fig. 4.1). The SPE serotype A is more similar to the staphylococcal enterotoxins B and C than to the other streptococcal or staphylococcal toxin serotypes (approximately 50% similarity), and with enterotoxins B and C and streptococcal superantigen comprise a subfamily within the larger toxin family [1].

The more recent observations for each of the streptococcal pyrogenic toxins will be discussed separately in the remainder of this review.

The gene for SPE A, speA, was cloned by Johnson and Schlievert [40] from Streptococcus pyogenes phage T12 into Escherichia coli. That SPE A is carried on a mobile genetic element

	SEB	SEC	SEA	SED	SEE	TSST-1	SPEB	SPEC
SPEA	50	45	30	35	35	25	20	30
SEB		70	35	35	35	25	20	25
SEC			30	35	30	20	20	20
SEA				50	70	25	20	30
SED					50	25	20	30
SEE						25	20	25
TSST-1							25	20
SPEB								20

Figure 4.1 Percent identity among aligned pyrogenic toxin superantigen primary amino acid sequences.

was first shown by the work of Frobisher and Brown [41], who made nonscarlatinal streptococci able to cause scarlet fever by exposing them to a filterable agent from scarlet fever strains. Several years later, the filterable agent was shown to be the lysogenic bacteriophage designated T12 [42,43], that Johnson and Schlievert [44] subsequently mapped and found to be 36 kb in size, terminally redundant, and circularly permuted. Subsequently, other *spe*A-bearing phages were identified from streptococcal isolates [45]. The genomes of these newly characterized phages are slightly different in size from T12, although they share sequences other than *spe*A with T12. As indicated above, the SPE A amino acid sequence is highly homologous to the staphylococcal enterotoxins B and C sequences (Fig. 4.1). Since *spe*A is carried on a phage and is located adjacent to the phage attachment site [45,46], it is thought that the *spe*A ancestor originated from a staphylococcal gene by imprecise excision of a phage and subsequent transfer across species. It is noteworthy that different phages of the *spe*A-bearing family may integrate into the bacterial chromosome at different sites [47].

SPE A is found in aqueous solutions primarily as a monomer with an approximate molecular weight of 26,000 Da. It is present in two forms, which can be converted into one form by a reducing agent [48]. When purified by isoelectric focusing, SPE A focuses as two distinct bands at pH 4.5 and 5.5 [1]. In our laboratory, SPE A is produced from a clone in *Staphylococcus aureus* strain RN 4220, and purified by ethanol precipitation of bacterial cultures grown to stationary phase at 37°C in a dialyzable beef heart medium [1]. The toxin is then dissolved in pyrogen-free water and purified to homogeneity by successive flat-bed isoelectric focusing separations in pH gradients of 3.5 to 10.0 and then 4.0 to 6.0.

The gene *spe*A was sequenced first by Weeks and Ferretti [49], and from the deduced amino acid sequence the peptide has a molecular weight of 29,244 Da. After cleavage of a 30 amino acid signal peptide, the mature toxin has a molecular weight of 25,787 Da, which is in agreement with previous physicochemical findings.

The high amino acid sequence similarity of enterotoxins B and C with SPE A allowed the generation of a three-dimensional structure model of SPE A by homology modeling (Fig. 4.2) [50], based on the coordinates of SEC1, whose crystal structure has been solved [51]. The SPE A structure appears to have all of the basic features associated with the pyrogenic toxin superantigen structures thus far solved, namely TSST-1, SPE C, and staphylococcal enterotoxins A, B, and C2, 3 [51–55]. The molecule is roughly divided in two domains: domain A is composed of a short portion of the N-terminal sequence and the entire C-terminal half of the molecule; domain B is composed of a continuous stretch of amino acids forming a series of antiparallel β-strands that fold to form a distinctive β-barrel structure or claw structure. A small cavity (top cavity) bordered by the top portion of domain B and by a short α-helix of the amino terminal region has been shown to be the site of interaction with TCR [56]. At least one of the residues in this cavity (Asp20) is also necessary for the toxin to be lethal in two animal models [57]. SPE A has three cysteine residues (Fig. 4.2) that are homologous to the cysteines forming a disulfide bridge in enterotoxins B and C. In the enterotoxins, the cysteine loop is thought to contribute to emetic activity and has been implicated in the binding of MHC class II. SPE A is devoid of emetic activity [58], even though several observations support the existence of a disulfide bridge between Cys 87 and Cys 98 [48,57,59]. Mutagenesis of either Cys 87 or 98 reduces superantigenicity of SPE A [57,59]. The β-barrel structure of domain B was shown to be the site of interaction with MHC class II receptors [59]. The integrity of residues on the side of the barrel is also necessary for lethality and full mitogenic activity [57].

SPE A biological activities are the most thoroughly characterized among the streptococcal exotoxins. That SPE A is a superantigen and stimulates T cells to proliferate in a Vβ-specific fashion was shown by Leonard et al. [14] and Tomai et al. [60]. Human T cells to which SPE A binds have TCRs with Vβ 2, 4, 8, 12, 14, and 15. Typical of superantigens, SPE A binds to MHC class II molecules and its T cell stimulatory activity is dependent on this binding. SPE A interacts best with HLA-DQ, less well with DR, and only marginally with DP [61].

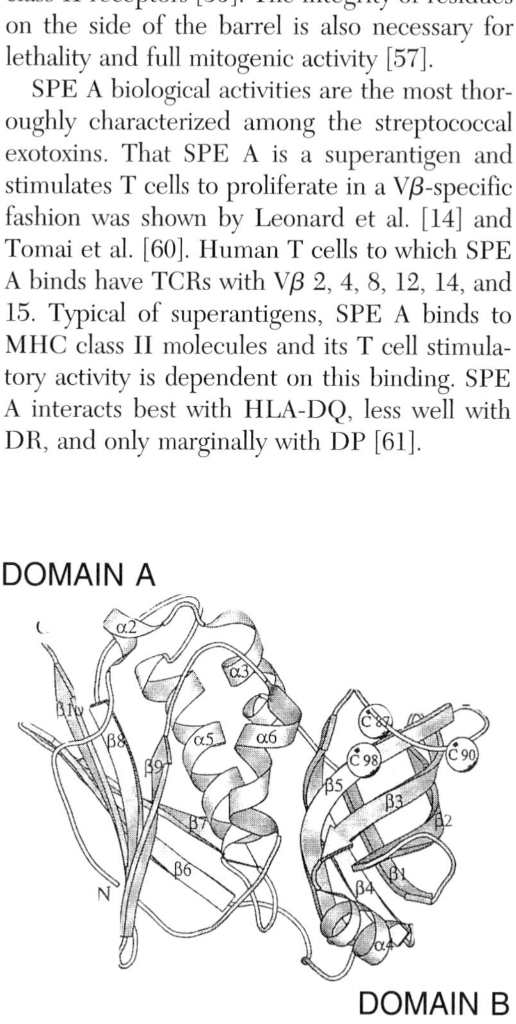

DOMAIN A

DOMAIN B

Figure 4.2 Ribbon diagram of the modeled structure of SPE A; the positions of the cysteine residues are highlighted.

SPE A was shown by Leonard and Schlievert [62] to bind tightly to the ketodeoxyoctanate (KDO) residues of the core region of lipopolysaccharide (LPS). The SPE A–LPS complex is lethal to T cells, and this property is separate from superantigenicity, since immune cell lethality is not dependent on the TCR and does not require antigen presenting cells. The immunolethality property of SPE A may in part contribute to the immune cell depletion detected late in TSS patients [62].

The role of SPE A in production of human disease was initially observed when investigators injected themselves and medical students with toxin and caused scarlet fever and TSS symptoms. Several animal models are also available. Among these, one of the most effective in reproducing the symptoms of TSS (except rash) is the subcutaneous implantation into rabbits of miniosmotic pumps, which deliver toxin in a constant amount over a period of 7 days [57,63,64]. Death in animals treated in this way can be prevented by fluid replacement therapy, which is consistent with TSS being a capillary leak syndrome [32]. In a study by Schlievert et al. [35], exponentially growing M1 or M3 group A streptococci were injected subcutaneously into SPE A–immunized rabbits and into a nonimmunized control group. All of the nonimmunized animals presented with symptoms of TSS, including both necrotizing fasciitis and a complete lack of inflammatory response in and near the site of injection. Most of the animals succumbed to the illness. Conversely, most of the SPE A–immune rabbits did not develop TSS and survived. Moreover, animals in the latter SPE A–immune group had large numbers of PMNs surrounding the injected streptococci. Collectively, the above studies indicate that SPE A has the ability to cause TSS. Furthermore, although SPE A alone does not cause necrotizing fasciitis, seen in many TSS patients, the toxin may establish conditions necessary to allow growth of the invading streptococci and production of virulence factors that cause the tissue necrosis.

Studies on environmental factors influencing expression and secretion of SPE A showed that SPE A production is maximal at slightly basic pH in buffered conditions and at temperatures between 37° and 39°C [65,66]. This is consistent with the expression of SPE A in deep-sited infections, and therefore with a role of this toxin in the pathogenesis of STSS and other severe infections [66].

Epidemiologic studies also reinforce the strong association between SPE A and TSS. Expression of SPE A is a variable trait, and is distributed among approximately 15% of general isolates of group A streptococci [67]. Several studies have shown that most isolates from TSS patients express SPE A or carry its gene [25,68–72]. SPE A is found most often associated with streptococcal serotypes M1, M3, and M18, in particular those strains carrying the invasive (inv+) genetic profile [35]. The increase in the last decade in prevalence of M1 and M3 types and of SPE A production corresponds to the increase in incidence and severity of serious streptococcal diseases [35].

Several pieces of evidence suggest that SPE B has an evolutionary origin different from the other SPEs [50]. The SPE B primary amino acid sequence bears little similarity to the other members of the pyrogenic toxins family (Fig. 4.1), SPE B is unique among pyrogenic toxin superantigens in that it is proteolytic, and finally, nearly all group A streptococci carry *spe*B, the gene encoding SPE B. *spe*B is localized on the chromosome and was first cloned by Bohach et al. [73] from a pharyngitis strain. The gene was cloned into *E. coli*, and the recombinant toxin reacted to SPE B antisera and conserved the mitogenic activity of the toxin from streptococci. However, its molecular weight was not in agreement with previous findings [74]. The discrepancy in size appears to be due to the toxin being present in two forms, one being a product of proteolytic cleavage. The toxin displays microheterogeneity when subjected to isoelectric focusing with isoelectric points [74] of 8.0, 8.3, and 9.0. SPE B can be obtained from *Streptococcus pyogenes* grown in dialyzable beef heart medium by ethanol precipitation, followed by solubilization in acetate buffered saline, and purification by isoelectric focusing separation in pH gradient 7.0 to 9.0 [1]. The toxin is not stably produced in *Staphylococcus aureus*.

The sequence of the gene *spe*B [75] predicts that the native SPE B is composed of 398 amino acids. After cleavage of the 27 residue signal peptide, the protein has a molecular weight of 40,314 Da. Further proteolysis originates a breakdown product with a molecular weight of 27,588 Da. The deduced amino acid sequence of SPE B is strikingly similar (84% identity) to the sequence of streptococcal proteinase precursor (SPP) [75], a cysteine protease secreted as an inactive zymogen by nearly all group A streptococci [76]. Hauser and Schlievert [75] were not able to show degradation of casein by SPE B and concluded that SPE B and SPP are variants of the same protein and that SPE B had lost proteolytic activity either because of mutation or as a result of the purification protocol. Later on, SPE B was purified from a different streptococcal strain and by a different procedure. This toxin preparation was shown to have proteolytic activity and was confirmed to be a cysteine protease [77]. At least in vitro, the low-molecular-weight cysteine protease can convert its own precursor to the active molecule [78,79]. Two groups independently inactivated *spe*B without affecting growth of the mutant strains, suggesting that SPE B proteolytic activity is not required for growth [80,81]. However, SPE B secretion occurs in response to nutrient deprivation, suggesting that streptococci facing starvation may secrete this protease to degrade host protein and gather nutrients [82].

Multiple examples of the protease activity of SPE B implicate the toxin as a virulence factor in the onset of invasive streptococcal infection, in particular of soft tissue infections. The protease was shown to degrade human vitronectin and cleave fibronectin [83] and to activate a host-cell matrix metalloprotease [84]. Kapur et al. [85] observed that the 27.5 kD form of SPE B can proteolyze IL-1β precursor to the active cytokine. SPE B can synergyze with streptolysin O (SLO) and streptococcal cell wall (SCW) antigen in a rat model of SLO- and SCW-induced acute lung injury [86]. M types 3 and 49 group A streptococci lacking a functional SPE B are unable to disseminate after intraperitoneal injection in mice, and are not lethal to animals [87,88]. Finally, SPE B was shown to contribute to streptococcal invasion of the epithelial cell line A-549 [81].

In addition to proteolytic activity, which is unique to SPE B in the pyrogenic toxin family, SPE B shares other biological activities of the family, such as pyrogenicity, cardiotoxicity, and superantigenicity, although this last property is still being debated. SPE B appears to expand T cell populations bearing the Vβ 8 receptor [60]. SPE B binds well to HLA DQ molecules on antigen-presenting cells (APCs), but binds with low affinity to the DR allele and probably does not bind to DP [61].

Although *speB* is carried by most streptococcal isolates [68], the toxin is detectable in the culture supernates of only approximately half of them. An explanation for this observation is that the expression of the gene may be regulated differently in different strains; alternatively, SPE B may be completely proteolytically degraded in some of the strains. Nonetheless, at least one report indicated that streptococcal strains from severe invasive infections are producer of higher levels of SPE B than strains from infections that are not deep sited [89]. Furthermore, M1 isolates of streptococci associated with TSS typically make high levels of SPE B. This makes the toxin an attractive candidate for contributing to the necrotizing fasciitis often seen in TSS cases.

Like *speA*, the gene for SPE C, designated *speC*, is contained on a circularly permuted, terminally redundant bacteriophage [43,90] within 1 kb of the phage attachment site. The gene *speC*, and thus SPE C, is a variable trait with approximately 50% of streptococci in general having the gene [91], but also like *speA*, *speC* is unevenly distributed among M types. For example, *speC* is present in nearly all M-type 18 organisms, but is much less common in M1 and M3 strains [68].

Goshorn et al. [92] cloned *speC* into *E. coli* and demonstrated the protein produced was biochemically and biologically similar to toxin made by streptococci. The gene has been cloned into *Staphylococcus aureus*, but the toxin is not stably produced. The nucleotide sequence of *speC* has been determined [93,94] and yields a protein of 235 amino acids that is processed to a 208 residue-secreted protein of 24,354 molecular weight after removal of a 27 residue signal peptide.

SPE C is most easily purified from M18 streptococci where yields of 100 μg/liter culture fluid are common. SPE C is purified from early stationary-phase cultures by ethanol precipitation, resolubilization in acetate-buffered saline, treatment with hyaluronidase to reduce the large amount of hyaluronic acid made by M18 organisms, and finally, preparative isoelectric focusing

[1]. In in vitro tests, SPE C is typically made by streptococci in amounts one-tenth those of SPE A.

SPE C shares only about 30% primary sequence similarity with SPE A and 20% with TSST-1 (Fig. 4.1). In spite of the low sequence similarity, SPE C shares the same biological properties as SPE A [1], and it is structurally very similar to TSST-1 [52,55]. The crystal structure of SPE C revealed that the same amino-terminal region of two molecules interact to form dimers [55]. This observation and binding studies [55,95] indicate that SPE C lacks the low-affinity binding site typical of all known superantigens (including TSST-1) with MHC class II receptors [96]. Rather, binding of SPE C to MHC class II resembles the high-affinity binding of the staphylococcal superantigen SEA that occurs at the C-terminal portion of the molecule and is mediated by coordination of a zinc atom [97,98]. Like SEA, SPE C also has at least one, possibly two, zinc coordination sites [55]. Although lacking one of the MHC class II binding regions, the SPE C dimer was suggested to bind two MHC and two T cell receptors [55]. This may explain the high potency of this superantigen.

Even though most steptococcal isolates obtained in the last decade from TSS patients express SPE A, a number of isolates are not associated with any of SPEs A, B, and C. For these reasons, searches for other streptococcal toxin superantigens have been initiated. Several novel superantigens have recently been identified. The best characterized are streptococcal superantigen (SSA) [99] and mitogenic factor (MF, SPE F) [100,101].

The SSA was initially identified as a class II–dependent T cell mitogen present in culture supernates of a group A streptococcal strain isolated from a fatal case of TSS [97]. After purification, the mitogenic activity was associated with a protein of approximately 28,000 molecular weight, whose amino terminus is very similar to, but distinct from, the staphylococcal enterotoxins B and C.

The gene for SSA, *ssa*, was cloned and expressed in *E. coli* [102]. The *ssa* transcript encodes a predicted peptide of 260 residues, of which the first 26 amino acids are the signal sequence. The calculated molecular weight of the mature protein is 26,892 Da. The predicted peptide is approximately 60% identical to SEB and SEC3 and shares significant but lesser similarity with SPE A (49% identity).

Purified SSA displays biological activities typical of superantigens. The toxin stimulates proliferation of a subset of T lymphocytes bearing receptors with Vβ 1, 3, 5.2, and 15 [99]. This subset is distinct from those stimulated by other pyrogenic toxins, indicating that in spite of sequence similarity, SSA is not an allele of other known streptococcal toxins. The stimulation of T lymphocytes by SSA, as for other superantigens, is dependent on the presence of class II MHC molecules, and precisely requires the alleles HLA-DR, -DQ, and H-2 I-E [99]. Mutational analysis and binding studies have revealed that SSA interacts with the T cell and MHC class II receptors differently from the other known superantigens, even the closely related SEB [103]. Another characteristic that distinguishes SSA from the other known superantigens is the post-translational modification of the molecule by addition of a yet unidentified biochemical moiety [104]. Because SSA is modified differently in streptococci and in *E coli*, the known biological properties of SSA secreted by the two bacterial hosts differ [104]. Other biological activities shared by other pyrogenic toxins have not been tested thus far in SSA.

Production of SSA is limited to group A streptococci and is mostly associated with M types 3 and 4, but not M1 [99]. SSA-positive M4 lineages are associated with cases of pharyngitis or scarlet fever rashes, but not to severe diseases, whereas M3 strains expressing SSA are associated with TSS or other severe invasive streptococcal diseases. These isolates are also positive for SPE A and often other SPEs, suggesting that the concomitant expression of SPEs and SSA may make those strains particularly virulent [99].

A novel factor with mitogenic activity on peripheral blood cells was identified by Yutsudo et al. [100] from supernates of *Streptococcus pyogenes* strain NY-5 cultures and later independently isolated by Norrby-Teglund et al. [101]. This protein is designated mitogenic factor (MF) or SPE F. The purified protein has a molecular weight of approximately 27,000. The gene encoding MF/SPE F (*mf*) was cloned in *E. coli* and sequenced [105]. The transcript is translated into a 271 residue peptide, which after cleavage of the 43 amino acid signal peptide becomes a mature protein with a calculated molecular weight of 23,363. The MF/SPE F amino acid sequence does not share similarity to the known SPEs.

The superantigenicity of MF/SPE F was tested on human peripheral blood cells. The toxin stimulates proliferation of subsets of T lymphocytes carrying Vβ 2, 4, 7, 8, 15, 18, 19, and 21 TCRs [101,106]. These Vβ specificites are unique to MF/SPE F. Binding of MF/SPE F to class II is not restricted, but preferentially occurs with HLA-DQ [101]. A later report indicated that MF/SPE F binds to HLA-DR [106]. MF/SPE F can also stimulate production of cytokines by lymphocytes; the cytokine secretion pattern is comparable, although not identical, to that induced by SPE A, SPE B [107], or SPE C [106]. Because of its superantigenicity and its ability to induce production of cytokines, MF was renamed SPE F. A recent report indicated that MF/SPE F has endonuclease activity displayed with ssDNA, dsDNA, and tRNA [108].

The distribution of MF/SPE F among group A and non–group A streptococcal strains was analyzed [101,109]. Of 370 group A streptococci general isolates analyzed 99.7% carried the *mf* gene, but none of the non–group A streptococci had *mf*. The large distribution of MF/SPE F in group A streptococci, which is comparable to the distribution of *spe*B, has a twofold significance. First, it can be speculated that like *spe*B, *mf* is carried on the *Streptococcus pyogenes* chromosome, rather than on a mobile element as *spe*A and *spe*C. In addition, detection by polymerase chain reaction (PCR) or by other methods of *mf* (as for *spe*B) in clinical isolates could be used as a diagnostic tool for group A streptococci.

Additional, less well–characterized streptococcal superantigens are also known. Streptococcal mitogenic exotoxin Z (SMEZ) [110] was isolated from strains T1 and NY-5. This factor, with mitogenic activity for human and rabbit lymphocytes, is predicted to have a moleculr weight of 25,254. The SMEZ appears to be distinct from the other known superantigens in its rabbit Vβ profile and its seroreactivity [110]. *Streptococcus pyogenes* mitogen-2 (SPM-2) [111] was initially isolated from *Streptococcus pyogenes* strain T12, but was subsequently found in supernates of other streptococcal strains. SPM-2 preferentially stimulates expansion of T cell subsets expressing Vβ 4, 7, and 8, and for this activity requires the presence of HLA-DR-bearing APCs [111]. A low-molecular-weight protein (8000 Da) with superantigenic activity (low-molecular-weight superantigen [LMWS]) was purified from a streptococcal isolate from a TSS case [112]. The LMWS isolectric point (pI) was approximately 7.2. This superantigen selectively expanded T cell populations expressing Vβs 4, 7, and 8 [112]. This superantigen induced the secretion from human peripheral blood cells of a cytokine profile similar to that induced by SPE A and C [113]. Finally, two novel superantigens were isolated by Newton and co-workers from strain JR from a TSS case [114]. These molecule had a molecular weight of approximately 30,000. The protein with a pI of 7.2 selectively expanded T cell–bearing Vβs 2 and 20; the protein with a pI of 8.0 expanded T cells bearing Vβs 3,12, 14, 15, and 20 [114].

STREPTOCOCCAL CYTOLYTIC TOXINS

The secreted, oxygen-sensitive streptolysin O (SLO) is part of a genetically related family of bacterial cytolytic toxins including staphylococcal α-toxin, listeriolysin O, pneumolysin, perfringolysin O, and others. The cell-associated, oxygen-stable streptolysin S (SLS) is less well understood, but is responsible for much of the hemolysis produced by group A streptococci (GAS) on blood-agar plates and is presumably related to SLS-like toxins generated by other organisms including *Treponema hyodysenteriae*, *Hemophilus pleuropneumonia*, *Streptococcus mutans*, and *Streptococcus agalactiae* [115]. More attention has recently been directed at SLO than SLS because isolation and purification of SLO is easier and because it is useful for the controlled permeabilization of cell membranes to introduce macromolecules or manipulate the intracellular milieu [116]. Several reviews summarize the understanding of these toxins through the mid-1980s [6–9]. Somewhat overshadowed by the superantigenic streptococcal pyrogenic exotoxins (SPEs), the role of SLO and SLS in GAS infec-

tions and their nonsuppurative sequelae continue to be ill defined.

Streptolysin O

Streptolysin O belongs to a family of "thiol-activated" toxins, so called because they are activated by reducing compounds. Streptolysin O is produced by most group A, C, and G streptococci [6]. Immunologically, functionally, and genetically, the oxygen-labile streptolysins isolated from groups A, C, and G streptococci are virtually identical [6,117,118]. Structural and sequence homology exists with other toxins in this family including listeriolysin and perfringolysin O [119,120]. Streptolysin O is the prototype of pore-forming cholesterol-binding cytolysins, of which staphylococcal α-toxin is the best characterized [121].

Streptococci produce the greatest amounts of SLO at the end of the log phase of growth. In solution SLO is inactivated by oxygen or prolonged storage. Obtaining pure, stable preparations of SLO has been problematic. After a long series of recovery steps, products are often contaminated with streptococcal enzymes. The traditional method is described by Alouf and Geoffroy [115]. Simpler methods of isolation are described in two more recent works [117,122]. Both appear to achieve fairly pure solutions of SLO. One procedure utilizes a silica gel column, ammonium sulfate precipitation, a hydroxyapatite column, and finally, a denaturing polyol column or isoelectric focusing to quickly obtain pure, stable SLO. The activity of SLO is quantified in hemolytic units (HU), which is the amount needed to achieve 50% lysis in a given system, as determined by dilution or colorimetric or spectrophotometric techniques. Specific activities from 100,000 to 750,000 HU/mg can be obtained. The *slo* gene has been cloned into *E. coli* but production of SLO has not been quantified [123].

Existing primarily in the extracellular fluid of streptococci, SLO is also found in the periplasmic space when expressed in *E. coli* [6,124]. Sulfhydryl (reducing) compounds reversibly activate or reactivate SLO. Heat, oxygen, cholesterol, serum lipid extracts, serum β-lipoprotein fractions, or red cell membranes inactivate or inhibit SLO [6,7]. Previously supposed to contain many cysteine residues involved in disulfide bonding and necessary for cytolytic activity, SLO is now known to contain only one cysteine. Once called the "essential cysteine," this residue is within a highly conserved 12 amino acid sequence [120]. Although oxidation or blocking of this cysteine results in toxin inactivation, it can be replaced with alanine or serine and retain hemolytic activity [125].

At least two active forms of SLO exist, having molecular weights of between 50,000 and 70,000 and isoelectric points primarily between 6.0–6.5 and 7.0–7.8 [6,122,126,127]. Active fragments of SLO exist and have been identified by several investigators [117,123]. Working with crude SLO preparations, one group found it to have a consistent molecular weight of 64,000, but a continuous range of isoelectric points from 5.4 to 8.3 [128]. The *slo* gene sequence is known. It predicts a 571 amino acid protein with a molecular weight of 63,645, which is probably cleaved prior to secretion, leaving a final product of about 57,000 molecular weight [119]. A report indicated that SLO can be cleaved in vitro by the streptococcal cysteine protease SPE B, but the significance of this observation in the context of host infection was not investigated [129]. The cleavage results in the loss of the 46 amino terminal residues of SLO, but full activity of SLO is conserved. Weller and co-workers also showed that the amino terminal region of SLO is not required for pore formation, and the amino terminal portion of the molecule is not likely to insert into the cytoplasmic membrane [130].

The understanding of SLO and its mechanism of action is presently much clearer because of recently performed, detailed structural analysis with electron microscopy (EM) and binding studies accompanied by mutational analysis. On the basis of EM studies, the individual SLO molecule is hypothesized to have hydrophobic and hydrophilic faces and consist of three parts: the "crown," the "neck," and the "base" [131]. Separate f (fixation) and t (toxic) sites are revealed by antigenic studies. They are required for cell binding and lysis, respectively [132]. The t site is necessary for polymerization of the cell membrane–bound SLO monomers [133]. A recent model of the SLO monomer, based on perfringolysin O structure [134], predicts that SLO

is composed of four domains, D1 through D4 [135]. The tryptophan-rich motif, which binds membrane cholesterol, is in D4. Following membrane insertion of D4, a change in conformation of domains D1 and D3 would allow SLO to oligomerize [135].

Ultrastructural studies disclose the presence of ring-, arc-, and rod-shaped structures on cell membranes (Fig. 4.3) [131]. These are oligomers of SLO that are stable, protease-resistant, cholesterol-free [136,137], and membrane protein–free [138]. A model of the SLO polymer has been advanced through EM studies [131]. This consists of two concentric rings of SLO monomers (internal and external) forming a double-layered, arc- or ring-shaped structure that spans the cell membrane. The hydrophilic faces of SLO molecules line the internal surface of the pore, and the hydrophobic faces are external, associated with the lipid membrane [137] (Fig. 4.4). The extent of the polymer may vary from an arc-shaped structure to a full ring. The holes produced by these structures are 20–40 nm in diameter [131], which differs considerably from the pore size of the related staphylococcal α-toxin and *E. coli* hemolysin (6–10 Å and 10–15 Å, respectively) [139]. The pores are stable and can be isolated in nondenaturing detergents [139].

Oligomerization of SLO in cell membranes and pore formation occur in a nonlinear two-step fashion as a function of SLO concentration. Streptolysin O monomers first bind to cholesterol in the cell membrane in a temperature-independent manner [138,139]. The 3β-OH group on cholesterol is thought to be necessary for binding. Streptolysin O will not bind to pure phosphatidylcholine membranes, but exhibits maximal binding with a cholesterol:phosphatidylcholine ratio of 1:1 [140]. The monomer must be in the reduced state for binding to take place. The binding step is inhibited by cholesterol or oxidation. The subsequent lytic step is temperature-dependent and inhibited by low pH, high ionic strength, divalent cations, or anti-streptolysin O (ASO) antibody. It is not inhibited by cholesterol. After the SLO monomer inserts its carboxyl-terminal end into the cell membrane, cholesterol plays no further role in pore formation. The monomers aggregate on the cell surface to form pores [131]. Initially, two membrane-bound monomers are thought to interact and form a dimer [141]. This rate-limiting

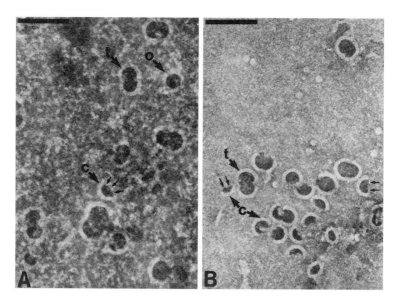

Figure 4.3 Lysis of erythrocytes by SLO seen by electron microscopy. (A) The RBC membrane without any special treatment. (B) The RBC membrane after removing extraneous material. Arrows show the free edge of the cell membrane. Twinned and circular configurations of the SLO pores are shown by (t) and (c), respectively. Bar, 100 nm (From Bhakdi et al. [137], with permission.)

nucleation process then proceeds quickly to the assembly of the transmembrane pore by sequential addition of membrane-bound monomers. First arc-shaped, then ring-shaped complexes form. Approximately 22 individual units are necessary for a functional pore. Streptolysin O monomers in solution do not aggregate, indicating that a conformational change of the monomer is necessary for aggregation to occur [139]. This conformational change may also provide the energy necessary to drive polymerization, since the process is ATP independent.

Streptolysin O can effect lysis of many cell types. On sensitive cells, cytolysis takes place

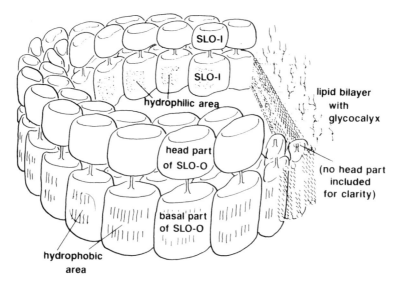

Figure 4.4 Hypothesized model of an SLO pore within a cell membrane. (From Sekiya et al. [131], with permission.)

even at low doses of toxin. However, activity varies with species and age of the cells and may vary with the actual pI of the SLO molecules [6,7,128,136]. The variable susceptibility of different cell types and of erythrocytes of different species is not dependent on binding and polymerization but could depend on the ability of the cell to tolerate pores or on the generation of nonfunctional pores [142]. The number of pores formed on cells varies even with the same preparation. Heat inactivation stops lysis but ring structures are still observed on the cells [123]. At low concentration SLO can be shed from cells without lysis. Nonetheless, permeabilization of the cell, once completed, is irreversible [142].

Streptolysin O induces swelling, degranulation, lysis, light emission, and impaired chemotaxis of polymorphonuclear leukocytes (PMNs). Leukotriene metabolism and response to leukotriene-inducing agents in neutrophils is also altered by SLO [143,144]. More than SPE A, SLO enhances CD11/CC18–mediated binding of PMNs to gelatin matrices [145]. It inhibits phagocytosis by macrophages and impairs lymphocyte response to mitogens. Streptolysin O damages intracellular organelles and platelets [6]. Monocytes are induced to produce TNF and IL-1β when exposed to SLO [17]. Functional SLO also increases secretion of IL-1β, IL-6, IL-8, and PGE2 by keratinocytes [146]. On monocytes, SLO also induces the shedding of CD14 and IL-6R, thus contributing to the inflammatory process [147]. Antigen-specific CD8$^+$ T cells were generated in rhesus monkeys in response to SLO [148]. However, SLO was unable to mediate the intracellular growth of *Bacillus subtilis* expressing SLO in contrast to listeriolysin O (LLO) and perfringolysin O (PFO), which could [149].

Streptolysin O is immunogenic. A fourfold rise in convalescent ASO antibody titer is helpful in confirming the diagnosis of streptococcal disease, including rheumatic fever and poststreptococcal glomerulonephritis. The maximal ASO titer occurs 3–6 weeks after infection [6]. False elevations in the ASO titer may be secondary to elevated serum β-lipoproteins (liver disease, hypercholesterolemia), serum contamination with growth products of *Bacillus cereus* or *Pseudomonas* spp., or oxidation of SLO. Serum cholesterol does not cause false-positive

ASO results as it is not in a state in serum that can interact with SLO. The ASO titer is not elevated during streptococcal skin infections, presumably because cholesterol in the epidermis is free and able to bind SLO [150]. False-positive and false-negative results may also occur because of the presence or absence of f- and t-site antibody [132]. The ASO titers vary with age, increasing rapidly from birth to age 12 then declining slowly to age 70 [151].

Sera from patients with streptococcal infections and high ASO titers have predominantly IgG1 antibody in contrast to anti-M-protein antibody, which is IgG1 and IgG3 [152]. Circulating immune complexes from patients with acute rheumatic fever contain antibody to SLO and antigens consistent with SLO that are not found in patients with pharyngitis or poststreptococcal acute glomerulonephritis [153,154]. Streptolysin O is able to activate the classical complement pathway but proceeds only through C5 in serum. When bound to red cells, activation will continue to the terminal attack complex, resulting in complement and SLO lesions on the cell surface. These effects are dependent on the presence of IgG [154].

Streptolysin O is a cardiac toxin. It brings about changes in myocardial contractility and affects the cardiac conduction system. Animals injected with lethal amounts of SLO (1–25 μg/kg [155]) have electrocardiogram (ECG) changes, but die without intravascular hemolysis [6]. In rats, SLO depresses hepatic microsomal enzymes and increases cytosolic N-acetyltransferase activity [156]. Isolated preparations of animal round-window membranes treated with SLO showed damage and destruction of the permeability barrier, thus implicating SLO as a possible etiologic agent in sensorineural hearing loss associated with chronic otitis media [157].

Streptolysin S

More than 95% of group A, B, C, and G streptococci and some of group E, H, and L streptococci produce SLS or an SLS-like hemolysin, with some interstrain variation in magnitude of SLS formation [126]. Streptolysin S has been difficult to isolate in pure form until recently. Production of SLS requires certain factors including maltose and a carrier. Streptolysin S is intimately associated with a stabilizing carrier molecule, which may be serum albumin, RNA, RNase-resistant core RNA, trypan blue, or a nonionic detergent. These carriers induce release of SLS from bacterial cells and can transfer SLS from one carrier to another [7]. Isolation of SLS in pure preparation unassociated with a carrier is one of the major obstacles to further investigation of this molecule that has now been overcome. The current method of purification of the carrier-free peptide is described by Alouf and Loridan [126,158]. This involves successive inductions of bacterial cells in appropriate culture media followed by a hydroxyapatite column, ultrafiltration, guanidine supplementation, a sephadex column, repeat ultrafiltration, and finally, isoelectric focusing. Although it is known that SLS causes osmotic hemolysis of red blood cells, the precise mechanism of cell lysis is not known. To date, no lesions have been observed on cell surfaces after exposure to SLS. Many questions remain concerning this molecule and its role in streptococcal disease.

The production of SLS is greatest in the late log or early stationary phase of growth. An iron concentration of 1.2 μg/ml is ideal [159]. Degradation quickly follows peak production and all activity disappears in the stationary phase unless stabilized with serum [159]. An inducer is required; the best is the RNase-resistant fraction of yeast RNA or lipotechoic acids. The inactivation of the streptococcal virulence regulator *mga* [160,161] causes an increase in SLS production [162]. This suggests that *mga*, which up-regulates cell-associated proteins (such as M protein), may be an inhibitor of SLS transcription.

Streptolysin S is estimated to consist of around 30 amino acids [6]. The purified protein has a pI of 9.2 and a molecular weight of about 1800 [126]. Intracellular hemolysin can be released from bacterial cells and is contained in the insoluble fraction, probably associated with the cell membrane [7,163]. Streptolysin S is inhibited by phospholipids, trypan blue, and ovolecithin [6,7,126]. Protease inhibitors prevent the production of SLS. Experiments involving cell fractions show that a precursor of SLS is in the insoluble fraction and that a necessary processing protease is in the supernate [163]. Liu et al. generated a mutant *Streptococcus pyogenes* with pleiotropic effects on SLS production

and riboflavin metabolism [164].This observation of a genetic linkage between riboflavin biosynthesis and SLS expression suggests a role of SLS in providing host-released growth factors to the infecting bacteria [165]. To date, the numerous efforts to clone the gene for SLS have not been successful.

A peptide has been identified from a bovine serum albumin (BSA)-pronase digest which appears to be necessary for the production of SLS in addition to maltose and an oligonucleotide carrier. The proposed primary structure consists of three peptides linked by two disulfide bonds, a pattern that occurs several times in BSA. The peptide is unable to induce SLS when the disulfide bonds are reduced. The calculated molecular weight of the peptide is 1046 [166,167].

Streptolysin S is one of the most potent hemolysins known with a specific activity, in purified form, of 3×10^6 HU/mg of protein. After exposure to SLS there is a lag phase during which red blood cells swell and then lyse secondary to the disruption of the osmotic barrier and the resultant flux of ions. No changes in the cell membrane are seen by electron microscopy. Streptolysin S is hypothesized to interact in some way with membrane phospholipid [6,7]. The first step, disruption of the cell membrane, is temperature-dependent. Streptolysin S may lyse eukaryotic cells, protoplasts, and L-forms. It can lyse erythrocytes, lymphocytes, PMNs, platelets, tissue culture cells, tumor cells, and intracellular organelles [126].

This toxin may be the cause of leukotoxic effects observed after ingestion of streptococci by phagocytes. White cells undergo degranulation, swelling, and bleb formation upon exposure to SLS [168]. It suppresses the T cell–dependent antibody response, T-helper function, and the lymphocyte response to mitogens [7].

When SLS is injected into rabbits, ECG changes and intravascular hemolysis take place prior to death [7]. The lethal dose in mice is about 25 μg/kg given intravenously [155]. Muscle necrosis occurs in animals after the injection of SLS [6]. One study showed that SLS had no effect when injected into rabbits and rats. This could have been due to suboptimal dosing [169]. A recent report describes two streptococcal Tn916 insertion mutants that have lost the ability to secrete SLS [170]. These mutants were much less effective than their respective parent strains in inducing subcutaneous infection in mice.

Because SLS is nonimmunogenic it has been suspected as a pathogenic factor in rheumatic fever. However, outbreaks have occurred through exposure to nonhemolytic group A streptococci and this makes its role uncertain [171]. Streptolysin S has not been implicated as an essential pathogenic factor in any streptococcal infection or their nonsuppurative sequelae.

This work was supported by Public Health Research Grant HL 36611 from the National Heart, Lung, and Blood Institute. Melodie Bahan is gratefully acknowledged for typing the manuscript.

REFERENCES

1. Bohach GA, Fast DJ, Nelson RD, Schlievert PM. Staphylococcal and streptococcal pyrogenic toxins involved in toxic shock syndrome and related illnesses. Crit Rev Microbiol 1989; 17:251–272.
2. Kim YB, Watson DW. Streptococcal exotoxins: biological and pathological properties. In: Wannamaker LW, Matsen JM (eds). Streptococci and Streptococcal Diseases. New York: Academic Press, New York 1972; 33–50.
3. Scherer MT, Ignatowitcz L, Winslow GM, Kappler JW, Marrack P. Superantigens: bacterial and viral proteins that manipulate the immune system. Annu Rev Cell Biol 1993; 9:101–128.
4. Schlievert PM, Johnson LP, Tomai MA, Handley JP. Characterization and genetics of group A streptococcal pyrogenic exotoxins. In: Ferretti JJ, Curtiss R III (eds). Streptococcal Genetics. Washington, DC: American Society for Microbiology, 1987; 136–142.
5. Watson DW, Kim YB. Erythrogenic toxins. In: Montie TC, Kadis S, Ajl SJ (eds). Microbial Toxins, Vol. III. Bacterial Protein Toxins. New York: Academic Press, 1970; 173–187.
6. Wannamaker LW, Schlievert PM. Exotoxins of the group A streptococci. In: Hardegree MC, Tu AT (eds). Handbook of Natural Toxins, Vol. 4. Bacterial Toxins. Marcel Dekker, New York: 1988; 267–295.
7. Wannamaker LW. Streptococcal toxins. Rev Infect Dis 1983; 5(Suppl 4):S723–S732.
8. Bhakdi S, Tranum-Jensen J. Membrane damage by channel-forming proteins: staphylococcal α-toxin, streptolysin-O and the C5b-9 complement complex. Biochem Soc Symp 1985; 50:221–233.
9. Alouf JE. Streptococcal toxin. Pharmacol Ther 1980; 11:661–717.
10. Dick GF, Dick GH. A skin test for susceptibility to scarlet fever. JAMA 1924; 82:265–266.
11. Watson DW. Host-parasite factors in group A streptococcal infections. Pyrogenic and other effects of immunologic distinct exotoxins related to scarlet fever toxins. J Exp Med 1960; 111:255–284.
12. Choi Y, Lafferty JA, Clements JR, Todd JK, Gelfand EW, Kappler J, Marrack P, Kotzin BL. Selective expansion of T cells expressing V beta 2 in toxic shock syndrome. J Exp Med 1990; 172:981–984.
13. Marrack P, Kappler JW. The staphylococcal enterotoxins and their relatives. Science 1990; 248:705–711.
14. Leonard BAB, Lee PK, Jenkins MK, Schlievert PM. Cell and receptor requirements for streptococcal pyrogenic exotoxin T cell mitogenicity. Infect Immun 1991; 59:1210–1214.
15. Fast DJ, Schlievert PM, Nelson RD. Toxic shock syndrome-associated staphylococcal and streptococcal pyrogenic toxins are potent inducers of tumor necrosis factor production. Infect Immun 1989; 57:291–294.
16. Nelson RD, Fast DJ, Schlievert PM. Pyrogenic toxin stimulation of TNF production by human mononuclear leukocytes and effect of TNF on neutrophil Ccemotaxis. In: Bonavida B, Granger G (eds). Tumor Necrosis Factor: Structure, Mechanism of Action, Role in Disease and Therapy. Basel: S. Karger, 1990; 177–186.
17. Hackett SP, Stevens DL. Streptococcal toxic shock syndrome: synthesis of tumor necrosis factor and interleukin-1 by monocytes stimulated with pyrogenic exotoxin A and streptolysin O. J Infect Dis 1992; 165:879–885.
18. Hackett SP, Stevens DL. Superantigens associated with staphylococcal and streptococcal toxic shock syndrome are potent inducers of tumor necrosis factor-β synthesis. J Infect Dis 1993; 168:232–235.
19. Muller-Alouf H, Alouf J, Gerlach D, Ozegowski J, Fitting C, Cavaillon J-M. Comparative study of cytokine release by human peripheral blood mononuclear cells stimulated with *Streptococcus pyogenes* superantigenic erythrogenic toxins, heat-killed, streptococci, and lipopolysaccharide. Infect Immun 1994; 62:4915–4921.
20. Norrby-Teglund A, Norgren M, Holm SE, Andersson U, Andersson J. Similar cytokine induction profiles of a novel streptococcal exotoxin, MF, and pyrogenic exotoxins A and B. Infect Immun 1994; 62:3731–3738.
21. Muller-Alouf H, Gerlach D, Desreumaux P, Leportier C, Alouf J, Capron M. Streptococcal pyrogenic exotoxin A (SPE A) superantigen induced production of hematopoietic cytokines, IL-12, and IL-13 by human peripheral blood mononuclear cells. Microb Pathog 1997; 23:265–272.
22. Ohara-Nemoto Y, Kaneko M. Expression of T-

cell receptor V beta 2 and type 1 helper T-cell-related cytokine mRNA in streptococcal pyrogenic exotoxin-C-activated human peripheral blood mononuclear cells. Can J Microbiol 1996; 42:1104–1111.

23. Sriskandan S, Evans TJ, Cohen J. Bacterial superantigen-induced human lymphocyte responses are nitric oxide dependent and mediated by IL-12 and IFN-gamma. J Immunol 1996; 156:2430–2435.

24. Cone LA, Woodard DR, Schlievert PM, Tomory GS. Clinical and bacteriologic observations of a toxic shock-like syndrome due to *Streptococcus pyogenes*. N Engl J Med 1987; 317:146–149.

25. Stevens DL, Tanner MH, Winship J, Swarts R, Ries KM, Schlievert PM, Kaplan EL. Reappearance of scarlet fever toxin A among streptococci in the Rocky Mountain West: association with severe streptococcal soft tissue infection, sepsis and the toxic shock-like syndrome. N Engl J Med 1989; 321:1–7.

26. Schlievert PM. The role of superantigens in human diseases. Curr Sci 1995; 8:170–174.

27. Parsonnet J. Mediators in the pathogenesis of toxic shock syndrome. Rev Infect Dis 1989; 11:S263–S269.

28. Stevens DL. Invasive group A streptococcus infections. Clin Infect Dis 1992; 14:2–13.

29. Kim YB, Watson DW. A purified group A streptococcal pyrogenic exotoxin. Physicochemical and biological properties including the enhancement of susceptibility to endotoxin lethal shock. J Exp Med 1970; 131:611–628.

30. Stone R, Schlievert PM. Evidence for the involvement of endotoxin in toxic-shock syndrome. J Infect Dis 1987; 155:682–689.

31. Schlievert PM, Bettin KM, Watson DW. Inhibition of ribonucleic acid synthesis by group A streptococcal pyrogenic exotoxins. Infect Immun 1979; 27:542–548.

32. Lee PK, Deringer JR, Kreiswirth BN, Novick RP, Schlievert PM. Fluid replacement and polymyxin B protection of rabbits challenged subcutaneously with toxic shock syndrome toxins. Infect Immun 1991; 59: 879–884.

33. Lee PK, Vercellotti GM, Deringer JR, Schlievert PM. Effects of staphylococcal toxic shock syndrome toxin-1 on aortic endothelial cells. J Infect Dis 1991; 164:711–719.

34. Cunnigham CM, Watson DW. Suppression of the antibody response by group A pyrogenic exotoxin and characterization of the cells involved. Infect Immun 1978; 19:470–476.

35. Schlievert PM, Assimacopoulos AP, Cleary PP. Severe invasive group A streptococcal disease: clinical description and mechanisms of pathogenesis. J Lab Clin Med 1996; 127:13–22.

36. Schlievert PM, Bettin KM, Watson DW. Reinterpretation of the Dick test: role of group A streptococcal pyrogenic exotoxin. Infect Immun 1979; 26:467–472.

37. Schwab JH, Watson DW, Cromartie WJ. Further studies of group A streptococcal factors with lethal and cardiotoxic properties. J Infect Dis 1955; 96:14–18.

38. Schlievert PM, Bettin KM, Watson DW. Pyrogenic exotoxin production by groups of streptococci: association with group A. J Infect Dis 1979; 140:676–681.

39. Schlievert PM, Watson DW. Group A streptococcal pyrogenic exotoxins: pyrogenicity, alteration of blood brain barrier, separation of sites for pyrogenicity and enhancement of lethal endotoxin shock. Infect Immun 1978; 21:753–763.

40. Johnson LP, Schlievert PM. Group A streptococcal bacteriophage T12 carries the structural genes for pyrogenic exotoxin type A. Mol Gen Genet 1984; 194:52–56.

41. Frobisher M Jr, Brown JH. Trasmissible toxigenicity of streptococci. Bull Johns Hopkins Hosp 1927; 41:167–173.

42. Zabriskie JB. The role of temperate bacteriophage in the production of erythrogenic toxin by group A streptococci. J Exp Med 1964; 119:761–780.

43. Johnson LP, Schlievert PM, Watson DW. Transfer of group A streptococcal pyrogenic exotoxin production to non-toxigenic strains by lysogenic conversion. Infect Immun 198l; 28:254–257.

44. Johnson LP, Schlievert PM. A physical map of the group A streptococcal pyrogenic exotoxin bacteriophage T12 genome. Mol Gen Genet 1983; 189:251–255.

45. Yu CE, Ferretti JJ. Molecular characterization of new group A streptococcal bacteriophages containing the gene for streptococcal erythrogenic toxin A (*spe*A). Mol Gen Genet 1991; 161–168.

46. Johnson LP, Tomai MA, Schlievert PM. Molecular analysis of bacteriophage involvement in group A streptococcal pyrogenic exotoxin A production. J Bacteriol 1986; 166:623–627.

47. McShan W, Ferretti JJ. Genetic diversity in temperate bacteriophages of *Streptococcus pyogenes*: identification of a second attachment site for phages carrying the erythrogenic toxin A. J Bacteriol 1997; 179:6509–6511.

48. Nauciel C, Blass J, Mangalo R, Raynaud M. Evidence for two molecular forms of streptococcal erythrogenic toxin. Conversion to a single form by 2-mercaptoethanol. Eur J Biochem 1969; 11:160–164.

49. Weeks CR, Ferretti JJ. Nucleotide sequence of the type A streptococcal exotoxin (erythrogenic toxin) gene from *Streptococcus pyogenes* bacteriophage T12. Infect Immun 1986; 52:144–150.

50. Hauser AR, Vath GM, Ohlendorf DH, Schlievert PM. Structural studies of streptococcal pyrogenic exotoxin superantigens. In: Thibodeau J, Sekaly R (eds). Bacterial Superantigens: Structure, Function and Therapeutic Potential. 1995; 39–48.

51. Hoffmann ML, Jablonski LM, Crum KK, Hackett SP, Chi YI, Stauffacher CV, Stevens DL, Bohach GA. Predictions of T cell receptor and major histocompatibility complex binding sites on staphylococcal enterotoxin C1. Infect Immun 1994; 62:3396–3407.

52. Prasad GS, Earhart CA, Murray DL, Novick RP, Schlievert PM, Ohlendorf DH. Structure of toxic shock syndrome toxin 1. Biochemistry 1993; 32:13761–13766.

53. Swaminathan S, Furey W, Pletcher J, Sax M. Crystal structure of staphylococcal enterotoxin B, a superantigen. Nature 1992; 359:801–806.

54. Schad EM, Zaitseva I, Zaitsev VN, Dohlsten M, Kalland T, Schlievert PM, Ohlendorf DH, Svensson LA. Crystal structure of the superantigen staphylococcal enterotoxin type A. EMBO J 1995; 14:3292–3301.

55. Roussel A, Anderson BF, Baker HM, Fraser JD, Baker EN. Crystal structure of the streptococcal superantigen SPE C: dimerization and zinc binding suggest a novel mode of interaction with MHC class II molecules. Nat Struct Biol 1997; 4:635–643.

56. Kline JB, Collins CM. Analysis of the interaction between the bacterial superantigen streptococcal pyrogenic exotoxin A (SPE A) and the human T cell receptor. Mol Microbiol 1997; 24:191–202.

57. Roggiani M, Stoehr JA, Leonard BAB, Schlievert PM. Analysis of toxicity of streptococcal pyrogenic exotoxin A mutants. Infect Immun 1997; 65:2868–2875.

58. Bohach G, Jablonski L, Roggiani M, Sadler I, Schlievert, P, Mitchell D, Ohlendorf D. Biological activity of pyrogenic toxins delivered at the mucosal surface. In: Arbuthnott JP, Furman B (eds). International Congress and Symposium Series No. 229. London: Royal Society of Medicine Press, 1998; 170–172.

59. Kline JB, Collins, CM. Analysis of the superantigenic activity of mutant and allelic forms of streptococcal pyrogenic exotoxin A. Infect Immun 1996; 64:861–869.

60. Tomai MA, Schlievert PM, Kotb M. Distinct T cell receptor Vβ gene usage by human T lymphocytes stimulated with streptococcal pyrogenic exotoxins and pep 5 M protein. Infect Immun 1992; 60:701–705.

61. Imanishi K, Igarashi H, Uchiyama T. Relative abilities of distinct isotypes of human major histocompatibility complex class II molecules to bind streptococcal pyrogenic exotoxin types A and B. Infect Immun 1992; 60:5025–5029.

62. Leonard BAB, Schlievert PM. Immune cell lethality induced by streptococcal pyrogenic exotoxin A and endotoxin. Infect Immun 1992; 60:3747–3755.

63. Parsonnet J, Gillis ZA, Richter G, Pier GB. A rabbit model of toxic shock syndrome that uses a constant, subcutaneous infusion of toxic shock syndrome toxin 1. Infect Immun 1987; 55:1070–1076.

64. Lee PK, Schlievert PM. Group A streptococcal pyrogenic exotoxins: quantification and toxicity in an animal model of toxic shock syndrome-like illness. J Clin Microbiol 1989; 27:1890–1892.

65. Xu S, Collins CM. Temperature regulation of the streptococcal pyrogenic exotoxin A–encoding gene (*spe*A). Infect Immun 1996; 64:5399–5402.

66. Chaussee MS, Liu J, Dtevens, DL, Ferretti JJ. Effects of environmental factors on streptococcal erythrogenic toxin A (SPE A) production by *Streptococcus pyogenes*. In: Horaud T, Bouvet A, Leclercq R, de Montclos H, Sicard M (eds). Streptococci and the Host. Adv Exp Med Biol 1997; 418:551–554.

67. Yu CE, Ferretti JJ. Molecular epidemiologic analysis of the type A streptococcal exotoxin (erythrogenic toxin) gene (*spe*A) in clinical *Streptococcus pyogenes* strains. Infect Immun 1989; 57:3715–3719.

68. Hauser AR, Stevens DL, Kaplan EL, Schlievert PM. Molecular analysis of pyrogenic exotoxins from *Streptococcus pyogenes* isolates associated with toxic shock-like syndrome. J Clin Microbiol 1991; 29:1562–1567.

69. Musser JM, Hauser AR, Kim M, Schlievert PM, Nelson K, Selander RK. *Streptococcus pyogenes* causing toxic shock-like syndrome and other invasive diseases: clonal diversity and pyrogenic exotoxin expression. Proc Natl Acad Sci USA 1991; 88:2668–2672.

70. Begovac J, Gmajnicki B, Schlievert PM, Johnson DR, Kaplan EL. Production of pyrogenic exotoxins in group A streptococci isolated from patients in Zagreb, Croatia. Eur J Clin Infect Dis 1992; 11:540–543.

71. Belani K, Schlievert PM, Kaplan EL, Ferrieri P. Association of exotoxin producing group A and severe disease in children. J Pediatr Infect Dis 1991; 10:351–354.

72. Talkington DF, Schwartz B, Black CM, Todd JK, Elliot J, Breiman RF, Facklam RR. Association of phenotypic and genotypic characteristics of invasive *Streptococcus pyogenes* isolates with clinical components of streptococcal toxic shock syndrome. Infect Immun 1993; 61:3369–3374.

73. Bohach GA, Hauser AR, Schlievert PM. Cloning of the gene, *spe*B, for streptococcal pyrogenic exotoxin type B in *Escherichia coli*. Infect Immun 1988; 56:1665–1667.

74. Barsumian EL, Cunningham CM, Schlievert PM, Watson DW. Heterogeneity of group A streptococcal pyrogenic exotoxin type B. Infect Immun 1978; 20:512–518.

75. Hauser AR, Schlievert PM. Nucleotide sequence of the streptococcal pyrogenic exotoxin type B gene and toxin relationship to streptococcal proteinase precursor. J Bacteriol 1990; 172: 4536–4542.

76. Elliott SD, Dole VP. An inactive precursor of streptococcal proteinase. J Exp Med 1947; 85: 305–320.

77. Ohara-Nemoto Y, Sasaki M, Kaneko M, Nemoto T, Ota M. Cysteine protease activity of streptococcal pyrogenic exotoxin B. Can J Microbiol 1994; 49:930–936.

78. Liu , Elliot SD. Streptococcal proteinase: the zymogen to enzyme transformation. J Biol Chem 1965; 240:1138–1142.

79. Gubba S, Low DE, Musser JM. Expression and characterization of group A streptococci extracellular cysteine protease recombinant mutant proteins and documentation of seroconversion during human invasive disease episodes. Infect Immun 1998; 66:765–770.

80. Chaussee MS, Gerlach D, Yu CE, Ferretti JJ. Inactivation of the streptococcal erythrogenic toxin B gene (speB) in Streptococcus pyogenes. Infect Immun 1993; 61:3719–3723.

81. Tsai P-J, Kuo C-F, Lin K-Y, Lin Y-S, Lei H-Y, Chen F-F, Wang J-R, Wu J-J. Effects of group A streptococcal cysteine protease on invasions of epithelial cells. Infect Immun 1998; 66:1460–1466.

82. Chaussee MS, Phillips ER, Ferretti JJ. Temporal production of streptococcal erythrogenic toxin B (streptococcal cysteine protease) in response to nutrient depletion. Infect Immun 1997; 65:1956–1959.

83. Kapur V, Topouzis S, Majesky MW, Li LL, Hamrick MR, Hamill RJ, Patti JM, Musser JM. A conserved Streptococcus pyogenes cysteine protease cleaves human fibronectin and degrades vitronectin. Microb Pathog 1993; 15:327–346.

84. Burns EH Jr, Marciel AM, Musser JM. Activation of a 66-kilodalton human endothelial cell matrix metalloprotease by Streptococcus pyogenes extracellular cysteine protease. Infect Immun 1996; 64:4744–4750.

85. Kapur V, Majesky MW, Li LL, Black RA, Musser JM. Cleavage of interleukin 1β (IL-1β) precursor to produce active IL-1β by a conserved extracellular cysteine protease from Streptococcus pyogenes. Proc Natl Acad Sci USA 1993; 90:7676–7680.

86. Shanley TP, Schrier D, Kapur V, Kehoe M, Musser JM, Ward PA. Streptococcal cysteine protease augments lung injury induced by products of group A streptococci. Infect Immun 1996; 64:870–877.

87. Lukomski S, Sreevatsan S, Amberg C, Reichardt W, Woischnik M, Podbielski A, Musser JM. Inactivation of Streptococcus pyogenes extracellular cysteine protease significantly decreases mouse lethality of serotype M3 and M49 strains. J Clin Invest 1997; 99:2574–2580.

88. Lukomski S, Burns EH, Wyde PR Jr, Podbielski A, Rurangirwa J, Moore-Poveda DK, Musser JM. Genetic inactivation of an extracellular cysteine protease (SpeB) expressed by Streptococcus pyogenes decreases resistance to phagocytosis and dissemination to organs. Infect Immun 1998; 66:771–776.

89. Simor AE, Louie L, Schwartz B, McGeer A, Scriver S, the Ontario GAS Study Project, Low DE. Association of protease activity with group A streptococcal (GAS) necrotizing fasciitis (NF). In: Program and Abstracts of the 33rd Interscience Conference on Antimicrobial Agents and Chemotherapy. Washington DC: American Society for Microbiology, 1993, Abstr 1164.

90. Goshorn SC, Schlievert PM. Phage association of streptococcal pyrogenic exotoxin type C. J Bacteriol 1989; 171:3068–3073.

91. Yu CE, Ferretti JJ. Frequency of the erythrogenic toxin B and C genes (speB and speC) among clinical isolates of group A streptococci. Infect Immun 1991; 59:211–215.

92. Goshorn SC, Bohach GA, Schlievert PM. Cloning and characterization of the gene, speC, for pyrogenic exotoxin type C from Streptococcus pyogenes. Mol Gen Genet 1988; 212:66–70.

93. Goshorn SC, Schlievert PM. Nucleotide sequence of streptococcal pyrogenic exotoxin type C. Infect Immun 1988; 56:2518–2520.

94. Kapur V, Nelson K, Schlievert PM, et al. Molecular population genetic evidence of horizontal spread of two alleles of the pyrogenic exotoxin C gene (speC) among pathogenic clones of Streptococcus pyogenes. Infect Immun 1992; 60:3513–3517.

95. Li P-L, Tiedemann RE, Moffat SL, Fraser JD, The superantigen streptococcal pyrogenic exotoxin C (SPE C) exhibits a novel mode of action. J Exp Med 1997; 186:375–383.

96. Fields BA, Malchiodi EL, Li H, Ysern X, Stauffacher CV, Schlievert PM, Karjalainen K, Mariuzza RA. Crystal structure of a T cell receptor β-chain complexed with a superantigen. Science 1996; 384:188–192.

97. Hudson KR, Tiedemann RE, Urban RG, Lowe SC, Strominger JL, Fraser, JD. Staphylococcal enterotoxin A has two cooperative binding sites on major histocompatibility complex class II. J Exp Med 1995; 182:711–720.

98. Fraser JD, Urban RG, Strominger JL, Robinson H. Zinc regulates the function of two superantigens. Proc Natl Acad Sci USA 1992; 89: 5507–5511.

99. Mollick JA, Miller GG, Musser JM, Cook RG, Grossman D, Rich RR. A novel superantigen isolated from pathogenic strains of Streptococcus pyogenes with aminoterminal homology to staphylococcal enterotoxins B and C. J Clin Invest 1993; 92:710–719.

100. Yutsudo T, Murai H, Gonzales J, Takao T, Shimonishi Y, Takeda Y, Igarashi H, Hinuma Y. A new type of mitogenic factor produced by Streptococcus pyogenes. FEBS Lett 1992; 308: 30–34.

101. Norrby-Teglund A, Newton D, Kotb M, Holm SE, Norgren M. Superantigenic properties of the group A streptococcal exotoxin SPE F (MF). Infect Immun 1994; 62:5227–5223.

102. Reda KB, Kapur V, Mollick JA, Lamphear JG, Musser JM, Rich RR. Molecular characterization and phylogenetic distribution of the streptococcal superantigen gene (*ssa*) from *Streptococcus pyogenes*. Infect Immun 1994; 62: 1867–1874.

103. Stevens KR, Van M, Lamphear JG, Rich RR. Altered orientation of streptococcal superantigen (SSA) on HLA-DR1 allows nonconventional regions to contribute to SSA V-beta specificity. J Immunol 1996; 157:4970–4978.

104. Stevens KR, Van M, Lamphear JG, Okriszewski RS, Ballard KD, Cook RG, Rich RR. Species-dependent post-translational modification and position 2 allelism: effects on streptococcal superantigen SSA structure and V beta specificity. J Immunol 1996; 157:2479–2487.

105. Iwasaki M, Igarashi H, Hinuma Y, Yutsudo T. Cloning, characterization and overexpression of a *Streptococcus pyogenes* gene encoding a new type of mitogenic factor. FEBS Lett 1993; 331:187–192.

106. Toyosaki T, Yoshioka T, Tsuruta Y, Yutsudo T, Iwasaki M, Suzuki R. Definition of the mitogenic factor (MF) as a novel streptococcal superantigen that is different from streptococcal pyrogenic exotoxin A, B, and C. Eur J Immunol 1996; 26:2693–2701.

107. Norrby-Teglund A, Norgren M, Holm SE, Andersson U, Andersson J. Similar cytokines induction profiles of a novel streptococcal exotoxin, MF, and pyrogenic exotoxins A and B. Infect Immun 1994; 62:3731–3738.

108. Iwasaki M, Igarashi H, Yutsudo T. Mitogenic factor secreted by *Streptococcus pyogenes* is a heat stable nuclease requiring His122 for activity. Microbiology 1997; 143:2449–2455.

109. Yutsudo T, Okumura K, Iwasaki M, Hara A, Kamitani S, Minamide W, Igarashi H, Hinuma Y. The gene encoding a new mitogenic factor in a *Streptococcus pyogenes* strain is distributed only in group A streptococci. Infect Immun 1994; 62:4000–4004.

110. Kamezawa Y, Nakahara T, Nakano S, Abe Y, Nozaki-Renard J, Isono T. Streptococcal mitogenic exotoxin Z, a novel superantigenic toxin produced by a T1 strain of *Streptococcus pyogenes*. Infect Immun 1997; 65:3828–3833.

111. Rikiishi H, Okamoto S, Sugawara S, Tamura K, Liu Z-K, Kumagai K. Superantigenicity of helper T-cell mitogen (SPM-2) isolated from culture supernatants of *Streptococcus pyogenes*. Immunology 1997; 91:406–413.

112. Geoffroy-Fauvet C, Müller-Alouf H, Champagne E, Cavaillon JM, Alouf JE. Identification of a new extracellular superantigenic mitogen from group A streptococci. In: Freer J, Aitken R, Alouf JE, Boulnois G, Falmagne P, Fehrenbach F, Montecucco C, Piemont Y, Rappuoli R, Wadstrom T, Witholt B (eds). Bacterial Protein Toxins. Zentralbl Bakteriol (Suppl) 1994; 24:90–91.

113. Müller-Alouf H, Capron M, Alouf JE, Geoffroy C, Gerlach D, Ozegowski JH, Fitting C, Cavaillon JM. Cytokine profile of human peripheral blood mononucleated cells stimulated with a novel streptococcal superantigen, SPE A, SPE C, and group A streptococcal cells. In: Horaud T, Bouvet A, Leclercq R, de Montclos H, Sicard M (eds). Streptococci and the Host. Adv Exp Med Biol 1997; 418:929–931.

114. Newton D, Norrby-Teglund A, McGeer A, Low DE, Schlievert PM, Kotb M. Novel superantigens from streptococcal toxic shock syndrome *Streptococcus pyogenes* isolates. In Horaud T, Bouvet A, Leclercq R, de Montclos H, Sicard M (eds). Streptococci and the Host. Adv Exp Med Biol 1997; 418:525–529.

115. Alouf JE, Geoffroy C. Production, purification, and assay of streptolysin O. Methods Enzymol 1988; 165:52–59.

116. Bhakdi S, Weller U, Walev I, Martin E, Jonas D, Palmer M. A guide to the use of pore-forming toxins for controlled permeabilization of cell membranes. Med Microbiol Immunol (Berl) 1993; 182:167–175.

117. Gerlach D, Köhler W, Günther E, Mann K. Purification and characterization of streptolysin O secreted by *Streptococcus equisimilis* (group C). Infect Immun 1993; 61:2727–2731.

118. Okumura K, Hara A, Tanaka T, Nishiguchi I, Minamide W, Igarashi H, Yutsudo T. Cloning and sequencing the streptolysin O genes of group C and group G streptococci. DNA Seq 1994; 4:325–328.

119. Kehoe MA, Miller L, Walker JA, Boulnois GJ. Nucleotide sequence of the streptolysin-O (*slo*) gene: structural homologies between SLO and other membrane-damaging, thiol-activated toxins. Infect Immun 1987; 55:3228–3232.

120. Tweten RK. Nucleotide sequences of the gene for perfringolysin O (theta-toxin) from *Clostridium perfringens*: significant homology with the genes for streptolysin O and pneumolysin. Infect Immun 1988; 56:3235–3240.

121. Alouf JE, Geoffrey C. The family of the antigenically related, cholesterol-binding ("sulphydryl-activated") cytolytic toxins. In: Slouf JE, Freer JH (eds). Sourcebook of Bacterial Protein Toxins. New York: Academic Press, 1991; 147–186.

122. Canalias F, Viver J, Beleta J, Gonzalez-Sastre F, Gella FJ. Purification and characterization of streptolysin O from *Streptococcus pyogenes*. Int J Biochem 1992; 24:1073–1079.

123. Kehoe M, Timmis KN. Cloning and expression in *Escherichia coli* of the streptolysin O determinant from *Streptococcus pyogenes*: character-

74   STREPTOCOCCAL INFECTIONS

ization of the cloned streptolysin O determinant and demonstration of the absence of substantial homology with determinants of other thiol-activated toxins. Infect Immun 1984; 43:804–810.

124. Calandra GB, Theodore TS. Cellular location of streptolysin O. Infect Immun 1975; 12:750–753.

125. Pinkney M, Beachey E, Kehoe M. The thiol-activated toxin streptolysin O does not require a thiol group for cytolytic activity. Infect Immun 1989; 57:2553–2558.

126. Alouf JE, Loridan C. Production, purification, and assay of streptolysin S. Methods Enzymol 1988; 165:59–64.

127. Bhakdi S, Roth M, Sziegoleit A, Tranum-Jensen J. Isolation and identification of two hemolytic forms of streptolysin-O. Infect Immun 1984; 46:394–400.

128. Suzuki J, Kobayashi S, Kagaya K, Fukazawa Y. Heterogeneity and hemolytic efficiency and isoelectric point of streptolysin O. Infect Immun 1988; 56:2474–2478.

129. Pinkney M, Kapur V, Smith J, Palmer M, Glanville M, Messner M, Musser JM, Bhakdi S, Kehoe MA. Different forms of streptolysin O produced by Streptococcus pyogenes and Escherichia coli expressing recombinant toxin: cleavage by streptococcal cysteine protease. Infect Immun 1995; 63:2776–2779.

130. Weller U, Müller L, Messner M, Palmer M, Valeva A, Tranum-Jensen J, Agrawal P, Biermann C, Döbereiner A, Kehoe MA, Bhakdi S. Expression of active streptolysin O in Escherichia coli as a maltose binding protein-streptolysin O fusion protein. Eur J Biochem 1996; 236:34–39.

131. Sekiya K, Satoh R, Danbara H, Futaesaku Y. A ring-shaped structure with a crown formed by streptolysin O on the erythrocyte membrane. J Bacteriol 1993; 175:5953–5961.

132. Watson KC, Kerr JC. Specificity of antibodies for t sites and f sites of streptolysin O. J Med Microbiol 1985; 19:1–7.

133. Hugo F, Reichwein J, Arvand M, Krämer S, Bhakdi S. Use of monoclonal antibody to determine the mode of transmembrane pore formation by streptolysin O. Infect Immun 1986; 54:641–645.

134. Rossjohn J, Feil SC, McKinstrey WJ, Tweten RK, Parker MW. Structure of a cholesterol-binding thiol-activated cytolysin and a model of its membrane form. Cell 1997; 89:685–692.

135. Palmer M, Vulicevic I, Saweljew P, Valeva A, Kehoe M, Bhakdi S. Streptolysin O: a proposed model of allosteric interaction between a pore-forming protein and its target lipid bilayer. Biochemistry 1998; 37:2378–2383.

136. Niedermeyer W. Interaction of streptolysin-O with biomembranes: kinetic and morphological studies on erythrocyte membranes. Toxicon 1985; 23:425–439.

137. Bhakdi S, Tranum-Jensen J, Sziegoleit A. Mech-

anism of membrane damage by streptolysin-O. Infect Immun 1985; 47:52–60.

138. Sekiya K, Danbara H, Yase K, Futaesaku Y. Electron microscopic evaluation of a two-step theory of pore formation by streptolysin O. J Bacteriol 1996; 178:6998–7002.

139. Bhakdi S, Bayley H, Valeva A, Walev I, Walker B, Weller U, Kehoe M, Palmer M. Staphylococcal alpha-toxin, streptolysin O, and Escherichia coli hemolysin: prototypes of pore-forming bacterial cytolysins. Arch Microbiol 1996; 165:73–79.

140. Alouf JE, Geoffroy C, Pattus F, Verger R. Surface properties of bacterial sulfhydryl-activated cytolytic toxins. Interaction with monomolecular films of phosphatidylcholine and various sterols. Eur J Biochem 1984; 141:205–210.

141. Palmer M, Valeva A, Kehoe M, Bhakdi S. Kinetics of streptolysin O assembly. Eur J Biochem 1995; 231:388–395.

142. Walev I, Palmer M, Valeva A, Weller U, Bhakdi S. Binding, oligomerization, and pore formation by streptolysin O in erythrocytes and fibroblast membranes: detection of nonlytic polymers. Infect Immun 1995; 63:1188–1194.

143. Bremm KD, König W, Thelestam M, Alouf JE. Modulation of granulocyte functions by bacterial exotoxin and endotoxins. Immunology 1987; l62:363–371.

144. Bremm KD, König W, Pfeiffer P, Rauschen I, Theobald K, Thelestam M, Alouf JE. Effect of thiol-activated toxins (streptolysin O, alveolysin, and theta toxin) on the generation of leukotrienes and leukotriene-inducing and -metabolizing enzymes from human polymorphonuclear granulocytes. Infect Immun 1985; 50:844–851.

145. Bryant AE, Kehoe MA, Stevens DL. Streptococcal pyrogenic exotoxin A and streptolysin O enhance polymorphonuclear leukocyte binding to gelatin matrixes. J Infect Dis 1992; 166:165–169.

146. Ruiz N, Wang B, Pentland A, Caparon M. Streptolysin O and adherence modulate proinflammatory responses of keratinocytes to group A streptococci. Mol Microbiol 1998; 27:337–346.

147. Walev I, Vollmer P, Palmer M, Bhakdi S, Stefan R-J. Pore-forming toxins trigger shedding of receptors for interleukin 6 and lipopolysaccharide. Proc Natl Acad Sci USA 1996; 93:7882–7887.

148. Chizzolini C, Millet PG, Olsen-Rasmussen MS, Collins WE. Induction of antigen-specific CD8[+] cytolytic T cells by the exogenous bacterial antigen streptolysin O in rhesus monkeys. Eur J Immunol 1991; 21:2727–2733.

149. Portnoy DA, Tweten RK, Kehoe M, Bieleck J. Capacity of listeriolysin O, streptolysin O, and perfringolysin O to mediate growth of Bacillus subtilis within mammalian cells. Infect Immun 1992; 60:2710–2717.

150. Burdash NM, Teti G, Hund P. Streptococcal an-

tibody test in rheumatic fever. Ann Clin Lab Sci 1986; 16:163–170.

151. Renneberg J, Söderström M, Prellner K, Frosgren A, Christensen P. Age-related variations in anti-streptococcal antibody levels. Eur J Clin Microbiol Infect Dis 1989; 8:792–795.

152. Falconer AE, Carson R, Johnstone R, Bird P, Kehoe M, Calvert JE. Distinct IgG1 and IgG3 subclass responses to two streptococcal protein antigens in man: analysis of antibodies to streptolysin O and M protein using standardized subclass-specific enzyme-linked immunosorbent assays. Immunology 1993; 79:89–94.

153. Gupta R, Badhwar AK, Bisno AL, Berrios X. Detection of C-reactive protein, streptolysin O, and anti-streptolysin O antibodies in immune complexes isolated from the sera of patients with acute rheumatic fever. J Immunol 1986; 137:2173–2179.

154. Bhakdi S, Tranum-Jensen J. Complement activation and attack on autologous cell membranes induced by streptolysin-O. Infect Immun 1985; 48:713–719.

155. Gill DM. Bacterial toxins: a table of lethal amounts. Microbiol Rev 1982; 46:86–94.

156. Hadasova E, Siegmund W, Franke G, Schneider T, Beyrich A, Bleyer H, Hübner G. Drug oxidation and *N*-acetylation in rats pretreated with subtoxic doses of streptolysin O. Biochem Pharmacol 1991; 42:702–704.

157. Engel F, Blatz R, Kellner J, Palmer M, Weller U, Bhakdi S. Breakdown of the round window membrane permeability barrier evoked by streptolysin O: possible etiologic role in development of sensorineural hearing loss in acute otitis media. Infect Immun 1995; 63:1305–1310.

158. Loridan C, Alouf JE. Purification of RNA-core induced streptolysin S, and isolation and haemolytic characteristics of the carrier-free toxin. J Gen Microbiol 1986; 132:307–315.

159. Griffiths BB, McClain O. The role of iron in the growth and hemolysin (streptolysin S) production in *Streptococcus pyogenes*. J Basic Microbiol 1988; 28:427–436.

160. Simpson WJ, LaPenta D, Chen D, Cleary PP. Coregulation of type 12 M protein and streptococcus C5a peptidase genes in group streptococci: evidence for a virulence regulon controlled by the *virR* locus. J Bacteriol 1990; 172:696–700.

161. Perez-Casal J, Caparon MG, Scott JR. *Mry*, a *trans*-acting positive regulator of the M protein gene of *Streptococcus pyogenes* with similarity to the receptor proteins of two-component regulatory systems. J Bacteriol 1991; 173:2617–2624.

162. Kihlberg B-M, Cooney J, Caparon MG, Olsén A, Björck L. Biological properties of a *Streptococcus pyogenes* mutant generated by Tn*916* insertion in *mga*. Microb Pathog 1995; 19:299–315.

163. Akao T, Akao T, Kobashi K, Lai CY. The role of protease in streptolysin S formation. Arch Biochem Biophys 1983; 223:556–561.

164. Liu S, Sela S, Cohen G, Jadoun J, Cheung A, Ofek I. Insertional inactivation of streptolysin S expression is associated with altered riboflavin metabolism in *Streptococcus pyogenes*. Microb Pathog 1997; 22:227–234.

165. Gargir A, Liu S, Sela S, Cohen G, Jadoun J, Cheung A, Ofek I. Biological significance of the genetic linkage between streptolysin S expression and riboflavin biosynthesis in *Streptococcus pyogenes*. In: Horaud T, Bouvet A, Leclercq R, de Montclos H, Sicard M (eds). Streptococci and the Host. Adv Exp Med Biol 1997; 418:987–989.

166. Akao T, Takahashi T, Kobashi K. Purification and characterization of a peptide essential for formation of streptolysin S by *Streptococcus pyogenes*. Infect Immun 1992; 60:4777–4780.

167. Akao T, Hironori T, Kobashi K. The essential factor for streptolysin S production by *Streptococcus pyogenes*. Chem Pharm Bull 1988; 36:3994–3999.

168. Ofek I, Bergner-Rabinowitz S, Ginsberg I. Oxygen-stable hemolysis of group A streptococci. VIII. Leukotoxic and antiphagocytic effects of streptolysins S and O. Infect Immun 1972; 6:459–464.

169. Griffiths BB, Rhee H. Effects of haemolysins of groups A and B streptococci on cardiovascular system. Microbiology 1992; 69:17–27.

170. Betschel SD, Borgia SM, Barg NL, Low DE, De Azavedo JCS. Reduced virulence of group A streptococcal Tn *916* mutants that do not produce streptolysin S. Infect Immun 1998; 66:1671–1679.

171. James L, McFarland RB. An epidemic of pharyngitis due to non-hemolytic group A streptococcus at Lowry Air Force Base. N Engl J Med 1971; 284:750–752.

5

Streptococcal Pharyngitis

STANFORD T. SHULMAN
ROBERT R. TANZ
MICHAEL A. GERBER

Infections of the pharynx and adjacent structures were described clearly in antiquity, antedating by many centuries recognition of their specific etiologies. It is not surprising that many of the early descriptions reflected considerable confusion between diphtheria and other (primarily streptococcal) infections of the pharyngeal region. The very earliest books on pediatric disorders included prominent mention of these infections.

HISTORICAL PERSPECTIVE

The first printed book on diseases of children, published in 1472 in Padua by Paolo Bagellardo a Flumine (?–1492), included a chapter entitled "On Abscesses of the Throat" [1]. It begins: "Children are also subject to abscesses around parts of the throat, such as are abscesses of the tonsils and are called commonly gaiones." Bagellardo referred to the much earlier writings of Johannes Mesuë (777–837), which included a section "On the Cure of Quinsey." The book published in 1484 by Cornelius Roelants of Mechlin, Belgium (1450–1525), *On Diseases of Infants*, included Chapter 31, entitled "On Apostema [abscess] of the Throat" [2].

Thomas Phaer (1510?–1560) is considered the father of English pediatrics because he pub-lished the first English-language pediatric book, *The Boke of Children*, in 1545 [3]. In the sec-tion "Quynsye, or Swelling of the Throte," he stated, "The quynsye is a dangerous sickness both in young and olde, called in latin angina, it is an inflammacion of the necke with swelling and great peyne, sometyme it lyeth in the verye throte. . . . Other whyles it breaketh out like a bonche on the one syde of the necke, and than also with verye great dyffycultye of breathynge . . . and it is more obediente to receive curacion. The signes are apparaunt to syghte, and besides that the chylde can not crye, neyther swallow downe his meat and drynke without payne."

Quinn has suggested that Hippocrates de-scribed illnesses consistent with scarlet fever in the fifth century, B.C. [4]. However, Thomas Sydenham (1624–1689) is most often credited with recognizing and describing scarlet fever (scarlatina) in 1676 and distinguishing it from measles, even though his description failed to note both the pharyngeal component of scarlet fever and its contagiousness [5]. Additional early descriptions of scarlet fever have been attributed to Gentile da Foligno (Padua, 14th century), In-grassia (Palermo, 1566), Horst (1624), Döring (Breslau, 1627), and Sennert (Wittenberg, 1628) [4]. The Swede Nils Rosen von Rosenstein (1706–1773) published a classic pediatric text in 1771 entitled *The Diseases of Children and Their*

Remedies [6]. Chapter XVI, "On The Scarlet Fever" recognized pharyngeal involvement and his description of an epidemic in Upsalla in 1741 is of interest:

"An exanthematic fever is sometimes epidemical among children, but seldom affects full grown persons; in it almost the whole body grows as red as scarlet cloth, and therefore it is called the scarlet fever (febris scarlativa). . . . I will here describe this fever according to the journal I kept of it in the year 1741, when it was to be met with almost in every house in Upsal, where children were to be found, affecting likewise some full grown persons. It was sometimes gentle, but sometimes very severe, so that of several children who lived under the same roof, it frequently happened that some of them were easily cured, whereas the others recovered with great difficulty. This scarlet fever began always with an indisposition in the throat . . . increasing quickly, so that some patients had their fauces and inside of their throat very red and inflamed within the first four-and-twenty hours. . . . Small red spots broke out generally on the second day . . . first on the face, after that on the neck, and then on the breast, lower part of the body, thighs, legs and feet . . . after four-and-twenty hours they had spread and dilated themselves so much that they made only one spot over the whole face. The same happened in the other parts of the body, especially in the flexures of the arms.

William Heberden (1767–1845) published *An Epitome of the Diseases Incident to Children* in 1804, drawing upon notes of his famous father, William Heberden, Sr. (1710–1801) [7]. This work includes Chapter 39, "Of the Ulcerated Sore Throat," and Chapter 40, "Of the Scarlet Fever." The latter chapter emphasizes that

most complain of soreness in the throat. Moreover, the glands under the ears, or elsewhere, often swell, and sometimes suppurate. . . . They who have once gone through the scarlet fever are generally secure for the rest of their lives. This disease, and the ulcerated sore throat, if they are not one and the same, at least require the same method of cure. . . . It is a point of great importance to determine how soon after this disease patients may be restored to their family without danger of communicating infection. I have known some children return to the society of their brothers and sisters the fifth day from the termination of the redness . . . and no harm has ensued.

The first American text to deal with children's health and diseases scientifically was *A Treatise on the Physical and Medical Treatment of Children*,

published by William P. Dewees (1768–1841) in 1825 [8]. Chapter XXXIV, "Of Scarlatina, or Scarlet Fever," highlighted the epidemiologic features of winter and spring predominance, the predilection for children, and its variable severity, but its contagiousness was doubted.

Bacteria were identified as causes of disease in the 1870s and 1880s. This finding was particularly influenced by Pasteur's efforts, but the relationship of streptococci to pharyngeal infections and scarlet fever slowly evolved over time. The first edition of Job Lewis Smith's classic text *Diseases of Infancy and Childhood* (1869) contained no mention of bacteria [9]. About a decade later, Edward Henoch's *Lectures on Diseases of Children* (1882) indicated that in attempting to distinguish between diphtheria and other inflammatory conditions of the pharynx, "microscopical examination will not decide the question, as bacteria are found in both affections" [10]. Henoch also stated that "the 'bacteria' doctrine has a very insecure foundation with regard to infectious diseases." The first edition of L. Emmett Holt's *The Diseases of Infancy and Childhood* (1897) [11] indicated that "acute primary pharyngitis is often attributed to cold and exposure, but it is probable that a large number of these cases will ultimately be shown to depend upon some form of infection. Certain children have a constitutional predisposition to attacks of pharyngitis, and contract it upon the slightest provocation. In some of them there is a strongly marked rheumatic diathesis." Regarding follicular tonsillitis, Holt writes, "the disease, in all probability, begins as an infectious inflammation at the bottom of the crypts, due to presence of streptococci or staphylococci, which readily enter from the mouth, and excute an attack whenever favorable conditions are present."

Holt's comments regarding scarlet fever highlight the confusion near the turn of the century:

Analogy leads to the belief that scarlet fever is due to a micro-organism, but as yet its nature has not been discovered. The complications are usually associated with the growth of the streptococcus pyogenes. Some have gone so far as to claim that this germ is the cause of the disease. From present knowledge, however, it appears rather to play the role of a secondary or accompanying infection. . . . To the streptococcus may be ascribed the membranous inflammations of the tonsils and pharynx, the otitis, the inflammations of the lymph nodes and the cellular tissue of the neck, and probably also the nephritis, pneumonia, and joint lesions. In many of the above conditions, the streptococcus is associated with other pyogenic germs, and in some cases with the diphtheria bacillus [11].

During the early decades of the 20th century, the etiologic relationship of what we now recognize as *Streptococcus pyogenes* to acute pharyngitis/tonsillitis and to scarlet fever became progressively more clear. In the 9th edition of *The Principles and Practice of Medicine* by Osler and McCrae (1923) [12], the importance of streptococcal infections of the mouth and throat in the etiology of acute septicemia was clearly acknowledged. Nevertheless, the specific cause of scarlet fever was said to be unknown, and "the trend of the work indicates that [the streptococcus] is only a secondary invader and that there is not a specific streptococcus." Acute tonsillitis, however, was recognized to be due to streptococci. This was largely on account of the series of epidemiologic studies carried out by Bloomfield and Felty at Johns Hopkins in the early 1920s [13]. Holt's 10th edition of *Diseases of Infancy and Childhood* (1939) stated that the great majority of acute tonsillitis was due to streptococci—either nonhemolytic, viridans, or beta-hemolytic—but acknowledged that most of the severe cases were due to beta-hemolytic organisms [14]. Scarlet fever was thought to be caused by a group of beta-hemolytic streptococci, the *Streptococcus scarlatinae*, that produced a soluble toxin.

The landmark development of the serologic grouping scheme for beta streptococci by Rebecca Lancefield subsequently established group A streptococci as the major specific agent of acute streptococcal tonsillitis/pharyngitis and scarlet fever [15].

CLINICAL EPIDEMIOLOGY

The clinical epidemiology of group A streptococcal pharyngitis is intertwined with the epidemiology of acute rheumatic fever (ARF). There is good reason for this: ARF was once a common and devastating complication of group A beta-hemolytic streptococcal (GABHS) pharyngitis in the United States, and efforts to understand and

prevent ARF required evidence that the two diseases were linked. Many early epidemiologic studies focused on ARF rather than on antecedent pharyngitis. Of course, studies could not distinguish group A streptococci from other beta-hemolytic groups until Lancefield's serogrouping was developed [15]. Many studies, especially those from the 1940s and 1950s, used the terms "infection," "colonization," and "carriage" interchangeably. All of these factors led to potentially misleading prevalence and incidence data. Although school-aged children and young adult military recruits were subjects of numerous studies, other age-groups were not studied as well.

The complaint of sore throat accounts for more than 7 million visits to pediatricians each year in the United States [16]. Streptococcal pharyngitis is diagnosed in 15%–20% of those patients.

Until the end of World War II, epidemics of streptococcal pharyngitis and subsequent epidemics of ARF were well known. Pharyngitis epidemics in U.S. military facilities afforded investigators opportunities to recognize clearly the relationship between streptococcal pharyngitis and ARF and to document the benefits of antibiotic therapy [17,18]. The importance of crowding in the transmission of streptococcal pharyngitis became evident in these military epidemics; for example, 100,000 cases of streptococcal pharyngitis and 2000 cases of ARF were diagnosed among recruits in 18 months at Farragut Naval Station in Idaho during World War II. Similar epidemics occurred at other military bases [19].

Evidence of the importance of crowding and close contact in the spread of GABHS exists in the modern era and in civilian populations. In a semi-closed community of 303 people living in an apartment building with a common dining room, 132 (43%) had GABHS isolated from throats within 6 weeks of recognition of an increase in numbers of patients with symptoms of pharyngitis and positive cultures [20]. Three M types accounted for most of the isolates; 75% were M type 58. In a kibbutz in Israel, 105 of 589 (21%) residents had symptomatic culture-positive pharyngitis in a 3-month period; all isolates were M type 62 [21]. In a boarding school in England 17% of 133 children 10–13 years old who lived in dormitories had M type 6 GABHS isolated from throats during a recent outbreak.

The recovery rate of GABHS among students who attended but did not live at the school was 7%. In this outbreak, 16 of 31 patients from whom GABHS was isolated were asymptomatic [22]. A day care center with 187 children and 27 adult staff experienced an outbreak of GABHS pharyngitis lasting 3 months. Three group A streptococcal serotypes accounted for 85% of the isolates [23]. In each of these outbreaks children were predominantly affected, but the experience in the U.S. military demonstrates that close living conditions favor the spread of GABHS even among adults.

Crowding is important because transmission occurs primarily by inhalation of organisms in large droplets or by direct contact with respiratory secretions. Streptococcal pharyngitis is particularly contagious early in the acute illness and for the first 2 weeks after the organism has been acquired (unless treated with antibiotics). The incubation period is 2 to 5 days. Appropriate antibiotic therapy rapidly eliminates GABHS from the throat. Brink et al. reported that fewer than 15% of penicillin-treated recruits harbored GABHS after 24 h of treatment [24]. Randolph et al. found that only 3% of appropriately treated children had positive throat cultures 18 to 24 h after treatment was begun [25]. Evidence that the elimination of GABHS from the throat prevents transmission was presented by Wannamaker et al. who showed that intramuscular or oral penicillin reduced the incidence of streptococcal disease on a military base [26]. More recent studies of outbreaks in schools [22], military bases [27], and on a kibbutz [21] confirm that appropriate antibiotic therapy halts transmission of GABHS and terminates outbreaks of pharyngitis.

Low socioeconomic status is a classic risk factor for development of ARF, but it is not clear if this relates to higher rates of streptococcal pharyngitis or to less access to appropriate medical care and treatment, or both. In developing nations and among certain ethnic groups such as the Maori of New Zealand and the Aboriginal peoples of Australia, increased transmission of GABHS because of substandard and crowded living conditions may interact with lack of available health care services and unawareness of the relationship of sore throat to ARF. However, the scant data that exist suggest that streptococcal pharyngitis is probably no more common in developing countries than it is in the U.S. [28]. Although methodologic differences undoubtedly exist, in India about 14% of patients with acute pharyngitis had GABHS isolated from the pharynx, in Egypt 19% had GABHS, and in Kuwait 22% were positive for GABHS, percentages that are comparable to those in Western countries.

Children 5 to 12 years old experience GABHS pharyngitis more frequently than those of other age-groups. Symptomatic GABHS pharyngitis is quite unusual in infancy, although it can occur. The age-related pattern of disease, with school-aged children most often affected, is readily apparent in community outbreaks [20,21]. Other age-groups are also affected, but the risk of subsequent ARF is markedly lower in those less than 3 years of age. Wherever it has been studied, cases of streptococcal pharyngitis generally peak in the late winter and early spring months [23,29,30].

Asymptomatic pharyngeal colonization by GABHS occurs frequently and appears to follow the age and seasonal pattern of pharyngitis. Colonization rates as high as 60% in school children have been reported in the U.S. [29]. Much more typical rates were found in a study in Philadelphia in 1955–57: average monthly rates of isolation of GABHS from asymptomatic children in three schools varied from 7.4% to 28.8% [30]. Higher rates of colonization were noted in the spring. More recently, in a private pediatric practice in Texas, 3.3% of healthy, asymptomatic children 3 months to 14 years old had GABHS isolated from the pharynx [31]. Isolation of GABHS was most common among children 5 to 7 years old (8.3%) and was absent in infants (3–12 months). There is evidence that, compared with children living in temperate regions, children living in the tropics are more likely to be asymptomatic carriers of beta-hemolytic streptococci [32]. However, group A streptococci predominate in temperate countries and groups C and G have been reported to be more commonly isolated in warmer regions.

Today streptococcal pharyngitis is endemic in the United States and other developed countries. The shift to endemic disease may have occurred because of improved sanitation and housing, the widespread use of antibiotics, or changes in GABHS.

Despite fairly high rates of asymptomatic pharyngeal colonization, epidemic GABHS pharyngitis has been unusual in recent years. Community or school surveillance cultures in endemic areas generally yield a variety of M serotypes. In contrast, epidemics of streptococcal pharyngitis tend to be associated with the predominance of a relatively limited number of the more than 80 M types, and strains with mucoid colonial morphology on sheep blood agar are overrepresented among those associated with epidemics. Recent outbreaks on U.S. military bases have followed this pattern; one to three M types characterized by mucoid colonies on blood agar were isolated in each of seven outbreaks that occurred between January 1984 and March 1994 [27]. Mass treatment of acute GABHS pharyngitis and mass prophylaxis with benzathine penicillin successfully controlled these military outbreaks. Such mucoid strains, which are probably more virulent than nonmucoid strains, were also noted in past military epidemics and were associated with some of the community outbreaks of ARF in the late 1980s and early 1990s in the United States [33,34].

An individual GABHS serotype enters and leaves a community fairly quickly [35]. Certain M types are overrepresented among pharyngeal isolates associated with ARF (e.g., M types 1, 3, 5, 6, and 18), while other M types are typically associated with uncomplicated pharyngitis (M types 4 and 12) [34]. Regional outbreaks or clusters of cases of ARF or of invasive GABHS infections may be related to certain M types becoming dominant in a community for a period of time. Nevertheless, by no means do all untreated GABHS pharyngeal infections caused by an ARF-associated M type result in development of ARF. Host factors are clearly important. Intratypic variability also occurs, so strains sharing the same M-protein can vary substantially in virulence. The basis of variations in virulence are poorly understood but probably relate to differences in genomic DNA [36].

When a strain of GABHS that produces erythrogenic or pyrogenic exotoxin A or C predominates in a community, some cases of streptococcal pharyngitis manifest as scarlet fever. The more common toxin, encoded by a lysogenized bacteriophage, is streptococcal pyrogenic exotoxin A (SPE A). Expression of the *spe*A gene appears to be variable; it can be associated with typical scarlet fever, with streptococcal toxic shock syndrome, or with simple pharyngitis [36].

Although they were unaware of the genetic basis for scarlet fever, Drs. George F. Dick and Gladys Henry Dick recognized in the 1930s that there were "varieties" of scarlet fever including "fulminating toxic or malignant scarlet fever" (toxic shock), "septic scarlet fever" (streptococcal sepsis), subclinical disease (virtually asymptomatic colonization with a scarlet fever-associated strain), and "scarlatina sine eruptione" (pharyngitis and fever without rash in a patient exposed to scarlet fever) [37]. The precise reasons for the variety of presentations of scarlet fever remain obscure but must involve host immune factors. However, pharyngitis without rash is probably the most common manifestation of acute pharyngeal infection with a SPE A–positive strain, and the same general epidemiologic characteristics exist as with streptococcal pharyngitis caused by a non–scarlet fever–associated strain.

Outbreaks of GABHS pharyngitis rarely may be food-borne. Serious milk-borne epidemics of sore throat and scarlet fever were once very common. For example, in the 1880s Dr. Emanuel Klein demonstrated that cows infected with streptococci were the source for several large outbreaks in England [38]. By the 1920s milk-borne epidemics of streptococcal pharyngitis were effectively eliminated in areas that routinely pasteurized milk. In the modern era, food prepared by a GABHS-infected or colonized cook occasionally leads to outbreaks of GABHS pharyngitis. Macaroni and cheese was implicated in an outbreak that occurred following an elementary school banquet [39]; the cook had a hand wound that yielded GABHS when cultured. In Italy, six restaurant staff colonized with the same strain of GABHS apparently served as the source in an outbreak linked to seafood [40]. A military unit in Israel experienced an outbreak of streptococcal pharyngitis associated with cabbage salad prepared by a cook who had GABHS pharyngitis [41]. Pharyngitis in food-borne outbreaks is usually marked by shorter-than-usual incubation times (less than 2 days), more severe acute symptoms, and predominance of a single M type.

CLINICAL FEATURES (TABLE 5.1)

Abrupt onset of fever and sore throat mark the typical case of streptococcal pharyngitis. Cough,

Table 5.1 Classic Features of Acute
Streptococcal Pharyngitis

Season	Late winter or early spring
Age	5 to 12 years
Symptoms	Sudden onset
	Sore throat
	Fever
	Headache
	Abdominal pain, nausea, vomiting
Signs	Pharyngeal erythema and exudation
	Tender, enlarged anterior cervical nodes
	Palatal petechiae
	Tonsillar hypertrophy
	Absence of cough, coryza, conjunctivitis, diarrhea

rhinorrhea, stridor, hoarseness, conjunctivitis, and diarrhea are quite unusual. Several nonspecific nonpharyngeal signs and symptoms are frequently associated with streptococcal pharyngitis, including headache, nausea, vomiting, malaise, and abdominal pain, especially in older children. The pharynx is erythematous. Petechiae may be seen on the soft palate. Tonsils, if present, are enlarged and erythematous, with patchy exudates on their surfaces. The papillae of the tongue may be red and swollen, leading to the designation "strawberry tongue." Tender, enlarged anterior cervical lymph nodes are often found. Younger children may have coryza with crusting below the nares, more generalized adenopathy, and a more chronic course, a syndrome called streptococcosis. Nasal cultures are positive in this syndrome.

Many patients with streptococcal pharyngitis exhibit signs and symptoms that are less severe than a "classic" case of this illness. Some of these patients have bona fide GABHS infection and others are merely colonized, with illnesses due to some other agent, most often a virus.

When a fine, diffuse red rash accompanies GABHS pharyngitis, the syndrome is called scarlet fever. Scarlet fever is rarely seen in children less than 3 years old and is less common in adults. The scarlet fever rash has a texture similar to fine sandpaper and blanches with pressure. Initially there is sore throat and fever. The face is flushed but without palpable rash. The area around the mouth remains pale in comparison to the extremely red cheeks, giving the ap-

pearance of "circumoral pallor." The rash is usually noticed initially on the upper chest about 24 h after onset of symptoms. The flexor skin creases, especially in the antecubital fossae, and may have more intense redness (Pastia's lines). Within Pastia's lines small petechiae can sometimes be seen and can be induced by placing a tourniquet on the upper arm (positive tourniquet test or Rumpel-Leeds phenomenon), evidence of capillary fragility. Erythema begins to fade within a few days with treatment, and within a week of onset desquamation may occur, first on the face, progressing downward, and often resembling that seen subsequent to a mild sunburn. Occasionally sheet-like desquamation may occur around the free margins of the fingernails, the palms, and the soles 7 to 10 days after onset.

The signs and symptoms of streptococcal pharyngitis are self-limited. In the absence of antibiotic treatment more than 50% of patients have resolution of fever and sore throat by the fourth day of the illness. By the sixth day of illness symptoms have resolved in nearly all patients. Symptoms resolve about 1 day earlier in patients treated with effective antibiotics [24,25,42,43].

DIAGNOSIS

Because the signs and symptoms of group A streptococcal pharyngitis can be nonspecific, establishing an accurate clinical diagnosis often remains difficult even for experienced physicians. Therefore it has become standard practice to seek bacteriologic confirmation of the diagnosis. Currently available laboratory methods include the many rapid streptococcal antigen detection tests currently marketed as well as the standard throat culture to aid in distinguishing those patients with streptococcal pharyngitis from those with other illnesses.

It is widely accepted that clinicians should seek to identify individuals with group A streptococcal pharyngitis from the larger number of patients who have pharyngitis caused by other (usually viral) agents. This traditional approach has persisted for more than 40 years since Breese and Disney pioneered the use of the throat swab cultured onto a sheep blood–agar plate in the physician's office to confirm the presence of GABHS [44]. The primary rationale for this approach has been the prevention of the major nonsuppurative sequela of streptococcal pharyngitis, acute rheumatic fever.

Currently it is at least as important for clinicians to identify the large fraction (70%–80%) of patients with complaint of sore throat who do *not* have GABHS infection and who therefore do not require antibiotic therapy as it is to identify those with GABHS infection [45]. This has become an increasingly important basis for clinical strategies involving management of acute pharyngitis patients as the threat of rheumatic fever gradually but steadily subsides. Antibiotics are associated with a finite risk of adverse reactions and can be costly, particularly the newly introduced antimicrobials. A staggering amount of money is expended annually in the United States for unnecessary antibiotics prescribed for acute nonbacterial infections, particularly upper respiratory infections of viral etiology. That this practice has serious consequences for society is emphasized by the relatively recent emergence of highly resistant gram-positive organisms in many countries, including strains of *Streptococcus pneumoniae* with high-level penicillin resistance (minimal inhibitory concentrations [MIC]>1.0 μg/ml) or with low-level penicillin resistance (MIC = 0.1 to 1.0 μg/ml) [46].

There are also recent reports of high rates of penicillin-resistant and low-level resistant alpha-streptococci (viridans streptococci), particularly from Europe [47], as well as evidence from several countries of high rates of erythromycin-resistant GABHS [48]. A direct correlation between the magnitude of antibiotic use and the emergence of resistant gram-positive organisms exists [49].

This alarming trend toward the development of resistant nasopharyngeal and oropharyngeal organisms, with their ability to cause serious infections including bacteremia, meningitis, and endocarditis, provides strong support for management strategies for acute pharyngitis that emphasize the identification of those individuals who do not have streptococcal pharyngitis and who therefore do not require antibiotic therapy. Such strategies will help reduce the selective pressure of antibiotics upon the microbial flora.

Clinical Diagnosis

It is well recognized that although characteristic or "classic" features of acute streptococcal pharyngitis can be appreciated, as discussed above, they are insufficiently precise to enable consistent, reliable, and accurate differentiation between patients with that entity and those with acute nonstreptococcal pharyngitis [50]. Several clinical scoring systems have been developed to aid in the diagnosis of acute streptococcal pharyngitis, but they have proved of limited usefulness, probably because of the confounding issues of streptococcal carriers (see below) and the fact that many or most patients with streptococcal pharyngitis lack a number of the classic features (see above). The best of the scoring systems was developed by Breese and Disney [44,51]. Because diagnoses based solely upon such formal or much more informal clinical assessments alone are not sufficiently precise, reliance upon a diagnostic laboratory test such as the throat culture or a rapid antigen detection test is necessary when one seriously entertains the diagnosis of acute streptococcal pharyngitis. It has been demonstrated that using clinical criteria alone, clinicians tend to overestimate the likelihood that patients have streptococcal infection [52].

It is important to note that the presence of certain signs and symptoms typical of acute viral infection should dissuade serious consideration of acute streptococcal pharyngitis and often dissuade performance of a laboratory test to rule out streptococcal pharyngitis. When classic signs and symptoms of viral illness such as rhinorrhea, hoarseness, cough, and diarrhea are present in a patient with pharyngitis, a diagnostic test for GABHS is much more likely to identify a chronic pharyngeal carrier of GABHS than a patient with bona fide acute streptococcal pharyngitis. Because chronic GABHS carriers appear to be at little or no risk for development of ARF or for dissemination of GABHS (see below), performing a diagnostic test in this circumstance is often unwarranted [45].

Throat Cultures

The reliability of the throat culture for detection of GABHS is subject to several technical variables. The most important variable is probably the quality of the technique of swabbing the patient's pharyngeal and tonsillar regions. Optimally, the throat swab should make contact with both tonsillar regions as well as with the posterior pharyngeal wall to ensure maximal recovery of GABHS.

Considerable debate has occurred regarding the most appropriate atmosphere of incubation for throat cultures for identification of GABHS. Anaerobic incubation conditions may increase the yield of GABHS by approximately 3% to 6% but also substantially increase the recovery of non–group A streptococcal organisms that must be differentiated from GABHS. It is not clear that the relatively small number of additional patients identified by anaerobic culture conditions represent those with bona fide acute streptococcal pharyngitis rather than with chronic streptococcal carriage. The overall conclusion of the several comparative studies that have assessed various incubation atmospheres is that anaerobic incubation is probably not justified or necessary in routine practice [53].

Selection of the most appropriate media for culture of GABHS has also generated considerable discussion. Some data suggest that use of sheep blood–agar containing trimethoprim/sulfamethoxazole may enhance the recovery of group A streptococci [54], but this has not been demonstrated conclusively. It is clear, however, that use of such selective media leads to substantially slower growth of GABHS and that maintaining and observing culture plates for 48–72 h becomes mandatory. At present the use of standard 5% sheep blood–agar plates without antibiotics appears to be the best recommendation for throat cultures; the increased cost and increased incubation time of selective media are not justified [53].

Use of the 0.04 U bacitracin disc for presumptive identification of GABHS is widespread because at least 95% of GABHS demonstrate a large zone of inhibition around the bacitracin disc, whereas 83% to 97% of non–group A beta streptococci do not [55]. This technique is most accurate when beta-hemolytic streptococci are subcultured from the primary plate onto a fresh blood-agar plate, the bacitracin disc is placed and the plate is evaluated after 18- to 24-h incubation for inhibition of growth. However, in most clinical settings the bacitracin disc is placed on the primary throat plate at the time of initial inoculation. Although subject to more potential misinterpretation, this technique is probably an acceptable and practical technique if the disc is placed in an area of at least moderate growth [53]. In general, subculturing individual colonies from the primary plate to another plate is beyond the capability of most office laboratories. Similarly, the utilization of more specific serogrouping procedures such as Lancefield's capillary precipitation technique or agglutination methods on isolated bacterial colonies is impractical for the office laboratory.

The accuracy of a single throat culture to yield GABHS has been the subject of a number of studies [44,53]. Perhaps the most informative of these investigations used duplicate throat swabs plated separately to investigate discordance rates. In summary, these studies demonstrated that a single throat culture is likely to be 90% to 97% sensitive in detecting the presence of GABHS and, therefore, that only 3% to 10% of individuals harboring GABHS in the pharynx may be missed by a single (well-performed) throat culture [56]. When one considers that in clinical practice there are several negative throat cultures for each positive one, the overall discordance rate for all throat cultures is approximately one-third to one-fourth of 3% to 10%, or 1% to 2%. Many with false-negative throat cultures likely harbor very small numbers of GABHS in the pharynx, and most are likely to be chronic streptococcal carriers rather than truly infected patients (see below). Overall, these considerations indicate that throat culture accuracy is within the range of acceptability for most diagnostic medical tests but point out that the throat culture, the so-called gold standard, does not always provide a totally accurate assessment [53].

Rapid Antigen Detection Tests

That 24 to 48 h may be required for throat culture results has stimulated the development of diagnostic tests that enable rapid identification of GABHS directly from throat swabs. The clinical use of these tests enables more timely therapeutic decisions that are based on the results of a diagnostic laboratory test.

All rapid tests for GABHS involve a brief acid-extraction step to solubilize GABHS cell-wall carbohydrate, with its subsequent identification by an immunologic reaction. The first rapid streptococcal antigen detection tests utilized latex agglutination methodology but had relatively ambiguous end points. Second generation tests based on enzyme immunoassay techniques offer the advantages of more sharply defined end points and greater sensitivity [57]. The most recent generation of rapid test is based on optical immunoassay (OIA) technology, with sharp end points, permanent results, and probably further increased sensitivity [58,59]. In general, current rapid antigen detection tests can be considered to have excellent specificity, i.e., positive tests are highly reliable indicators of the presence of group A streptococci, and therapeutic decisions can be based upon them with confidence. However, the sensitivity of these assays, i.e., their ability to detect true positives, is more variable and is not high enough that a negative rapid test can be relied upon to rule out the presence of GABHS. The OIA test may be a notable exception to this, as suggested in our recent large study [59].

The advantage of rapid diagnostic tests, of course, is the speed of obtaining a result—generally within 10 to 20 min after obtaining the throat swab. This facilities earlier institution of therapy, perhaps more prompt clearance of symptoms, and earlier return of patients to school and to work. Although it has been suggested that early therapy may blunt the immune response and predispose patients to more frequent infections with GABHS [60], this was not verified [61], and physicians should not be deterred from instituting early therapy for patients confirmed to have GABHS infection. The disadvantages of the rapid streptococcal antigen tests are their expense and the need, because of relatively low sensitivity rates, to confirm negative rapid tests with a conventional throat culture, with the possible exception of the OIA test [59].

Several factors can affect the results obtained with rapid streptococcal antigen tests, including the level of training of the individual chosen to perform these tests. Studies have demonstrated that when a clinician who has evaluated an individual patient also performs a rapid antigen detection test, a strong observer bias can be apparent. That is, when a clinician strongly suspects that a patient has acute streptococcal pharyngitis, the clinician may be more likely to overread a rapid streptococcal antigen test as positive [62]. Therefore, rapid antigen tests must have objective end points to prevent such bias.

Rapid tests are intended for the diagnosis of acute streptococcal pharyngitis rather than for evaluation of the effectiveness of therapy. A positive result in an asymptomatic patient does not distinguish among infection, colonization (carriage), or the presence of nonviable organisms (for example, following effective therapy).

Serologic Tests

Seeking serological evidence of an antibody response to extracellular products or cellular components of group A streptococci (such as streptolysin O) is not useful for diagnosis of acute pharyngitis. Because serum antibody levels require at least 10 to 14 days to rise, streptococcal antibody tests are valid only for determining past infection. Antibodies often measured when evaluating a possible poststreptococcal illness include anti-streptolysin O (ASO), anti-DNase B, and anti-hyaluronidase (AHT). Performance of more than one of these tests improves sensitivity to detect a response to a recent (but not current) GABHS infection. However, the Streptozyme® test (Wampole Laboratories, Cranbury, NJ), an assay that uses latex particles coated with group A streptococcus broth culture supernates, has been shown to be poorly standardized and therefore cannot be recommended [63].

Diagnostic Practices

Several surveys have examined the strategies actually used by physicians to diagnose streptococcal pharyngitis. Cochi et al. surveyed primary care physicians in December 1982 and January 1983, before rapid tests were available, and found that approximately 25% of the respondents always or nearly always obtained throat cultures from patients with sore throat, but that cultures were never or almost never obtained by 23% of those surveyed [64]. Pediatricians were more likely than internists or family/general practitioners to use throat cultures. In 1993,

Schwartz et al. surveyed pediatricians about their diagnostic approaches to children with pharyngitis [65]. An optimal approach, defined as use of culture alone or as a backup to a negative rapid antigen test for at least 80% of patients, was used by only 44% of pediatricians who responded to the survey. Seventeen percent reported using clinical findings or rapid test without culture for most children with pharyngitis. We obtained similar results from a recent national survey of U.S. pediatricians; 64% used rapid tests at least some of the time, 42% used throat cultures when the rapid test was negative, 38% used cultures alone, and 20% used strategies that are not recommended [66]. Thus, it appears that many physicians do not follow recommended guidelines for diagnosing streptococcal pharyngitis.

THERAPY

Treatment in the Early Antibiotic Era

The value of penicillin in treatment of acute streptococcal pharyngitis was established in the late 1940s and early 1950s. That many nonpenicillin antimicrobial agents also are active in vitro and in vivo against group A streptococci was established during subsequent decades, prompting re-evaluation of whether penicillin should remain the treatment of choice. Nevertheless, authoritative bodies continue to recommend that penicillin be the drug of choice for acute pharyngitis in non-penicillin-allergic individuals

[67–69]. The evolution of antibiotic treatment of streptococcal pharyngitis is reviewed here.

After the initial demonstration that sulfonamides could prevent streptococcal infections [70–72], the treatment of streptococcal pharyngitis and epidemic scarlet fever with antibiotics began immediately after World War II. The studies of Jersild in Copenhagen [73] compared twice- or thrice-daily injections of 40,000–150,000 U crystalline penicillin for 3 or 6 days to oral sulfanilamide for 8 days. These studies concluded that 3 days of penicillin was inadequate to eradicate streptococci and that 6 days of treatment shortened the febrile period by 2–3 days, reduced culture-positive rates at days 2–5 and weeks 2–4 after therapy, markedly reduced the incidence of suppurative complications (especially otitis media and need for mastoidectomy) then so frequent, shortened hospital stay, and appeared to prevent poststreptococcal nephritis (rheumatic fever was not mentioned). Sulfanilamide therapy was very ineffective in eradicating streptococci (Table 5.2).

Shortly thereafter, an historic series of studies at the Fort Warren Air Force Base, Wyoming, was carried out in recruits with acute streptococcal pharyngitis, using a depot intramuscular preparation of crystalline procaine penicillin G in peanut or sesame oil [17,24,26,74]. It was found that a single dose of 6×10^5 U, providing 4–6 days of antistreptococcal activity (regimen 3 in Table 5.3), reduced post-treatment culture positivity to 31% (compared to 57% in untreated controls). A three-dose regimen of 3×10^5 U at time 0 and at 48 h and 6×10^5 U at 96 h (regimen 1 in Table 5.3) providing 9–10 days of ac-

Table 5.2 Copenhagen Penicillin Studies (1945–1947)

Acute Scarlet Fever	IM Penicillin 90,000–150,000 U BID ×6 Days	PO Sulfanilamide ×8 Days
Fever duration	4.5 days	7.0 days
Culture positive after treatment	4%	73%
Suppurative complications	5.5%	49.5%
Suppurative otitis media	0%	4%
Acute Suppurative Otitis with Scarlet Fever	IM Penicillin 90,000–150,000 U BID–TID ×6–23 days	PO Sulfanilamide
Mastoidectomy required	3.5%	21%–38%

Adapted from Jersild [73].

Table 5.3 Warren AFB Studies of Streptococcal Pharyngitis Treated with Procaine Penicillin G in Oil

	Regimen 1 vs Controls		Regimen 2 vs Controls		Regimen 3 vs Controls	
Number	516	487	200	239	262	270
Percent positive GABHS at follow-up	13%	52%	18%	44%	31%	57%
Percent with typeable GABHS with same serotype at follow-up	7%	35%	8%	30%	29%	60%
No. definite ARF	2	20	0	4	0	4
No. possible ARF	1	2	1	4	1	1

Regimen 1, 300,000 U stat and at 48 h, 600,000 U at 96 h. Regimen 2, 300,000 U stat and at 72 h. Regimen 3, 600,000 U stat.
Adapted from Wannamaker [74].

tivity lowered postculture positivity to only 13%. With the latter three-dose regimen, Wannamaker et al. demonstrated 93% eradication of the original GABHS serotype and 90% prevention of ARF (Table 5.3; [74]). When benzathine penicillin G, a better depot preparation, became available, even higher rates of eradication of GABHS and prevention of ARF were achieved [75].

The classic investigations carried out at Fort Warren in 1949 and 1950 are the major placebo-controlled studies that document the efficacy of an antimicrobial agent to prevent ARF. They form the basis for the current assumption that other agents that reliably eradicate GABHS from the upper respiratory tract, including the oral regimens commonly used today, also prevent this nonsuppurative complication. Studies by Brink and by Houser in the early 1950s, also at Fort Warren, demonstrated that the three-dose intramuscular (IM) penicillin regimen or oral aureomycin (tetracycline) for 4 days initiated within the first 24 h of acute pharyngitis

symptoms reduced fever and prevented otitis, but that aureomycin did not eradicate streptococci effectively or prevent recurrences [24]. In 1953, Houser also reported that oral aureomycin for 4–6 days reduced ARF compared to untreated controls but not as effectively as penicillin [76]. When it became clear that effective prevention of ARF required streptococcal eradication, acceptable treatment regimens for streptococcal pharyngitis had to meet this requirement, and the initial 1955 American Heart Association recommendations for primary prevention of ARF population focused exclusively on penicillin [77].

The active pediatric group of Burtis Breese and Frank Disney in Rochester, NY, performed a large number of treatment studies of streptococcal pharyngitis over a period of more than 30 years. In a series of over 1200 pediatric infections, they initially showed that a single injection of 600,000 U benzathine penicillin G was the best regimen, eradicating GABHS in 93%; 95% had no clinical recurrence by 31 days (Table 5.4;

Table 5.4 Breese's Streptococcal Treatment Studies in Children 1947–1952

Regimen	n	Clinical Recurrence <31 days (%)	Bacteriologic Recurrence <31 days (%)
Symptomatic	52	15	73
Oral sulfonamides × 5–8 days	101	21	68
Oral aureomycin × 8–12 days	87	25	26
Oral penicillin 1.2–3.6 × 10^6 U over 8–10 days	89	17	25
IM procaine penicillin G 300,000 U × 1	115	32	41
IM procaine penicillin G 300,000 U day 0 + day 3	131	17	25
IM procaine penicillin G 300,000 U days 0, 3, 6	206	8	17
IM procaine penicillin G 300,000 U day 0, then oral penicillin 2.4–3.6 × 10^6 U on days 3–10	169	14	18
IM bicillin G 600,000 1 × 10^6 U ×1	108	5	7

Adapted from Breese [78].

Table 5.5 Comparison of IM Benzathine Penicillin and 4 Oral Regimens

	600,000 U IM benz.	800,000 U/day Benz. Pen. G PO × 10 days	800,000 U/day Pen. V PO × 10 days	800,000 U/day Buff. Pot. Pen. G PO × 10 days	250,000 U Buff. Pot. Pen. G +250 mg Probenecid TID × 10 days	250,000 U Buff. Pot. Pen. G +500 mg Probenecid BID × 10 days
Patients	122	115	122	114	66	72
Bacteriologic cure[a]	93%	87%	89%	85%	82%	90%
Recurrence with same streptococcus <25 days	2.8%	9.3%	4.8%	9.6%	7.4%	4.0%
Hives or rash	2.5%	0	2.5%	0.9%	18.2%	15.3%

Benz., benzathine; Buff. Pot., buffered potassium; Pen., penicillin.

[a]The authors adjusted the cure rates to indicate that 60% of bacteriologic failures represent new strains of streptococci.

Adapted from Breese and Disney [81].

[78]). ARF and acute glomerulonephritis did not occur in treated patients. In subsequent studies, post-treatment acquisition of a new streptococcal strain was shown to be common, but less so after treatment with benzathine penicillin G [79]. This group also compared 600,000 U IM benzathine penicillin G to four oral benzathine penicillin G regimens, 150,000 U three times daily for 8 days, 200,000 U three times daily for 8 or 10 days, or 200,000 U four times daily for 10 days [80]. The intramuscular regimen and 10 days of oral penicillin four times per day were comparable and were considered superior to thrice-daily therapy for 8 or 10 days. When various 10-day oral penicillin regimens were compared to IM benzathine penicillin, the latter performed slightly better (Table 5.5) [81]. In yet another well-designed study, these investigators compared IM benzathine penicillin G to five different oral penicillin G 10-day regimens (200,000 U QID; 400,000 U BID; 400,000 U QID; 800,000 U QD and 800,000 U BID); one-month bacteriologic cure rates were comparable (83%–89%) for all oral regimens except once daily penicillin G, with a significantly higher cure rate with IM benzathine (95%) [82]. Once-daily penicillin G was clearly associated with an unacceptably high failure rate. The clinical recurrence rate also was lowest (1%) in the IM group (Table 5.6).

The pain and limp associated with benzathine penicillin G injections also prompted studies with preparations that combined procaine penicillin, or 5 mg prednisolone with 600,000 U IM benzathine penicillin G. Both additives were effective [83]. Studies by Bass et al. found the bacteriologic cure rates associated with 900,000 U benzathine combined with 300,000 U procaine penicillin G; with 600,000 U benzathine penicillin combined with 600,000 U procaine penicillin G; and with 1,200,000 U benzathine penicillin G alone to be comparable and superior to that achieved with 600,000 U benzathine penicillin G alone. Overall, the 900/300 regimen was associated with the highest cure rate [84].

Stillerman and Bernstein compared 125 mg and 250 mg doses of oral penicillin V (a better absorbed preparation) in children, each given thrice daily, and found a significantly higher cure

Table 5.6 Oral Penicillin G for Streptococcal Pharyngitis

	800,000 U QD	200,000 U QID	400,000 U BID	400,000 U QID	800,000 U BID	600,000 U Benzathine Penicillin IM
Number	50	92	95	95	98	97
Bacteriologic cure	58%	89%	83%	84%	85%	95%
Recurrence	14%	6%	3%	7%	10%	1%

Adapted from Disney [82].

rate with the higher dose regimen (89% vs. 77%, $P < 0.001$) [85]. Rosenstein and colleagues found 400,000 U (250 mg) oral penicillin V twice daily to be highly effective and that oral nafcillin was no better [86].

Early studies of streptococcal pharyngitis among penicillin-allergic individuals focused on erythromycin. Haight compared twice-daily IM procaine penicillin for 10 days to 200 mg oral erythromycin six times daily for 10 days in U.S. naval recruits and found virtually identical eradication rates and rapid clinical improvement [87]. The earliest pediatric studies showed lower eradication rates with oral erythromycin than with oral penicillin [88], but using improved formulations with better absorption, oral erythromycin was comparable to oral penicillin [89–91]. In those studies, 40 mg/kg/day of erythromycin appeared to be superior to 20 mg/kg/day.

During the 1970s, a number of studies compared erythromycin estolate in various schedules (20–40 mg/kg/day in 2–4 daily doses) to oral phenoxymethyl penicillin V and reported 1-month bacteriologic cure rates of 83%–94%, without significant differences among drugs or schedules [92–97]. Most studies comparing various erythromycin salts did not demonstrate significant differences, although Ryan et al. reported a 96% 1-month bacteriologic cure rate with estolate and 84% with stearate ($P < 0.05$) [98]. However, Janicki et al. found no differences among stearate (30 mg/kg/day), estolate (30 mg/kg/day), and ethylsuccinate (50 mg/kg/day) (91%–96% cures) [99], and Derrick and Dillon obtained comparable results with estolate (30 mg/kg/day) and ethyl succinate (40 mg/kg/day) [100].

Initial studies of oral cephalosporins for streptococcal pharyngitis in the early 1970s evaluated cephalexin and yielded results comparable to, or marginally superior to, those achieved with oral or IM penicillin [101–104]. The consensus conclusion based on these studies was that the additional expense of the cephalosporins compared to that of penicillin could not be justified by marginally higher bacteriologic cure rates [105]. Stillerman reviewed this issue in 1986, however, and disagreed on the basis of his five relatively small comparative clinical trials [106].

Contemporary Treatment

Despite its more than four-decade role as the therapy of choice for acute streptococcal pharyngitis as reviewed above, penicillin continues to be challenged in this regard. Penicillin is currently recommended by both the American Heart Association and The Committee on Infectious Diseases of the American Academy of Pediatrics as well as by the World Health Organization as the drug of choice for treatment of streptococcal pharyngitis [67–69], with oral penicillin V largely replacing IM benzathine penicillin G in areas with little ARF.

As new antimicrobial agents continue to be developed, periodic reassessment of therapeutic options for this major infectious disease appears appropriate. Likewise, it is important to consider whether the clinical effectiveness of penicillin for acute streptococcal pharyngitis has changed over its long period of usage.

Several reports have suggested that bacteriologic failure rates following 10 days of oral penicillin treatment have increased in recent years. Markowitz and colleagues carefully analyzed the streptococcal pharyngitis bacteriologic failure rates associated with oral penicillin in reports published during the period 1953 to 1993 [107]. These authors evaluated 51 published treatment studies that met defined criteria to ensure comparability of the protocols employed. In 32 of 51 studies, serotyping of GABHS isolates had been performed to assess whether pretreatment and post-treatment isolates were identical. The results of this very careful analysis are summarized in Table 5.7. No significant difference in bacteriologic failure rates was observed when studies reported from 1953 to 1979 and those reported from 1980 to 1993 were compared, regardless of whether the follow-up period analyzed was 1–14 days (with failure rates = 10.5%–12.5%) or 1–60 days (with failure rates = 14%–16.9%) after completion of treatment. On the basis of these data, the authors concluded that oral penicillin is as effective as it was 40 years ago for treatment of streptococcal pharyngitis and that it remains the therapy of choice [107]. In vitro support for that view has come from Jelinkova and co-workers, who reported that the penicillin sensitivity of GABHS strains isolated from 1951

Table 5.7 Bacteriologic Failure Rates After Oral Penicillin for Streptococcal Pharyngitis

	No. Studies	Mean Failure Rates (%)	
		Days 1–14	Days 1–60
Including all studies			
Entire period (1953–1993)	51	11.6	17.3
1953–1979	29	11.1	16.9
1980–1993	22	12.4	17.7
Including studies with serotyping			
Entire period (1953–1993)	32	11.3	15.2
1953–1979	18	10.5	14.0
1980–1993	14	12.0	19.9

Adapted from Markowitz [107].

to 1992 in Prague, Czechoslovakia, had not changed [108], and from the report of Macris and colleagues who reported no change in penicillin sensitivity in a collection of GABHS from 1917 to 1997 [109].

A large number of more recent clinical trials have demonstrated that oral cephalosporins are effective clinically and bacteriologically in treatment of streptococcal pharyngitis. These include cefadroxil, cefaclor, cefixime, cefprozil, cefuroxime axetil, loracarbef, ceftibuten, and cefpodoxime proxetil. It has been inferred that they likely prevent ARF because they eradicate GABHS effectively. The cephalosporins appear to be satisfactory alternatives to penicillin, particularly for patients who are allergic (without anaphylaxis) to penicillin. Of course, these agents are substantially more expensive than oral penicillin or amoxicillin, and this cost differential generally precludes their routine use.

The question of whether oral cephalosporins are superior to penicillin for acute streptococcal pharyngitis has been raised. Stillerman's 1986 review is noted above [106]. Several more recent clinical trials that compared oral penicillin V to an oral cephalosporin reported significantly higher rates of pharyngeal eradication of GABHS by the latter agents; occasionally higher clinical cure rates were also reported. In a meta-analysis of 19 such comparative studies [110] and in a subsequent commentary [111]. Pichichero concluded that the cephalosporins could replace penicillin as the treatment of choice for streptococcal pharyngitis. We pointed out in extensive detail the many flaws of this meta-analysis [112].

A very important confounder in streptococcal pharyngitis treatment trials is the inadvertent enrollment of chronic streptococcal carriers who are experiencing an intercurrent pharyngitis of other etiology, as discussed below. It is inevitable that some "contamination" of the treatment group by such carriers will occur in clinical studies. Because penicillin is very ineffective, and other antibiotics with broader antimicrobial spectra may be more effective, in eradicating streptococcal carriage, such carrier contamination of enrollees in comparative trials disfavors penicillin and inflates apparent penicillin bacteriologic failure rates. The slightly lower bacteriologic failure rates often observed with oral cephalosporins may reflect the efficacy of cephalosporins in treatment of chronic carriage rather than in treatment of bona fide acute pharyngitis.

This was confirmed in our recent study in which no difference in bacteriologic eradication between cefadroxil- and penicillin-treated patients was found in those patients likely to have bona fide GABHS pharyngitis. In contrast, much higher eradication rates were observed in the cefadroxil group among patients likely to be streptococcal carriers [113].

This is illustrated by comparing the two studies shown in Table 5.8. In trial I [114], great care was exercised to exclude chronic carriers based on their history and/or presenting signs and symptoms, including those with history of frequent episodes of pharyngitis with positive throat cultures and those with upper respiratory infection symptoms. Bacteriologic failure rates were quite low (2.3% for penicillin V and 6.5% for amoxicillin-clavulanate) and were not significantly different. In trial II [115], substantially higher bacteriologic failure rates were found—

Table 5.8 Bacteriologic Failure Rates in
Two Trials

		Failure Rate (%)
Trial I[a]	Penicillin V	2.3
	Amoxicillin-clavulanate	6.5
Trial II[b]	Penicillin V	19
	Cephalexin	10

[a]Data from Tanz et al., [114].

[b]Data from Disney et al., [115].

19% for penicillin V and 10% for cephalexin—
a statistically significant difference. It is noteworthy that subjects in trial II included 12% who
lacked sore throat, 22% who lacked fever, and
25% who lacked pharyngeal erythema, with dis-
proportionately more in the penicillin group
lacking each of these features [115]. This
strongly suggests that trial II included many who
were chronic carriers rather than experiencing
acute streptococcal pharyngitis, with relatively
more carriers in the penicillin group. These features likely account both for overall higher bacteriologic failure rates and for the less favorable
results observed with penicillin. Substantial carrier contamination appears likely in most studies included in the above-noted meta-analysis
[110]. We strongly recommend that careful attempts be made to exclude likely carriers from
clinical trials of acute streptococcal pharyngitis,
to avoid erroneous conclusions.

For several decades erythromycin has remained the recommended first oral alternate to
penicillin V for streptococcal pharyngitis [67,68].
The early studies in the 1950s and 1960s that established its clinical and bacteriologic efficacy
are noted above. However, the substantial gastrointestinal intolerance associated with the various erythromycin preparations prompted development of other macrolides. Newer agents in
this class such as josamycin, clarithromycin, and
azithromycin have in vitro activity against
GABHS comparable to that of erythromycin but
are associated with substantially less gastrointestinal distress [116]. The two newer agents
now available in the United States, clarithromycin and azithromycin, are effective in
treating streptococcal pharyngitis. It must be
noted that 2%–4% of GABHS are resistant to
this class of agents in most areas, with much

higher resistance rates reported from areas of
the world with excessive nonprescription use of
these antimicrobials.

Clarithromycin is well absorbed orally, independent of food ingestion, can be given twice
daily, and achieves good concentrations in tonsillar tissues. Excellent clinical and bacteriologic
results have been demonstrated with 10-day
treatment courses [117,118]. Although the incidence of adverse gastrointestinal reactions associated with clarithromycin is higher than with
penicillin, this was considerably lower than occurs with erythromycin. Most reports have been
in patients at least 12 years old, but this agent is
now approved for treatment of streptococcal
pharyngitis in children under 12 years as well.

Azithromycin is also well absorbed after oral
ingestion but should be taken an hour before or
2 h after meals because food impairs its absorption. Its serum half-life is 11–14 h, allowing for
once-daily dosing. The drug is highly concentrated within polymorphonuclear leukocytes
(PMNs), tonsils, sinus, and middle ear fluids
[119]. At least six clinical trials of azithromycin
for streptococcal pharyngitis are of note. Hooten
reported data from a U.S. multicenter trial of
subjects at least 16 years old given either 10 days
of penicillin V or a loading dose of 500 mg
azithromycin followed by 250 mg once daily for
4 days [120]. Azithromycin-resistant GABHS
were isolated from only 2.2% of patients; these
patients were considered unevaluable and were
omitted from analysis. In each group, 99% were
considered clinically cured or improved. Eradication of GABHS was achieved in 91% of
azithromycin and in 96% of penicillin-treated
patients. Adverse reactions, usually mild to moderate gastrointestinal complaints, occurred in
16.6% of azithromycin and 1.7% of penicillin recipients ($P < 0.001$).

Hamill reported a U.K. study of 3 days of
azithromycin compared to 10 days of penicillin
V in children 2–12 years old with group A streptococcal pharyngitis [121]. Bacteriologic eradication at day 11 was 95% in each group, and the
drugs were well tolerated. In a similar study from
Austria, Weippl compared erythromycin ethyl
succinate three times per day for 10 days to
azithromycin once daily for 3 days in children
2–12 years [122]. Bacteriologic eradication was
91% and 98% for azithromycin and eryth-

romycin, respectively, at day 12 after onset of therapy. Other assessments were comparable, with 14% azithromycin and 13% erythromycin recipients reporting gastrointestinal side effects. Three other studies of 3-day azithromycin regimens (one daily 10 mg/kg dose) in children have been published [123–125]. Two of these three studies found 3-day treatment to not reliably result in clinical and bacteriologic cure [124,125]. Currently, azithromycin is approved in the U.S. for 5-day treatment of children ≥2 years old with streptococcal pharyngitis at 12 mg/kg in a single daily dose.

Other Once-Daily Antibiotic Regimens

In addition to the azithromycin studies noted above, several clinical trials to evaluate once-daily therapy of streptococcal pharyngitis for 10 days utilizing other agents have been reported. In the 1960s there were several reports of single-daily dose oral penicillin that proved unsatisfactory, as noted above [82]. At least eight published trials have reported results with once-daily oral cefadroxil, cefixime, or cefprozil comparable to those with oral penicillin usually administered three to four times daily [126]. Despite the expected improved adherence to once-daily regimens, the cost of these nonpenicillin agents even as a single daily dose has inhibited their recommendation or widespread adoption as standard therapy for streptococcal pharyngitis.

Svartzman et al. reported a clinical trial of streptococcal pharyngitis in 1993, using once-daily amoxicillin, a much less expensive drug, for 10 days, compared to penicillin V given three to four times daily [127]. The dose of amoxicillin in this trial was 750 mg for adults and 50 mg/kg for children. Subjects included 77 children less than 10 years old, 45 11- to 20-year olds, and 22 subjects more than 20 years of age with initial positive throat cultures. No differences were observed in clinical responses, days lost from school or work, or positive cultures after 2 days of therapy (6/82 or 7% with penicillin and 3/75 or 4% with amoxicillin). At 14–21 days after starting antibiotics, 5/82 (6%) of those receiving penicillin and 0/75 (0%) receiving amoxicillin had positive throat cultures ($P < 0.004$). Unfortunately, no serotyping of organisms was performed, and the three amoxicillin recipients with

positive cultures at 2 days were crossed to penicillin treatment; it is unclear how they were classified in follow-up. Although the numbers studied in this imperfect trial were limited, this suggests that once-daily amoxicillin, which is relatively inexpensive, may be effective in streptococcal pharyngitis. A more recent study has also found that once-daily amoxicillin is effective when given for 10 days [128]. More studies of this issue are warranted.

Other Short-Duration Therapeutic Regimens

Since the Warren Air Force Base studies of the late 1940s reviewed above, 10 days of therapy has been standard for streptococcal pharyngitis to maximize eradication of GABHS [67,74]. Several trials of shorter courses of penicillin, 7 days by Schwartz et al. [129] and 5 days by Gerber et al. [130], were associated with unacceptably higher bacteriologic failure rates compared to 10-day regimens. Short-course (3 or 5 days) experience with azithromycin is reviewed above, and several reported trials have utilized 4 or 5 days of an oral cephalosporin. Milatovic compared 10 days of oral penicillin to 5 days of cefadroxil, with about 100 children in each group [131]. Bacteriologic failure rates of 11.5% with penicillin and 16% with cefadroxil were observed, a difference that was not statistically significant; an 8% failure rate had been observed with 10 days of cefadroxil by the same investigators in two other clinical trials. Portier and colleagues investigated 5 days of cefuroxime axetil or cefpodoxime proxetil twice daily in comparison to penicillin V thrice daily for 10 days in French adults with group A streptococcal pharyngitis [132]. Bacteriologic cure at completion of therapy was achieved in 8/10 (80%) cefuroxime axetil patients, 69/72 (97%) cefpodoxime proxetil recipients, and 94% of those treated with oral penicillin. Aujard et al. found that results from cefuroxime axetil (20 mg/kg/day) in two daily doses for 4 days were comparable to those for penicillin (45 mg/kg/day) in three daily doses for 10 days [133]. Additional recent studies have demonstrated satisfactory responses to a 5-day course of Cefdinir given twice daily [134], a 6-day course of amoxicillin given twice daily [135], and 5 days of cefpodoxime given twice daily [136] in patients with streptococcal pharyngitis. The cost of the cephalosporins remains an important deterrent even with abbreviated courses.

Adjunctive Therapy

The effect of anti-inflammatory or other therapy as an adjunct to antibiotics for streptococcal pharyngitis has not been explored fully. Krugman et al. showed that addition of 5 mg cortisone or 2 mg 9-alpha-fluorohydrocortisone to 600,000 U benzathine penicillin did not reduce local discomfort but that adding 5 mg prednisolone or an equal amount of aqueous procaine penicillin reduced the pain and local reactions associated with the injection without reducing the efficacy of penicillin to eradicate streptococci [137,138]. As noted above, Breese et al. reported that addition of 5 mg prednisolone was more effective than procaine in reducing injection pain and local reaction; no additional benefit was observed with 10 mg prednisolone [83]. Prednisolone also appeared to be associated with a speedier return to health as assessed by mothers.

In a trial of adjunctive therapy, O'Brien et al. studied the addition of 10 mg dexamethasone or placebo to oral erythromycin for adult streptococcal pharyngitis associated with "severe dysphagia or odynophagia" [139]. Although they reported clinical benefit without untoward effects, this therapy should not be recommended for routine use as it has not been confirmed nor evaluated in children.

Therapeutic Conclusions

Recommended treatment regimens are shown in Table 5.9. Oral penicillin V for 10 days continues to be the treatment of choice for streptococcal pharyngitis and the oral standard against which other proposed treatments must be measured. The efficacy of IM benzathine penicillin G as a single dose for acute streptococcal pharyngitis remains unchallenged as well. Nonpenicillin agents may be associated with slightly higher bacteriologic eradication rates compared to oral penicillin, probably as a result of higher rates of eradication of chronic carriage, but the additional cost appears to make use of these

Table 5.9 Recommended Treatment Regimens for Acute Streptococcal Pharyngitis

Standard	Weight <27 kg	Weight ≥27 kg	Route	Duration
Penicillin V	250 mg BID or TID	250 mg TID or 500 mg BID	Oral	10 days
Benzathine penicillin G	600,000 U	1.2 million U	IM	Once
Benzathine penicillin G + **Procaine penicillin G**	900,000 U + 300,000 U	900,000 Units[a] + 300,000 U	IM	Once
Amoxicillin	Weight <15 kg: 125 mg TID	Weight ≥ 15 kg: 250 mg TID	Oral	10 days

Penicillin-Allergic Patients	Dose	Route	Duration
Erythromycin			
Ethylsuccinate[b]	40–50 mg/kg/day BID or TID	Oral	10 days
Estolate[b]	20–40 mg/kg/day BID or TID	Oral	10 days
Clarithromycin	Children: 7.5 mg/kg/dose BID Adults: 250 mg BID	Oral	10 days
Azithromycin	Children: 12 mg/kg QD × 5 Adults: 500 mg first day, then 250 mg QD × 4	Oral	5 days
Clindamycin[c]	10–20 mg/kg/day TID	Oral	10 days
Cephalosporins[d]	Varies with antibiotic chosen	Oral	10 days

[a]Efficacy of this regimen in larger adolescents or adults is not fully established.

[b]Maximum dose is 1000 mg/day.

[c]Usual maximum dose is 450 mg/dose.

[d]First-generation cephalosporins are preferred (examples: cephalexin, cefadroxil); dosage and frequency of administration vary among agents. Avoid use in patients with history of immediate (anaphylactic) hypersensitivity to penicillin or other β-lactam antibiotics.

agents unwarranted. Additional carefully conducted clinical trials are needed, particularly involving once-daily or short-course regimens, and we have proposed principles to guide such future trials (Table 5.10) [112]. Efforts to minimize enrollment of carriers in treatment trials of acute streptococcal pharyngitis are especially important, since they seriously confound the data.

TREATMENT FAILURES, CHRONIC CARRIAGE, AND RECURRENCES

Antimicrobial treatment failures with GABHS pharyngitis are generally classified as either clinical or bacteriologic failures. However, the significance of a *clinical* treatment failure (usually defined as persistent or recurrent signs or symptoms of apparent GABHS pharyngitis) is difficult to determine in that GABHS pharyngitis is a self-limited illness even without therapy [24,42]. Without repeat isolation of the infecting strain of GABHS (i.e., true bacteriologic treatment failure), it is particularly difficult to determine the clinical significance of persistent or recurrent signs or symptoms of apparent GABHS pharyngitis.

Bacteriologic treatment failure can be classified as either a true or an apparent failure. *True* bacteriologic treatment failure is the persistence of the specific strain of GABHS that caused an acute episode of pharyngitis despite a complete course of appropriate antimicrobial therapy. *Ap-*

Table 5.10 Recommendations for Future Treatment Trials

Minimize carrier enrollment by excluding patients with viral symptoms of rhinorrhea, cough, hoarseness, or history of recurrent streptococcal isolates

Randomized controlled design, with blinded evaluations

Inclusion of patients with positive throat cultures including 1+ positives

Documentation of drug compliance

Establishment of definitions of treatment failure and success prior to enrollment

Serotyping of group A streptococci when post-therapy culture(s) are positive to assess homology

Follow-up cultures should be obtained within 14 days after completion of therapy to minimize risk of re-acquisition

Adapted from Shulman et al. [112].

parent bacteriologic treatment failure, on the other hand, occurs in a variety of situations.

Patients who have become streptococcal pharyngeal carriers (i.e., with presence of GABHS in the upper respiratory tract for prolonged periods of time without illness or evidence of an immunologic response) are the most common form of *apparent* bacteriologic treatment failures. The vast majority of asymptomatic patients who harbor GABHS in their upper respiratory tracts following a complete course of appropriate antibiotic therapy are streptococcal carriers. Streptococcal carriers are unlikely to spread the GABHS to their close contacts and are at very low risk, if any, for developing suppurative (e.g., peritonsillar abscess) or nonsuppurative (e.g., ARF) complications [140]. Chronic pharyngeal carriage of GABHS can last for 6 to 12 months or more, and the precise mechanism(s) that lead to this condition remain obscure. During the winter and spring in temperate climates, more than 20% of asymptomatic school-aged children may be GABHS carriers [29–31,140,141]. Presumably, a similar proportion of school-aged children with acute viral pharyngitis are also streptococcal carriers. Therefore, the major practical problem posed by streptococcal carriage is the difficulty prospectively of distinguishing children with true acute GABHS pharyngitis from those who are streptococcal carriers with symptoms related to intercurrent viral pharyngitis [142]. Streptococcal antibody titers are often elevated in carriers (from prior infections), and neither they nor quantitative throat cultures have proved useful to distinguish between streptococcal carriage and true infection with GABHS.

An *apparent* bacteriologic failure also can occur when a newly acquired GABHS strain is mistaken for the original infecting strain of GABHS. Serotyping of GABHS isolates, which is performed only in research settings, is necessary to evaluate this possibility. In addition, patients with acute GABHS pharyngitis from whom the infecting strain has been eradicated from the upper respiratory tract may reacquire the same strain of GABHS from a family member or other close contact and appear to be a bacteriologic failure. Finally, poor compliance with oral antimicrobials can produce an *apparent* bacteriologic treatment failure, i.e., one that erroneously suggests ineffectiveness of the antibiotic used for treatment.

Several explanations for *true* bacteriologic failures with penicillin therapy for acute GABHS pharyngitis have been proposed. It has been suggested that some GABHS may have become less sensitive to penicillin; however, there is no evidence to support this hypothesis [108,109], and no penicillin-resistant strain of GABHS has yet been identified [143]. It has also been suggested that some strains of GABHS may have developed penicillin tolerance (i.e., a discordance between the concentrations of penicillin required to inhibit and to kill the organisms). Although there are reports indicating that some strains of GABHS may be penicillin-tolerant, the role, if any, of penicillin tolerance in *true* bacteriologic treatment failure has not been established [144,145]. It has also been suggested that bacterial species within the normal pharyngeal flora can interfere with the colonization and growth of GABHS in the upper respiratory tract and influence the outcome of penicillin treatment of GABHS pharyngitis [146]. Absence of bacterial interference, therefore, might promote persistence of GABHS, but a role for the absence of such bacterial interference in *true* bacteriologic treatment failures remains unestablished [113,146–148]. Finally, it has been suggested that a variety of bacteria present in the normal pharyngeal flora produce β-lactamases that may contribute to penicillin treatment failures by inactivation of the penicillin in the upper respiratory tract. Although several investigations have addressed this issue, the findings have been inconsistent and inconclusive [113,114,144,147].

Although the specific reason(s) for bacteriologic treatment failures have yet to be determined, it has been suggested that the incidence of bacteriologic treatment failures with oral penicillin has increased in recent years [110,111]. As discussed above, however, careful analysis shows that there is little evidence to support this hypothesis [107].

Although most chronic streptococcal carriers require no medical intervention, there are specific situations in which identification and eradication of streptococcal carriage is desirable. These include the following: (1) when there is a personal or family history of ARF or rheumatic heart disease; (2) when "ping-pong" spread has occurred within a family; (3) when a family has an inordinate amount of anxiety about GABHS that can not be dispelled by counseling; (4) when outbreaks of GABHS pharyngitis occur in closed or semi-closed communities; (5) in communities with outbreaks of ARF, invasive GABHS infections, or poststreptococcal acute glomerulonephritis; and (6) when tonsillectomy is being considered seriously because of chronic carriage of GABHS or suspected recurrent streptococcal pharyngitis.

Streptococcal carriage is very difficult to eliminate with conventional penicillin therapy and, in most circumstances, therapy is not warranted. A short course of rifampin, in conjunction with penicillin, has been shown to be effective in most patients [149,150]. Rifampin can be given as a 10 mg/kg (maximum 600 mg/day) dose every 12 h for eight doses with one dose of intramuscular benzathine penicillin G [149]. A 20 mg/kg (maximum 600 mg/day) dose of rifampin every 24 h for four doses during the last 4 days of a 10-day course of oral penicillin for acute streptococcal pharyngitis decreases bacteriologic failures, perhaps by eradicating chronic carriage [150]. More recently, we reported that oral clindamycin at 20 mg/kg/day in three doses per day (maximum 450 mg/day) for 10 days is highly effective in eradicating the streptococcal carrier state [151]. Successful eradication of the carrier state makes evaluation of subsequent episodes of acute pharyngitis much easier; however, chronic carriage may recur upon re-exposure to GABHS. When a chronic carrier develops an episode of acute pharyngitis, the patient should be managed as if the carrier state were not present, i.e., if symptoms of acute streptococcal pharyngitis are present, the patient should be evaluated and treated with penicillin if the diagnosis is confirmed.

The child who experiences repeated episodes of symptomatic acute pharyngitis associated with a positive laboratory test for GABHS is a relatively common and difficult problem for the practicing physician. The fundamental question that must be addressed is whether the patient is having repeated episodes of acute GABHS pharyngitis or, alternatively, is a chronic streptococcal carrier experiencing repeated episodes of intercurrent viral pharyngitis. Such a patient is more likely to be a streptococcal carrier when

(1) the specific clinical findings (rhinorrhea, hoarseness, etc.) suggest a viral etiology; (2) the epidemiologic findings (e.g., age, season) suggest a viral etiology; (3) there is little clinical response to appropriate antimicrobial therapy; (4) throat cultures are also positive between episodes of acute pharyngitis; and (5) there is no serologic response (rising titers) to GABHS extracellular antigens (e.g., anti-streptolysin O, anti-deoxyribonuclease B). Serotyping of serial isolates of GABHS cannot be obtained easily; however, if performed in a chronic carrier, it demonstrates that all of the isolates are the same serotype. Once it has been determined that a patient experiencing repeated episodes of acute pharyngitis associated with positive throat cultures or rapid tests for GABHS is actually a chronic streptococcal carrier, the management of that patient is as described above; most do not warrant treatment.

The patient with repeated episodes of symptomatic acute pharyngitis associated with positive throat cultures or rapid tests for GABHS is likely to be experiencing repeated episodes of bona fide acute GABHS pharyngitis when (1) the clinical findings (e.g., absence of viral symptoms) suggest GABHS as the etiology; (2) the epidemiologic findings (season, age) suggest GABHS as the etiology; (3) there is the expected prompt clinical response to antibiotic therapy with each episode; (4) throat cultures are negative between episodes of pharyngitis; and (5) there is a serologic response to GABHS extracellular antigens. If serotyping of the GABHS isolates can be performed, it demonstrates that the isolates are different. Some practitioners have suggested that once it has been determined that a patient is experiencing repeated episodes of GABHS pharyngitis, prophylactic oral penicillin V (250 mg given twice daily) be given during the winter and early spring, but the efficacy of this regimen in this circumstance is unproven. In addition, tonsillectomy has been considered and has been suggested to be beneficial only in patients who meet stringent criteria: seven streptococcal pharyngitis episodes within 1 year, five episodes within each of 2 years, or three episodes within each of 3 years, with all episodes consisting of specific clinical findings [152]. A relatively small group of patients meet these criteria and may possibly benefit from tonsillectomy; any

benefit can be expected to be relatively short-lived and persist for only a 2-year period following tonsillectomy [152]. In general, we strongly discourage tonsillectomy for this indication.

COMPLICATIONS

Suppurative complications from the spread of GABHS to adjacent structures were very common before antimicrobials became available; they usually appeared within 1 week after onset of the pharyngitis. Antimicrobial therapy of GABHS pharyngitis has greatly reduced the frequency of suppurative complications caused by the spread of GABHS from the pharynx to adjacent structures. Peritonsillar abscess ("quinsy") is a suppurative complication of GABHS pharyngitis that presents with fever, severe throat pain, dysphagia, "hot potato voice," pain referred to the ear, and bulging of the peritonsillar area with asymmetry of the tonsils and displacement of the uvula. Occasionally, peritonsillar cellulitis without a well-defined abscess occurs. When a peritonsillar abscess is identified, either clinically or by imaging studies (e.g., computed tomography scan), surgical drainage is indicated. A retropharyngeal abscess may arise from extension of a GABHS infection of the pharynx or peritonsillar region into the retropharyngeal (prevertebral) space. Fever, dysphagia, drooling, stridor, extension of the neck, and a mass in the posterior pharyngeal wall may be noted. Surgical drainage is required if frank suppuration has occurred. Spread of GABHS from the pharynx via lymphatics to regional lymph nodes can cause cervical lymphadenitis that can suppurate. Otitis media, mastoiditis, and sinusitis also may occur as complications of GABHS pharyngitis.

The nonsuppurative sequelae of ARF, acute poststreptococcal glomerulonephritis, and probably reactive arthritis/synovitis are well-recognized complications of GABHS infections, although the pathogenetic mechanisms involved are still poorly understood. ARF occurs only after GABHS infection of the upper respiratory tract and not after GABHS infection of the skin. Therapy with an appropriate antimicrobial begun within 9 days after the onset of symptoms is highly effective in preventing this complication. The latent period between GABHS infection of the upper respiratory tract and the onset of ARF varies from 2 to 4 weeks. The current risk of developing ARF following an untreated episode of GABHS pharyngitis is not known precisely but appears quite low, at least in developed countries. In the early 1950s, during epidemic outbreaks of GABHS pharyngitis, the attack rate was as high as 3%. The incidence of ARF had been declining in the United States over recent decades. However, beginning in 1985, several unexpected local and regional clusters of ARF were reported, beginning with an outbreak in the Salt Lake City area [33,153]. In contrast with earlier outbreaks in this country, most of the patients were white, middle-class children from rural and suburban communities. Although it was once thought that all GABHS had equal potential to cause ARF, certain strains now appear to be particularly rheumatogenic. The reasons for the local resurgence of ARF remain to be fully elucidated but may be related to local presence of these highly rheumatogenic strains of GABHS.

In contrast to ARF, poststreptococcal acute glomerulonephritis does not appear to be prevented by antimicrobial treatment of the antecedent GABHS infection and can occur after either a GABHS infection of the skin or upper respiratory tract. The latent period for glomerulonephritis is approximately 3 weeks after a skin infection and 10 days after an upper respiratory tract infection. The incidence of acute glomerulonephritis also has been declining in the United States in recent years. This varies at least in part with the prevalence of nephritogenic strains of GABHS in the community. In pharyngitis or pyoderma outbreaks associated with nephritogenic strains, the incidence of nephritis varies from 10% to 15%.

In the absence of other features of ARF, poststreptococcal reactive arthritis (analogous to other postinfectious arthritides) probably occurs. The relationship of this entity to ARF is unclear, but it may represent *form fruste* or incomplete ARF. Those patients who fulfill the Jones criteria should be considered to have ARF [154], after other diagnoses have been excluded, and should be managed accordingly.

pp. 134-137

REFERENCES

1. Bagellardo P. Libellus de Egritudinibus Infantium, Padua, 1472. Quoted in Ruhräh J. Pediatrics of the Past. New York: Paul B. Hoeber, 1925, 28–70.
2. Roelants C. On Diseases of Infants. Louvain, 1484. Quoted in Rührah J. Pediatrics of the Past. New York: Paul B. Hoeker, 1925, 99–134.
3. Phaer T. The Boke of Children. 1545. Quoted in Ruhräh J. Pediatrics of the Past. New York: Paul B. Hoeber, 1925, 147–195.
4. Quinn RW: Did scarlet fever and rheumatic fever exist in Hippocrates' time? Rev Infect Dis 1991, 13:1243–1244.
5. Sydenham T. Medical Observations Concerning the History and Cure of Acute Diseases. London, 1676.
6. Rosen von Rosenstein N. The Diseases of Children and Their Remedies. 1771; published in English, 1776, London: T. Cadell.
7. Heberden W. An Epitome of the Diseases Incident to Children. London, 1804. Quoted in Ruhräh J. Pediatrics of the Past. New York: Paul B. Hoeber, 1925, 519–555.
8. Dewees WP. A Treatise on the Physical and Medical Treatment of Children. Philadelphia: H.C. Carey & I. Lea, 1825.
9. Smith JL. Diseases of Infancy and Childhood. Philadelphia: Henry C. Lea, 1869.
10. Henoch E. Lectures on Diseases of Children. New York: William Wood, 1882.
11. Holt LE. The Diseases of Infancy and Childhood. New York: Appleton, 1897.
12. Osler W, McCrae T. The Principles and Practices of Medicine, 9th ed. New York: Appleton, 1923.
13. Bloomfield AL, Felty AR. Bacteriologic observations on acute tonsillitis with reference to epidemiology and susceptibility. Arch Intern Med 1923; 32:483–490.
14. Holt LE. The Diseases and Infancy and Childhood, 10th ed., New York: Appleton, 1936.
15. Lancefield RC. A serologic differentiation of human and other groups of hemolytic streptococci. J Exp Med 1933; 57:571–595.
16. Woodwell D. Office visits to pediatric specialists, 1989. In: Advance Data from Vital and Health Statistics, no. 208. Hyattsville, MD: National Center for Health Statistics, 1992.
17. Denny FW, Wannamaker LW, Brink WR, Rammelkamp CH Jr, Custer EA. Prevention of rheumatic fever: treatment of the preceding streptococcic infection. N Engl J Med 1950; 143:151–153.
18. Catanzaro FJ, Stetson CA, Morris LJ, Chamovitz R, Rammelkamp CH, Stolzer BL, Perry WD. Symposium on rheumatic fever and rheumatic heart disease: the role of the streptococcus in the pathogenesis of rheumatic fever. Am J Med 1954; 17:749–756.

19. Quie PG. Development of effective programs for control of epidemic streptococcal infections. Pediatr Infect Dis J 1991; 10(Suppl):S7–S10.
20. Gastanaduy AS, Kaplan EL, Huwe BB, McKay C, Wannamaker LW. Failure of penicillin to eradicate group A streptococci during an outbreak of pharyngitis. Lancet 1980; 2:498–502.
21. Dagan R, Ferne M, Sheinis M, Alkan M, Katzenelson E. An epidemic of penicillin-tolerant group A streptococcal pharyngitis in children living in a closed community. J Infect Dis 1987; 156:514–516.
22. Rushdy AA, Cooke RPD, Iverson AM, Pickering BJ. Boarding school outbreak of group A streptococcal pharyngitis. Commun Dis Report 1995; 5:R106–R108.
23. Smith TD, Wilkinson V, Kaplan EL. Group a streptococcus-associated upper respiratory tract infections in a day-care center. Pediatrics 1989; 83:380–384.
24. Brink WR, Rammelkamp CH Jr, Denny FW, Wannamaker LW. Effect of penicillin and aureomycin on the natural course of streptococcal tonsillitis and pharyngitis. Am J Med 1951; 10:300–308.
25. Randolph MF, Gerber MA, DeMeo KK, Wright L. Effect of antibiotic therapy on the clinical course of streptococcal pharyngitis. J Pediatr 1985; 106:870–875.
26. Wannamaker LW, Denny FW, Perry WD, Rammelkamp CH, Eckhardt GC, Houser H, Hahn EO. The effect of penicillin prophylaxis on streptococcal disease rates and the carrier state. N Engl J Med 1953; 249:1–7.
27. Brundage JF, Gunzenhauser JD, Longfield JN, Rubertone MV, Ludwig SL, Rubin FA, Kaplan EL. Epidemiology and control of acute respiratory diseases with emphasis on group A betathemolytic streptococcus: a decade of U.S. Army experience. Pediatrics 1996; 97:964–970.
28. Taranta A, Markowitz M. Rheumatic Fever, 2nd ed. London: Kluwer, 1989.
29. Quinn RW, Denny FW, Riley HD. Natural occurrence of hemolytic streptococci in normal school children. Am J Public Health 1957; 47:995–1009.
30. Cornfeld D, Warner G, Weaver R, Bellows MT, Hubbard JP. Streptococcal infection in a school population: preliminary report. Ann Intern Med 1958; 49:1305–1319.
31. Ginsburg CM, McCracken GH, Crow SD, Lancaster K. Seroepidemiology of the group A streptococcal carriage state in a private pediatric practice. Am J Dis Child 1985; 139:614–617.
32. Karoui R, Majeed HA, Yousof AM, Hussain K. Hemolytic streptococci and streptococcal antibodies in normal school children in Kuwait. Am J Epidemiol 1982; 116:709–721.
33. Veasey LG, Wiedmeier SE, Orsmond GS, Ruttenberg MM, Hill HR. Resurgence of acute rheumatic fever in the intermountain area of the United States. N Engl J Med 1987; 316:421–427.
34. Kaplan EL. Recent epidemiology of group A streptococcal infections in North America and abroad: an overview. Pediatrics 1996; 97:945–948.
35. Anthony B, Kaplan E, Wannamaker L, Chapman S. The dynamics of streptococcal infections in defined population of children: serotypes associated with skin and respiratory infections. Am J Epidemiol 1976; 104:652–666.
36. Cleary PP, Kaplan EL, Handley JP, Schlievert PM. Clonal basis for resurgence of serious Streptococcus pyogenes disease in the 1980s. Lancet 1992; 339:518–521.
37. Dick GF, Dick GH. Scarlet Fever. Chicago: Yearbook Medical, 1938.
38. Wilson LG. The historical riddle of milk-borne scarlet fever. Bull Hist Med 1986; 60:321–342.
39. Farley TA, Wilson SA, Mahoney F, Kelso KY, Johnson DR, Kaplan EL. Direct inoculation of food as the cause of an outbreak of group A streptococcal pharyngitis. J Infect Dis 1993; 167:1232–1235.
40. Gallo G, Berzero R, Caftai N, Orefici G. An outbreak of group A food-borne streptococcal pharyngitis. Eur J Epidemiol 1992; 18:292–297.
41. Shemesh E, Fischel T, Goldstein N, Alkan M, Livneh A. An outbreak of foodborne streptococcal throat infection. Isr J Med Sci 1994; 30:275–278.
42. Denny FW, Wannamaker LW, Hahn EO. Comparative effects of penicillin, aureomycin and terramycin on streptococcal tonsillitis and pharyngitis. Pediatrics 1953; 11:7–14.
43. Denny FW. Effect of treatment on streptococcal pharyngitis: is the issue really settled? Pediatr Infect Dis J 1985; 4:352–354.
44. Breese BB, Disney FW. The accuracy of diagnosis of beta streptococcal infections on clinical grounds. J Pediatr 1954; 44:670–673.
45. Shulman ST. Streptococcal pharyngitis: diagnostic considerations. Pediatr Infect Dis J 1994; 13:567–571.
46. Edwards KM. Resisting the urge to prescribe. J Pediatr 1996; 128:729–730.
47. Wilcox MH, Winstanley TG, Douglas CWI, Spencer RC. Susceptibility of α-haemolytic streptococci causing endocarditis. J Antimicrob Chemother 1993; 32:63–69.
48. Seppala H, Nissinen A, Jarvinen H, Huovinen P. Resistance to erythromycin in group A streptococci. N Engl J Med 1992; 326:292–297.
49. Baquero F, Martinez-Beltran J, Loza E. A review of antibiotic resistance patterns of Streptococcus pneumoniae in Europe. J Antimicrob Chemother 1991; 28(Suppi C):31–38.
50. Wannamaker LW. Diagnosis of pharyngitis: clinical and epidemiologic features. In: Shulman ST (ed). Pharyngitis: Management in an Era of

Declining Rheumatic Fever. New York: Praeger, 1984; 33–46.

51. Breese BB. A simple scorecard for the tentative diagnosis of streptococcal pharyngitis. Am J Dis Child 1977; 131:514–517.

52. Poses RM, Cebul RD, Collins M, Fager SS. The accuracy of experienced physicians' probability estimates for patients with sore throats. JAMA 1985; 254:925–929.

53. Gerber MA. Diagnosis of pharyngitis: methodology of throat culture. In: Shulman ST (ed). Pharyngitis: Management in an Era of Declining Rheumatic Fever. New York: Praeger, 1984; 61–72.

54. Gunn BA. SXT and Taxo A disks for presumptive identification of group A and G streptococci in throat cultures. J Clin Microbiol 1976; 4:192–194.

55. Murray PR, Wold AD, Hall MM, Washington JA. Bacitracin differentiation for presumptive identification of group A beta-hemolytic streptococci: comparison of primary and purified plate testing. J Pediatr 1976; 89:576–579.

56. Gerber MA. Comparison of throat cultures and rapid strep tests for diagnosis of streptococcal pharyngitis. Pediatr Infect Dis J 1989; 8:820–824.

57. Dobkin D, Shulman ST. Evaluation of an ELISA for group A streptococcal antigen for diagnosis of pharyngitis. J Pediatr 1987; 110:566–569.

58. Harbeck RJ, Teague J, Crossen GR, Maul DM, Childers PL. Novel rapid optical immunoassay technique for detection for group A streptococci from pharyngeal specimens: comparison with standard culture methods. J Clin Microbiol 1993; 31:839–844.

59. Gerber MA, Tanz RR, Kabat W, Dennis E, Bell G, Kaplan EL, Shulman ST. Optical immunoassay test for group A beta hemolytic streptococcal pharyngitis. JAMA 1997; 277:899–903.

60. Pichichero ME, Disney FA, Talpey WB, Hoekelman RA. Adverse and beneficial effects of immediate treatment of group A beta-hemolytic streptococcal pharyngitis with penicillin. Pediatr Infect Dis J 1987; 635–643.

61. Gerber MA, Randolph MF, DeMeo KK, Kaplan EL. Lack of impact of early antibiotic therapy for streptococcal pharyngitis on recurrence rates. J Pediatr 1990; 117:653–658.

62. Henderson EL, Meier FA, Fortner CA, Zanga JR. Physician bias and the interpretation of rapid tests for group A streptococcal pharyngitis. Am J Dis Child 1988; 142:405–406.

63. Kaplan EL, Howe BH. The sensitivity and specificity of an agglutination test for antibodies to streptococcal extracellular antigens. Pediatrics 1980; 96:367–373.

64. Cochi SL, Fraser DW, Hightower AW, Facklam RR, Broome CV. Diagnosis and treatment of streptococcal pharyngitis: survey of U.S. medical practitioners. In: Shulman ST (ed). Pharyngitis: Management in an Era of Declining Rheumatic Fever. New York: Praeger, 1984.

65. Schwartz B, Fries S, Fitzgibbon AM, Lipman H. Pediatricians' diagnostic approach to pharyngitis and impact of CLIA 1988 on office diagnostic tests. JAMA 1994; 271:234–238.

66. Hofer C, Binns HJ, Tanz RR. Strategies for managing group A streptococcal (GABHS) pharyngitis: a survey of board certified pediatricians. Arch Pediatr Adolesc Med 1997; 151:824–839.

67. Dajani A, Taubert K, Ferrieri P, Peter G, Shulman ST. Treatment of acute streptococcal pharyngitis and prevention of rheumatic fever. Pediatrics 1995; 96:758–765.

68. Committee on Infectious Diseases, American Academy of Pediatrics. 1997 Redbook, 24th ed. Elk Grove Village, IL, AAP: 1997.

69. World Health Organization. Rheumatic Fever. WHO Technical Report Series #764. Geneva: World Health Organization, 1988.

70. Coburn AF. Prevention of respiratory tract bacterial infections by sulfadiazine prophylaxis in United States Navy. JAMA 1944; 126:88–92.

71. Kuttner AG, Reyersbach G. The prevention of streptococcal upper respiratory infections and rheumatic fever recurrences in rheumatic children by prophylactic sulfanilamide. J Clin Invest 1943; 22:77–85.

72. Hodges RG. The use of sulfadiazine as a prophylactic against respiratory disease. N Engl J Med 1944; 231:817–820.

73. Jersild T. Penicillin therapy in scarlet fever and complicating otitis. Lancet 1948; 1:671–673.

74. Wannamaker LW, Rammelkamp CH, Denny FW, Brink WR, Houser HB, Hahn EO. Prophylaxis of acute rheumatic fever. Am J Med 1951; 10:673–695.

75. Chamovitz R, Catanzaro FJ, Stetson CA, Rammelkamp CH. Prevention of rheumatic fever by treatment of previous streptococcal infections. N Engl J Med 1954; 251:466–470.

76. Houser HB, Eckhardt GC, Hahn EO, Denny FW, Wannamaker LW, Rammelkamp CH. Effect of aureomycin treatment of streptococcal sore throat on the streptococcal carrier state, the immunologic response of the host, and the incidence of acute rheumatic fever. Pediatrics 1953; 12:593–606.

77. Jones TD. Prevention of rheumatic fever and bacterial endocarditis through control of streptococcal infections. Circulation 1955; 11:317–320.

78. Breese BB. Treatment of beta-hemolytic streptococcic infections in the home. JAMA 1953; 152:10–14.

79. Breese BB, Disney FA. The successful treatment of beta-hemolytic streptococcal infections in children with a single injection of repository penicillin. Pediatrics 1955; 15:516–519.

80. Breese BB, Disney FA. A comparison of intramuscular and oral benzathine penicillin G in the treatment of streptococcal infections in children. J Pediatr 1957; 51:157–162.
81. Breese BB, Disney FA. Penicillin in the treatment of streptococcal infections. N Engl J Med 1958; 259:57–62.
82. Breese BB, Disney FA, Talpey WB. Penicillin in streptococcal infections. Am J Dis Child 1965; 110:125–130.
83. Breese BB, Disney FA, Talpey WB. Improvement in local tolerance and therapeutic effectiveness of benzathine penicillin. Am J Dis Child 1960; 99:149–153.
84. Bass JW, Crast FW, Knowles CP, Onufer CN. Streptococcal pharyngitis in children: comparison of four treatment schedules with intramuscular penicillin G benzathine. JAMA 1976; 235:1112–1116.
85. Stillerman M, Bernstein SH. Streptococcal pharyngitis therapy. Am J Dis Child 1964; 197:35–46.
86. Rosenstein BJ, Markowitz M, Goldstein E, Kramer I, O'Mansky B, Seidel H, Sigler A, Tramer A. Factors involved in treatment failures following oral penicillin therapy of streptococcal pharyngitis. J Pediatr 1968; 73:513–520.
87. Haight TH. Erythromycin therapy of respiratory infections: I. Controlled studies on the comparative efficacy of erythromycin and penicillin in scarlet fever. J Lab Clin Med 1954; 43:15–30.
88. Stillerman M, Bernstein SH, Smith ML, Gittelson SB, Karelitz S. Antibiotics in the treatment of beta-hemolytic streptococcal pharyngitis: factors influencing the results. Pediatrics 1960; 25:27–34.
89. Stillerman M, Bernstein SH, Smith ML, Gorvey JD. Erythromycin propionate and potassium penicillin V in the treatment of group A streptococcal pharyngitis. Pediatrics 1963; 31:22–28.
90. Moffett HL, Cramblett HG, Black JP. Erythromycin estolate and phenoxymethyl penicillin in the treatment of streptococcal pharyngitis. Antimicrob Agents Chemother 1963; 3:759–763.
91. Breese BB, Disney FA, Talpey WB. Beta-hemolytic streptococcal illness: a comparison of the effectiveness of penicillin G, triacetyloleandomycin and erythromycin estolate. Am J Dis Child 1966; 111:128–130.
92. Howie VM, Ploussard JH. Compliance dose-response relationships in streptococcal pharyngitis. Am J Dis Child 1976; 123:18–20.
93. Levine MK, Berman JD. A comparison of clindamycin and erythromycin in beta-hemolytic streptococcal infections. J Med Assoc Ga 1972; 61:108–111.
94. Shapera RM, Hable KA, Matsen JM. Erythromycin therapy twice daily for streptococcal pharyngitis. JAMA 1973; 226:531–535.
95. Breese BB, Disney FA, Talpey WB, Green JL, Tobin J. Streptococcal infections in children: comparison of the therapeutic effectiveness of erythromycin administered twice-daily with erythromycin, penicillin phenoxymethyl and clindamycin administered three times daily. Am J Dis Child 1974; 128:457–460.
96. Derrick CW, Dillon HC. Erythromycin therapy for streptococcal pharyngitis. Am J Dis Child 1976; 130:175–178.
97. Breese BB, Disney FA, Green JL, Talpey WB. The treatment of beta-hemolytic streptococcal pharyngitis: comparison of amoxicillin, erythromycin estolate and penicillin V. Clin Pediatr (Phila) 1977; 16:460–463.
98. Ryan D, Dreher GH, Hurst JA. Estolate and stearate forms of erythromycin in the treatment of acute beta-hemolytic streptococcal pharyngitis. Med J Aust 1973; 1:20–24.
99. Janicki RS, Garnham JC, Worland MC, Grundy WE, Thomas JR. Comparison of erythromycin ethylsuccinate, stearate and estolate treatments of group A streptococcal infections of the upper respiratory tract. Clin Pediatr (Phila) 1975; 14:1098–1107.
100. Derrick CW, Dillon HC. Streptococcal pharyngitis therapy: a comparison of two erythromycin formulations. Am J Dis Child 1979; 133:1146–1148.
101. Disney FA, Breese BB, Green JL, Talpey WB, Towbin JR. Cephalexin and penicillin therapy of childhood beta-hemolytic streptococcal infections. Postgrad Med J 1971; 47:47–51.
102. Stillerman M, Isenberg HD. Streptococcal pharyngitis therapy: comparison of cyclacillin, cephalexin and potassium penicillin V. Antimicrob Agents Chemother 1970; 10:270–273.
103. Matsen JM, Torstenson O, Siegel SE, Bacaner H. Use of available dosage forms of cephalexin in clinical comparison with phenoxymethyl penicillin and benzathine penicillin in the treatment of streptococcal pharyngitis in children. Antimicrob Agents Chemother 1974; 6:501–506.
104. Derrick CW, Dillon HC. Therapy for prevention of acute rheumatic fever. Circulation 1974; 50:38–40.
105. Dillon HC. Antibiotic therapy: influence of duration, frequency, route of administration and compliance. In: Shulman ST (ed). Pharyngitis: Management in an Era of Declining Rheumatic Fever. New York: Praeger, 1984; 133–151.
106. Stillerman M. Comparison of oral cephalosporins with penicillin therapy for group A streptococcal pharyngitis. Pediatr Infect Dis J 1986; 5:649–654.
107. Markowitz M, Gerber MA, Kaplan EL. Treatment of streptococcal pharyngotonsillitis: reports of penicillin's demise are premature. J Pediatr 1993; 123:679–685.
108. Jelinkova J, Urbaskova P, Motlova J, Jelinek J, Krizova P. Long-term follow-up of susceptibil-

ity of *Streptococcus pyogenes* to penicillin. In: Totolian A (ed). Pathogenic Streptococci: Present and Future. St. Petersburg: Lancer, 1994; 59–61.

109. Macris MH, Hartman N, Murray B, Klein RF, Roberts RB, Kaplan EL, Horn D, Zabriskie JB. Studies of the continuing susceptibility of group A streptococcal strains to penicillin during eight decades. Pediatr Infect Dis J 1998; 17:377–381.

110. Pichichero ME, Margolis PA. A comparison of cephalosporins and penicillins in the treatment of group A beta-hemolytic streptococcal pharyngitis. Pediatr Infect Dis J 1991; 10:275–281.

111. Pichichero ME. Cephalosporins are superior to penicillin for treatment of streptococcal tonsillopharyngitis. Pediatr Infect Dis J 1993; 12:268–274.

112. Shulman ST, Gerber MA, Tanz RR, Markowitz M. Streptococcal pharyngitis. The case for penicillin therapy. Pediatr Infect Dis J 1994; 13:1–7.

113. Gerber MA, Tanz RR, Kabat W, Bell GL, Siddiqui PN, Lerer TJ, Lepow ML, Kaplan EL, Shulman ST. Potential mechanisms for failure to eradicate group A streptococci from the pharynx. Pediatrics 1999 (in press).

114. Tanz RR, Shulman ST, Sroka PA, Marubio S, Brook I, Yogev R. Lack of influence of beta-lactamase-producing flora on recovery of group A streptococci after treatment of acute pharyngitis. J Pediatr 1990; 117:859–863.

115. Disney FA, Dillon H, Blumer JL, Dudding BA, McLinn SE, Nelson DB, Selbst SM. Cephalexin and penicillin in the treatment of group A beta-hemolytic streptococcal throat infections. Am J Dis Child 1992; 146:1324–1327.

116. Neu HC. Clinical microbiology of azithromycin. Am J Med 1991; 91:(Suppl.3A):12S–18S.

117. Stein GE, Christensen S, Mummaw N. Comparative study of clarithromycin and penicillin V in the treatment of streptococcal pharyngitis. Eur J Clin Microbiol Infect Dis 1991; 10:949–953.

118. Schrock CG. Clarithromycin vs. penicillin in the treatment of streptococcal pharyngitis. J Fam Pract 1992; 35:622–626.

119. Karma P, Pukander J, Pentilla M. Azithromycin concentrations in sinus fluid and mucosa after oral administration. Eur J Clin Microbiol Infect Dis 1991; 10:856–859.

120. Hooten TM. Comparison of azithromycin and penicillin V for the treatment of streptococcal pharyngitis. Am J Med 1991; 91(Suppl. 3A):23S–26S.

121. Hamill J. Multicentre evaluation of azithromycin and penicillin V in the treatment of acute streptococcal pharyngitis and tonsillitis in children. J Antimicrob Chemother 1993; 31(Suppl E):89–94.

122. Weippl G. Multicentre comparison of azithromycin vs. erythromycin in the treatment of paediatric

pharyngitis or tonsillitis caused by group A streptococci. J Antimicrob Chemother 1993; 31(Suppl E):95–101.

123. O'Doherty B. Azithromycin versus penicillin V in treatment of pediatric pharyngitis. Eur J Microb Infect Dis 1996; 15:718–724.

124. Schaad UB, Heynen G. Evaluation of the efficacy, safety and toleration of azithromycin vs. penicillin V in streptococcal pharyngitis. Pediatr Infect Dis J 1996; 15:791–795.

125. Pacifico L, Scopetti F, Ranucci A, Chiesa C. Comparative efficacy and safety of 3-day azithromycin and 10-day penicillin V in streptococcal pharyngitis. Antimicrob Agents Chemother 1996; 40:1005–1008.

126. McCarthy JM. Comparative efficacy and safety of cefprozil versus penicillin, cefaclor and erythromycin in the treatment of streptococcal pharyngitis and tonsillitis. Eur J Clin Microbiol Infect Dis 1994; 13:846–850.

127. Svartzman P, Tabenkin H, Rosentzwaig A, Dolginov F. Treatment of streptococcal pharyngitis with amoxicillin once a day. BMJ 1993; 306:1170–1172.

128. Feder HM, Gerber MA, Randolph MF, Kaplan EL. Once daily amoxicillin therapy for the treatment of group A streptococcal pharyngitis [Abstract]. Pediatr Res 1997; 41:119a.

129. Schwartz RH, Wientzen RL Jr, Pedreira F, Guandolo VL. Penicillin V for group A streptococcal pharyngitis: a randomized trial of seven vs. ten days' therapy. JAMA 1981; 246:1790–1795.

130. Gerber MA, Randolph MF, Chanatry J, Kaplan EL. Five vs. ten days of penicillin V therapy for streptococcal pharyngitis. Am J Dis Child 1987; 141:224–227.

131. Milatovic D. Evaluation of cefadroxil, penicillin and erythromycin in the treatment of streptococcal tonsillopharyngitis. Pediatr Infect Dis J 1991;10:S61–S63.

132. Portier H, Chavanet P, Gouyon JB, Guetat F. Five day treatment of pharyngitis with cefpodoxime proxetil. J Antimicrob Chemother 1990; 26:(Suppl E):79–85.

133. Aujard Y, Boucot I, Brahami N, Bingen E. Comparative efficacy and safety of four day cefuroxime axetil and ten day penicillin treatment of group A beta-hemolytic streptococcal pharyngitis in children. Pediatr Infect Dis J 1995; 14:295–300.

134. Tack KJ, Hedrick JA, Rothstein E, Keyserling C. Study of 5-day cefdinir treatment for streptococcal pharyngitis. Arch Pediatr Adolesc Med 1997; 151:45–49.

135. Cohen R, Levy C, Doit C, De La Rocque F, Bingen E. Six-day amoxicillin vs. ten-day penicillin V therapy for group A streptococcal tonsillopharyngitis. Pediatr Infect Dis J 1996; 15:678–682.

136. Dajani AS. Pharyngitis/tonsillitis: European and U.S. experience with cefpodoxime proxetil. Pediatr Infect Dis J 1995; 14(4 Suppl):S7–S11.

137. Krugman S, Ebin EV. Improved local tolerance to benzathine penicillin G. Pediatrics 1958; 21:243–246.

138. Krugman S, Powell VE. Local tolerance to penicillin. J Pediatr 1956; 49:699–702.

139. O'Brien JF, Meade JL, Flak JL. Dexamethasone as adjuvant therapy for severe acute pharyngitis. Ann Emerg Med 1993; 22:212–215.

140. Kaplan EL. The group A streptococcal carrier state: an enigma. J Pediatr 1980; 97:337–345.

141. Quinn RW, Federspiel CF. The occurrence of streptococci in school children in Nashville, Tennessee, 1961–1967. Am J Epidemiol 1973; 97:22–33.

142. Kaplan EL, Gastanaduy AS, Huwe B. The role of the carrier in treatment failures after therapy for group A streptococci in the upper respiratory tract. J Lab Clin Med 1981; 98:326–335.

143. Coonan KM, Kaplan EL. In vitro susceptibility of recent North American group A streptococcal isolates to eleven oral antibiotics. Pediatr Infect Dis J 1994; 13:630–635.

144. Smith TD, Huskins WC, Kim KS, Kaplan EL. Efficacy of beta-lactamase-resistant penicillin and influence of penicillin tolerance in eradicating streptococci from the pharynx after failure of penicillin therapy for group A streptococcal pharyngitis. J Pediatr 1987; 110:777–782.

145. Kim KS, Kaplan EL. Association of penicillin tolerance with failure to eradicate group A streptococci from patients with pharyngitis. J Pediatr 1985; 107:681–684.

146. Crowe CC, Sanders WE Jr, Longley S. Bacterial interference. Role of the normal throat flora in prevention of colonization of group A streptococcus. J Infect Dis 1973; 128:527–532.

147. Roos K, Grahn E, Holm SE. Evaluation of beta-lactamase activity and microbial interference in treatment failures of acute streptococcal tonsillitis. Scand J Infect Dis 1986; 18:313–319.

148. Huskins WC, Kaplan EL. Inhibitory substances produced by *Streptococcus salivarius* and colonization of the upper respiratory tract with group A streptococci. Epidemiol Infect 1989; 102:401–412.

149. Tanz RR, Shulman ST, Barthel MJ, Willert C, Yogev R. Penicillin plus rifampin eradicates pharyngeal carriage of group A streptococci. J Pediatr 1985; 106:876–880.

150. Chaudhary S, Bilinsky SA, Hennessy JL, Bisno AL. Penicillin V and rifampin for the treatment of group A streptococcal pharyngitis: a randomized trial of 10 days penicillin vs. 10 days penicillin with rifampin during the final 4 days of therapy. J Pediatr 1985; 106:481–486.

151. Tanz RR, Poncher JR, Corydon KE, Kabat W, Yogev R, Shulman ST. Clindamycin treatment of chronic pharyngeal carriage of group A streptococci. J Pediatr 1991; 119:123–136.

152. Paradise JL, Bluestone CD, Bachman RZ, Colborn DK. Efficacy of tonsillectomy for recurrent throat infection in severely affected children. N Engl J Med 1984; 310:674–683.

153. Veasy LG, Tani LY, Hill HR. Persistence of acute rheumatic fever in the intermountain area of the United States. J Pediatr 1994; 124:9–16.

154. Ayoub EM, Ahmed S. Update on complications of group A streptococcal infections. Curr Prob Pediatr 1997; 27:90–101.

6

Rheumatic Fever Pathogenesis

ELIA M. AYOUB
MALAK KOTB
MADELEINE W. CUNNINGHAM

Rheumatic fever can be classified as an autoimmune collagen-vascular disease or a postinfectious connective tissue disorder. The disease manifests after a latency period of about 3 weeks following group A streptococcal infection of the upper respiratory tract. During the latency period, the affected individual is asymptomatic. The disease is expressed then as a nonpurulent inflammation of certain organs, mainly the joints, the heart, or the brain.

Knowledge of the association of rheumatic fever and rheumatic heart disease with group A streptococcal infection dates back to the early part of the twentieth century. Intense efforts by a number of investigators over the past five decades have helped clarify certain facets of the pathogenesis of rheumatic fever. However, the exact mechanism by which infection with the group A streptococcus leads to this unique complication in certain individuals is still an enigma. The current hypothesis of the pathogenesis of rheumatic fever is outlined in Figure 6.1. A fundamental component of this hypothesis is the uniqueness of the host and the organism initiating the disease: only certain individuals are prone to this disease and only certain strains of group A streptococci are capable of initiating the inflammatory reaction that leads to the expression of the disease in the susceptible human host. The mechanism underlying this inflammatory process

appears to be immune mediated and may be related either to the formation of antibodies directed against streptococcal antigens that cross-react with tissue components in the affected organs or to the stimulation of cell-mediated immune reactivity that is noxious to these tissues. The characteristics of the group A streptococcus and the susceptible host, as well as the mechanism leading to tissue inflammation and injury will be described in this chapter.

FACTORS INVOLVED IN HOST SUSCEPTIBILITY TO RHEUMATIC FEVER

Evidence that indirectly supports the concept of susceptibility to rheumatic fever can be divided into two categories: epidemiologic and immunologic. Recent data on the molecular genetics of the human leukocyte antigens provide more direct support for a genetic basis for susceptibility to this disease. However, it can be stated that to date, no single trait has been identified that can be used to cull out individuals susceptible to rheumatic fever from among a general population. Several reasons account for this problem. These include the fact that the pathogenesis of rheumatic fever involves factors peculiar to the inciting infectious agent and the

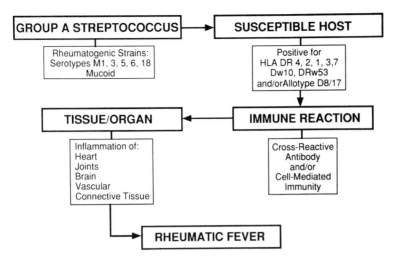

Figure 6.1 Pathogenesis of rheumatic fever. (From Moss and Adams [208], with permission.)

host and that to date, we have been unable to establish an animal model for this disease. Unfortunately, the only definitive criterion that is currently available for susceptibility to rheumatic fever is that the individual has been afflicted by the disease.

Epidemiological Evidence

Studies by Newsholme, reported one century ago on the epidemiology of rheumatic fever, were first to provide a clue regarding the "hereditary" nature of this disease [1]. Subsequent observations on the attack rates of rheumatic fever, its familiar incidence, and racial or ethnic differences in incidence and clinical expression of the disease have lent support to this concept. It is well documented that rheumatic fever occurs in 2%–3% of previously normal individuals following proven group A streptococcal pharyngitis. However, this attack rate is markedly higher (30%–80%) for individuals who have had a previous attack of rheumatic fever. Observations on the high incidence of rheumatic fever in families was well described in surveys made by the British Medical Council [2]. One of the most impressive examples of such a family was reported by Pickles, who documented rheumatic fever or mitral stenosis in 23 of 53 descendants of a man who had rheumatic fever [3]. These observations prompted further studies on the familial incidence of this disease. Read et al. [4] and Schwent-

ker [5] revealed that rheumatic fever occurred 4 to 8 times more frequently in relatives of patients with this disease. On the basis of these observations and those reported by Wilson and Schweitzer [6], it was concluded that susceptibility to rheumatic fever was inherited through a recessive autosomal gene.

In an attempt to exclude the influence of environmental factors on the above observations, DiSciascio and Taranta examined the incidence of rheumatic fever in monozygotic and dyzygotic twins [7]. The concordance rate for disease was 19% in monozygotic twins and 2.5% in dyzygotic twins. Additional studies showed that genetic factors appear to play a more prominent role in determining the clinical manifestations of the disease. Arthritis and Sydenham's chorea were more concordant in monozygotic than in dyzygotic twins [7]. These observations suggest that genetic factors may play a minor role in susceptibility to rheumatic fever, but a stronger role in determining the manifestations of the disease in patients who acquire rheumatic fever.

Increased incidence of rheumatic fever in certain ethnic populations or racial extractions was recorded by several investigators. Early studies suggested that the incidence of rheumatic fever was higher in the Irish population of New York [8]. More recently, a higher incidence of the disease was reported in African Americans, Hispanics, and Native American Indians. In addition, patients from these ethnic groups tend to have a more severe illness when they acquire rheumatic fever than their Caucasian counterparts [9–11] Similar observations on racial susceptibility have been reported from other countries. In Hawaii, the risk for acquiring rheumatic fever is 88 times more in Samoan children than in the Caucasian population of those islands [12,13]. Studies on the incidence of the disease in New Zealand revealed that the incidence in the Maori population is 60 to 100 times greater than in the Caucasian population of that country and 20 times higher than its incidence in the American African population in the United States [11–14]. Some of these differences could be ascribed to socioeconomic conditions. However, two observations tend to minimize the role of this variable. The first is that the increased incidence of rheumatic fever in the Maori population in New Zealand is seen at all socioeconomic strata [14]. The second is the finding of an increased incidence of rheumatic fever in African-American children in Miami compared to the Caucasian population of the same socioeconomic status in that city [15]. These findings suggest that hereditary factors indigent to those ethnic groups influence susceptibility to rheumatic fever.

Immunologic Evidence

Several investigators have proposed that an innate state of hyperimmune responsiveness is the underlying mechanism in the pathogenesis of rheumatic fever. To ascertain this possibility, many of these investigators looked for evidence of immune hyperresponsiveness to nonstreptococcal and to streptococcal antigens.

Immune Response to Nonstreptococcal Antigens

Initial studies compared the immune response of patients with rheumatic fever with the response of nonrheumatic controls to a variety of antigens, including isologous red blood cells, influenza A and B virus vaccines, typhoid vaccine, pneumococcal polysaccharide, and diphtheria toxoid. No consistent differences could be documented between the immunologic response of patients with rheumatic fever and their controls.

The first study to provide evidence for a "hyperimmune status" in patients with rheumatic fever was conducted by Rejholec [16]. In this prospective study, 998 school children were immunized with *Brucella abortus* vaccine and the immune response determined by measuring the serum antibody titer to the brucella antigen. The children were followed for 9 months and the incidence of streptococcal pharyngitis and acute rheumatic fever in that population was documented. Twelve patients in this cohort developed rheumatic fever following streptococcal pharyngitis. The occurrence of rheumatic fever in these children was then correlated with their brucella antibody titer. This correlation revealed that children who acquired rheumatic fever belonged to a group that had the highest antibody response to the brucella vaccine. Subsequent studies by Meiselas et al. [17] confirmed the hyperimmune response of patients with rheumatic fever to brucella antigen. Although these findings support the concept of hyperimmune responsiveness of patients who develop rheumatic fever to the brucella antigen, no explanation has been offered to date for the hyperimmune response of these patients to this specific antigen.

Immune Response to Streptococcal Antigens

The first description of the occurrence of hyperresponsiveness to streptococcal antigens in patients with rheumatic fever was based on the finding that patients with this disease had significantly higher levels of antibodies to the extracellular group A streptococcal antigens (ASO, antistreptokinase, antihyaluronidase) than patients with uncomplicated group A streptococcal infections [18]. Our studies on the antibody response to the extracellular streptococcal antigens (ASO, anti-DNase, B, anti-NADase) failed to show a consistent difference between patients with acute rheumatic fever and patients with poststreptococcal glomerulonephritis [19]. Evidence for an exaggerated response to a streptococcal antigen was obtained from studies on the response of patients with rheumatic fever to a streptococcal cellular antigen, the group-specific carbohydrate. Although a comparison of the titers of this antibody during the acute disease revealed no differences between patients with rheumatic fever and those with glomerulonephritis, significant differences were found in the titers of antibody to this antigen during the subacute and chronic phase of the disease [20–22]. While antibody to the group-specific carbohydrate declined to normal levels within 1 to 2 years in patients who had glomerulonephritis and also in patients with rheumatic fever who did not have mitral valve involvement, the level of this antibody remained elevated in patients with residual mitral valve disease. No such difference was encountered in the pattern of the antibody response to the extracellular antigens. These findings indicate that patients with rheumatic mitral valve disease have a peculiar hyperimmune response to the group A streptococcal carbohydrate.

The above observation is of particular significance because of studies revealing that the immune response of laboratory animals to the group A streptococcal carbohydrate is under genetic control. Certain animals are hyperresponders to this antigen while others are not and inbreeding studies show that this trait is maintained in the offspring of these animals [23,24]. Further evidence for genetic control of the response to the streptococcal cell-wall carbohydrate in animals was obtained in studies showing that genetically related animals produce idiotypically related antibodies to this antigen, that the idiotypic determinants of this antibody segregate in a Mendelian fashion, and that the clonotypes of the IgG form of the antibodies remain constant and are predetermined [25–27]. Similar observations on the genetic control of antibody to the streptococcal carbohydrate in humans were reported by Sasazuki et al. [28] who also found high and low responders to this antigen in humans. The high and low antibody responders were segregated to different families. Pedigree studies of these families suggested that the high response to this antigen was controlled by a single recessive gene whereas the low response was controlled by a dominant gene. Interestingly, the analysis of these data indicated that the gene controlling the low response to the streptococcal cell-wall antigen was closely linked to an HLA gene.

Evidence Derived from Studies of Genetic Markers

Early studies on the secretor status of ABO blood group substances in saliva had suggested an association of nonsecretor status with susceptibility to rheumatic fever. This observation could not be confirmed in subsequent studies [29–32]. These studies and the above observations were instrumental in redirecting the search for genetic markers of susceptibility to rheumatic fever to a potential association with genes within the major histocompatibility locus. The advent of data on the linkage between inheritance of human leukocyte antigens and genetic predisposition to certain diseases prompted investigators to examine the association of rheumatic fever with inheritance of HLA antigens. HLA molecules are encoded by genes present on the short arm of the sixth chromosome. These molecules are divided into class I (HLA-A, -B, and -C) and class II antigens (HLA-DR, -DQ, and -DP). The class I antigens are expressed on non-nucleated cells while the class II antigens are present on outer membrane of antigen-presenting cells and B lymphocytes where they function as antigen receptors. Because of the described association of ankylosing spondylitis with a class I antigen, HLA-B27, initial studies focused on examining an association between rheumatic fever and class I antigens. Positive associations between a number of alleles, including HLA-A3, -A10, -A23, -A25, -A29, -Aw30/31, -Aw33, -B5, -B7, -B8, -Bw17, and -Bw41, and negative associations with some of these and other alleles, HLA-A2, -A3, -A10, -A28, and -Bw16, were described [33–38].

The inconsistency of these findings prompted subsequent investigators to refocus attention on the association of rheumatic fever with class II antigens (Table 6.1). One of the first studies to address this association was reported from our laboratory [39,40]. The study, which was conducted on Caucasian-American and African-American subjects, revealed a positive association of HLA-DR4 with susceptibility to rheumatic fever in the Caucasian population and an association of DR2 with rheumatic fever in the African-American population. HLA-DR1 showed a significant association in the latter pop-

Table 6.1 Significant Associations of HLA-DR Antigens with Rheumatic Fever

Study	Location	No. Patients	Ethnicity	HLA Class II Antigen Association	Positive (%)	
					Controls	Patients
Ayoub et al. [40]	Florida, USA	24	Caucasian	DR4	32	63
		48	African American	DR2	23	54
Anastasiou-Nana et al. [41]	Utah, USA	33	Caucasian	DR4	32	52
Jhinghan et al. [43]	New Delhi, India	134	Indian	DR3	26	50
Rajapakse et al. [42]	Saudi Arabia	40	Arab	DR4	12	65
Maharaj et al. [48]	Durban, South Africa	120	Black South African	DR1	3	13
Taneja et al. [44]	India	54	Indian	DQw2	32	63
Guilherme et al. [46]	Sao Paulo, Brazil	40	Brazilian	DR7	26	58
				DRw53	39	73
Ozkan et al. [45]	Turkey	107	Turkish	DR3	23	49
				DR7	33	57
Weidebach et al. [47]	Sao Paulo, Brazil	24	Brazilian	DR16 DRw53	34	83

ulation with Sydenham's chorea. This observation was the first indication of a racial difference in the association of rheumatic fever with HLA antigens. Other studies confirmed this difference. Anastasiou-Nand et al. [41] and Rajapakse et al. [42] confirmed the positive association of rheumatic fever with DR4 in Caucasian patients. Jhinghan et al. [43] and Taneja et al. [44] found a positive association between DR3 and a negative association between DR2 and this disease in Hindu patients. Ozkan et al. [45] reported highly significant associations between DR3 and DR7 and a negative association with DR5 in Turkish patients with rheumatic fever. The association of DR7 with susceptibility to rheumatic fever was also encountered in Brazilian patients who were characterized as highly mixed white or light mulatto [46]. In this study, a significant association with the DRw53 antigen was also found. This latter observation is of interest because the DRw53 antigen is encoded by the DRβ4 gene and is co-expressed with the DR4, DR7, and DR9 antigens.

Although the latter finding appears to support the association of the DR4 and DR7 alleles with susceptibility to rheumatic fever, the question regarding the lack of a universal association of susceptibility to this disease with a specific allele it still left unanswered. Because most of the studies to date have utilized the microcytotoxicity method for identifying the class II antigens, other methods have been explored to determine

if a more defined relationship between susceptibility to rheumatic fever and an HLA-DR allele could be established. The use of primer-specific amplification in the polymerase chain reaction (PCR) and oligonucleotide hybridization techniques have allowed the identification of subtypes or splits of the DR alleles. Using this approach, investigators have now established a more defined association with a subtype when previous studies had shown an association with the major DR allele of that subtype. Using the primer-specific PCR amplification in our laboratory, we have found that the previously described association of rheumatic fever in American-Caucasian patients with DR4 was not significant when assessed by this technique [46a]. Instead, a more significant association with DR16 was found. This allele is a split of the DR2, which has two subtypes, DR15 and DR16. The specificity of this association was reflected by the absence of an association with DR15, the other subtype of the DR2 allele [46a].

Recognizing the limitations involved in HLA-DR typing, Weidebach et al. [47] used restriction fragment-length polymorphism in re-examining the association of class II antigens with rheumatic fever. They were able to identify a DNA fragment, which they designated a 13.81 kb fragment, that was present in 83% of the Brazilian patients with rheumatic fever and in only one-third of the controls. This DNA fragment appears to be associated with DR53 and

DR16. As noted above, HLA-DR53 comprises sequences that are shared in common with DR4, DR7, and DR9 while DR16 is a subtype of DR2. This finding, while again asserting the association of DR2, DR4, and DR7 with rheumatic fever, still points to the diversity of the alleles that appear to be associated with this disease. In the above study, Weidebach and co-workers tried to define a nucleotide sequence that is common to these alleles and that would carry a more specific association with susceptibility to rheumatic fever. These investigators were unable to define a sequence or single allele that carried a specific association with susceptibility to this disease.

Recently, Kotb and colleagues studied the association of class II [47a] alleles in Egyptian patients with rheumatic heart disease (RHD) using the primer-specific PCR amplification technique. They found an increased frequency of DRB1*0701 and DQA1*0201 alleles and DRB1*0701-DQA1*0201 and DRB1*13-DQA1*0501-3-DQB1*0301 haplotypes in patients compared to ethnic controls. The finding of an association with DRB1*0701-, DR6-, and DQB1*0201-related haplotypes is in agreement with the reported associations in Turkish [45], Brazilian [46], Mexican [47b], Japanese [47c], and South African [48] RHD patients. These data indicate that certain class II alleles and haplotypes are associated with RHD, and that this association appears to be stronger and more consistent when analyzed in patients with one of the major manifestations of rheumatic fever.

The above findings appear to question the association of rheumatic fever with a specific class II allele. In fact, these findings seem to suggest an association with a "susceptibility gene" that is closely allied to the DR locus. Certain findings by Zabriskie and co-workers provide support for this possibility [49]. These investigators have described an alloantigen identified by a monoclonal antibody (MAb) designated D8/17 that is present on the surface of B cells of almost all the patients with rheumatic fever they evaluated and on the B cells of about 14% of the controls. This antigen does not appear to be associated with any of the known HLA antigens. Recent observations in our laboratory have identified yet another molecule that is present on the B cells of most patients with rheumatic fever and on the cells of all but a minority of normal controls.

Studies performed with lymphoblastoid B cell lines derived from patients with rheumatic fever and from normal controls have led to the identification of a molecule of about 70 kDa that, when solubilized from these cells and incubated with a MAb with specificity for HLA-DR antigens, coprecipitates with the HLA-DR molecules [50]. This molecule was found in the immunoprecipitates of B cells of 75% of all patients with rheumatic fever, in 83% of the B cell lines of patients with rheumatic heart disease, but in 26% of the cells of normal controls. Healthy mothers of patients with rheumatic fever were similarly tested and half of those were found to have this marker on their cells. This finding suggests that this 70 kDa molecule is closely associated with the HLA-DR locus and that it is not an acquired antigen, since it is found in a higher frequency on the cells of mothers of the patients than in normal controls.

The above findings, while falling short of identifying a specific major histocompatibility complex (MHC) molecule that can specifically identify individuals who are susceptible to rheumatic fever, suggest the presence of such a molecule in the proximity of the MHC region. The data on the phenotypic distribution of the D8/17 molecule discussed above have been interpreted as consistent with an autosomal recessive mode of inheritance and are indicative of at least one genetic factor for susceptibility to rheumatic fever [49]. Current progress in research promises to identify the gene responsible for this susceptibility and to clarify the role of such a gene in the immunopathogenesis of this disease in the not too distant future.

ROLE OF CELL-MEDIATED IMMUNITY TO GROUP A STREPTOCOCCAL ANTIGENS IN PATHOGENESIS OF RHEUMATIC FEVER

Clinical and Experimental Evidence Supporting the Role of Cell-Mediated Immunity in Rheumatic Fever and Rheumatic Heart Disease

The role of cellular immunity in rheumatic fever and rheumatic heart disease was suggested many years ago by observations indicating that the disease is rare prior to 3–4 years of age and that recurrent infection with group A streptococci appear to be a prerequisite for the development of that disease [51]. It is now generally accepted that molecular mimicry between a number of streptococcal components and cardiac proteins triggers humoral and cellular reactions that contribute to the pathogenesis of this disease [52–58]. However, despite extensive investigations into the nature of host proteins that cross-react with streptococcal components, and the finding by numerous investigators of heart cross-reactive autoantibodies in the sera of patients with rheumatic fever and rheumatic heart disease, the pathogenic significance of these heart cross-reactive autoantibodies has remained unclear. In fact, the level of autoantibodies often shows little correlation with clinical and/or histopathological manifestations. Many patients who contract streptococcal pharyngitis develop antibodies against cardiac tissue and yet most have no evidence of rheumatic fever or cardiac injury [55,59–61]. Furthermore, in experimental models of autoimmune myocarditis, it is well documented that adoptive transfer of disease can be accomplished with T cells and not autoantibodies from affected animals [62,63]. A suggestion that the same may be true in rheumatic fever was provided by earlier studies of Lawrence [64,65], who observed that delayed cutaneous reactivity to group A streptococcal antigens can be transferred with peripheral leukocytes in humans.

Mounting clinical and experimental evidence suggests that cell-mediated immune responses play a pivotal role in the pathogenesis of rheumatic fever. This evidence dates back to the 1940s when Humphrey and Pagel [66] observed that patients with rheumatic fever have heightened skin reactivity to streptococcal antigens as compared to nonrheumatic controls. In the ensuing years, the phenomenon of hypersensitivity to streptococcal antigens was confirmed and further investigated by several groups [67–75]. A number of studies have demonstrated a significant increase in activated CD4 T cells and streptococcal antigen-reactive T cells in peripheral blood of rheumatic fever patients and rheumatics with active carditis [76–78]. Others, however, have reported depressed lymphocyte proliferative responses to streptococcal antigens and mitogens in children with rheumatic fever [79–83]. It is possible that this depression is mediated by high titers of autoantibodies present in the sera of patients during the acute attack. Such antibodies have been shown to block the proliferation and differentiation of lymphocytes in response to streptococcal antigens [84,85]. This view is supported by the finding of Benatar et al., who documented the presence of serum suppressor factors during the acute phase of the disease [86]. The suppression of lymphocyte responses seen in these few reports is transient and the response usually returns to normal levels as the acute symptoms subside [70,76,86]. Thus, variations in the level and/or type of antibodies found in patients during the acute phase of the disease may account for the apparent discrepancies regarding changes in T cell subsets and function during this phase of the disease. Alternatively, a retrospective evaluation of studies that reported depressed responses to streptococcal antigens suggests that the stimulation with these antigens, some of which are now known to be superantigens, was conducted under conditions that might have resulted in overstimulation, apoptosis, and death of responsive T cells in culture. Thus, what might have appeared as a depressed response may in fact have been a very potent response to this particular stimulus. In light of recent knowledge regarding the mode of activation of immune cells by streptococcal antigens and the sophistication of immunological techniques, it may be necessary to re-evaluate changes in immune responses that occur in patients during active and quiescent disease.

Remarkable differences in cellular immune response to streptococcal antigens effecting lymphocyte migration inhibition and blastogenesis transformation have been noted between rheumatic fever patients and nonrheumatic subjects [69,72–75]. Interestingly, these differences were significant only when pharyngeal streptococcal isolates from patients with rheumatic fever, but not skin isolates from patients with impetigo, were used to stimulate lymphocytes from patients and controls, suggesting that rheumatic fever strains may possess unique antigens that are highly stimulatory to lymphocytes of rheumatic fever individuals [73,74]. Although this increased cellular reactivity was seen in response to streptococcal cell walls and membranes, the response to strepto-coccal membrane antigens was greater and longer lasting, persisting for up to 2–3 years after the attack. That this hyperreactivity is genetically determined was suggested by the studies of Hafez et al. [69], who found a significant correlation between the level of cellular responsiveness in HLA identical siblings and concluded that an inherited recessive gene, closely associated with HLA genes, is responsible for the phenomenon of hyperresponsiveness to streptococcal antigens.

The importance of cell-mediated immune responses to streptococcal antigens in rheumatic fever was further highlighted by the finding that cytotoxic immune cross-reactions occur between streptococcal antigens and mammalian tissues [85,87–91]. One of the earliest indications came from studies that showed accelerated allograft rejection in animals hyperimmunized with group A streptococcal antigens [87]. However, more direct evidence was provided by the studies of Friedman et al. [88], who showed that lymphocytes sensitized to group A streptococci exerted a cytopathic effect on heart tissue cultures. Similarly, Senitzer et al. [91] found that an autoimmune response to syngeneic cardiac determinants can be induced in BALB/c mice by immunization with group A streptococcal cell membranes. These findings were confirmed by Yang et al. [92], who demonstrated that membrane antigens from group A, but not group C, streptococci can induce guinea pig T cells to differentiate into cytotoxic T lymphocytes (CTL) capable of destroying allogeneic cardiac heart cells. The target specificity of this CTL population was demonstrated by the lack of cytotoxicity toward other tissues such as skeletal muscle, skin fibroblasts, and liver cells, and heart cross-reactive antibodies failed to either mediate or augment the killing of cardiac cells. The existence of this phenomenon in humans was demonstrated by the study of Hutto and Ayoub [85], who documented the presence of circulating heart-reactive CTL in blood of patients with active rheumatic carditis. Interestingly, this cytotoxic activity was blocked by the patients' plasma, suggesting that heart cross-reactive autoantibodies may have a protective role in this disease.

In addition to the above studies, direct histopathologic examination of heart tissues provided strong evidence that cell-mediated immunity has an active role in the pathogenesis of rheumatic carditis. Marboe et al. [93] analyzed an endomyocardial biopsy from patients with rheumatic heart disease and observed a heterogeneous infiltrate composed of T cells, macrophages, B cells, and mast cells. The predominant cells were T lymphocytes with twice as many CD4 cells as CD8 T cells. Following treatment, the cellular infiltrate diminished and the ratio of CD4:CD8 T cells declined to 0.59. Similar findings were reported by Raizada et al. [94], who examined valvular tissue removed from patients 10 to 20 years following the initial attack and noted that the majority of T cells in the pathogenic lesion belonged to the CD4 subset. In a subsequent study, Kemeny et al. [95] found that the cellular infiltrate consisted primarily of T cells and macrophages, and noted an increase in HLA DR expression on most of the infiltrating cells as well as on the vascular endothelium. Aberrant expression of class II molecules in heart tissues, which was also noted on valvular fibroblasts by Amoils et al. [96], may have an important role in disease pathogenesis because it can allow the presentation of sequestered self-antigens to T cells by nonprofessional antigen-presenting cells. This mode of presentation can potentially induce the activation of autoreactive T cells that can, in turn, mediate the autoimmune destruction of myocardial tissues and heart valves.

Although the above studies suggested a strong role for streptococcal antigen-responsive T cells in rheumatic carditis, direct evidence was provided by Guilherme et al. [90] who generated T cell clones from valvular tissues of rheumatic heart disease patients and demonstrated that these clones were responsive to specific epitopes of type 5 M proteins. In addition, recent studies in our laboratory show that stimulation with streptococcal antigens enhances the ability of T cells to recognize specific myocardial proteins [97,97a]. However, our ability to decipher the exact role of cellular immunity to streptococcal antigens in the pathogenesis of rheumatic fever has been greatly hampered by the lack of knowledge regarding the target autoantigen in this disease.

Streptococcal Virulence Factors Mediating Cellular Immune Responses

Group A streptococci produce a variety of virulence factors that are capable of eliciting humoral and cellular immune responses in the mammalian host. The surface M protein is considered one of the major virulence factors for these organisms because it protects the bacteria from phagocytic cells [98,99] and elicits immune responses that are believed to play a central role in the pathogenesis of rheumatic fever and rheumatic heart disease [52,57,84,100–105]. Over 100 different M protein serotypes have been identified, but not all are associated with these sequelae. Serotypes that show association with rheumatic fever are casually called rheumatogenic, and those that are associated with glomerulonephritis are considered nephritogenic [101,106]. Extensive studies have been devoted to gain a better understanding of the differences between these serotypes and to deduce the structure–function relation of M proteins. Because most of these studies are detailed elsewhere in this book, we will focus on those points that are relevant to our discussion of cell-mediated immune responses.

One of the first indications that M proteins elicit cellular immunity came from the work of Lawrence [64,65], who demonstrated passive transfer of delayed cutaneous hypersensitivity to nonreactive subjects by injecting viable leukocytes from individuals presensitized to crude M type 1 protein. Later, Fox et al. [68] observed that a significant number of adults reacted to intercutaneous injection of acid extracts of M types 12 and 24 group A streptococci. However, in as much as the hot acid extracts used in these studies were crude preparations, it was difficult to determine whether this cellular reactivity was mediated by the M protein or by other streptococcal components such as pyrogenic exotoxins. To address this concern, Beachey and colleagues generated highly purified pepsin-extracted M proteins (pep M), demonstrated that these preparations were devoid of toxin activity, and studied the effects of pure pep M proteins on cell-mediated immune responses in humans [67,107–111].

Studies by Dale et al. [111] demonstrated that human T cells respond briefly to purified pep M preparations. Cord blood lymphocytes responded in a similar fashion, indicating that the response was not merely due to prior exposure to streptococcal infections [111]. Unlike the response to streptococcal pyrogenic exotoxins, none of the lymphocytes from nonimmunized laboratory animals, including those from mice and rabbits, responded to in vitro stimulation with pep M-5, pep M-6, or pep M-24, suggesting the existence of species-specific responses to these proteins. Antibodies to peptide fragments of the M protein precipitated out the mitogenic activity, thereby providing evidence that the response was mediated by the pep M proteins and not by minute contaminants of pyrogenic toxins [111]. These findings suggested that M protein may be a polyclonal T cell mitogen. However, biochemical studies reveal that this protein does not behave like a typical mitogen [112,113]. Further investigations have revealed that pep M proteins, including recombinant pep M-5 protein [114–116], belong to the family of microbial superantigens that stimulate T cells by interacting with specific elements within the variable region of the T cell receptor (TCR) β chain, designated Vβ elements. A number of "rheumatogenic serotypes," including M types 5, 6, 18, 19, and 24, were found to be superantigens to human T cells [116]. Although each serotype had a unique pattern of Vβ specificity, the specificity for Vβ4 was shared among the rheumatogenic M proteins tested, but not by the nonrheumatogenic pep M-2 serotype that stimulated only Vβ2-bearing T cells. The significance of this finding to the pathogenesis of rheumatic heart disease remains to be elucidated.

There is compelling direct and indirect evidence to suggest that superantigens may contribute to the initiation and/or exacerbation of certain autoimmune diseases believed to have an infectious etiology (reviewed in refs. [117–125]). Superantigens are unique because they are bifunctional, interacting with at least two types of receptors expressed on different mononuclear cells of the immune system. The receptor for superantigens on T cells is the TCR, and it is well documented that MHC class II molecules expressed primarily on B cells, monocytes, and dendritic cells serve as receptors for these proteins. The binding of superantigens to the TCR and/or to class II molecules can trigger intracellular biochemical signals which in turn program a cascade of events leading to cell activation, differentiation, proliferation, and the release of inflammatory cytokines (reviewed in refs. [121,122]). Activation of T cells based on their Vβ type and regardless of the antigenic specificity of the TCR can potentially cause expansion of autoreactive T cells.

In addition, the interaction between superantigens and T cells can cause the release of TH1 cytokines, including interferon γ (IFN-γ), which in turn synergizes with superantigens to induce the production of other inflammatory cytokines by T cells, B cells, and monocytes (reviewed in refs. [120–122]). High levels of inflammatory cytokines can cause tissue destruction, upregulation of MHC molecules, and costimulatory ligands, thereby facilitating the exposure and presentation of sequestered self-antigens. Therefore, the aberrant expression of class II molecules on heart tissues of rheumatic carditis patients [95,96,126] may have been induced by inflammatory reactions elicited by the M protein as well as by other streptococcal superantigens or toxins, such as streptolysin O and lipoteichoic acid, that are known to induce the release of inflammatory cytokines [127–132]. We believe that the local inflammatory responses may have an important role in the pathogenesis of rheumatic fever and rheumatic heart disease, and current work in our laboratory is designed to address this issue.

Besides their ability to activate large numbers of T cells and elicit the production of inflammatory cytokines [130,133], certain serotypes of pep M protein, namely pep M-5, M-6, and M-19, were found to induce the differentiation of CTL with the capacity of killing cultured myocardial cells [84,134]. Consistent with superantigen-activated CTL, pep M–activated CTL included both CD4 and CD8 cells that kill their targets in an MHC nonrestricted fashion [84]. The cytotoxicity elicited by pep M proteins against cultured myocardial cells was partially neutralized by heart cross-reactive antibodies raised against type 5 M protein, suggesting, as previously noted also by Hutto and Ayoub [85], that these antibodies may have a protective role in disease pathogenesis [84].

It should be noted that M proteins are not the only streptococcal component that induce cytotoxic activity of human lymphocytes, and that other streptococcal antigens and superantigens are also capable of inducing this activity [135–137]. Gray et al. [136] reported that another streptococcal superantigen, streptococcal pyrogenic exotoxin A (SPE A), augments natural killer cell activity and that this effect is significantly greater on mononuclear cells from rheumatic heart disease patients. Despite these intriguing findings, studies that directly examine the role of streptococcal-induced CTL activity in the pathogenesis of rheumatic fever are lacking, and the mechanism of autoimmune destruction in these diseases remains an enigma.

Role of Shared Streptococcal and Heart T Cell Epitopes in Pathogenesis of Rheumatic Fever and Rheumatic Heart Disease

In an attempt to understand the basis for organ specificity in rheumatic heart disease, shared T cell epitopes between heart tissues and M proteins have been investigated both in vitro [138] and in vivo [90]. Studies by Guilherme et al. [90] showed that T cells isolated from valvular tissues of rheumatic heart disease patients respond to specific sequences of the streptococcal M-5 protein, as well as to heart proteins. The highest response was elicited by 43–65 kDa valvular proteins and by amino acid residues 163–177 of the M-5 protein. Interestingly, we have reported that this region of the M-5 protein is important for its ability to stimulate T cells [139] and that it harbors an amino acid sequence motif that is shared by other superantigens as well as by the human invariant chain for class II molecules [140]. Furthermore, this region of the M-5 molecule contains a myosin cross-reactive epitope [141]. This finding prompted us to examine whether stimulation of human T cells with pep M-5 would enhance their ability to recognize cardiac myosin. Purified myosin failed to stimulate resting human T cells to proliferate; however, when T cells were first primed with pep M-5 they recognized the myosin epitopes and proliferated in response to cardiac but not skeletal muscle myosin (Fig. 6.2). Priming with the polyclonal T cell mitogen, anti-CD3, failed to induce this effect [97]. It is possible, therefore, that the superantigenic properties of pep M-5 allow it to act as an adjuvant that enhances the ability of autoreactive T cells to respond to heart cross-reactive T cell epitopes expressed by the

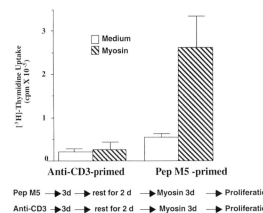

Pep M5 ─▶3d ─▶ rest for 2 d ─▶Myosin 3d ─▶ Proliferation

Anti-CD3 ─▶3d ─▶ rest for 2 d ─▶ Myosin 3d ─▶ Proliferation

Figure 6.2 Effect of priming T cells with pep M-5 on their response to cardiac myosin. T cells (2×10^6/ml) were stimulated with either 1 μg/ml anti-CD3 MAb or 0.5 μg/ml of pep M-5 protein. After 3 days in culture, the cells were washed and placed in fresh RPMI-complete medium for 48 h to rest. Recovered cells (0.6×10^5) were then incubated in 96-well plates with either medium alone or 0.2 μg purified cardiac myosin in a final volume of 200 μl. Proliferation was measured 3 days later by determining [^{3}H]-thymidine uptake. The data are presented as mean cpm of triplicate cultures ± SEM.

M protein or any other streptococcal molecule. Once activated beyond a certain threshold, these cells may home onto the heart where they can be further stimulated by self-antigens that are presented by class II molecules expressed on activated endothelial cells and heart-infiltrating leukocytes. Clearly, additional studies are required to test this attractive hypothesis.

To summarize, considerable progress has been made toward our understanding of cell-mediated immune responses to streptococcal antigens and their possible role in the pathogenesis of rheumatic fever and rheumatic heart disease. Although evidence supports the role of M proteins in the pathogenesis of rheumatic fever and rheumatic heart disease, it is highly unlikely that these molecules act alone in mediating disease pathogenesis. The contribution of other streptococcal components such as streptococcal carbohydrates, pyrogenic exotoxins, and other extracellular products should be investigated. It is clear also from the above discussion that we cannot simply extrapolate in vitro findings to stage events that actually take place in the host. Therefore, to decipher the pathogene-

sis of rheumatic fever and rheumatic heart disease, we need a better understanding of host factors that contribute to disease susceptibility and potentiate immune responses to the pathogen. This can only be achieved by directly analyzing patient samples, characterizing the specificity and function of immune cells isolated from pathological lesions, and identifying heart antigens that are target to autoimmune recognition in these diseases.

A PERSPECTIVE ON IMMUNE MECHANISMS OF TISSUE INJURY

Background

As described previously in this chapter, infection of the susceptible host with certain M protein serotypes of group A streptococci leads to the production of acute rheumatic fever (ARF) [142, 143]. The clinical manifestations of ARF [144,145] are thought to result from an antigenic mimicry between certain streptococcal and self-antigens. Hyperimmune responses by the host against the streptococcal antigens leads to a cross-reaction with those host antigens that are located in the heart, joints, skin, or brain [74,146]. The streptococcal and host antigens associated with immunological cross-reactivity between the group A streptococci and host tissues are the subject of this review.

Historically, immunological cross-reactivity of antistreptococcal antibodies with host tissues and streptococcal antigens was noted in the 1960s when investigators found antibodies against host tissues after immunization of rabbits with streptococcal membranes [55,147,148], whole streptococci, and cell-wall extracts [54,149–153]. Group A streptococcal carbohydrate, the C polysaccharide, was shown to react with antibodies against valvular heart tissue [154], and a C polysaccharide peptidoglycan complex or cell wall particles were shown to produce connective tissue lesions and arthritis in animals [155,156]. Studies in humans with ARF demonstrated that autoantibodies against heart tissue were present in the sera of patients with the disease [157]. In immunofluorescence tests, antibody was found deposited in the hearts of patients who had died from rheumatic carditis [158], and sera from patients with ARF reacted with heart tissues [55,61]. Patients with rheumatic carditis and valvulitis had persistently high levels of anti-group A carbohydrate antibody that correlated with the presence of valvular heart disease [20]. These early studies strongly suggested that anti-streptococcal/anti-heart antibodies could react with heart tissues and deposit in the hearts of patients with ARF. Evidence for antibody deposition in cardiac tissues in humans suggested that cross-reactive antibodies play a role in the pathogenesis of the disease, although direct proof of this hypothesis in animal models has not yet been demonstrated.

Heart Cross-reactive Antistreptococcal Monoclonal Antibodies: Identification of Myosin as Autoantigen

To prove the hypothesis that the antistreptococcal/anti-heart antibodies were truly cross-reactive antibody molecules, human and mouse MAbs were produced from BALB/c mice immunized with streptococcal antigens and from humans with ARF [141,159–163]. Human and mouse antistreptococcal/anti-heart MAbs were used to identify the autoantigens, streptococcal antigens, and the epitopes that are involved in the immunological cross-reactions in ARF.

Mouse Monoclonal Antibodies

The first studies of cross-reactive mouse antistreptococcal MAbs (36.2.2, 49.8.9, and 54.2.8) led to the discovery that the antistreptococcal antibodies reacted with myosin, a major protein constituent of heart tissue [159]. Subsequently, it was reported that immunization of animals with cardiac myosin could induce myocarditis [164,165]. Affinity purification of ARF sera on myosin columns led to the identification of myosin-specific antibodies in ARF that reacted with streptococcal M protein [141,162]. Studies of the anti-myosin antibodies in ARF sera confirmed that the specificities of the human and mouse MAbs were similar to those found in patients with rheumatic fever. The investigation of mouse MAbs 36.2.2, 49.8.9, and 54.2.8 yielded a wealth of important information about the specificities recognized by cross-reactive anti-streptococcal MAbs [160,161]. The MAbs 36.2.2

and 54.2.8 were readily inhibited by myosin and its proteolytic subfragments, heavy (HMM) or light meromyosin (LMM). The MAb 49.8.9 was not inhibited by any of these molecules. The MAb 36.2.2 reacted with actin and keratin [160,161] and was inhibited by the LMM fragment of myosin [160]. The MAb 54.2.8 not only reacted with myosin but reacted strongly with DNA and synthetic polynucleotides [161] and was shown to be a strong antinuclear antibody with specificities similar to those reported for sera from mice or humans with systemic lupus erythematosus (Fig. 6.3). The characteristics of MAbs 36.2.2 and 54.2.8 divided antistreptococcal cross-reactive antibodies into two groups on the basis of cross-reactivity with DNA. However, in the study of the human MAbs, no antinuclear reactivity was observed as described below. This

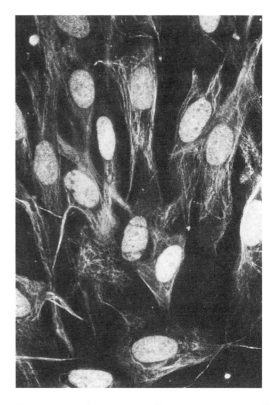

Figure 6.3 Indirect immunofluorescence staining of acetone-fixed fibroblasts after reaction with anti-streptococcal MAb 54.2.8. The strong reaction of the MAb 54.2.8 with the fibroblasts shows the intense antinuclear reactivity and the staining of the cytoskeleton. (From Cunningham and Swerlick [161], with permission from the *Journal of Experimental Medicine*.)

was not surprising since no antinuclear antibody is observed in the sera of patients with ARF.

Cross-reactive mouse antistreptococcal MAbs were also produced by Fitzsimons and Lange [166], who showed that their panel of antistreptococcal membrane MAbs cross-reacted with lung, kidney, and heart tissues. One of their antistreptococcal membrane MAbs destroyed lung tissue and was lethal to mice [166]. Some of the MAbs in the panel were reactive with myosin and actin in vitro and reacted with Z-bands in heart tissue when injected in vivo into mice [167].

In another study, a large panel of antistreptococcal murine MAbs was produced by Fenderson et al. [168]. BALB/c mice were immunized with either streptococcal membranes, PepM-5, or lysin-extracted M-5 protein in incomplete Freund's adjuvant. All mouse MAbs produced against streptococcal components were from streptococci grown in a chemically defined medium to avoid any contamination of streptococcal preparations with tissue proteins. In this panel of murine MAbs [168], several MAbs were found to cross-react with group A streptococcal M protein and tropomyosin (Table 6.2). Tropomyosin is an α-helical coiled-coil molecule similar in structure to myosin. It was strongly recognized by antistreptococcal MAbs 27.4.1 and 112.2.2 [168]. Tropomyosin was shown by Manjula and Fischetti to have amino acid sequence homology with M proteins [169,170]. An example of the amino acid sequence homology between tropomyosin and M-6 protein is shown in Figure 6.4. Similar α-helical structural homologies are observed between streptococcal M proteins of various serotypes and host α-helical coiled molecules such as myosin, tropomyosin, keratin, or laminin [171].

Similarities between the α-helical structures of M protein and myosin may lead to aberrant immune responses in the susceptible host. Immunization of animals with cardiac myosin induced myocarditis, whereas immunization with skeletal myosin did not [164]. The immune response against cardiac myosin–specific epitopes has been suggested to be the cause of myosin-induced myocarditis in animals [164,172,173]. Mouse antistreptococcal MAbs have been investigated for their reaction with purified human cardiac myosin and its subfragments, LMM, S1, and S2, and the sites of MAb reactivity have been identified. Figure 6.5 illustrates the myosin molecule and its subfragments with the locations of the MAb reactivity as described previously by Dell et al. [174].

Studies by Shikhman et al. [163,175,176] have defined a third group of heart and tissue cross-reactive antistreptococcal MAbs that react with the group A streptococcal carbohydrate moiety N-acetyl-β-D-glucosamine (GlcNAc). These antistreptococcal MAbs reacted with GlcNAc, myosin, keratin, vimentin, or other α-helical molecules. The anti-GlcNAc antibodies characterized to date do not react with DNA or the cell nucleus and clearly comprise a separate group of cross-reactive antistreptococcal antibodies. Immunological cross-reactivity between N-acetylglucosamine and heart tissue was also reported previously by Goldstein et al. [154]. It has been

Table 6.2 Cross-reactivy of Antistreptococcal Mouse Monoclonal Antibodies

Monoclonal Antibody	Antigen Specificity	Reference
6.5.1	Actin/vimentin/keratin/GlcNac[a]	[168,175]
8.5.1	Keratin/vimentin/GlcNac[a]	[168,175]
27.4.1	Myosin/tropomyosin/keratin/M5/M6	[168]
36.2.2	Myosin/tropomyosin/actin/keratin /laminin/PepM1,5,6	[159–162,171]
49.8.9	Vimentin/actin/keratin/M5/M6/GlcNac[a]	[168,175]
54.2.8	Myosin/tropomyosin/vimentin/DNA[b] Keratin/M5/M6	[159–162,168]
101.4.1	Myosin/vimentin/actin/keratin/M5/M6/GlcNac[a]	[168,175]
112.2.2	Myosin/tropomyosin/actin	[168]
654.1.1	Myosin/tropomyosin/DNA[b]/M5/M6	[168]
10B6	Myosin/class I M proteins	[143,177,189]

[a]GlcNac, N-acetyl-glucosamine.

[b]DNA, anti-nuclear antibody.

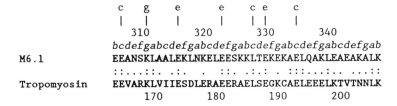

```
              c   g     e       e    c e    c
              |   |     |       |    | |    |
             310        320         330        340
           bcdefgabcdefgabcdefgabcdefgabcdefgabcdefgab
M6.1       EEANSKLAALEKLNKELEESKKLTEKEKAELQAKLEAEAKALK
           ::....::. .::.   .   ::. .:.: . :::....:.  ....::
Tropomyosin EEVARKLVIIESDLERAEERAELSEGKCAELEEELKTVTNNLK
             170        180         190        200
```

Figure 6.4 Sequence alignment of M-6 protein and human cardiac tropomyosin in a region exhibiting significant homology. Lower-case letters a to g directly above the sequence designate the position of these amino acids within the 7-residue pattern (a-b-c-d-e-f-g) in both segments based on previous analysis. Lower case letters b, c, g, e, and f identify identities in these external locations in the heptad repeat. Double dots indicate identities and single dots are conservative substitutions. (From Fenderson et al. [168], with permission from the *Journal of Immunology*.)

demonstrated that antibodies against the group A streptococcal carbohydrate, a polymer containing rhamnose and *N*-acetyl-glucosamine, remained elevated for prolonged time periods in patients with rheumatic valvulitis [20]. Table 6.3 summarizes the 3 major groups of antistreptococcal heart cross-reactive antibodies and Table 6.2 summarizes the known mouse antistreptococcal MAb cross-reactivities. One of the MAbs listed is MAb 10.B6, which recognizes the class I epitope of M protein [143,177].

Human Monoclonal Antibodies

All human antistreptococcal heart cross-reactive MAbs that have been characterized are in group

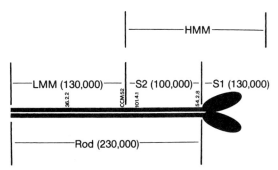

Figure 6.5 Diagram of the myosin molecule containing heavy and light chains. The diagram illustrates the light meromyosin (LMM) tail and the heavy meromyosin (HMM) fragment containing the S2 rod region and the S1 globular head. The epitopes recognized by antistreptococcal MAbs 36.2.2, 101.4.1, and 54.2.8 are positioned in the rod region. Antimyosin MAb CCM-52 is also shown. (From Dell et al. [174], with permission from the *European Heart Journal*.)

3 and react strongly with GlcNac (Table 6.4). Human cross-reactive MAbs from rheumatic carditis patients were reactive with GlcNAc, myosin, or other cytoskeletal proteins [163]. It is becoming evident that antimyosin antibody responses are linked to the anti-*N*-acetyl-glucosamine (GlcNAc) antibody response. It is not surprising that the human MAbs do not react with DNA, since in ARF there are no antinuclear antibodies detected in patient sera. Thus, the human MAbs follow the reactivity pattern observed for the human ARF sera [141,162]. Affinity-purified antimyosin antibody from ARF sera reacts distinctly with human cardiac myosin heavy chain at 200 kDa [141,162]. The affinity-purified antimyosin antibody also reacts with M protein and GlcNAc. Mimicry between GlcNAc and α-helical proteins has been shown to utilize synthetic peptides that behave like GlcNAc [176].

To summarize, the mouse and human MAbs have been invaluable in identification of the antigens in tissues that may play a role in ARF. The cross-reactive antibodies are most certainly markers of the disease process in ARF, and may also deposit in tissues and bring about inflammation. The α-helical coiled-coil proteins present in the

Table 6.3 Cross-reactive Antistreptococcal Antibody Groups

Group 1	Reactivity with myosin and other α-helical coiled-coil proteins
Group 2	Reactivity with DNA and cell nucleus and α-helical coiled-coil proteins
Group 3	Reactivity with *N*-acetyl-glucosamine (GLcNac) and α-helical coiled-coil proteins

Table 6.4 Human Antistreptococcal Monoclonal Antibody Specificities

Monoclonal Antibody	Antigen Specificity	Reference
10.2.3	Myosin/keratin/vimentin/actin /M5/M6/GlcNac[a]	[141,192]
1.C8	Myosin/vimentin/keratin/GlcNac	[163]
1.H9	Myosin/keratin/GlcNac	[163]
4.F2	Myosin/keratin/GlcNac	[163]
5.G7	Heat aggregated IgG/myosin/keratin/GlcNac	[163]
5.G3	Keratin/GlcNac	[163]
1.C3	Laminin/keratin/GlcNac	[163]
9.B12	Keratin/GlcNac	[163]
2.H11	Keratin/GlcNac	[163]
3.B6	Myosin/tropomyosin/vimentin/actin	(Not published)

[a]GlcNac, N-acetyl-glucosamine.

heart, joints, and skin, such as myosin [159,160], tropomyosin [167], vimentin, [161,178], keratin [175,176,179], or related molecules, are recognized by the cross-reactive antibodies that may deposit in tissues and lead to disease symptoms of carditis, arthritis, or erythema marginatum. Future studies in animal models will be important in understanding the role of antibody in the pathogenesis of the disease.

Molecular Analysis of Myosin Cross-reactive Epitopes of Streptococcal M Proteins: Specificity of Anti-Myosin Antibodies in ARF for Sites in Streptococcal M Protein

Studies of Synthetic Peptides

Investigation of the streptococcal M proteins over the past 15 years has provided important information about the sequence and primary structure of the molecule [169,170,180–182]. Manjula and Fischetti first identified the α-helical coiled-coil structure characteristic of the M protein [169,170]. Their studies showed structural homology between M protein and α-helical coiled-coil molecules such as tropomyosin and the desmin-keratin family [168,183]. Dale and Beachey [184] showed that antimyosin antibody was produced in rabbits immunized with M protein, and that an epitope reactive with the antimyosin antibodies was present in M-6 and M-19 proteins. Mouse antistreptococcal/antimyosin MAbs 36.2.2, 54.2.8, and 654.1.1 reacted with PepM-5 in Western immunoblots, whereas the other cross-reactive mouse MAbs reacted with the intact recombinant M-5 or M-6 protein [168,175]. Studies by Kraus et al. [178] demonstrated a vimentin cross-reactive epitope present in the M-12 protein, and M protein peptides containing brain cross-reactive epitopes were localized to the M-5 protein sequence 134–184 and the M-19 sequence 1–24 [185]. Table 6.5 summarizes these previously identified tissue cross-reactive sites.

Table 6.5 Summary of Tissue Cross-reactive Epitopes of Streptococcal M Proteins

M Type	Sequence	Autoantigen/Tissue [Reference]
M-1 (1–26)	NGDGNPREVIEDLAANNPAIQNIRLR	Myocardium Kidney/vimentin [178]
M-5 (84–116)	KQQRDTLSTQKETLEREVQNIQYNNETLKIKNG	Myosin [141,184]
M-5 (164–197)	TIGTLKKILDETVKDKLAKEQKSKQNIGALKQEL	Sarcolemma [186] Myosin [141] Brain [185]
M-5 (183–189)	EQKSKQN	Myosin [141]
M-5 (134–163)	QESKEEKALNELLEKTVKDKLAKEQENKE	Brain [185]
M-5 (175–184)	TVKDKLAKE	Brain [185]
M-12 (1–25)	DHSDLVAEKQRLEDLGQKFERLKQR	Vimentin [178]
M-19 (1–14)	VRYSRESPEDKLKK	Myocardium/ sarcolemma [187]
M-19 (1–24)	VRYSRESPEDKLKKIIDDLDAKEN	Brain [185]

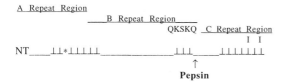

Figure 6.6 Myosin cross-reactive sites in M-5 protein A-, B-, and C-Repeat regions. Sites marked (⊥) within the A-repeat region induce anti-myosin antibodies in BALB/c mice (187a). Previous reports suggested that M-5 sequences 84–116 in the A-repeat region and 164–197 [141] in the B-repeat region react with anti-heart antibodies. The * marks the location of the sequence (NT4) that produces myocarditis in autoimmune strains of mice [188]. Site QKSKQ reacts with anti-myosin antibody from ARF [141] and induces antibody against myosin in BALB/c mice [187a]. Sites marked in the C-repeat region react with anti-myosin antibody from ARF sera [190] and induce anti-myosin antibodies in BALB/c mice [187a]. The C-repeat sites that are recognized as the class I epitope are marked with an I (see Table 6.6 for amino acid sequences).

Previous epitope mapping of M protein sites recognized by antimyosin antibodies in ARF utilized a set of synthetic peptides spanning the PepM5 molecule [141]. Affinity-purified antimyosin antibodies were obtained from ARF sera and reacted with the peptides in ELISA competitive inhibition assays. A site recognized by antimyosin antibody was located near the pepsin cleavage site of M-5 protein and contained the amino acid sequence Gln-Lys-Ser-Lys-Gln (M5 residues 184–188). Additionally, several cross-reactive mouse MAbs and human MAbs 10.2.3 and 10.2.5 reacted with peptides containing this sequence [141]. M-5 residues 164–197 induced antibodies against the sarcolemmal membrane of heart tissue [186], and residues 84–116 induced heart reactive antibody and also reacted with antimyosin antibodies from one of the ARF patients studied [141,186]. An amino terminal sequence in M-19 was found to induce heart cross-reactive antibody [187]. A summary of the currently known myosin cross-reactive antibody binding sites in M-5 protein is shown in Figure 6.6 and Table 6.5 summarizes sequences from several M proteins.

More recent studies in our laboratory have utilized a set of overlapping 18-mer synthetic peptides spanning the A-, B-, and C-repeat regions of the M-5 protein (Table 6.6). Immunization of BALB/c mice with each of these peptides has revealed that M-5 peptides NT3-NT7, B2B3B, and C1A–C3 induce antimyosin antibodies [187a].

Table 6.6 Overlapping Synthetic Peptides of Streptococcal M-5 Protein[a]

Peptide	Sequence	Amino Acid Residue
NT1	AVTRGTINDPQRAKEALD	1–18
NT2	KEALDKYELENHDLKTKN	14–31
NT3	LKTKNEGLKTENEGLKTE	27–44
NT4	GLKTENEGLKTENEGLKTE	40–58
NT5	KKEHEAENDKLKQQRDTL	59–76
NT6	QRDTLSTQKETLEREVQN	72–89
NT7	REVQNTQYNNETLKIKNG	85–102
NT8	KIKNGDLTKELNKTRQEL	98–115
B1A	TRQELANKQQESKENEKAL	111–129
B1B	ENEKALNELLEKTVKDKI	124–141
B1B2	VKDKTAKEQENKETIGTL	137–154
B2	TIGTLKKILDETVKDKIA	150–167
B2B3A	KDKIAKEQENKETIGTLK	163–180
B3A	IGTLKKILDETVKDKLAK	176–193
B2B3B	DKISKEQKSKQNIGALKQ	189–206
B3B	GALKQELAKKDEANKISD	202–219
C1A	NKISDASRKGLRRDLDAS	215–232
C1B	DLDASREAKKQLEAEHQK	228–245
C1C2	AEHQKLEEQNKISEASRK	241–258
C2A	EASRKGLRRDLDASREAK	254–271
C2B	SREAKKQLEAEQQKLEEQ	267–284
C2C3	KLEEQNKTSEASRKGLRR	280–297
C3	KGLRRDLDASREAKKQ	293–308

[a]Sequence is from reference [52]. Numerical order is from the start of the mature protein.

The anti-M-5 peptide response was 10 times greater against cardiac myosin than against skeletal myosin, tropomyosin, vimentin, and laminin as measured by titration in the ELISA. These data suggested a cardiac myosin–directed response against certain M-5 peptides in BALB/c mice. Mice developed mild lymphocytic infiltrates in the heart when immunized with NT4, NT5, NT6, B1A, and B3B (see Table 6.6 for peptide sequences) [187a]. Table 6.7 contains a summary of the M protein sites observed to induce antimyosin or inflammatory responses in mice. M-5 peptide B2B3B (Table 6.7) contained the Gln-Lys-Ser-Lys-Gln (QKSKQ) sequence that had previously been shown to inhibit antimyosin antibodies in ARF [141]. The B2B3B peptide induced immune responses to cardiac or skeletal myosin and the LMM fragment of myosin. This evidence further supported previous findings indicating that the QKSKQ sequence is important in the immune-mediated cross-reactions to myosin in ARF [141].

More than one M-5 peptide has been shown to react with a single heart cross-reactive MAb (M.W. Cunningham, unpublished data). The cross-reactivity of a single MAb with several peptides is most likely due to overlapping sequences and structural homologies within the synthetic peptides. The amino acid heptad repeat pattern

```
NT4        GLKTENEG--LKTENEG--LKTE
           |  | | |       |  | | |      |  | |
MYO        KLQTENGE   LQTENGE   LQTE
```

Figure 6.7 Sequence homology between M-5 sequence from the NT4 peptide shown in Table 6.6 and a sequence in human cardiac myosin. The entire sequence of the NT4 peptide is shown and the sequence in cardiac myosin is repeated to show the similarity with the repeats in the peptide. The homologous sequence is repeated four times in the M-5 protein and is present only once in cardiac myosin. The myosin sequence is conserved among cardiac myosins. Repeated sequences in M proteins may be important in inducing autoimmune responses against the heart. The NT4 peptide produced myocarditis in MRL/++ mice [188] and inflammation in hearts of BALB/c mice [187a].

necessary to maintain the α-helical coiled-coil structure and the homology within repeated regions in the primary amino acid sequence are likely to be contributing factors in the binding of M protein and myosin by the cross-reactive MAbs. In addition, there may be multiple binding sites on M protein by the cross-reactive MAbs as indicated by the binding of several peptides by a single MAb. Repeated regions may also influence the production of heart or myosin cross-reactive antibodies when repeated regions have homology with myosin or other host proteins. Homologies have been found between specific amino acid sequence repeats in M proteins and myosin or tropomyosin [180,188]. One of the most notable homologies includes a sequence located in the NT4 peptide of M-5 that contains a sequence 80% identical to a site in cardiac myosins. The NT4 peptide produced myocarditis in autoimmune prone MRL/++ mice [188]. Figure 6.7 illustrates the homology between the MS NT4 sequence and cardiac myosin.

Anti-Myosin Antibodies in ARF React with the C-Repeat Region and Class I Epitope of M Protein

Studies by Bessen and colleagues have demonstrated that M proteins can be classified into two groups on the basis of reactivity with anti-M protein MAb 10.B6 [143]. Class I M protein serotypes react with MAb 10.B6 and are primarily group A streptococcal strains associated

Table 6.7 M Protein Sites Associated with Anti-Myosin Antibody Production and Inflammation in BALB/c Mice

Peptide[a]	Reaction
NT2	Anaphylaxis/allergy
NT3	Anti-myosin antibody
NT4	Anti-myosin antibody/inflammation[b]
NTS	Anti-myosin antibody/inflammation
NT6	Anti-myosin antibody/inflammation
NT7	Anti-myosin antibody
B1A	Inflammation
B3B	Inflammation
B2B3B	Anti-myosin antibody
C1A	Anti-myosin antibody
C1B	Anti-myosin antibody
C1C2	Anti-myosin antibody
C2A	Anti-myosin antibody/class I epitope
C2B	Anti-myosin antibody
C2C3	Anti-myosin antibody
C3	Anti-myosin antibody/class I epitope

[a]Peptide sequences are shown in Table 6.6.
[b]Inflammation is mild lymphocytic infiltrate in the heart.

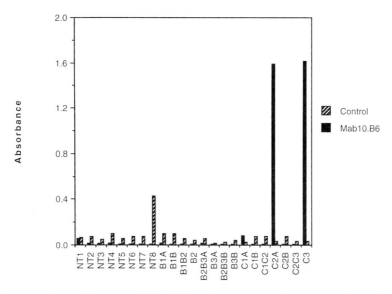

Figure 6.8 Reaction of anti-M protein MAb 10.B6 with streptococcal M-5 peptides in the ELISA. MAb 10.B6 (10 μg/ml), an anti-M protein MAb that recognizes a rheumatic fever–associated M protein epitope, was reacted with M-5 peptides as shown in Table 6.6. The MAb 10.B6 reacted with M-5 peptides C2A and C3. A control antibody did not react with these peptides [190].

with pharyngitis and rheumatic fever. Additional evidence has demonstrated that patients with ARF respond more strongly than patients with uncomplicated disease to the class I epitope [189,190]. The anti-M protein MAb 10.B6, which recognizes the class I epitope, was found to react with M-5 peptides C2A and C3 (Fig. 6.8). Antibodies against the peptide C3 were affinity purified from ARF sera, and the anti-C3 antibodies were shown to react with myosin [190]. Figure 6.9 shows the sequence homology between the amino acid sequence of peptide C3 and myosin. The identical sequence RRDL is conserved in both skeletal and cardiac myosins and is located in the HMM subfragment of myosin heavy chain. The MAb 10.B6, which reacted with the class 1 M protein serotypes, recognized M-5 peptides C2A and C3 and was found to react with myosin in Western immunoblots and ELISAs. The cross-reactivity between antibodies recognizing the class I epitope and myosin may lead to a better understanding of how rheumatogenic serotypes induce autoimmune responses in the susceptible host. Although peptides C2A and C3 contain the class I epitope and induce antimyosin antibody, they do not induce heart inflammation in rats or mice [187a].

Molecular Basis of Cross-reactive Antibody in Acute Rheumatic Fever: Idiotypes and Immunoglobulin Genes

The antibody produced in ARF has been analyzed in two ways. First, the antibodies were investigated to determine if a particular idiotype was present on anti-myosin antibodies in ARF. To do this, the anti-myosin antibodies were affinity purified from ARF sera and used to immunize rabbits for production of anti-idiotypic antibody. The result was the development of an anti-idiotypic serum that identified the anti-myosin antibodies in ARF [191]. The anti-idiotypic reagent was presumably specific for the antigen-combining site on the anti-myosin antibody present in ARF [191]. Studies of normal sera, ARF sera, sera from uncomplicated streptococcal infections, acute poststreptococcal glo-

```
QKMRRDLE                HUMAN CARDIAC MYOSIN [1168-1175]
  . :::::.
KGLRRDLDASREAK          M5 PEPTIDE C3 [282-299]
```

Figure 6.9 Sequence homology between the M-5 C3 peptide and human cardiac myosin. The C3 peptide contains the class I M protein epitope. The homologous sequence is highly conserved among cardiac and skeletal myosins [190].

merulonephritis (AGN), systemic lupus erythematosus (SLE), Sjogren's syndrome (SS), Chagas disease, myocarditis, and IgA nephropathy revealed that the Myl idiotype was elevated in ARF, AGN, SS, and SLE. The other diseases demonstrated normal levels of the Myl idiotype. These data linked the Myl idiotype and ARF with other autoimmune diseases and with cross-reactive anti-myosin antibody production.

The second method of analysis of the cross-reactive antibodies was the determination of the nucleotide sequence of the V-D-J genes of the cross-reactive human immunoglobulin molecules. Although our work is in progress, many of the VH and VL genes that have been utilized in encoding the human cross-reactive antibodies have been identifiable autoantibody germline genes [191a]. The first study was published on human MAb 10.2.3 which was shown to be encoded by a VH 26 germline gene [192]. The VH 26 gene is often used in anti-DNA antibodies and rheumatoid factors. Gene rearrangements encoding the highly cross-reactive immunoglobulin genes may be critical in the development of pathogenic antibody. Human antibodies are under investigation for their cytotoxicity and potential to deposit in tissues and to produce tissue inflammation.

Potential Role of Antibody in Tissue Injury: Investigation of Cytotoxic Antistreptococcal MAb 36.2.2

Defining the role of the heart-reactive antibody in ARF is important in understanding the mechanisms of tissue injury in the disease. If the previous studies by Kaplan et al. [151,158] demonstrating antibody deposition in the hearts of patients with ARF are correct, they support a role for antibody in the pathogenesis of the disease. Although cross-reactive antibodies react with the intracellular cytoskeletal protein, myosin, the antibodies may also react with the cell surface and bind complement, which would permit antibody and complement deposition with cellular damage. Investigation of mouse antistreptococcal MAbs for cytotoxicity on heart cells in the presence of complement revealed that mouse antistreptococcal MAb 36.2.2 was highly cytotoxic in chromium-51 release assays [193]. In addition, MAb 36.2.2 was found to react with the surface of rat heart cells in indirect immunofluorescence assays (Fig. 6.10). An unusual characteristic of MAb 36.2.2 was its reaction with laminin, an extracellular matrix protein surrounding the rat heart cells [193a]. It is not known whether the strong cytotoxicity was a re-

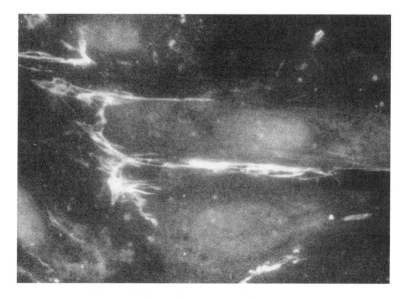

Figure 6.10 Reaction of cytotoxic antistreptococcal MAb 36.2.2 with the surface of rat heart cells in an indirect immunofluorescence assay. The MAb 36.2.2 was cytotoxic at concentrations of <1 μg [193,193a]. (From Antone et al. [193a], with permission from the *Journal of Immunology*.)

sult of MAb 36.2.2 reactivity with laminin, but it is highly suggestive that antistreptococcal MAbs that react with the extracellular matrix and/or cell surface proteins may have the potential for tissue damage. Two human cross-reactive MAbs, 1.H9 and 3.B6, have been found to be cytotoxic [193a] (Galvin JE and Cunningham MW, unpublished data). A recent report described the deposition of anti-myosin antibodies in the extracellular matrix of DBA/2 mice [172]. Administration of anti-myosin antibodies to mice led to deposition of antibodies and to cellular infiltration and inflammation in their hearts. Parallel studies of anti-myosin or anti-heart antibodies from ARF or myocarditis have not yet been reported.

An alternative explanation for antibody deposition in ARF may be that the antibody reacts in tissues with exposed myosin from damaged myocardial cells. Antibody is then allowed to penetrate the cell membrane or to react with cell contents already extruded during tissue necrosis. This is certainly a possibility, since the reports by Kaplan et al. [158] recognized that antibody in the rheumatic heart was deposited within myocardial cells as well as around them. If the cells were dead and myosin exposed, this might explain what was observed years ago. This hypothesis does not exclude the presence of cytotoxic antibodies in ARF. It would, however, explain some of the observations made by Kaplan and Svec [151].

Heart-Reactive Antistreptococcal Antibodies and T Cells in Valvular Injury in Acute Rheumatic Fever

The most serious pathological hallmark of ARF is valvular injury which leaves the valve(s) damaged and deformed. To determine if antistreptococcal MAbs reacted with heart valves, Gulizia et al. reacted MAbs 36.2.2, 49.8.9, and 54.2.8 with human heart valvular tissue sections [194]. The antistreptococcal MAbs reacted strongly with valvular endothelium and valvular interstitial cells within the valve matrix. Endothelium can become highly responsive in the presence of cytokines and in inflammatory situations, with enhanced expression of cell adhesion molecules that promote cellular infiltration [195–198]. Antibody and complement deposition on the vascular and valvular endothe-

lium would affect vascular permeability and induce endothelial changes. Heart or myosin cross-reactive antistreptococcal MAbs are shown to react strongly with the valvular endothelium (Fig. 6.11). Once the endothelium is activated, there would be cellular infiltration of the valve and myocardium by activated T lymphocytes. Injury and loss of valvular endothelium would expose subendothelial structures.

None of the antistreptococcal antibodies reacted with collagen in the valve, suggesting that collagenous structures were not the target of the heart cross-reactive antibodies. However, cross-reactive MAbs did react with the tentacular valvular interstitial cells buried in the valvular stroma. Valvular interstitial cells were found in increased numbers in rheumatic valves compared with normal valves [194]. The valve tissue

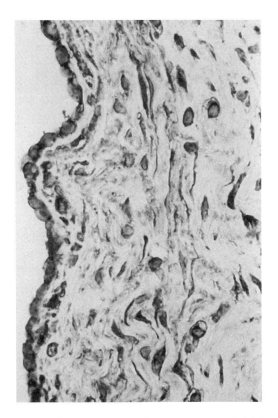

Figure 6.11 Reaction of antistreptococcal MAb 54.2.8 with a human valve section. The MAb 54.2.8 reacted strongly with the endothelium and with proteins and valvular interstitial cells in the valve matrix. No reaction was observed with the collagen matrix. (From Gulizia et al. [194], with permission from the *American Journal of Pathology*.)

responds to the inflammation and immune injury by proliferation and elaboration of connective tissue components, resulting in valvular scarring which leads to cardiac insufficiency.

In recent studies, human T cell lines/clones were developed from surgical heart valve specimens of rheumatic carditis patients previously infected with the M-5 serotype [90]. Lymphocytes were taken from mitral valves, papillary muscle, and left atrium and cultured in vitro. The T lymphocyte clones proliferated to streptococcal M-5 protein peptides and heart tissue extracts or fractions of cardiac proteins. Therefore, the T cells cloned from the rheumatic valves cross-reacted with M-5 peptides and heart proteins. It was not certain if the heart proteins were myosin. The M-5 peptides that caused proliferation of the T cell clones included M-5 residues 1–25 (TVTRGTISDPQRAKEALDKYELENH), 81–96 (DKLKQQRDTLSTQKETL EREVQNI), and 163–177 (ETIGTLKIDLDETVK). In this particular study [90], peptides from the C-repeat region of M protein were not investigated. The specific cardiac proteins that produced proliferation of the T cell clones were not identified [90]. The T cell clones were found to be CD4+ except for one clone that was CD8+, but the studies of the valvular lymphocyte clones did not identify if the T cells were cytotoxic. The presence of cytotoxic CD8+ T cells in ARF were first reported by Hutto and Ayoub in peripheral blood lymphocytes from ARF patients [85]. Dale and Beachey reported that human lymphocytes stimulated with pep M-5 protein were cytotoxic for heart cells in vitro [84]. The presence of cytotoxic T cell clones in heart tissues would be tissue damaging, and the CD8+ lymphocytes would be even more effective in the presence of inflammatory CD4+ cells.

Myosin Cross-reactive T Cell Epitopes of Streptococcal M-5 Protein

T cells from ARF patients have been shown to be highly reactive to streptococcal antigens in comparison with T cells from patients with uncomplicated streptococcal infections or normal individuals [74,80,199,200,201]. Some reports have suggested that lymphocytes from ARF patients or from animals sensitized to streptococcal antigens were cytotoxic to cardiac cells in vitro [85,88,92]. Human lymphocytes stimulated

with pep M-5 protein were cytotoxic for cells in vitro [84].

In more recent studies, pep M proteins and erythrogenic toxins A and C have been reported to be superantigens [114,115,202,203]. Superantigens differ from typical antigens in that they can function as a mitogenic stimulus for certain subsets of T cells. The general hyperresponsiveness observed in the susceptible host may be due to the exposure of T (and B) lymphocytes to superantigenic molecules. Expansion of T lymphocytes by specific protein sequences presented in the conventional way to T cells may further influence the development of tissue-damaging T cells.

Only a few studies have investigated the myosin cross-reactive T cell epitopes of M-5 protein [90,138,205]. One study described above investigated the T cells in rheumatic valvular lesions and response of the valvular T cell clones to M-5 peptides [90]. Another study of human T cell clones investigated carboxy-terminal segments of the streptococcal M-5, M-6, and M-24 proteins and identified epitopes that cross-reacted with cardiac and skeletal myosins [138]. Peptides from human cardiac myosin, human perinatal myosin, and human skeletal myosin were investigated. Two cross-reactive human T cell lines/clones were obtained from a normal individual and one from a rheumatic fever patient [138]. The two myosin cross-reactive clones from the normal individual proliferated to sequences in the M-5 protein carboxy-terminal region, residues 337–356 (LRRDLDASREAKKQVEK ALE) and 347–366 (AKKQVEKALEEANSKLAALE). The residues are reported in this study from the beginning of the leader sequence instead of from the beginning of the mature M protein. A myosin cross-reactive T cell clone from an individual with ARF proliferated to the M-5 sequence 397–416 (LKEQLAKQAEELAKLRAGKA), which is a sequence also located in the C-terminal region of M-5. Four myosin peptides produced responses from the T cell clones [138], although little consensus sequence among the peptides was observed. Table 6.8 summarizes the T cell epitopes of M-5 protein that may play a role in immune cross-reactions with myosin or heart antigens that can stimulate T cells that may infiltrate the valve or myocardium.

Table 6.8 Summary of Myosin or Heart Cross-reactive T Cell Epitopes of M-5 Protein

Peptide	Sequence[a]	Origin of T Cell Clone or Response[b] [Reference]
1–25	TVTRGTISDPQRAKEALDKYELENH	ARF/valve [46]
81–96	DKLKQQRDTLSTQKETLEREVQNI	ARF/valve [46]
163–177	ETIGTLKKILDETVK	ARF/valve [46]
337–356	LRRDLDASREAKKQVE KALE	Normal/PBL [138]
347–366	AKKQVEKALEEANSKLAALE	Normal/PBL [138]
397–416	LKEQLAKQAEELAKLRAGKA	ARF/PBL [138]
NT5 59–76	KKEHEAENDKLKQQRDTL	BALB/c/lymph node[c]
B1B2 137–154	VKDKIAKEQENKETIGTL	
B2 150–167	TIGTLKKILDETVKDKIA	
C2A 254–271	EASRKGLRRDLDASREAK	
C3 293–308	KGLRRDLDASREAKKQ	
B1A 111–129	TRQELANKQQESKENEKAL	Lewis rat/myocardium[d]
B1B 124–141	ENEKALNELLEKTVKDKI	
B1B2 137–154	VKDKLAKEQENKETIGTL	
B2 150–167	TIGTLKKILDETVKDKIA	
C1C2 241–258	AEHQKLEEQNKISEASRK	
C3 293–308	KGLRRDLDASREAKKQ	

[a]Underlined sequences are those found repeatedly in several of the studies.

[b]ARF, acute rheumatic fever; PBL, peripheral blood lymphocytes.

[c]BALB/c mice were immunized with purified human cardiac myosin and the recovered lymph node lymphocytes were stimulated with each of the peptides in tritiated thymidine uptake assays.

[d]Myosin reactive T cell line was from Lewis rat myocardium from episode of myosin-induced myocarditis.

Recent studies in our laboratory have investigated the M-5 peptides that stimulated lymphocytes from BALB/c mice sensitized to human cardiac myosin. In these studies, animals were immunized with human cardiac myosin and lymphocytes isolated from the lymph nodes were reacted with each of the M-5 peptides shown in Table 6.6. The M-5 peptides that stimulated lymphocytes from the human cardiac myosin–immunized mice were NT3, NT4, NT5, NT6, and NT7 in the A-repeat region, B1B2, B2, and B3A in the B-repeat region, and C1A, C2A, and C3 in the C-repeat region [204]. The most dominant sites observed in five separate experiments were NT5, B1B2/B2, C2A, and C3. Some of these sites contained sequences reported to stimulate T cell clones from ARF valves or peripheral blood. Myosin-reactive T cells cloned from myocarditic hearts of Lewis rats were stimulated by peptides in the B- and C-repeat region of M-5 protein (Table 6.8) [190]. These studies show that specific sites exist in the M-5 protein that stimulate lymphocytes or their T cell clones/lines from ARF or from animals immunized with human cardiac myosin.

Molecular Mimicry: Breaking Tolerance

Molecular mimicry between the microorganism and the host has been proposed as a mechanism for the development of autoimmune diseases [55,205,206]. Evidence suggests that microorganisms contain proteins that are similar enough to host proteins that they can stimulate B or T cells to respond to self proteins. The breaking of tolerance to cardiac myosin epitopes by a streptococcal antigen may explain the development of B and T cell autoimmunity against the heart in ARF. The hypothesis that M proteins or other streptococcal components, such as the group A streptococcal carbohydrate, could influence an autoimmune response against myosin in the susceptible host is based on an accumulation of evidence collected over the past 10 years. These data show that antistreptococcal and anti-myosin antibodies cross-react with streptococcal and host antigens including M proteins and myosins with the identification of homologous regions between the two proteins [141,160,161,170,174, 175,179,188,190,192,193,207]. In addition, the group A carbohydrate epitope *N*-acetyl-glucosamine mimics peptide sequences from α-helical molecules such as myosin, keratin, and the M protein [163,175,176]. Anti-myosin antibody can target the heart, producing antibody deposition, inflammation, and tissue damage [172].

Studies suggest that myosin and M protein cross-reactive T cells exist [90,138] and are likely to produce lesions in the heart in ARF [90]. The pathogenic response by the susceptible host most likely involves the recognition of streptococcal/myosin epitopes by MHC antigens that present these epitopes to inflammatory (TH1, CD4$^+$) and cytotoxic (CD8$^+$) T cell subsets. The streptococcal infection brings about the production of large quantities of influential cytokines that would up-regulate expression of MHC class I and II molecules in tissues and would determine the T cell subsets involved in the immune response in the susceptible host. Activated T cells would migrate into target tissues such as the heart by infiltration through activated vascular endothelium into the tissues. Activation of autoreactive T cells may be affected by streptococcal superantigens [114,115,202,203] and other mitogens produced by the infection. Activated lymphocytes that target the heart are probably the CD4$^+$ TH1 subset and the CD8$^+$ cytotoxic subset. The inflammatory CD4$^+$ T cells would produce tissue inflammation and scarring while the cytotoxic CD8$^+$ subset would be important in destruction of myocardial cells in the heart. The CD4$^+$ lymphocytes produce cytokines such as IFN-γ which would influence the CD8$^+$ T cells to become more effective cytotoxic lymphocytes.

If M protein mimics cardiac myosin, then it should be possible to produce cardiac lesions with the M protein. The Lewis is an established rat model of myosin induced myocarditis [165]. The Lewis rat model was used to determine if the M protein could substitute for cardiac myosin [190]. Immunization of the Lewis rat with the recombinant M-6 protein resulted in 50% of the animals developing small foci of myocarditis and two out of six animals developing valvulitis (Quin T, and Cunningham MW, manuscript in preparation). Positive control animals developed myocarditis lesions following immunization with human cardiac myosin. A T cell clone, developed from lymph nodes of animals immunized with the recombinant M-6 protein,

reacted to recombinant M-6 protein, skeletal and cardiac myosins, and light meromyosin. The clone was CD4$^+$ and produced IL-2 and IFN-γ. The T cell clone/line was TH0 or TH1 clone. TH1 clones could direct inflammatory responses against the heart. Studies are in progress to determine if the T cell clone can transfer disease. Animal models of valvulitis such as the Lewis rat will be important in understanding the steps in the pathogenesis of ARF.

REFERENCES

1. Newsholme A. The Milroy lectures on the natural history and affinities of rheumatic fever: a study in epidemiology. Lancet 1895; 1:589–592.
2. Paul JR. The rheumatic family. In: The Epidemiology of Rheumatic Fever. New York: American Heart Association, 1957; 125–130.
3. Pickles WN. A rheumatic family. Lancet 1943; 2:241.
4. Read FEM, Ciocco A, Taussig HB. Frequency of rheumatic manifestations among siblings, parents, uncles, aunts and grandparents of rheumatic and control patients. Am J Hyg 1938; 27:719–737.
5. Schwentker FF. The epidemiology of rheumatic fever. In: Thomas L (ed). Rheumatic Fever. Minneapolis: University of Minnesota Press, 1952; 17–27.
6. Wilson MG, Schweitzer M. Pattern of hereditary susceptibility in rheumatic fever. Circulation 1954; 10:699–704.
7. DiSciascio G, Taranta A. Rheumatic fever in children. Am Heart J 1980; 99:635–658.
8. Paul JR. Age, sex and racial relationships. In: The Epidemiology of Rheumatic Fever. New York: The American Heart Association, 1957; 81–92.
9. Bison A. The rise and fall of rheumatic fever. JAMA 1985; 254:538–541.
10. Pope RM. Rheumatic fever in the 1980s. Bull Rheum Dis 1989; 38:1–8.
11. Markowitz M. The decline of rheumatic fever: role of medical intervention. The Lewis W. Wannamaker Memorial Lecture. J Pediatr 1985; 106:545–550.
12. Chun LT, Reddy DV, Yamamoto LG. Rheumatic fever in children and adolescents in Hawaii. Pediatrics 1987; 79:549–552.
13. Chun LT, Reddy V, Rhoads GG. Occurrence and prevention of rheumatic fever among ethnic groups of Hawaii. Am J Dis Child 1984; 138:476–478.
14. Wannamaker LW. Changes and changing concepts in the biology of group A streptococci and in the epidemiology of streptococcal infections. Rev Infect Dis 1979; 1:967–975.

15. Ferguson GW, Shultz JM, Bisno AL. Epidemiology of acute rheumatic fever in a multiethnic, multiracial urban community: the Miami-Dade County experience. J Infect Dis 1991; 164:720–725.

16. Rejholec V. Incidence of rheumatic fever in relation to immunologic reactivity. Ann Rheum Dis 1957; 16:23–30.

17. Meiselas LE, Zingale SB, Lee SL, Richman S, Siegel M. Antibody production in rheumatic diseases: the effect of brucella antigen. J Clin Invest 1961; 40:1872–1881.

18. Stetson CA. The relation of antibody response to rheumatic fever. In: McCarty M (ed). Streptococcal Infections. New York: Columbia University Press, 1954; 208–218.

19. Wannamaker LW, Ayoub EM. Antibody titers in acute rheumatic fever. Circulation 1960; 21:598–614.

20. Dudding BA, Ayoub EM. Persistence of streptococcal group A antibody in patients with rheumatic valvular disease. J Exp Med 1968; 128:1081–1098.

21. Shulman ST, Ayoub EM, Victorica BE. Differences in antibody response to streptococcal antigens in children with rheumatic and nonrheumatic mitral valve disease. Circulation 1974; 50:1244–1251.

22. Ayoub EM, Shulman ST. Pattern of antibody response to the streptococcal group A carbohydrate in rheumatic patients with or without carditis. In: Read SE, Zabriskie JB (eds). Streptococcal Disease and the Immune Response. New York: Academic Press, 1980; 649–659.

23. Braun DG, Eichmann K, Krause RM. Rabbit antibodies to streptococcal carbohydrates: influence of primary and secondary immunization and of possible genetic factors on the antibody response. J Exp Med 1969; 129:809–830.

24. Leslie GA, Carwile HF. Immune response of rats to group A streptococcal vaccine. Infect Immun 1973; 7:781–785.

25. Briles DE, Krause RM. Mouse strain-specific idiotypy and interstrain idiotype cross-reactions. J Immunol 1973; 113:522–530.

26. Braun DG, Kelus AS. Idiotypic specificity of rabbit antibodies to streptococcal group polysaccharides. J Exp Med 1973; 138:1248–1265.

27. Braun DG, Quintans J, Luzzati AL, Lefkovits I, Read SE. Antibody response of rabbit blood lymphocytes in vitro: kinetics, clone size, and clonotype analysis in response to streptococcal group A polysaccharide antigens. J Exp Med 1976; 143:360–371.

28. Saszuki T, Kaneoka H, Nishimura Y, Kaneoka R, Hayama M, Ohkuni H. An HLA-linked immune suppression gene in man. J Exp Med 1980; 152:297S–313S.

29. Glynn AA, Glynn LE, Holborow EJ. Secretion of blood-group substances in rheumatic fever. BMJ 1959; 2:266–270.

30. Clarke CA, McConnell RB, Sheppard PM. ABO blood groups and secretor character in rheumatic carditis. BMJ 1960; 1:21–23.

31. Dublin TD, Bernanke AD, Pitt EL, Massell BF, Allen FH, Amezcua F. Red blood cell groups and ABH secretor system as genetic indicators of susceptibility to rheumatic fever and rheumatic heart disease. BMJ 1964; 2:775–779.

32. Haverkorn van Rijsewijk MJ, Goslings WRO. Secretor status of streptococcus pyogenes group A carriers and patients with rheumatic heart disease or acute glomerulonephritis. BMJ 1963; 2:542–543.

33. McDermott M, McDevitt H. The immunogenetics of rheumatic diseases. Bull Rheum Dis 1988; 38:1–10.

34. Falk JA, Fleischman JL, Zabriskie JB, Falk RE. A study of HL-A antigen phenotype in rheumatic fever and rheumatic heart disease. Tissue Antigens 1973; 3:173–178.

35. Murray GC, Montiel MM, Persellin RH. A study of antigens in adults with acute rheumatic fever. Arthritis Rheum 1978; 21:652–656.

36. Greenberg LJ, Gray ED, Yunis EJ. Association of HL-A5 and immune responsiveness in vitro to streptococcal antigens. J Exp Med 1975; 141:935–943.

37. Yoshinoya S, Pope RM. Detection of immune complexes in acute rheumatic fever and their relationship to HLA-B5. J Clin Invest 1980; 65:136–145.

38. Leirisalo M, Koivuranta P, Laitinen O. Rheumatic fever and its sequels in children: a follow-up study with HLA analysis. J Rheumatol 1980; 7:506–514.

39. Ayoub EM. The search for host determinants of susceptibility of rheumatic fever: the missing link. Circulation 1984; 69:197–201.

40. Ayoub EM, Barrett DJ, Maclaren NK, Krischer JP. Association of class II human histocompatibility leukocyte antigens with rheumatic fever. J Clin Invest 1986; 77:2019–2025.

41. Anastasiou-Nana MI, Anderson JL, Carlquist JF, Nanas JN. HLA-DR typing and lymphocyte subset evaluation in rheumatic heart disease: a search for immune response factors. Am Heart J 1986; 112:992–997.

42. Rajapakse CNA, Halim K, Al-Orainey I, Al-Nozha M, Al-Aska AK. A genetic marker for rheumatic heart disease. Br Heart J 1987; 58:659–662.

43. Jhinghan B, Mehra NK, Reddy KS, Taneja V, Vaidya MC, Bhatia ML. HLA, blood groups and secretor status in patients with established rheumatic fever and rheumatic heart disease. Tissue Antigens 1986; 27:172–178.

44. Taneja V, Mehra NK, Reddy KS, Narula J, Tandon R, Vaidya MC, Bhatia ML. HLA-DR/DQ and reactivity to B cell alloantigen D8/17 in Indian patients with rheumatic heart disease. Circulation 1989; 80:335–340.

45. Ozkan M, Carin M, Sonmez G, Senocak M,

Ozdemir M, Yakut C. HLA antigens in Turkish race with rheumatic heart disease. Circulation 1993; 87:1974–1978.

46. Guilherme L, Weidebach W, Kiss MH, Snitcowsky R, Kalil J. Association of human leukocyte class II antigens with rheumatic fever or rheumatic heart disease in a Brazilian population. Circulation 1991; 83:1995–1998.

46a. Ahmed S, Ayoub EM, Scornik JC, Wang CY, She JX. Poststreptococcal reactive arthritis. Clinical characteristics and association with HLA-DR alleles. Arthritis Rheum 1998; 41:1096–1102.

47. Weidebach W, Goldberg AC, Chiarella JM, Guilherme L, Snitcowsky R, Pileggi F, Kalil J. HLA class II antigens in rheumatic fever: analysis of the DR locus by restriction fragment polymorphism and oligotyping. Hum Immunol 1994; 40:253–258.

47a. Guédez Y, Kotby A, El-Demellawy M, Galal A, Thomson A, Zaher A, Samir Kassem S, and Kotb M. 1999. HLA class II associations with rheumatic heart disease are more evident and consistent among clinically homogeneous patients. Circulation (in press).

47b. Debaz H, Olivo A, Perez-Luque E, Vasquez-Garcia MN, Burguete A, Chavez-Negrete A, Velasco C, Arguero R, Gorodeszky C. DNA analysis of class II alleles in rheumatic heart disease in Mexicans. 22nd Annual ASHI Meeting Abstracts. Kansas City: 1996; 49:63.

47c. Koyanagi T, Koga Y, Nishi H, Toshima H, Sasazuki T, Imaizumi T, Kimura A. DNA typing of HLA class II genes in Japanese patients with rheumatic heart disease. J Mol Cell Cardiol 1996; 28:259–261.

48. Maharaj B, Hammond MG, Appadoo B, Leary WP, Puditin DJ. HLA-A, B, DR, and DQ antigens in black patients with severe chronic rheumatic heart disease. Circulation 1987; 76:259–261.

49. Khanna AK, Buskirk DR, Williams RC, Gibofsky A, Crow MK, Menon A, Fotino M, Reid HM, Poon-King T, Rubinstein P, Zabriskie JB. Presence of a non-HLA B cell antigen in rheumatic fever patients and their families as defined by a monoclonal antibody. J Clin Invest 1989; 83:1710–1716.

50. Ayoub EM, Atkinson MA, Alsaeid K, Schiffenbauer J. Association of 70 Kd molecule with HLA-DR of rheumatic fever patients. Zentralbl Bakteriol 1992; 22S:528–530.

51. Rantz La, Maroney M, Di Caprio JM. Hemolytic streptococcal infection in childhood. Pediatrics 1953; 12:498–515.

52. Beachey EH, Majumdar G, Tomai M, Kotb M. Molecular aspects of autoimmune responses to streptococcal M proteins. In: Gallin FA (ed). Advances in Host Defense Mechanisms. New York: Raven Press, 1990; 83–95.

53. Kaplan MH, Frengley JD. Autoimmunity to the heart in cardiac disease. Current concepts of the relation of autoimmunity to rheumatic fever postcardiotomy and postinfarction syndromes and cardiomyopathies. Am J Cardiol 1969; 24:459–473.

54. Kaplan MH, Suchy ML. Immunologic relation of streptococcal and tissue antigens II. Crossreactions of antisera to mammalian heat tissue and the cell wall constituent of certain strains of group A streptococci. J Exp Med 1964; 119:643–650.

55. Zabriskie JB. Mimetic relationships between group A streptococci and mammalian tissues. Adv Immunol 1966; 7:147–188.

56. Ayoub EM. Immune response to group A streptococcal infections. Pediatr Infect Dis J 1991; 10(Suppl):S15–S19.

57. Dell A, Antone SM, Gauntt CJ, Crossley CA, Clark WA, Cunningham MW. Autoimmune determinants of rheumatic carditis: localization of epitopes in human cardiac myosin. Eur Heart J 1991; 12:158–162.

58. Vashishtha A, Fischett VA. Surface-exposed conserved region of the streptococcal M protein induces antibodies cross-reactive with denatured forms of myosin. J Immunol 1993; 150:4693–4701.

59. Ayoub EM, Kaplan EL. Host-parasite interaction in the pathogenesis of rheumatic fever. J Rheumatol 1991; 18(Suppl 30):6–13.

60. Bahr GM, Yousof AM, Majeed H, Chedid L, Behbehani K. Antibodies to a streptococcal cell wall adjuvant structure persist in patient with chronic rheumatic heart disease. J Mol Cell Cardiol 1989; 21:61–66.

61. Zabriskie JB, Hsu KC, Seegal BC. Heart-reactive antibody associated with rheumatic fever: characterization and diagnostic significance. Clin Exp Immunol 1970; 7:147–159.

62. Neu N, Ploier B, Ofner C. Cardiac myosin-induced myocarditis. J Immunol 1990; 145:4094–4100.

63. Smith SC, Allen PM. The role of T cells in myosin-induced autoimmune myocarditis. Clin Immunol Immunopathol 1993; 68:100–106.

64. Lawrence HS. The cellular transfer in humans of delayed cutaneous reactivity to hemolytic streptococci. J Immunol 1952; 68:159–178.

65. Lawrence HS. Transfer of skin reactivity to streptococcal products. In: McCarty M (ed). Streptococcal Infections. New York: Columbia University Press, 1954; 143–156.

66. Humphrey JH, Pagel WB. The tissue response to heat-killed streptococci in the skin of normal subjects and in persons with rheumatic fever, rheumatoid arthritis, subacute bacterial endocarditis and erythema nodosum. Br J Exp Pathol 1949; 30:282–288.

67. Beachey EH, Stollerman GH, Johnson RH, Ofek I, Bisno AL. Human immune response to immunization with a structurally defined polypep-

tide fragment of streptococcal M protein. J Exp Med 1979; 150:862–877.

68. Fox EN, Wittner MK, Dorfman A. Antigenicity of the M proteins of group A hemolytic streptococci. J Exp Med 1966; 124:1135–1151.

69. Hafez M, Abdalla A, El-Shannawy F, Al-Tonbary Y, Sheaishaa A, El-Morsi Z, Tawfik S, Settien A, Abou-El Khair M. Immunogenetic study of the response to streptococcal carbohydrate antigen of the cell wall in rheumatic fever. Ann Rheum Dis 1990; 49:708–714.

70. Hafez M, El-Shannawy F, El-Salab S, El-Morsi Z, El-Ziny M, Al-Tonbary Y, Abdalla A, Abou-El Enein A. Studies of peripheral blood 1 lymphocytes in assessment of disease activity in rheumatic fever. Br J Rheumatol 1988; 27:181–186.

71. Pachman LM, Fox EN. Cellular and antibody reactions to streptococcal M protein types 1, 3, 6, and 12. J Immunol 1970; 105:898–907.

72. Read SE, Fischetti VA, Utermohlen V, Falk R, Zabriskie JB. Cellular reactivity studies to streptococcal antigens. Migration inhibition studies in patients with streptococcal infections and rheumatic fever. J Clin Invest 1974; 54:439–450.

73. Read SE, Reid HFM, Fischetti VA, Poon-King T, Ramkisson R, McDowell M, Zabriskie JB. Serial studies on the cellular immune response to streptococcal antigens in acute and convalescent rheumatic fever patients in Trinidad. J Clin Immunol 1986; 6:433–441.

74. Reid HGM, Read SE, Poon-King T, Zabriskie JB. Lymphocyte response to streptococcal antigens in rheumatic fever patients in Trinidad. In: Read SE, Zabriskie JB (eds). Streptococcal Diseases and the Immune Response. New York: Academic Press, 1980; 681–693.

75. Sapru RP, Ganguly NK, Sharma S, Chandani RE, Gupta AK. Cellular reaction to group A beta hemolytic streptococcal membrane antigen and its relation to complement levels in patients with rheumatic heart disease. BMJ 1977; 2:422–424.

76. Bhatia R, Narula J, Reddy KS, Koicha M, Malaviya AN, Pothineni RB, Tandon R, Bhatia ML. Lymphocyte subsets in acute rheumatic fever and rheumatic heart disease. Clin Cardiol 1989; 12:34–38.

77. Morris K, Mohan C, Wahi PL, Anand IS, Ganguly NK. Increase in activated T cells and reduction in suppressor/cytotoxic T cells in acute rheumatic fever and active rheumatic heart disease: a longitudinal study. J Infect Dis 1993; 167:979–983.

78. Williams RCJ, Zabriskie JB, Mahros F, Hassaballa F, Abdin ZH. Lymphocyte surface markers in acute rheumatic fever and post-streptococcal acute glomerulonephritis. Clin Exp Immunol 1977; 27:135–142.

79. Bahr GM, Yousof AM, Behbehani K, Majeed HA, Sakkalah S, Souan K, Jarrad I, Geoffroy C, Alouf JE. Antibody levels and in vitro lympho-proliferative responses to Streptococcus pyogenes erythrogenic toxin A and mitogen of patients with rheumatic fever. J Clin Microbiol 1991; 29:1789–1794.

80. Gray ED, Wannamaker LW, Ayoub EM, el-Kholy A, Abdin ZH. Cellular immune responses to extracellular streptococcal products in rheumatic heart disease. J Clin Invest 1981; 68:665–671.

81. Hirschorn K, Schribman RR, Verbo S, Gruskin RH. The action of streptolysin S on peripheral lymphocytes of normal subjects and patients with acute rheumatic fever. Proc Natl Acad Sci USA 1964; 52:1151–1157.

82. Lueker RD, Abdin ZH, Williams RCJ. Peripheral blood T and B lymphocytes during acute rheumatic fever. J Clin Invest 1975; 55:975–985.

83. Lueker RD, Williams RC Jr. Decreased reactivity of lymphocytesin mixed-leukocyte culture from patients with rheumatic fever. Circulation 1972; 46:655–660.

84. Dale JB, Beachey EH. Human cytotoxic lymphocytes evoked by group A streptococcal M protein. J Exp Med 1987; 166:1825–1835.

85. Hutto J, Ayoub EM. Cytotoxicity of lymphocytes from patients with rheumatic carditis to cardiac cells in vitro. In: Read SE, Zabriskie JB (eds). Streptococcal diseases and the immune response. New York: Academic Press 1980; 733–738.

86. Benatar A, Beatty DW, Human DG. Immunological abnormalities in children with acute rheumatic carditis and acute post-streptococcal glomerulonephritis. Int J Cardiol 1988; 21:51–58.

87. Chase RMJ, Rapaport FT. The bacterial induction of homograft sensitivity. I. Effects of sensitization with group A streptococci. J Exp Med 1965; 122:721–731.

88. Friedman I, Laufer A, Ron N, Davies AM. Experimental myocarditis: in vitro and in vivo studies of lymphocytes sensitized to heart extracts and group A streptococci. Immunology 1971; 20:225–232.

89. Gowrishanker R, Agarwal SC. Leukocyte migration inhibition with human heart valve glycoproteins and group A streptococcal ribonucleic acid proteins in rheumatic heart disease and post-streptococcal glomerulonephritis. Clin Exp Immunol 1980; 39:519–525.

90. Guilherme L, Cunha-Neto E, Coelho V, Snitcowsky R, Pomerantzeff PMA, Assis RV, Pedra F, Neumann J, Goldberg A, Patarroyo ME, Pileggi F, Kalil J. Human heart-infiltrating T cell clones from rheumatic heart disease patients recognize both streptococcal and cardiac proteins. Circulation 1995; 92:415–420.

91. Senitzer D, Cafruny W, Pansky B, Freimer E. Spontaneous and induced cell-mediated reactivity to syngeneic cells. Nature 1977; 268:158–159.

92. Yang LC, Soprey PR, Wittner MK, Fox EN. Streptococcal induced cell mediated immune destruction of cardiac myofibers in vitro. J Exp Med 1977; 146:344–360.

93. Marboe CC, Knowles D, Weiss MB, Fenoglio JJ. Monoclonal antibody identification of mononuclear cells in endomyocardial biopsy specimens from a patient with rheumatic carditis. Hum Pathol 1985; 16:332–338.

94. Raizada V, Williams RCJ, Chopra P, Copinath N. Tissue distribution of lymphocytes in rheumatic heart valves as defined by monoclonal anti–T cell antibodies. Am J Med 1983; 74:90–96.

95. Kemeny E, Grieve T, Marcus R, Sareti P, Zabriskie JB. Identification of mononuclear cells and T cell subsets in rheumatic valvulitis. Clin Immunol Immunopathol 1989; 52: 225–237.

96. Amoils B, Morrison RC, Wadee AA, Marcus R, Ninin D, King P, Sareli P, Levin S, Rabson AR. Aberrant expression of HLA-DR antigen on valvular fibroblasts from patients with active rheumatic carditis. Clin Exp Immunol 1986; 66:88–94.

97. Kotb M. Post-streptococcal autoimmune sequelae: a link between infection and autoimmunity. In: Dalgleish AG, Albertini A, Paoletti R (eds). The Impact of Biotechnology on Autoimmunity. 1994;

97a. El-Demellawy M, El-Ridi R, Guirguis N, Abdel-Alim M, Kotby A, Kotb M. Preferential Recognition of Human Myocardial Antigens by T-lymphocytes from Rheumatic Fever and Rheumatic Heart Disease Patients. Infect. Immun. 1997; 65:2197–2205.

98. Horstmann RD, Sievertsen HJ, Knobloch J, Fischett VA. Antiphagocytic activity of streptococcal M protein: selective binding of complement control protein factor H. Proc Natl Acad Sci USA 1988; 85:1657–1661.

99. Whitnak E, Beachey EH. Inhibition of complement-mediated opsonization and phagocytosis of streptococcus pyogenes by D fragments and fibrin bound to cell-surface M protein. J Exp Med 1985; 162:1983–1997.

100. Beachey EH, Bronze M, Dale JB, Kraus W, Poirier T, Sargent S. Protective and autoimmune epitopes of streptococcal M proteins. Vaccine 1988; 6:192–196.

101. Bisno AL. Group A streptococcal infections and acute rheumatic fever. N Engl J Med 1991; 325:783–793.

102. Dale JB, Beachey EH. Multiple heart-cross-reactive epitopes of streptococcal M proteins. J Exp Med 1985; 161:113–122.

103. Fischetti VA. Streptococcal M protein. Sci Am 1991; 264:58–65.

104. Robinson JH, Kehoe MA. Group A streptococcal M proteins: virulence factors and protective antigens. Immunol Today 1992; 13:362–367.

105. Stollerman GH. Rheumatogenic streptococci and autoimmunity. Clin Immunol Immunopathol 1991; 61:131–142.

106. Stollerman GH. Nephritogenic and rheumatogenic group A streptococci. J Infect Dis 1969; 120:258–263.

107. Beachey EH, Alberti H, Stollerman GH. Delayed hypersensitivity to purified streptococcal M protein in guinea pigs and in man. J Immunol 1969; 102:42–52.

108. Beachey EH, Seyer JM, Dale JB, Simpson WA, Kang AH. Type-specific protective immunity evoked by synthetic peptide of Streptococcus pyogenes M protein. Nature 1981; 292: 457–459.

109. Beachey EH, Seyer JM, Kang AH. Repeating covalent structure of streptococcal M protein. Proc Natl Acad Sci USA 1978; 75:3163–3167.

110. Beachey EH, Stollerman G, Chiang EY, Chiang TM, Seyer JM, Kang AH. Purification and properties of M protein extracted from group A streptococci with pepsin: covalent structure of the amino terminal region of type 24 M antigen. J Exp Med 1977; 145:1469–1483.

111. Dale J, Simpson W, Ofek I, Beachey E. Blastogenic responses of human lymphocytes to structurally defined polypeptide fragments of streptococcal M protein. J Immunol 1981; 126:1499–1505.

112. Kotb M, Dale JB, Beachey EH. Stimulation of S-adenosylmethionine synthetase in human lymphocytes by streptococcal M protein. J Immunol 1987; 139:202–206.

113. Majumdar G, Beachey EH, Tomai MA, Kotb M. Differential signal requirements in T-cell activation by mitogen and superantigen. Cell Signal 1991; 2:521–530.

114. Tomai M, Kotb M, Majundar G, Beachey EH. Superantigenicity of streptococcal M protein. J Exp Med 1990; 172:359–362.

115. Tomai M, Aileon JA, Dockter ME, Majumdar G, Spinella DG, Kotb M. T cell receptor V gene usage by human T cells stimulated with the superantigen streptococcal M protein. J Exp Med 1991; 174:285–288.

116. Watanabe-Ohnishi R, Aelion J, Le Gros HL, Tomai MA, Sokurenko EV, Newton D, Takahara J, Irino S, Rashed S, Kotb M. Characterization of unique human TCR β specificities for a family of streptococcal superantigens represented by rheumatogenic serotypes of M protein. J Immunol 1994; 152:2066–2073.

117. Cole BC, Atkin CL. The Mycoplasma arthritidis T-cell mitogen, MAM: a model superantigen. Immunol Today 1991; 12:271–276.

118. Friedman SM, Tumang JR, Crow MK. Microbial superantigens as etiopathogenic agents in autoimmunity. Rheum Dis Clin North Am 1993; 19:207–222.

119. Johnson DR, Stevens DL, Kaplan EL. Epidemiologic analysis of group A streptococcal serotypes associated with severe systemic infec-

tions, rheumatic fever or uncomplicated pharyn-gitis. J Infect Dis 1992; 166:374–382.

120. Kotb M. Role of superantigens in the patho-genesis of infectious diseases and their seque-lae. Curr Opin Infect Dis 1992; 5:364–374.

121. Kotb M. Bacterial exotoxins as superantigens. Clin Microbiol Rev 1995; 8:411–426.

122. Kotb M. Infection and immunity: a story of the host, the pathogen, and the copathogen. Clin Immunol Immunopathol 1995; 74:10–22.

123. Kotzin BL, Leung DY, Kappler J, Marrack P. Superantigens and their potential role in human disease. Adv Immunol 1993; 54:99–166.

124. Marrack P, Kappler J. The staphylococcal en-terotoxins and their relatives. Science 1990; 248:705–711.

125. Schlievert PM. Role of superantigens in human diseases. J Infect Dis 1993; 167:997–1002.

126. Narula J, Chopra P, Talwar KK, Sachdev S, Bha-tia R, Reddy KS, Malaviya AN, Tandon R, Bha-tia ML. Histopathological and immunohisto-chemical studies in acute rheumatic myocarditis in man: a prospective endomyocardial biopsy study. Circulation 1988; 78(Suppl II):SII–440. (Abstract)

127. Andersson J, Nagy S, Bjork L, Abrams J, Holm S, Andersson U. Bacterial toxin-induced cy-tokine production studied at the single-cell level. Immunol Rev 1992; 127:69–96.

128. Fast DJ, Schlievert PM, Nelson RD. Toxic shock syndrome-associated staphylococcal and strep-tococcal pyrogenic toxins are potent inducers of tumor necrosis factor production. Infect Immun 1989; 57:291–294.

129. Hackett SP, Stevens DL. Streptococcal toxic shock syndrome: synthesis of tumor necrosis fac-tor and interleukin-1 by monocytes stimulated with pyrogenic exotoxin A and streptolysin O. J Infect Dis 1992; 165:879–885.

130. Kotb M, Ohnishi H, Majumdar G, Hackett S, Bryant A, Higgins G, Stevens D. Temporal re-lationship of cytokine release by peripheral blood mononuclear cells stimulated by the strep-tococcal superantigen pep M5. Infect Immun 1993; 61:1194–1201.

131. Muller-Alouf H, Alouf JE, Gerlach D, Fitting C, Cavaillon JM. Cytokine production by murine cells activated by erythrogenic toxin type A su-perantigen of *Streptococcus pyogenes*. Im-munobiology 1992; 186:435–448.

132. Muller-Alouf H, Alouf JE, Gerlach D, Oze-gowski JH, Fitting C, Cavaillon JM. Compara-tive study of cytokine release by human periph-eral blood mononuclear cells stimulated with *Streptococcus pyogenes* superantigenic eryth-rogenic toxins, heat-killed streptococci, and lipopolysaccharide. Infect Immun 1994; 62: 4915–4921.

133. Kotb M, Watanbe-Ohnishi R, Wang B, Tomai MA, Le Gros L, Schlievert P, El Demellawy M, Geller A. Analysis of the TCR Vβ specificities of

bacterial superantigens using PCR. Immuno-methods 1983; 2:33–40.

134. Kotb M, Courtney H, Dale JB, Beachey EH. Cellular and biochemical responses of human T lymphocytes by streptococcal M proteins. J Im-munol 1989; 142:966–970.

135. Dohlsten M, Lando PA, Hedlund G, Trowsdale J, Kalland T. Targeting of human cytotoxic T lymphocytes to MHC class II-expressing cells by staphylococcal enterotoxins. Immunology 1990; 71:96–100.

136. Gray ED, Abdin ZH, el-Kholy A, Mansour M, Miller LC, Zaher S, Kamel R, Regelmann WE. Augmentation of cytotoxic activity by mitogens in rheumatic heart disease. J Rheumatol 1988; 15:1672–1676.

137. Uchida A, Mickshe M. Lysis of fresh human tu-mor cells by autologous peripheral blood lym-phocytes and pleural effusion. J Natl Cancer Inst 1983; 71:673.

138. Pruksakorn S, Currie B, Brandt E, Phorn-phutkul C, Hunsakunachai S, Manmontri A, Robinson JH, Kehoe MA, Galbraith A, Good MF. Identification of T cell autoepitopes that cross-react with the C-terminal segment of the M protein of group A streptococci. Int Immunol 1994; 6:1235–1244.

139. Wang B, Schlievert PM, Gaber AO, Kotb M. Lo-calization of an immunologically functional re-gion of the streptococcal superantigen pepsin-extracted fragment of type 5 M protein. J Immunol 1993; 151:1419–1429.

140. Claesson L, Larhammar D, Rask L, Peterson PA. cDNA clone for the human invariant Y chain of class II histocompatibility antigens and its im-plications for the protein structure. Proc Natl Acad Sci USA 1983; 80:7395–7404.

141. Cunningham MW, McCormack MW, Fender-son PG, Ho MK, Beachey EH, Dale JB. Human and murine antibodies cross-reactive with streptococcal M protein and myosin recognized the sequence Gln-Lys-Ser-Lys-Gln in M protein. J Immunol 1989; 143: 2677–2683.

142. Bisno A. The concept of rheumatogenic and non-rheumatogenic group A streptococci. In: Read SE, Zabriskie JB (eds). Streptococcal Dis-eases and the Immune Response. New York: Academic Press, 1980; 789–803.

143. Bessen D, Jones KF, Fischetti VA: Evidence for two distinct classes of streptococcal M protein and their relationship to rheumatic fever. J Exp Med 1989; 169:269–283.

144. Dajani AS, Ayoub EM, Bierman FZ, Bisno AL, Denny FW, Durack DT, Ferrieri P, Freed M, Gerber M, Kaplan EL, Karchmer AW, Markowitz M, Rahimtoola SH, Shulman ST, Stollerman G, Masato T, Taranta A, Taubert KA, Wilson W. Guidelines for the diagnosis of rheumatic fever: Jones criteria, updated 1992. JAMA 1992; 87:302–307.

145. Jones TD. The diagnosis of rheumatic fever. JAMA 1944; 126:481–484.

146. Anderson HC, Kunkel HC, McCarty M. Quantitative anti-streptokinase studies in patients infected with group A hemolytic streptococci: a comparison with serum antistreptolysin and gamma globulin levels with special reference to the occurrence of rheumatic fever. J Clin Invest 1948; 27:425–434.

147. Zabriskie JB, Freimer EH. An immunological relationship between group A streptococci and mammalian muscle. J Exp Med 1966; 124:661–668.

148. Van de Rijn I, Zabriskie JB, McCarty M. Group A streptococcal antigens cross reactive with myocardium. Purification of heart reactive antibody and isolation and characterization of the streptococcal antigen. J Exp Med 1977; 146:579–599.

149. Kaplan MH, Meyeserian M. An immunological cross-reaction between group A streptococcal cells and human heart tissue. Lancet 1962; 1:706–710.

150. Kaplan MH. Immunologic relation of streptococcal and tissues antigens. I. Properties of an antigen in certain strains of group A streptococci exhibiting an immunologic cross-reaction with human heart tissue. J lmmunol 1963; 90:595–606.

151. Kaplan MH, Svec KH. Immunological relation of streptococcal and tissue antigens. J Exp Med 1964; 119:651–666.

152. Lyampert IM, Vvedenskaya OI, Danilova TA. Study on streptococcus group A antigens common with heart tissue elements. Immunol 1966; 11:313–320.

153. Lyampert IM, Beletskrya LV, Ugryumova GA. The reaction of heart and other organ extracts with the sera of animals immunized with group A streptococci. Immunol 1968; 15:845–854.

154. Goldstein I, Halpern B, Robert L. Immunologic relation between streptococcus A polysaccharide and the structural glycoproteins of heart valve. Nature 1967; 213:44–47.

155. Schwab JH. Biological properties of streptococcal cell wall particles. I. Determinants of the chronic nodular lesions of connective tissue. J Bacteriol 1965; 90:1405–1411.

156. Cromartie WJ, CraddockJG, SchwabJH, Anderle SK, Yang CH. Arthritis in rats after systemic injecion of streptococcal cells or cell walls. J Exp Med 1977; 146:1585–1602.

157. Cavelti PA. Autoantibodies in rheumatic fever. Proc Soc Exp Biol Med 1945; 60:379–381.

158. Kaplan MH, Bolande R, Rakita L, Blair J. Presence of bound immunoglobulins and complement in the myocardium in acute rheumatic fever. N Engl J Med 1964; 271:637–645.

159. Krisher K, Cunningham MW. Myosin: a link between streptococci and heart. Science 1985; 227:413–415.

160. Cunningham MW, Hall NK, Krisher KK, Spanier AM. A study of anti-group A streptococcal monoclonal antibodies cross-reactive with myosin. J Immunol 1986; 136:293–298.

161. Cunningham MW, Swerlick RA. Polyspecificity of anti-streptococcal murine monoclonal antibodies and their implications in autoimmunity. J Exp Med 1986; 164:998–1012.

162. Cunningham MW, McCormack JM, Talaber LR. Human monoclonal antibodies reactive with antigens of the group A streptococcus and human heart. J Immunol 1988; 141:2760–2766.

163. Shikhman AR, Cunningham MW. Immunological mimicry between N-acetyl-B-D-glucosamine and cytokeratin peptides. J Immunol 1994; 152:4375–4387.

164. Neu N, Rose NR, Beisel KW, Herskowitz A, Gurri-Glass G, Craig SW. Cardiac myosin induces myocarditis in genetically predisposed mice. J Immunol 1987; 139:3630–3636.

165. Kodama M, Matsumoto Y, Fujiwara M, Massani M, Izumi T, Shibota A. A novel experimental model of giant cell myocarditis induced in rats by immunization with cardiac myosin fraction. Clin Immunol Immunopathol 1991; 57:250–262.

166. Fitzsimons E, Lange CF. Hybridomas to specific streptococcal antigen induced tissue pathology in vivo: autoimmune mechanism for poststreptococcal sequelae. Autoimmunity 1991; 10:115–124.

167. Lange CF. Localization of [C¹⁴] labeled anti-streptococcal cell membrane monoclonal antibodies (anti-SCM mAb) in mice. Autoimmunity 1994; 19:179–191.

168. Fenderson PG, Fischetti VA, Cunningham MW. Tropomyosin shares immunologic epitopes with group A streptococcal M proteins. J Immunol 1989; 142:2475–2481.

169. Manjula BN, Fischetti VA. Tropomyosin-like seven residue periodicity in three immunologically distinct streptococcal M proteins and its implication for the antiphagocytic property of the molecule. J Exp Med 1980; 151:695–708.

170. Manjula BN, Trus BL, Fischetti VA. Presence of two distinct regions in the coiled-coil structure of the streptococcal PepM5 protein: relationship to mammalian coiled-coil proteins and implications to its biological properties. Proc Natl Acad Sci USA 1985; 82:1064–1068.

171. Cunningham MW, Antone SM, Gulizia JM, McManus BA, Gauntt CJ. α-helical coiled-coil molecules: a role in autoimmunity against the heart. Clin Immunol Immunopathol 1993; 68:118–123.

172. Liao L, Sindhwani R, Rojkind M, Factor S, Leinwand L, Diamond B. Antibody-mediated autoimmune myocarditis depends on genetically determined target organ sensitivity. J Exp Med 1995; 187:1123–1131.

173. Donermeyer DL, Beisel KW, Allen PM, Smith SC. Myocarditis-inducing epitope of myosin

binds constitutive and stably to I-AK on antigen presenting cells in the heart. J Exp Med 1995; 182:1291–1300.

174. Dell VA, Antone SM, Gauntt CJ, Clark WA, Cunningham MW. Autoimmune determinants of rheumatic carditis: localization of epitopes in human cardiac myosin. Eur Heart J 1991; 12:158–162.

175. Shikhman AR, Greenspan AR, Cunningham MW. A subset of mouse monoclonal antibodies cross-reactive with cytoskeletal proteins and group A streptococcal M proteins recognizes N-acetyl-β-D-glucosamine. J Immunol 1993; 151: 3902–3914.

176. Shikhman AR, Greenspan NS, Cunningham MW. Cytokeratin peptide SFFGSGFGGGY mimics N-acetyl-β-N-D-glucosamine in reaction with antibodies and lectins, and induces in vivo anti-carbohydrate antibody response. J Immunol 1994; 153:5593–5606.

177. Jones KF, Fischetti VA. The importance of the location of antibody binding on the M6 protein for opsonization and phagocytosis of group A M6 streptococci. J Exp Med 1988; 167: 1114–1123.

178. Krauss W, Seyer M, Beachey EH. Vimentin-cross-reactive epitope of type 12 streptococcal M protein. Infect Immun 1989; 57:2457–2461.

179. Swerlick RA, Hall NK, Cunningham MW. Monoclonal antibodies cross-reactive with group A streptococci and normal and psoriatic human skin. J Invest Dermatol 1986; 87:367–371.

180. Fischetti VA. Streptococcal M protein: molecular design and biological behavior. Clin Microbiol Rev 1989; 2:286–314.

181. Bisno AL, Craven DE, McCabe WR. M proteins of group G streptococci isolated from bacteremic human infection. Infect Immun 1987; 55:753–757.

182. Hollingshead SK, Fischetti VA, Scott JR. A highly conserved region present in transcripts encoding heterologous M proteins of group A streptococcus. Infect Immun 1987; 55:3237–3239.

183. Manjula BN, Fischetti VA. Sequence homology of group A streptococcal PepM5 protein with other coiled-coil proteins. Biochem Biophys Res Commun 1986; 140:684–690.

184. Dale JB, Beachey EH. Sequence of myosin-crossreactive epitopes of streptococcal M protein. J Exp Med 1986; 164:1785–1790.

185. Bronze MS, Dale JB. Epitopes of streptococcal M proteins that evoke antibodies that cross-react with human brain. J Immunol 1993; 151: 2820–2828.

186. Sargent SJ, Beachey EH, Corbett CE, Dale JB. Sequence of protective epitopes of streptococcal M proteins shared with cardiac sarcolemmal membranes. J Immunol 1987; 139:1285–1290.

187. Bronze MS, Beachey EH, Dale JB. Protective and heart-crossreactive epitopes located within

the N-terminus of type 19 streptococcal M protein. J Exp Med 1988; 167:1849–1859.

187a. Cunningham MW, Antone SM, Smart M, Liu R, Kosanke S. Molecular analysis of human cardiac myosin-cross-reactive B- and T-cell epitopes of the group A streptococcal M5 protein. Infect Immun 1997; 65:3913–3923.

188. Huber SA, Cunningham MW. Streptococcal M protein peptide with similarity to myosin induces CD4$^+$ T cell dependent myocarditis in MRL/++ mice and induces tolerance against coxsackieviral myocarditis. J Immunol 1996; 156: 3528–3534.

189. Bessen DE, Veasy LG, Hill HR, Augustine NH, Fischetti VA. Serologic evidence for a class I group A streptococcal infection among rheumatic fever patients. J Infect Dis 1995; 172:1608–1611.

190. Quinn A, Kent W, Fischetti, VA, Hemric M, Cunningham MW. Immunological relationship between the class I epitope of streptococcal M protein and myosin. Infect Immun 1998; 66:4418–4424.

191. McCormack JM, Crossley CA, Ayoub EM, Harley JB, Cunningham MW. Poststreptococcal anti-myosin antibody marker associated with systemic lupus erythematosus and Sjogren's syndrome. J Infect Dis 1993; 168:915–921.

191a. Adderson, EE, Shikhman, AR, Ward, KE, Cunningham, MW. Molecular analysis of polyreactive monoclonal antibodies from rheumatic carditis: human anti-N-acetyl-glucosamine/anti-myosin antibody V region genes. J Immunol 1998; 161:2020–2031.

192. Quinn A, Adderson EE, Shackleford PG, Carroll WL, Cunningham MW. Autoantibody germline gene segment encodes VH and VL regions of a human anti-streptococcal Mab recognizing streptococcal M protein and human cardiac myosin epitopes. J Immunol 1995; 154: 4203–4212.

193. Cunningham MW, Antone SM, Gulizia JM, McManus BM, Fischetti VA, Gauntt CJ. Cytotoxic and viral neutralizing antibodies crossreact with streptococcal M protein, enteroviruses and human cardiac myosin. Proc Natl Acad Sci USA 1992; 89:1320–1324.

193a. Antone, SM, Adderson, EE, Mertens, NMJ, Cunningham, MW. Molecular analysis of V gene sequences encoding cytotoxic anti-streptococcal/anti-myosin mAb 36.2.2 which recognizes the heart cell surface protein laminin. J Immunol 1997; 159:5422–5430.

194. Gulizia JM, Cunningham MW, McManus BA. Immunoreactivity of anti-streptococcal monoclonal antibodies to human heart valves: evidence for multiple cross-reactive epitopes. Am J Pathol 1991; 138:285–301.

195. Springer TA. Traffic signals for lymphocyte recirculation and leukocyte emigration: the multistep paradigm. Cell 1994; 76:301–314.

196. Kuchroo VK, Das MP, Brown JA, Ranger AM, Zamvil SS, Sobel RA, Weiner HL, Nabavi N, Glimcher L. B7-1 and B7-2 costimulatory molecules activate differentially the Th1/Th2 developmental pathways: application to autoimmune disease therapy. Cell 1995; 80:707–718.

197. Shimizu Y, Newmann W, Tanka Y, Shaw S. Lymphocyte interactins with endothelial cells. Immunol Today 1992; 13:106–112.

198. Toyama-Sorimachi N, Miyake K, Miyasaka M. Activation of CD44 induces ICAM-1/LFA-1 independent CA++, Mg++ independent adhesion pathway in lymphocyte–endothelial cell interaction. Eur J Immunol 1993; 23:439–446.

199. Read SE, Zabriskie JB. Immunological concepts in rheumatic fever pathogenesis. In: Miescher PA, Muller-Eberhard HJ (eds). Textbook of Immunopathology. New York: Grune and Stratton, 1976; 471–487.

200. Read SE, Zabriskie JB, Fischetti VA, Utermohlen V, Falk R. Cellular reactivity studies to streptococcal antigens in patients with streptococcal infections and their sequelae. J Clin Invest 1974; 54:439–450.

201. Gibofsky A, Williams RC, Zabriskie JB. Immunological aspects of acute rheumatic fever. Clin Immunol Allergy 1987; 1:577–590.

202. Abe J, Forrester J, Nakahara T, Lafferty JA, Kotzin BL. Selective stimulation of human cells with streptococcal erythrogenic toxins A and B. J Immunol 1991; 146:3747–3750.

203. Hauser AR, Stevens DL, Kaplan EL, Schlievert PM. Molecular analysis of pyrogenic exotoxins from *Streptococcus pyogenes* isolates associated with toxic shock syndrome. J Clin Microbiol 1991; 29:1562–1567.

204. Cunningham MW, Antone SM, Smart M, Liu R, Rosanke S. Molecular analysis of human cardiac myosin-cross-reactive B- and T-cell epitopes of the group A streptococcal M5 protein. Infect. Immun. 1997; 65:3913–3923.

205. Cunningham MW. Molecular mimicry: bacterial antigen mimicry. In: Bona CA, Siminovitch K, Theophilopoulos AN, Zanetti M (eds). The Molecular Pathology of Autoimmunity. New York: Harwood Academic Press, 1993; 245–256.

206. Oldstone MBA. Overview: infectious agents as etiological triggers of autoimmune disease. Curr Top Microimmunol 1989; 145:1–3.

207. Dillon HC, Jr. Streptococcal infections and glomerulonephritis. In: Hoeprick PD, Jordan MC (eds). Infectious Diseases, 4th ed. Philadelphia: JB Lippincott and Co. 1989; 994–1001.

208. Ayoub EM. Acute rheumatic fever. In: Emmanouilides GC, Allen HD, Riemenschneider TA, Gutgesell HP (eds). Moss and Adams Heart Disease in Infants, Children, and Adolescents Including the Fetus and Young Adult, 5th ed. Baltimore: Williams and Wilkins, 1995; 1400–1416.

7

Rheumatic Fever

MILTON MARKOWITZ
EDWARD L. KAPLAN

Acute rheumatic fever, a nonsuppurative inflammatory disease, is the result of a group A beta-hemolytic streptococcal infection of the upper respiratory tract. However, the pathogenetic mechanism(s) that leads to rheumatic fever remains incompletely defined (see Chapter 6). It is generally agreed, however, that the clinical manifestations of rheumatic fever are the result of an abnormal host immune response to one or more as yet undefined group A streptococcal antigens. Rheumatic fever consists of a number of clinical manifestations that may occur singly or in combination. The most common manifestation is arthritis; the most serious, carditis; the most curious, chorea; the most rare and inconsequential, erythema marginatum and subcutaneous nodules. These manifestations were originally described independently of each other; it was Cheadle who, over 100 years ago, put together these divergent manifestations of rheumatic fever into a single clinical syndrome. These findings have remained essentially unchanged to the present time [1]. The incorrect diagnosis of rheumatic fever was prevalent prior to the formulation of diagnostic criteria by T. Duckett Jones more than 50 years ago [2]. These criteria have been revised periodically and are widely accepted.

Rheumatic fever occurs in all parts of the world, including both industrialized and developing countries [3]. Although the incidence of rheumatic fever and the prevalence of rheumatic heart disease decreased remarkably in North America and in Western Europe and Japan after the Second World War (incidence approximately 0.5–2.0/100,000/year) [4,5], a well-documented resurgence of rheumatic fever in middle-class families and among military recruits in the United States in the 1980s and 1990s has confirmed that increased standard of living and more widely available medical care cannot always effectively control the disease [6–10].

The incidence of rheumatic fever in many developing countries continues to be very high [11]. Consequently, rheumatic fever remains the leading cause of heart disease in children and young adults in these countries. Published data have indicated that as many as half of all children seen with cardiovascular disease are those with rheumatic fever and rheumatic heart disease in developing countries [12]. A curious and unique epidemiological observation has been the remarkably high incidence of acute rheumatic fever in the Aboriginal population in northern Australia where incidence rates of 650/100,000 population/year have been described [13]. The reasons for this remain incompletely defined. Whether this is related to living conditions or to a genetic propensity as in the case of the Maoris in New Zealand is unclear.

Thus, despite more than 50 years of understanding how this sequel to group A streptococcal infection can be prevented, it still remains a very significant illness in developing countries of the world. The resurgence of acute rheumatic fever in the United States, especially that documented in Utah, gives further evidence that this is not simply a disease of developing countries but that the potential for this complication remains worldwide at the end of the twentieth century.

Rheumatic fever is an important disease because carditis may cause permanent damage to the heart (rheumatic valvular heart disease). One of the most striking characteristics of rheumatic fever is its tendency to recur following subsequent group A streptococcal infections. Recurrent attacks are the major cause of deaths and disabilities from rheumatic heart disease. Fortunately, recurrences can be virtually eliminated by continuous antibiotic administration ("secondary" prophylaxis) to prevent streptococcal infections; many countries throughout the world have established prevention programs [3].

CLINICAL MANIFESTATIONS OF RHEUMATIC FEVER

There is an average latent period of 10–20 days between the preceding group A streptococcal upper-respiratory tract infection and the onset of acute rheumatic fever. This interval is the same length in first attacks and in recurrences. There is no evidence of clinical manifestations during the latent period.

Specific clinical manifestations of acute rheumatic fever are found with high enough frequency to make them diagnostically important. This observation is what led T. Duckett Jones to propose the Jones criteria in 1944 [2].

These more frequent clinical findings have been designated *major manifestations*. They include carditis, migratory polyarthritis, chorea, subcutaneous nodules, and erythema marginatum. There are other less specific signs, symptoms, and laboratory findings that, while nonspecific, may still be helpful in recognizing the disease. These are known as *minor manifestations* and include, arthralgia, fever, elevated acute phase reactants, and prolongation of the PR interval on the electrocardiogram.

A third and separate category of findings is required to confirm the diagnosis but is not truly a part of the clinical spectrum. This is evidence of a preceding group A streptococcal infection, either by history, by culture (or rapid antigen test determination), or by elevated or rising streptococcal antibody titers such as antistreptolysin O or anti-deoxyribonuclease B.

The clinical onset of rheumatic fever varies from patient to patient. When arthritis is the initial manifestation, the onset is characteristically acute. If carditis is also present, there may be no symptoms referable to the heart, unless pericarditis or congestive failure is present. If carditis is the only manifestation, especially in an initial attack, the onset is often insidious with pallor, malaise, and fatigue as the only gradually developing symptoms. With Sydenham's chorea, the onset may appear to be acute, but there is usually a history of lack of coordination and behavioral changes noted days or even weeks earlier.

Recurrent attacks of rheumatic fever are often difficult to recognize in patients with underlying rheumatic heart disease resulting from previous attacks. Similarly, infective endocarditis may be confused with a recurrent attack in a patient with underlying rheumatic heart disease.

DIAGNOSIS

The Jones Criteria

In 1944, T. Duckett Jones, concerned by the frequency of the incorrect diagnosis of rheumatic fever, proposed diagnostic guidelines based on combinations of clinical manifestations and laboratory findings according to their diagnostic usefulness [2]. These guidelines have become known as the Jones criteria. Jones designated clinical signs that are most useful major manifestations and the less specific signs and symptoms were called minor manifestations. According to the Jones scheme, two major criteria or one major and two minor criteria indicate a high probability of acute rheumatic fever.

Major Criteria for Diagnosis of Rheumatic Fever

Carditis

Carditis is the most important clinical manifestation of rheumatic fever. In its most fulminant form, it may cause death during the acute stage, or as happens more often, it may result in subsequent disability from its chronic sequel, rheumatic valvular heart disease. During the period of declining incidence in economically developed countries, the incidence and severity of carditis also declined. However, during the outbreaks of rheumatic fever in the United States in the late 1980s and 1990s, clinically severe acute rheumatic fever was not rare. For example, in one of these outbreaks, 72% of the patients had clinical evidence of carditis, and of these, 19% were in heart failure (Table 7.1; [6]). Of considerable pathogenetic importance is the echocardiographic evidence that valvular involvement in patients with acute rheumatic fever may be subclinical in some instances [6]. Although still somewhat controversial, because of this, the possibility that all patients with rheumatic fever in fact have valvular involvement has been considered. Much has been made of the antigenic mimicry between the myocardium and somatic moieties of the group A streptococcus. Yet, despite the hypothesis that this mimicry is pathogenetically responsible for myocardial involvement and despite the presence of Aschoff bodies in myocardium, clinical myocarditis is not as clinically significant as the myocarditis of, for example, viral infection. Furthermore, chronic myocardial involvement is not a significant part of chronic rheumatic heart disease. In the latter case, when myocardial dysfunction occurs, it usually is a consequence of the valvular damage.

Rheumatic carditis is usually associated with a significant heart murmur. Since the mitral valve is the most common site of rheumatic inflammation (mitral valvulitis), a blowing holosystolic murmur is audible at the cardiac apex. It may be soft, but it is usually grade 3 (on a scale of 6). This murmur of mitral regurgitation is often accompanied by an apical mid-diastolic murmur (Carey Coombs murmur). This diastolic murmur is low-pitched, localized to a small area of the apex, and should not be mistaken for the murmur of mitral stenosis, which is "rumbling", of long duration in the cardiac cycle, and harsher. Less frequent than apical murmurs is the basal diastolic murmur of aortic regurgitation. It is a high-pitched, decrescendo murmur, which in the early stages of the disease may be short, faint, and easily missed. It is best heard along the left sternal border with the patient sitting up. Aortic valvulitis may occur alone or with mitral valvulitis. However, isolated aortic valve involvement is quite unusual in patients with acute rheumatic fever or those with rheumatic heart disease. Before echocardiography was available, aortic valve involvement was often likely confused with congenital aortic valve deformities (bicuspid aortic valves or aortic stenosis).

Clinically evident pericarditis is among the least common of the clinical findings in patients with acute rheumatic carditis. It should be suspected if chest pain is present, but is often discovered by chance when a precordial friction rub is heard. The rub is usually heard in both phases of the cardiac cycle. Rheumatic pericarditis is rarely an isolated cardiac finding; a loud rub can obscure heart murmurs early in the course of an attack.

Congestive heart failure is the most serious clinical manifestation of rheumatic carditis and

Table 7.1 Frequency of Major Manifestations in Outbreaks of Acute Rheumatic Fever in the United States, 1987–88[a]

Reference	Carditis	Arthritis	Syndenham's Chorea	Erythema Marginatum	Subcutaneous Nodules
Veasy et al. [6]	72	56	32	3	8
Wald et al. [7]	59	47	30	0	0
Hosier et al. [8]	50	65	18	10	3
Congeni et al. [9]	30	78	9	13	0

[a]Percent of patients with manifestations

may occur at any time during the course of an attack of active carditis. Patients should be examined frequently for evidence of this complication. The conventional findings of shortness of breath and peripheral edema are less common in children, even though hepatomegaly is frequent. A gallop rhythm and basilar rales are often present. Other cardiac findings include tachycardia disproportionate to the fever. Diminution of the intensity of the first heart sound is a frequent finding and is a clue that a first-degree heart block is present. Cardiac enlargement is a common finding in patients with acute carditis. Cardiomegaly is due mainly to dilatation of the left ventricle, which can be determined by chest X-ray or by echocardiography.

Arthritis

Arthritis is the most common clinical manifestation of rheumatic fever, and from which the disease gets its name. It is one of the earliest manifestations of acute onset of rheumatic fever. It is the clinical manifestation that is most likely to bring the patient to medical attention because of the severe pain and accompanying fever, which is almost always present in patients with arthritis.

In rheumatic fever the joint involvement varies from mild joint pain without objective signs (arthralgia) to signs of severe inflammation with swelling, heat, and tenderness. The arthritis of rheumatic fever affects several of the larger joints of the extremities, usually one after the other, hence the term "migratory" polyarthritis. The migratory aspect is an extremely important clinical finding in patients suspected of having acute rheumatic fever. Rarely, only a single joint is involved.

The small joints of the hands and feet are seldom involved in those with rheumatic fever. This, in addition to the absence of morning stiffness in rheumatic fever, is very helpful in differentiating this from other forms of arthritis in young children, especially juvenile rheumatoid arthritis.

Characteristically, the affected joint is exquisitely painful. The pain is out of proportion to swelling and other signs of inflammation. The duration of involvement of each affected joint varies from a few days to a week, and all joint symptoms usually spontaneously subside in 2 to 4 weeks, even without anti-inflammatory treatment. There appears to be an inverse relation between the severity of polyarthritis and the degree of cardiac involvement. Patients who have carditis as their only clinical manifestation often have a history of arthralgias. Rheumatic fever arthritis never causes permanent deformities of the joints. The arthritis of rheumatic fever is not infrequently masked when anti-inflammatory medications are taken prior to allowing the process to define itself.

Chorea

Sydenham's chorea is one of the most unique aspects of the rheumatic fever syndrome. Its latent period following the streptococcal infection is considerably longer than that of the other major manifestations. Several months may elapse between the infection and the onset, making association with the group A streptococcal infection more difficult. It was a much less frequent finding in patients with rheumatic fever in the 1970s and early 1980s in North America, but during the resurgence of rheumatic fever it was found in almost one-third of patients (Table 7.1).

Chorea is characterized by involuntary movements, muscular weakness, and emotional disturbances. The movements are abrupt, purposeless, and nonrepetitive. They may affect all voluntary muscles, but involvement of the upper extremities and the face are most obvious. The speech is often slurred and facial grimaces are present. Emotional changes are manifested by outbursts of inappropriate behavior. There may be diffuse hypotonia and the handwriting becomes changed and may become illegible. The onset is usually insidious. Sydenham's chorea may be either bilateral (more common) or unilateral.

In most patients with chorea there may be no other clinical signs of rheumatic fever ("pure" chorea). While active arthritis rarely occurs concurrently with chorea, there may be subclinical, transient signs of carditis. As many as 25% of patients with so-called pure chorea ultimately have evidence of rheumatic heart disease [14]. Chorea may last from 2 to 4 months, occasionally up to 1 year.

Subcutaneous Nodules

Sometimes, round, firm swellings varying in size from 0.5 to 2.0 cm may occur singly or in crops. They are usually found over the bony prominences, occiput, and tendons. They appear from 1 to several weeks after the onset of the onset of an attack of rheumatic fever, and generally are limited to patients with severe carditis. Since the swellings are painless, the patient is usually unaware of them. They can be easily missed, unless the examiner is careful. Nodules rarely last more than a month. Rheumatic fever nodules remain a clinical curiosity at the present time.

Erythema Marginatum

The skin rash of rheumatic fever begins as a bright pink spot, the center of which fades as the periphery spreads with a sharp outer edge forming an irregular ring. The rash appears almost entirely on the trunk, less often on the extremities and never on the face [15]. The lesions are very evanescent and can be brought out after a warm bath. Erythema marginatum is an uncommon manifestation of rheumatic fever, usually appearing early in the course of an attack in patients with carditis. The rash can persist or recur for many months after other signs of acute rheumatic fever have abated.

Minor Criteria for Diagnosis of Rheumatic Fever

The minor criteria are much less specific findings in patients with rheumatic fever. In fact, their presence is only used as supportive evidence. For example, fever, arthralgia, and elevated acute-phase reactants are especially common in tropical countries and are present in many and varied disease processes. Similarly, since streptococcal infections are very prevalent among the pediatric age-group, the presence of minor criteria and an elevated streptococcal antibody should be viewed with caution.

Fever is almost always present at the onset of an acute attack of rheumatic fever. It usually ranges from 38° to 40°C. Higher temperature elevations are often present when polyarthritis is the mode of onset. Patients with insidious-onset carditis may have had a low-grade fever for several weeks before they come to medical attention. Children with "pure" chorea are usually afebrile. High fever rarely lasts for more than a week or two even without medication, and may become low grade thereafter. However, in most instances, the fever of rheumatic fever is not as chaotic as that seen in juvenile rheumatoid arthritis.

Arthralgia (i.e., joint pain without objective findings) is a common complaint in patients with active rheumatic fever. The joint manifestations may be limited to arthralgia, or arthritis may be present in some joints and arthralgia in others. Patients with insidious-onset carditis often have a history of recurrent joint pain over a period of days or several weeks. Arthralgia is frequently mistaken for arthritis in patients with acute rheumatic fever. One of the reasons for this may be related to the fact that for patients with suggestions of rheumatic fever, salicylates are often prescribed and the symptoms resolve before frank arthritis develops. Arthralgia due to other causes and the arthritis or arthralgia associated with otherwise uncomplicated streptococcal infection make this diagnosis more difficult to evaluate.

Other Diagnostic Considerations

Rheumatic fever may affect a number of organs and tissues, singly or in combination. No single manifestation, with the exception of "pure" chorea, is characteristic enough to be diagnostic. Furthermore, there is no single or specific laboratory test that is diagnostic of rheumatic fever. Therefore, the diagnosis of acute rheumatic fever is a clinical one.

During the past half-century there have been four revisions of the criteria [16–19]. However, the basic principles used by Jones for the original criteria have remained useful. The first two revisions strengthened the criteria by emphasizing the importance of the antecedent streptococcal infection. In 1956, evidence of a recent streptococcal infection was added to the list of minor manifestations [16]. Evidence of such an infection could be based on a history of scarlet fever, a positive culture of the throat for group A beta-hemolytic streptococci, or an elevated or rising antistreptolysin O titer. In the 1965 revision, the diagnostic rule of two major or one major and two minor manifestations was retained, but supporting evidence of a preceding group A streptococcal infection was required [17]. This change was based on reducing the chance of incorrectly diagnosing rheumatic fever in patients with clinical syndromes that might fulfill the clinical criteria, but were due to nonstreptococcal causes. Sydenham's chorea and insidious-onset carditis are two exceptions to this additional requirement, because in these patients, rheumatic fever is often considered and diagnosed after a prolonged interval from the precipitating infection. In such patients the chances of either recovering the organism by throat culture or demonstrated antibody evidence of the preceding infection are significantly reduced.

The latest revision of the Jones criteria (1992) did not alter the diagnostic rule, but for the first time stated that this should only apply to the initial attack of acute rheumatic fever (Table 7.2; [19]). This change was made because for some patients with a past history of rheumatic fever or rheumatic heart disease, the signs and symptoms may be less apparent and insufficient to completely fulfill the Jones criteria. There

should be a strong suspicion of a rheumatic recurrence in such cases, but only if there is supporting evidence of a recent group A streptococcal infection [14].

The 1992 revision of the Jones criteria also made clear that there are two other circumstances in which the diagnosis of rheumatic fever can be made without strict adherence to the Jones criteria. Chorea may occur as the only manifestation of rheumatic fever. Similarly, insidious-onset carditis may be the only sign of active rheumatic fever in patients who come to medical attention months after the onset of the disease. This latter change was made in consideration of the experience of many physicians in developing countries where patients who present with indolent carditis are frequently seen [3,20]. The Jones criteria have endured and are valued by clinicians and investigators for providing consistency in diagnosing acute rheumatic fever. The criteria are also useful for educators, providing a readily recalled framework for instructing health-care professionals about this important cause of cardiovascular disease.

Differential Diagnosis of Rheumatic Fever

The frequent occurrence of combinations of clinical and laboratory manifestations of acute rheumatic fever makes the diagnosis straightforward in most instances. On the other hand, when major manifestations or combinations of the minor manifestations appear as isolated features early in the course of the disease, problems with the diagnosis often occur.

Carditis

The finding of a precordial murmur in children with fever and ill-defined extremity pain is a frequent source of over-diagnosis of acute rheumatic fever. The likelihood that such a murmur is functional is great since innocent murmurs are so common in children and may appear "new," not having been previously recorded. The innocent murmur is short and generally has a pure-tone musical or vibratory quality. It is usually heard along the upper or the lower left sternal border and seldom radiates. Although a functional or innocent murmur can be prominent, especially in

Table 7.2 Guidelines for Diagnosis of Initial Attack of Rheumatic Fever: (1992) [19]

Major manifestations

Carditis
Polyarthritis
Chorea
Erythema marginatum
Subcutaneous nodules

Minor manifestations

Clinical findings
Arthralgia
Fever
Laboratory findings
Elevated acute phase reactants
Erythrocyte sedimentation rate
C-reactive protein
Prolonged PR interval

Supporting evidence of antecedent Group A streptococcal infections

Positive throat culture or rapid streptococcal antigen test

Elevated or rising streptococcal antibody titer

If supported by evidence of preceding group A streptococcal infection, the presence of two major manifestations or of one major and two minor manifestations indicates a high probability of acute rheumatic fever. There are two exceptions to this rule: chorea and indolent carditis.

a thin child, it can be readily distinguished from the apical location and blowing quality of the systolic murmur of rheumatic mitral regurgitation.

Isolated pericarditis is rarely due to acute rheumatic fever; a viral etiology is much more likely. However, a friction rub can obscure heart murmurs that become more evident after the pericarditis begins to subside. In contrast to viral myocarditis, rheumatic carditis is essentially always accompanied by evidence of valvular disease and a significant and characteristic murmur. Echocardiography can be very useful in this aspect of confirming a correct diagnosis.

Acute rheumatic carditis is rarely mistaken for congenital heart disease, but chronic rheumatic valvular disease can be confused with congenital defects of the heart. Atrial septal defects associated with a deformed mitral valve (atrioventricular canal defects) as well as isolated defects of the mitral valve are often impossible to distinguish clinically from rheumatic mitral regurgitation, especially in the absence of a history of rheumatic fever. Mitral valve prolapse is still another cause of a murmur of mitral valve regurgitation. It can be distinguished from rheumatic valvular disease by the characteristic systolic click and late systolic murmur. The differential diagnosis of aortic regurgitation in children can be difficult since congenital aortic valve deformities are also common. Again, echocardiography has been important in the differentiation.

Infective endocarditis may be mistaken for a recurrent attack of rheumatic fever in patients with established rheumatic heart disease. Confusion is easy because infective endocarditis often affects the joints as well as the heart [21]. Other extracardiac manifestations are useful in the differential diagnosis, but tend to appear late in the course of the disease. Blood cultures should be obtained whenever there is any clinical suspicion of infective endocarditis.

Arthritis

When arthritis is the sole clinical manifestation of rheumatic fever, a number of other musculoskeletal conditions have to be considered before arriving at a diagnosis. Monoarticular arthritis is a relatively rare initial manifestation of rheumatic fever. However, when a patient with a single inflamed joint is encountered, septic arthritis must be excluded by appropriate studies. Polyarthritis occurs in rheumatoid arthritis, but it is less likely to be migratory than in patients with rheumatic fever. The age of onset may provide a clue because when polyarthritis occurs in children under 3 years of age, juvenile rheumatoid arthritis is a much more likely cause than rheumatic fever. However, there are times when the distinction between these two diseases can only be made by observing the difference between the rapid resolution of the joint findings in rheumatic fever and the more prolonged course in individuals with rheumatoid arthritis. Arthralgia/arthritis can also be the initial manifestation in lupus erythematosus and should be considered, especially in adolescents.

Arthralgia is a genuine rheumatic symptom, but all too often the term "arthralgia" is applied loosely to describe limb pain of almost any kind. The most common complaints of this kind in children are the so-called growing pains. The latter are limited to the muscles of the lower extremities, occur at the end of the day or soon after falling asleep, and have no other clinical or laboratory signs of rheumatic fever.

"Reactive arthritis" is a term used to describe pain and swelling of the joints caused by infections elsewhere in the body. Shigella, salmonella, and Yersinia enterocolitica are among the infectious agents known to cause a sterile arthritis. The group A beta-hemolytic streptococcus has also been reported to be a cause of reactive arthritis [22]. Usually, these are patients with only one major and one minor manifestation, and hence do not fulfill the Jones criteria. Some have considered poststreptococcal reactive arthritis to be an entity distinct from rheumatic fever [17]. However, a review of several series of such patients reported that a significant number developed valvular heart disease. It was recommended that such patients be placed on antistreptococcal antibiotic prophylaxis [23].

Other conditions with musculoskeletal signs and symptoms that can mimic rheumatic fever include Lyme disease, serum sickness, and hematologic disorders such as sickle-cell disease, leukemia, and Henoch-Schönlein purpura. Appropriate clinical observation and laboratory studies can help to separate these patients and resolve the clinical confusion.

Chorea

In the fully developed clinical syndrome, the diagnosis of Sydenham's chorea is usually quite straightforward. Multiple tics can be readily distinguished from choreiform movements by the repetitive nature of the tics and their lack of interference with coordination. Mild choreiform movements can be seen in children with acquired or congenital central nervous system defects, but other neurologic signs are also usually present. Huntington's chorea rarely begins in childhood. There is often a family history and the movements tend to be choreoathetoid. Choreiform movements have been described in association with lupus erythematosus and Wilson's disease. The diagnosis of Sydenham's chorea often becomes a diagnosis of exclusion, requiring the elimination of other considerations from the differential diagnosis.

Protracted low-grade fever may lead to a suspicion of rheumatic fever, especially as noted earlier, if accompanied by vague extremity pain. However, patients with fever of undetermined origin (FUO) are rarely found to have rheumatic fever.

Patients with illnesses that resemble rheumatic fever often by chance have an elevated antistreptolysin O titer. This is because group A streptococcal infections are very prevalent in the age-group most likely to develop rheumatic fever. While an elevated titer is proof of a recent streptococcal infection, it is not in itself sufficient to establish the diagnosis of rheumatic fever. Similarly, elevated acute phase reactants (erythrocyte sedimentation rate or C-reactive protein) are not specific for rheumatic fever. Streptococcal antibody titers and acute-phase reactants must be evaluated in conjunction with a careful history and physical examination.

Echocardiography has been very effective in separating several forms of congenital heart disease (e.g., cleft mitral valves, bicuspid aortic valves) from rheumatic valvular heart disease. The precise use of echocardiography to evaluate "subclinical" mitral regurgitation has remained somewhat controversial [24–27], mainly because of the lack of comprehensive and prospective longitudinal studies. However, this controversy should soon be settled and the efficacy of echocardiographic evaluation in all patients in whom a diagnosis of rheumatic fever is being considered can then be more confidently documented.

TREATMENT OF PATIENTS WITH RHEUMATIC FEVER

There are no drugs that have been shown to either prevent or eradicate the immune-mediated inflammatory process in either myocardium or valve tissue, thereby preventing rheumatic heart disease. However, there are effective anti-inflammatory agents that can control joint pain and fever. Inotropic agents are effective should congestive heart failure occur. Furthermore, many patients heal spontaneously after an initial attack of rheumatic fever and remain well [28].

Patients with acute rheumatic fever should be placed at bed rest. Frequently, hospitalization is initially required so that patients can be evaluated continuously. The duration of bed rest varies with the severity of the attack. Ideally, 1 to 2 weeks of bed rest and close observation are desirable. If clinically significant carditis occurs, it usually does so within that time. Afterwards, if there are no signs of cardiac involvement and the fever and joint symptoms are under control, ambulation can be increased steadily over the next 2 weeks. By 1 month after the attack, if there is no clinical or laboratory evidence of rheumatic activity after discontinuing anti-inflammatory medications, the patient can resume his or her usual activities.

Patients with mild carditis (i.e., no cardiac enlargement), should be kept at rest until the heart sounds are of good quality, the intensity of the murmur(s) has stabilized, the resting pulse rate is normal, and the acute-phase reactants have returned to or are near normal. Four to six weeks of bed rest may be required followed by progressive ambulation which can be initiated during the next month. If after the end of this period the physical findings are stable, the patient can return to school, but should avoid excessive physical activities for at least the following 2 to 3 months.

Patients with cardiac enlargement (with or without congestive failure) should be kept at strict rest until the heart size has decreased or has become stabilized, the sleeping pulse is below 100/min, and the acute-phase reactants have returned to normal. A minimum of 3 months may be required, and then increasing physical activities be introduced gradually if guided by pulse rate and heart size.

Antimicrobial Treatment for Patients with Rheumatic Fever

Once the diagnosis of rheumatic fever has been established, the patient should be given therapeutic doses of penicillin to eradicate residual group A streptococci, either by a single injection of 1.2 million units of benzathine penicillin G or 250 mg of oral penicillin V twice a day for 10 days. (A more complete discussion of the treatment of group A streptococcal upper-respiratory tract infections is presented in Chapter 5.) After this initial course of antibiotic therapy, long-term secondary antistreptococcal prophylaxis should be started immediately. For patients with documented allergy to penicillin, erythromycin has been the antibiotic of choice.

Anti-inflammatory Therapy for Acute Rheumatic Fever

Salicylates and steroids are very effective in suppressing the acute manifestations of rheumatic fever, but neither has been shown to prevent chronic valvular rheumatic heart disease. They should be withheld until the diagnosis is confirmed if arthralgia or questionable arthritis are the only indications for suspecting rheumatic fever. Analgesics such as acetaminophen or even codeine can be used to control pain and will not interfere with the full development of migratory polyarthritis, the appearance of which may certify the diagnosis of rheumatic fever. There are no controlled or comprehensive studies evaluating the effectiveness of nonsteroidal anti-inflammatory drugs for treatment of acute rheumatic fever.

Patients with definite clinical evidence of arthritis should be treated with aspirin. The starting total dose is 100 mg/kg/day in divided doses for the first 2 weeks. The dosage can then be reduced to 75 mg/kg/day for the next 2 to 4 weeks, or until all laboratory manifestations of inflammatory disease have returned to normal. It is not unusual for acute-phase reactants to "re-bound" after salicylates are discontinued. Retreatment is not usually advised unless there is also evidence of a clinical rebound.

Corticosteriod therapy is reserved for patients with significant carditis, especially if there is cardiomegaly or congestive heart failure. Such patients tolerate steroids better and clinically improve more rapidly than only with salicylates. The effect of steroids on the long-term outcome with respect to cardiac sequelae was the subject of many studies following their introduction. Controlled studies using average- or large-dose regimens, and short or long courses of treatment, showed that corticosteroids were not more effective than salicylates in reducing the incidence of residual valvular damage [14–29].

Prednisone is the drug of choice, starting with a dose of 2 mg/kg/day in divided doses not to exceed a total dose of 80 mg/day. After 2 to 3 weeks of treatment, Prednisone may be slowly withdrawn, decreasing the daily dose at the rate of 5 mg every 2 to 3 days. When tapering is started, aspirin at 75 mg/kg/day should be added and continued for about 6 weeks after prednisone is stopped. Overlapping treatment in this way reduces the chance of post-therapeutic rebounds and the reappearance of clinical manifestations. Mild rebounds usually subside spontaneously in a few days and do not require retreatment. If the rebound includes further increase in cardiomegaly and return of congestive heart failure, a short course of steroid therapy should be reinstituted, once again overlapping with salicylates. The use of nonsteroid anti-inflammatory drugs has not been carefully studied in patients with rebound.

Treatment of Congestive Heart Failure

Congestive heart failure of rheumatic carditis is often controlled with bed rest, oxygen, and steroids. If there is no improvement within 24 h, digitalis is indicated. It is no longer believed that the incidence of digitalis toxicity is higher in patients with active carditis than in inactive rheumatic heart disease. Digoxin has been the preparation of choice. However, in the severely ill child other inotropic agents have been used. Diuretics are rarely needed in children with heart failure early in the course of their first attack, but diuretics may be used.

Treatment of Sydenham's Chorea

Patients with chorea should be placed in a quiet atmosphere at home, or initially in a hospital until the chorea can be controlled. Bed rest is indicated for severe attacks and precautions should be taken to prevent bruising and falling out of bed. Steroids have been reported to be of value in treating chorea, but most experienced clinicians believe that steroids do not appear to influence the symptoms or the clinical course of patients with chorea, and do not recommend their use. Phenobarbital is an often-used sedative for mildly affected patients. In severely affected patients, chlorpromazine was recommended in the past. More recently, haloperidol has been successfully used. It should also be emphasized that patients with chorea, even in the absence of other rheumatic fever manifestations, require long-term antistreptococcal prophylaxis.

LONG-TERM MANAGEMENT OF RHEUMATIC FEVER

The long-term prognosis of individuals who have experienced an attack of acute rheumatic fever remains unclear. There can be little doubt that recurrent attacks enhance the chances of developing rheumatic heart disease. On the other hand, studies have suggested that individuals who receive consistent long-term prophylaxis are likely to lose their murmur over a period of years [28]. The studies showing this were based upon careful clinical observation. Long-term prospective evaluations utilizing echocardiography will be required to assist in more accurately defining the prognosis of patients with rheumatic heart disease, especially those with minimal involvement.

Because of the inherent dangers of recurrent attacks, prophylaxis with either intramuscular (IM) benzathine penicillin G, oral penicillin V, or oral sulfadiazine has been the recommendation worldwide. Previous studies have indicated that IM benzathine penicillin G is most effective [30]. This undoubtedly is related to the issue of compliance in taking oral medications. Although concern has been expressed about the possibility of anaphylaxis in patients receiving IM benzathine penicillin G for secondary prophylaxis, data suggest that the likelihood of anaphylaxis is less than the risk of recurrence of rheumatic fever [31].

The duration of secondary prophylaxis for prevention of recurrent attacks of rheumatic fever is controversial. While some believe that individuals with documented rheumatic valvular heart disease should be given antistreptococcal prophylaxis for life, many believe that as the risk of recurrent attacks decreases with time or in those individuals whose living and working conditions indicate a low risk, this prophylaxis may be stopped 5 years after the most recent attack. Most authorities in the field believe that the duration of long-term secondary prophylaxis is best recommended for each individual case. Patients who have had documented Sydenham's chorea should be given secondary prophylaxis similar to those individuals who have experienced the arthritis or carditis of acute rheumatic fever.

The most effective interval between injections of benzathine penicillin G injections has been debated. Classically, injections have been administered every 4 weeks, but recent data have reported a reduction in both streptococcal infections and rheumatic recurrences when injections are given every 3 weeks [32]. Many authorities and authoritative groups have recommended IM injections of 1.2 million units of benzathine penicillin G every 4 weeks for most patients, but have agreed that injections may be given every 3 weeks in patients deemed to be at increased risk of rheumatic fever recurrences.

REFERENCES

1. Cheadle WB. Various Manifestations of the Rheumatic State as Exemplified in Childhood and Early Life. London: Smith, Elder, 1889.
2. Jones TD. The diagnosis of rheumatic fever. JAMA 1944; 126:481–484.
3. World Health Organization. Rheumatic fever and rheumatic heart disease: a report of a WHO Study Group. World Health Organ Tech Rep Ser 1988; 764:21–25.
4. Gordis L. The virtual disappearance of rheumatic fever in the United States: lessons in the fall and rise of disease. T. Duckett Jones Memorial Lecture. Circulation 1985; 72:1155–1162.
5. Kaplan EL. Global assessment of rheumatic fever and rheumatic heart disease at the close of the century. Influences and dynamics of populations and pathogens: a failure to realize prevention? T.

Duckett Jones Memorial Lecture. Circulation 1993; 88:1964–1972.

6. Veasy LG, Weidmeier SE, Orsmond GS, Ruttenberg HD, Boucek MM, Roth SJ, Tait VF, Thompson JA, Daly JA, Kaplan CL, Hill HR. Resurgence of acute rheumatic fever in the intermountain area of the United States. N Engl J Med 1987; 316:421–427.

7. Wald ER, Dashefsky B, Feidt C, Chiponis D, Byers C. Acute rheumatic fever in western Pennsylvania and the tristate area. Pediatrics 1987; 80:371–374.

8. Hosier DM, Craenen JM, Teske DW, Wheller JJ. Resurgence of rheumatic fever. Am J Dis Child 1987; 141:730–733.

9. Congeni B, Rizzo C, Congeni J, Sreenivasan W. Outbreak of acute rheumatic fever in northeast Ohio. J Pediatr 1987; 111:176–179.

10. Veasy LG, Tani LY, Hill HR. Persistence of acute rheumatic fever in the intermountain area of the United States. J Pediatr 1994; 125:673–674.

11. Vijaykumar M, Narula J, Reddy KS, Kaplan EL. Incidence of rheumatic fever and prevalence of rheumatic heart disease in India. Int J Cardiol 1994; 43:221–228.

12. Daniel E, Abegaz B. Profile of cardiac disease in an out-patient cardiac clinic. Trop Geogr Med 1993; 45:121–123.

13. Carapetis JR, Wolff DR, Currie BJ. Acute rheumatic fever and rheumatic heart disease in the Top End of Australia's Northern Territory. Med J Aust 1996; 164:146–149.

14. Markowitz M, Gordis L. Rheumatic Fever, 2nd ed. Philadelphia: W.B. Saunders, 1972.

15. Perry CB. Erythema marginatum (rheumaticum). Arch Dis Child 1937; 12:233–238.

16. Rutstein DD, Bauer W, Dorfman A, Gross RE, Lichty JA, Taussig HB, Whittemore R. Jones criteria (modified) for guidance in the diagnosis of rheumatic fever. Circulation 1956; L3:617–620.

17. Stollerman GH, Markowitz M, Taranta A, Wannamaker LW, Whittemore R. Jones criteria (revised) for guidance in the diagnosis of rheumatic fever. Circulation 1965; 32:664–668.

18. Committee on Rheumatic Fever and Bacterial Endocarditis of The American Heart Association. Jones criteria (revised) for guidance in the diagnosis of rheumatic fever. Circulation 1984; 69:203A–208A.

19. Special Writing Group of the Committee on Rheumatic Fever, Endocarditis, and Kawasaki Disease of the American Heart Association. Guidelines for the diagnosis of rheumatic fever: Jones criteria, 1992 update. JAMA 1992; 268:2069–2073.

20. Okuni M. Problems in the clinical application of revised Jones diagnostic criteria for rheumatic fever. Jpn Heart J 1971; 12:436–441.

21. Doyle EF, Taranta A, Markowitz M, Spagnuolo M, Kuttner AG. The risk of bacterial endocarditis during anti-rheumatic prophylaxis JAMA 1967; 201:807–812.

22. Herold BC, Shulman ST. Poststreptococcal arthritis. Pediatr Infect Dis 1988; 2:681–682.

23. Schaffer FM, Agarwal R, Helm J, Gingell RL, Roland JM, O'Neil KM. Poststreptococcal reactive arthritis and silent carditis: a case report and review of the literature. Pediatrics 1994; 93:837–839.

24. Marcus RH, Sareli P, Pocock WA, Meyer TE, Antunes MJ, Magalhaes MP, Barlow JB, Grieve T. Functional anatomy of severe mitral regurgitation in active rheumatic carditis. Am J Cardiol 1989; 63:577–584.

25. Folger GM, Hajar R, Robida A, Hajar HA. Occurrence of valvular disease in acute rheumatic fever without evidence of carditis; colour flow Doppler identification. Fr Heart J 1992; 67:434–438.

26. Abernathy M, Bass N, Sharpe N, Grant C, Greaves S, Whalley G, Neutze J, Lennon D, Clarkson P, Snow S. Doppler echocardiography and the early diagnosis of carditis in acute rheumatic fever. Aust N Z J Med 1994; 24:530–535.

27. Minich LL, Tani LY, Pagotto LT, Shaddy RE, Veasy LG. Doppler echocardiography distinguishes between physiologic and pathologic "silent" mitral regurgitation in patients with rheumatic fever. Clin Cardiol 1997; 20:924–926.

28. Tompkins DG, Boxerbaum B, Liebman J. Long term prognosis of rheumatic fever patients receiving regular intramuscular benzathine penicillin. Circulation 1972; 45:543–551.

29. Albert DA, Harel L, Karrison T. The treatment of rheumatic carditis: a review and meta-analysis. Medicine 1995; 24:1–12.

30. Wood HF, Feinstein AR, Taranta A, Epstein JA, Simpson R. Rheumatic fever in children and adolescents. III. Comparative effectiveness of three prophylaxis regimens in preventing streptococcal infections and rheumatic recurrences. Ann Intern Med 1964; 60(Suppl 5):31–43.

31. Markowitz M, Kaplan EL, Cuttica R, Berrios X, Huang Z, Rao X, Wahi P, Bali HK, Millard D, Choi JY, Hong CY, Majeed HA, Clarkson P, Neutze J, Lue HC, Vongprateep C, Phornphutk C, Munoz S. Allergic reactions to long-term benzathine penicillin prophylaxis for rheumatic fever. Lancet 1991; 337:1308–1310.

32. Lue HC, Wu MH, Wang JK, Wu FF, Wu YN. Three versus four week administration of benzathine penicillin G: effects on incidence of streptococcal infections and recurrences of rheumatic fever. Pediatrics 1996; 97:984–988.

8

Streptococcal Pyoderma

BASCOM F. ANTHONY

Although the role of the streptococcus in superficial skin infections has been recognized for years, much of the current understanding of streptococcal pyoderma and its complications was generated in clinical studies conducted in the 1960s and 1970s in such diverse locations as Alabama, northern Minnesota, rural Mississippi, and Trinidad. A remarkable range of findings emerged from these studies of an infection that was essentially confined to a few superficial layers of cornified squamous epithelium: (1) the documentation that acute rheumatic fever is not a complication of streptococcal skin infection and that acute glomerulonephritis is, even in the absence of pharyngitis, provided the appropriate nephritogenic streptococci are present; (2) the differentiation of impetigo and respiratory group A streptococci; (3) the establishment of a secondary role for the staphylococcus in nonbullous impetigo, at least for the time being; (4) the definition of the natural history, epidemiology, and immune responses in streptococcal pyoderma; and (5) the development of effective treatment and prophylactic regimens. Many of these observations are summarized in excellent contemporaneous reviews [1–3]. Despite a dearth of clinical studies of streptococcal skin infections in recent decades, molecular studies in the 1990s have shed new light on the pathogenesis of pyoderma from the perspective of the group A streptococcus and the cells of the human skin.

The focus of this chapter is on the role of the streptococcus in infections of the epidermis and dermis. Since the earliest descriptions of impetigo, there has been controversy over the contributions of the group A streptococcus and *Staphylococcus aureus* to nonbullous impetigo. That controversy cannot be totally avoided here.

PYODERMA: DEFINITIONS AND CLINICAL APPEARANCE

Pyoderma as discussed in this review refers to bacterial infection of the dermis and epidermis. Histopathologically, the lesion of *impetigo contagiosa* is limited to the deeper layers of the epidermis, where a bacteria-rich pustule develops. The only subepidermal abnormality is the accumulation of neutrophiles and other inflammatory cells in the papillary dermis underlying the subcorneal focus of infection. If the pustule and resulting ulceration extend into the dermis, *ecthyma* ensues and with it the likelihood of subsequent scarring [4]. Impetigo develops in individuals with normal skin who live under certain conditions, most importantly exposure to minor cutaneous insults that disrupt the stratum corneum and to group A streptococci that are capable of causing pyoderma. *Impetiginization* refers to the development of impetigo-like lesions in individuals with an underlying skin abnormality, e.g., eczema. Chronic skin disorders and poor hygiene are especially likely to lead to ecthyma, scarring, and other disabling complications.

The earliest clinical lesion in impetigo is a vesicle containing clear fluid (see Plate 5); this is transient and often unnoticed and rapidly changes into a pustule with a moderately thick and tenacious crust that is golden or reddish-black in color. The lesion is often surrounded by an erythematous halo. Systemic manifestations are mild or absent and, except for itching, local symptoms are minimal. Enlargement and tenderness of the regional lymph nodes are common, but lymphadenitis and lymphangitis are unusual presenting complaints [1,2]. Streptococcal impetigo most commonly affects the extremities, especially the lower extremities, probably because of the importance of minor trauma. Lesions on the trunk are next in frequency. The face and scalp may be involved but facial impetigo is distinctive from the circumoral and perinasal lesions that occur in some young children with group A streptococcal nasopharyngitis.

Streptococcal impetigo is clearly distinguishable from bullous impetigo, with its relatively clear fluid and thin, varnish-like crusts. Bullous impetigo is a well-defined entity within the broader clinical spectrum of the staphylococcal scalded skin syndrome. The responsible staphylococci (usually phage type 71 or another member of phage group II), the exfoliative toxin, and the mechanism of toxin action in the pathogenesis of the characteristic lesions have been well described and characterized [5].

MICROBIOLOGY AND PATHOGENESIS

Impetigo lesions can occasionally be shown to harbor beta-hemolytic streptococci of groups B, C, and G [6,7]. Group A strains that are better known for their association with pharyngitis are also rarely isolated from these lesions [8]. Typically, however, these superficial skin lesions are infected with "impetigo strains" of group A streptococci. In 1955, Parker et al. [9] and Barrow [10] reported that group A streptococci from impetigo lesions differ from other group A isolates. Most of their impetigo isolates lacked an identifiable M protein and, when typed by agglutination of the T protein complex, fell into three T patterns (3/13/B3264, 8/25/Imp19, and 5/11/12/27/44) that were unusual among non-skin isolates throughout Britain.

More extensive studies from Minnesota and Alabama expanded the number of prevalent T patterns isolated from skin lesions. However, most impetigo isolates still could not be M typed in the earlier studies [6,7]. With further development of new typing sera, it became clear that impetigo streptococci possess M protein with regularity [11–14], usually in a unique combination with a particular T protein pattern. Some M proteins assigned to impetigo strains were previously known, e.g., M types 2, 8, 22, 33, 39, and 41, but many were new and were assigned higher type numbers in the 50s and 60s [14]. With some exceptions, impetigo or skin M types tend to produce a serotypic serum opacity factor or lipoproteinase, whereas M types associated with pharyngitis generally do not [15]. Two useful tabulations of M and T type associations and their relationship to the pathogenic potential of group A streptococci have recently been published [15,16].

The group A streptococcus is clearly not a member of the "resident" or long-term flora of the skin [17]. Following observations suggesting that these streptococci may be "transient" skin flora that precede the development of pyoderma and later appear in the respiratory tract [18], an intensive study was conducted by Ferrieri et al. in a small group of children and their families on the Red Lake Indian Reservation [19]. This confirmed the regular appearance of group A streptococci on intact skin a mean of 10 days (range 2–33) before the development of impetigo lesions. The source of the streptococci on normal skin was not always clear, whether from the skin lesions or respiratory tracts of other individuals. With or without the intervening development of impetigo, the streptococcus subsequently appeared in the nose a mean of 14 days after detection on normal skin and could be isolated from the throat about a week later [19]. These observations indicate that the key pathogenic factor for impetigo streptococci is the ability to persist on normal skin for a substantial period of time; pyoderma lesions develop when the epidermis is traumatized, even minimally.

These findings clash with considerable evidence that group A streptococci survive poorly on normal skin because of the antistreptococcal effect of skin lipids [20,21]. A more recent study that may reconcile this apparent conflict suggests that repeated deposition of streptococci on the surface is a more likely event than actual streptococcal multiplication on the skin; the same study also confirms the capacity of group A streptococci on the skin surface to produce lesions when the superficial stratum corneum is disrupted [22].

It has been shown that impetigo streptococci adhere to skin better than to buccal epithelium and that throat strains demonstrate the opposite affinity [23]. Binding to fibronectin has been thought to play a role in streptococcal respiratory infections [24]. Recent studies propose a dual adhesin system in skin infection whereby M protein attaches to keratinocytes (the stratified squamous epithelial cells of the skin) and the fibronectin-binding protein (protein F) binds to Langerhans cells (the antigen-processing cells of the stratum granulosum) [25]. In vitro studies also suggest that differentiation of keratinocytes is essential for the adherence of group A streptococci [26] and that keratinocytes are up-regulated by adherent streptococci to produce an array of cytokines [27]. Thus, the interactions of impetigo streptococci with specific cells of the epidermis may control the characteristic inflammatory and immune responses of impetigo.

The migration of streptococci from normal skin to lesion to respiratory tract helps to explain the complex findings when children with a high rate of streptococcal pyoderma are monitored with clinical observations and cultures of skin lesions and the respiratory tract. Such a group of Native American children at Red Lake, Minnesota, was followed year round for 2 years. Based on sites and relative frequency of isolation, it was possible to identify M types of respiratory streptococci with little or no capacity to produce pyoderma lesions. An additional set of impetigo M types was observed that demonstrated the capacity to produce skin lesions and inhabit the respiratory tract [8]. There is a limited number of strains that have been shown to be capable of producing both impetigo and pharyngitis. One of these is type 49, the original

Red Lake nephritogenic strain [28]. Another is type 65, a non-nephritogenic strain described by Dillon et al. [29].

In a recent study of over 100 group A streptococci of different M types collected from different locales and clinical sources over many years, strains were classified on the basis of the sequences of the gene segments encoding the peptidoglycan-spanning domains of the M proteins and other surface proteins that probably play a role in virulence. The patterns of gene sequences between most impetigo and pharyngeal strains were quite different [30], providing genetic confirmation 40 years later of the 1955 reports of Parker et al. [9] and of Barrow [10].

IMMUNE RESPONSE IN STREPTOCOCCAL PYODERMA

Patients with streptococcal skin infections mount a vigorous antibody response to some extracellular antigens of the group A streptococcus, such as anti-DNAseB and antihyaluronidase. However, the antistreptolysin O (ASO) response is absent or feeble in individuals with uncomplicated impetigo [31,32] as well as patients with acute glomerulonephritis (AGN) complicating impetigo [33]. Kaplan and Wannamaker showed this to be due to the inhibitory effect of skin lipids, including cholesterol, on the immunogenicity as well as other biological properties of streptolysin O [34]. The practical effect of this phenomenon is that the ASO antibody test is not a reliable indicator of a recent group A streptococcal infection of the skin.

The development of type-specific immunity or antibody to the homologous M protein has been demonstrated in a few patients with streptococcal pyoderma [35]. When a group of children at Red Lake was followed closely, the most consistent M antibody response was in children harboring a pharyngeal strain (type M-6); two-thirds of those with positive throat cultures developed type 6 antibody. The antibody responses of children to "impetigo" strains (M-31 and M-49) was less consistent (42%–54% of children), but occurred after either skin infection or positive throat cultures and was unrelated to duration of exposure to the strain [36]. During the Viet Nam conflict, the incidence of streptococcal ecthyma was significantly greater in white

U.S. soldiers than in African-American troops. Pyoderma is more common in black than in Caucasian children in the United States, raising the possibility of long-term immunity to impetigo streptococci as a result of childhood skin infection [37].

ROLE OF STAPHYLOCOCCUS IN NONBULLOUS IMPETIGO

Since the first description of impetigo 130 years ago, both streptococci and *Staphylococcus aureus* have been commonly recovered from skin lesions and opinion has fluctuated between which of these is the primary pathogen.

Several potential technical problems exist that could affect isolation rates of streptococci and staphylococci and further confuse this issue. One is the tendency for larger, intensely hemolytic staphylococcal colonies to obscure smaller colonies of beta-hemolytic streptococci. Although some investigators have incorporated staphylococcal inhibitors into the primary culture medium, we observed no significant advantage in the use of selective sheep blood agar over nonselective medium in the Red Lake studies (E.L. Kaplan and B.F. Anthony, unpublished data). An additional potential problem in identifying streptococci in mixed cultures is the production of a bacteriocin-like substance by staphylococci. The production of such a substance is characteristic of staphylococci associated with bullous impetigo. The substance is highly active in vitro against group A streptococci [38] and appears to have some activity in vivo against streptococci in an animal model of impetigo [39]. However, there is no evidence that staphylococcal strains commonly isolated from nonbullous impetigo produce such inhibitors.

A strong case was made in the 1960s and 1970s for the streptococcus as the primary pathogen in impetigo, with the staphylococcus as a secondary contaminant. Group A streptococci were isolated substantially more commonly than staphylococci from skin lesions and, in some studies, cultures of early lesions more often yielded pure streptococcal growth [7,40,41]. In an intensive study that included serial cultures of the same skin lesions, a single streptococcal strain was shown to persist 85% of the time; in contrast, a change in phage type of the staphylococcal strain could be shown in 57% of lesions that were cultured repeatedly [40]. Staphylococci isolated from nonbullous lesions have not been reported to express any unique characteristics or phage patterns. The responses of impetigo to penicillin therapy were also consistent with a primary streptococcal lesion; clinical cure rates were high and not influenced by the presence of β-lactamase producing staphylococci in impetigo cultures [42].

Many reports of impetigo that have appeared since 1980 have recorded higher rates of staphylococcal than of streptococcal isolations from skin lesions [43–49] and several authors have concluded that there has been a significant change in the epidemiology of impetigo. However, outpatients attending a clinic or emergency room are not ideal for comparison with selected populations under aggressive, prospective surveillance. In Dillon's last study of impetigo, published in 1985 and based in a rural day-care center in Alabama, he and his colleagues observed what was clearly an outbreak of streptococcal impetigo [50]. Therefore, while staphylococcal isolates from nonbullous impetigo lesions have increased in recent reports, it is not clear that this applies to the populations that experienced streptococcal pyoderma in the preceding two decades. It is unfortunate that there are no new insights on pathogenesis or epidemiology to accompany the expanding rates of staphylococcal isolation.

There is no characterization of staphylococcal isolates to accompany the reputed change in the etiology of impetigo to *Staphylococcus aureus*. Most authors make no clinical distinction between the clinical appearance of nonbullous impetigo ascribed to a streptococcal or staphylococcal etiology. Lookingbill, however, reported differences between nonbullous impetigo that he attributed to the group A streptococcus and to the staphylococcus [45]. Staphylococcal lesions were more common on the face whereas streptococcal impetigo was more often located on the lower extremities. Staphylococcal crusts were honey-colored and thinner than the yellow or brown crusts attributed to streptococcal impetigo. Removal of staphylococcal crusts revealed a shallow glistening base and removal of streptococcal crusts often led to bleeding and a deeper, ecthymatous lesion. The streptococcal lesion, but not the staphylococcal lesion, was surrounded by an area of erythema. These observations have not been confirmed by others. At Red Lake, Dajani et al. observed nonbullous lesions that yielded only staphylococci on repeated cultures and observed that the crusts were thin, light brown, and varnish-like and suggested the possibility that such lesions spontaneously healed at a faster rate than the more typical streptococcal pyoderma [40]. An additional development in impetigo consists of reports of poorer responses to penicillin therapy than described in earlier decades and poorer than observed with regimens that are more effective against the staphylococcus [43,46–48].

EPIDEMIOLOGY OF IMPETIGO

Impetigo has historically been an affliction of persons living in warm and humid environments. Reports from the southeastern United States have documented the frequency of impetigo and its dominant role in that region as the antecedent infection preceding AGN [51–53]. Taplin et al. compared the prevalence of streptococcal pyoderma at three locations in Colombia. Although the populations (children and soldiers) and hygienic conditions were not ideal for comparison, the prevalence of streptococcal pyderma was inversely related to altitude and directly related to humidity [54]. Despite the importance of warmth and humidity as risk factors for impetigo, outbreaks of skin infection and AGN have been documented in colder and even arctic climates [6,55].

In the southeastern U.S., impetigo is a disease of the summer and fall, the incidence rising after mid-July and declining in mid-October [7]. At Red Lake, Minnesota, the same seasonal trends described in the Southeast prevail, although skin infections at Red Lake have been documented throughout the year and were observed in as many as 12% of a group of young children in one January [8]. In pediatric populations, impetigo occurs at the same rates in boys and girls [41]. It appears to be most prevalent in pre-school children (2 to 5 years), but close observations have indicated that in this age-group skin lesions are also more extensive and may cause the greatest concern to parents and hence may be reported more often to health-care personnel [41].

Adult contacts of children with endemic impetigo infrequently contract lesions, but adult outbreaks of pyoderma in military personnel [56] and athletic teams [57,58] are well known. The regular occurrence of minor skin trauma, poor hygienic conditions, and impetigo streptococci are clearly important factors in such populations. During the Viet Nam conflict, streptococcal ecthyma of the feet and ankles in military personnel exposed continuously to wet feet and jungle combat was commonplace, severe, and disabling, a problem previously encountered in World War II as "jungle sores" [37].

The incidence of impetigo is striking in populations that have been studied closely. Presumably, this reflects the spread of impetigo streptococci in children who are constantly experiencing minor skin trauma. When Native American children at Red Lake were followed closely during three summers, 81% experienced one or more episodes of impetigo [19]. The rate was even higher when a similar population was followed the year round [8].

COMPLICATIONS OF STREPTOCOCCAL IMPETIGO

Acute rheumatic fever is not a complication of streptococcal pyoderma, but AGN is an important and common sequel. The most important determinant is infection with an impetigo strain with nephritogenic potential. Of such streptococci, type M-49 has enjoyed the widest global distribution. The specificity of combinations of M and T antigens is quite striking. For example, type M-2 with the 8/25/Imp19 T complex was a common pyoderma antecedent of AGN in Alabama [59] while M-2/T-2 strains were associated with scarlet fever and AGN in a California classroom outbreak [60]. Similarly, M-4/T-4 strains have historically been associated with pharyngitis and AGN, but M-60/T-4 was an important pyoderma-AGN strain in Alabama [59].

When studied prospectively, the attack rates for AGN following pyoderma in children infected with M-49 or acute pharyngitis due to nephritogenic M-12 in Navy personnel were remarkably similar at 12% [61,62]. However, in the pyoderma study in school-age children, the attack rate was almost 10 times higher (43%) in children under 6.5 years than in older children (5%) [62].

There appear to be no important differences in clinical severity or manifestions of AGN following pharyngitis or pyoderma [1,2]. However, the mean latent period between infection and first evidence of AGN is substantially longer following pyoderma (21 days) than pharyngitis (10 days) [63]. In prospective studies of streptococcal pyoderma, where asymptomatic subjects were screened for evidence of AGN with serum complement determinations or urinalysis, the ratio of clinical to subclinical AGN varied between roughly 1:1 and 3.5:1 [62,64]. (See Chapter 9.)

Suppurative complications such as cellulitis, lymphangitis, and lymphadenitis occur with streptococcal pyoderma, particularly if it is severe or neglected. Metastatic infections and invasive disease are unusual. Life-threatening, "toxic" streptococcal disease often involves the skin, but rarely if ever is preceded by impetigo, apparently because skin strains of group A streptococci lack the requisite virulence genes [30]. (See Chapter 10.)

TREATMENT AND PROPHYLAXIS OF STREPTOCOCCAL IMPETIGO

The treatment of choice for streptococcal impetigo is penicillin, which may be given as a single injection of benzathine penicillin G or as a 7-day course of oral penicillin V. If the etiology is in doubt, alternative systemic therapy with an antistaphylococcal β-lactam or cephalosporin or erythromycin is appropriate. Topical therapy alone is recommended only when lesions are minimal in extent or number and is not effective for scalp lesions [65]. Mupirocin, a natural product of *Pseudomonas fluorescens*, is an effective but costly topical agent. Penicillin is also recommended for eradication and prevention of further spread of nephritogenic streptococci to family members or other close contacts, but the prevention of AGN in the individual infected with a nephritogenic skin streptococcus cannot be expected with any confidence.

The most effective prophylaxis of streptococcal pyoderma includes cleanliness, good hygiene, and prompt, appropriate care of cuts and abrasions, measures either unavailable or impractical in populations with endemic infection. Injections of benzathine penicillin have been shown to prevent streptococcal pyoderma for several weeks [66] and may be considered under special circumstances.

REFERENCES

1. Wannamaker LW. Differences between streptococcal infections of the throat and the skin. New Engl J Med 1970; 282:23–30,78–85.
2. Dillon HC. Streptococcal infections of the skin and their complications: impetigo and nephritis. In: Wannamaker LW, Matsen JM (eds). Streptococci and Streptococcal Diseases. New York: Academic Press, 1972; 571–587.
3. Peter G, Smith AL. Group A streptococcal infections of the skin and pharynx. New Engl J Med 1977; 297:311–317,365–370.
4. Hood AF, Kwan TH, Mihm MC, Horn TC. Primer of Dermatopathology, 2nd ed. Boston: Little, Brown, 1993.
5. Melish ME. Staphylococci, streptococci and the skin. Semin Dermatol 1982; 1:101–109.
6. Anthony BF, Perlman LV, Wannamaker LW. Skin infections and acute nephritis in American Indian children. Pediatrics 1967; 39:263–279.
7. Dillon HC. Impetigo contagiosa. Suppurative and nonsuppurative complications. Am J Dis Child 1968, 115:530–541.
8. Anthony BF, Kaplan EL, Wannamaker LW, Chapman SS. The dynamics of streptococcal infections in a defined population of children: serotypes associated with skin and respiratory infections. Am J Epidemiol 1976; 104:652–666.
9. Parker MT, Tomlinson AJH, Williams REO. The association of certain types of *Staphylococcus aureus* and of *Streptococcus pyogenes* with superficial skin infections. J Hyg 1955; 53:458–473.
10. Barrow GI. Clinical and bacteriological aspects of impetigo contagiosa. J Hyg 1955; 53:495–508.
11. Top FH, Wannamaker LW, Maxted WR, Anthony BF. M antigens among group A streptococci isolated from skin lesions. J Exp Med 1967; 126:667–685.
12. Johnson JC, Baskin RC, Beachey EH, Stollerman GH. Virulence of skin strains of nephritogenic group A streptococci: new M protein serotypes. J Immunol 1968; 101:187–191.
13. Dillon HC, Dillon MSA. New streptococcal serotypes causing pyoderma and acute glomerulonephritis: types 59, 60, and 61. Infect Immun 1971; 9:1070–1078.

14. Dillon HC, Derrick CW, Dillon MS. M-antigens common to pyoderma and acute glomerulonephritis. J Infect Dis 1974; 130:257–267.
15. Johnson DR, Kaplan EL. A review of the correlation of T-agglutination patterns and M-protein typing and opacity factor production in the identification of group A streptococci. J Med Microbiol 1993; 38:311–315.
16. Ayoub EM, Ferrieri P. Group A streptococcal diseases. In: Hoeprich PD, Jordan MC, Ronald AR (eds). Infectious Diseases, 5th ed. Philadelphia: J.B. Lippincott, 1994; 349–366.
17. Roth RR, James WD. Microbiology of the skin: resident flora, ecology and infection. J Am Acad Dermatol 1989; 20:367–390.
18. Dudding BA, Burnett JW, Chapman SS, Wannamaker LW. The role of normal skin in the spread of streptococcal pyoderma. J Hyg 1970; 68:19–28.
19. Ferrieri P, Dajani AS, Wannamaker LW, Chapman SS: Natural history of impetigo: site sequence of acquisition and familial patterns of spread of cutaneous streptococci. J Clin Invest 1972; 51:2851–2862.
20. Ricketts CR, Squire JR, Topley E. Human skin lipids with particular reference to the self-sterilising power of the skin. Clin Sci 1951; 10:89–111.
21. Speert DP, Wannamaker LW, Gray ED, Clawson CC. Bactericidal effect of oleic acid on group A streptococci: mechanism of action. Infect Immun 1979; 26:1202–1210.
22. Leyden JJ, Stewart R, Kligman AM. Experimental infections with group A streptococci in humans. J Invest Dermatol 1980; 75:196–201.
23. Alkan M, Ofek I, Beachey EH. Adherence of pharyngeal and skin strains of group A streptococci to human skin and oral epithelial cells. Infect Immun 1977; 18:555–557.
24. Hanski E, Caparon M. Protein F, a fibronectin-binding protein, is an adhesin of the group A streptococcus *Streptococcus pyogenes.* Proc Natl Acad Sci USA 1992; 89:6172–6176.
25. Okada N, Pentland AP, Falk P, Caparon MG. M protein and protein F act as important determinants of cell-specific tropism of *Streptococcus pyogenes* in skin tissue. J Clin Invest 1994; 94:965–977.
26. Darnstadt GL, Fleckman P, Jonas M, Chi E, Rubens CE. Differentiation of cultured keratinocytes promotes the adherence of *Streptococcus pyogenes.* J Clin Invest 1998; 101:128–136.
27. Wang B, Ruiz N, Pentland A, Caparon M. Keratinocyte proinflammatory response to adherent and nonadherent group A streptococci. Infect Immun 1997; 65:2119–2126.
28. Maxted WR, Fraser CAM, Parker MT. *Streptococcus pyogenes,* type 49. A nephritogenic streptococcus with a wide geographical distribution. Lancet 1967; 1:641–644.
29. Dillon HC, Derrick CW, Gooch PE. A new M-type of group A streptoccus of clinical importance in pyoderma and pharyngitis. J Gen Microbiol 1975; 91:119–126.
30. Bessen DE, Sotir CM, Readdy TL, Hollingshead SK. Genetic correlates of throat and skin isolates of group A streptococci. J Infect Dis 1996; 173:896–900.
31. Kaplan EL, Anthony BF, Chapman SS, Ayoub EM, Wannamaker LW. The influence of the site of infection on the immune response to group A streptococci. J Clin Invest 1970; 49:1405–1414.
32. Bisno A, Nelson KE, Waytz P, Brunt J. Factors influencing serum antibody responses in streptoccal pyoderma. J Lab Clin Med 1973; 81:410–420.
33. Dillon HC, Reeves MS. Streptococcal immune response in nephritis after skin infections. Am J Med 1974; 56:333–346.
34. Kaplan EL, Wannamaker LW. Suppression of the antistreptolysin O response by cholesterol and by lipid extracts of rabbit skin. J Exp Med 1976; 144:754–767.
35. Bisno AL, Nelson KE. Type-specific opsonic antibodies in streptococcal pyoderma. Infect Immun 1974; 10:1356–1361.
36. Flores AE, Johnson DR, Kaplan EL, Wannamaker LW. Factors influencing antibody responses to streptococcal M protein in humans. J Infect Dis 1983; 147:1–15.
37. Allen AM, Taplin D, Twigg L. Cutaneous streptococcal infections in Vietnam. Arch Dermatol 1971; 104:271–280.
38. Dajani AS, Wannamaker LW, Demonstration of a bactericidal substance against beta-hemolytic streptococci in supernatant fluids of staphylococcal cultures. J Bacteriol 1969; 97:985–991.
39. Dajani AS, Wannamaker LW. Experimental infection of the skin in the hamster simulating human impetigo. J Exp Med 1971; 134:588–599.
40. Dajani AS, Ferrieri P, Wannamaker LW. Natural history of impetigo. J Clin Invest 1972; 51:2863–2868.
41. Dajani AS, Ferrieri P, Wannamaker LW. Endemic superficial pyoderma in children. Arch Dermatol 1973; 108:517–521.
42. Dillon HC Jr. The treatment of streptococcal skin infections. J Pediatr 1970; 76:676–684.
43. Schachner L, Taplin D, Scott GB, Morrison M. A therapeutic update on superficial skin infections. Pediatr Clin North Am 1983; 30:397–404.
44. Tunnessen, WW. Practical aspects of bacterial skin infections in children. Pediatr Dermatol 1985; 2:255–256.
45. Lookingbill DP. Impetigo. Pediatr Rev 1985; 7:177–181.
46. Barton LL, Friedman AD. Impetigo: a reassessment of etiology and therapy. Pediatr Dermatol 1987; 3:185–188.
47. Demidovich CW, Wittler RR, Ruff ME, Bass JW, Browning WC. Impetigo; current etiology and comparison of penicillin, erythromycin and cephalexin therapies. Am J Dis Child 1990; 144:1313–1315.
48. Dagan R. Impetigo in childhood. Changing epi-

demiology and new treatments. Pediatr Ann 1993; 22:235–240.

49. Darmstadt GL, Lane AT. Impetigo: an overview. Pediatr Dermatol 1994; 11:293–303.

50. Maddox JS, Ware JC, Dillon HC Jr. The natural history of streptococcal skin infection: prevention with topical antibiotics. J Am Acad Dermatol 1985; 13:207–212.

51. Blumberg RW, Feldman DB. Observations on acute glomerulonephritis associated with impetigo. J Pediatr 1962; 60: 677–685.

52. Markowitz M, Bruton D, Kuttner AG, Cluff LE. The bacteriologic findings, streptococcal immune response, and renal complications in children with impetigo. Pediatrics 1965; 35:393–404.

53. Hall WD, Blumberg RW, Moody MD. Studies in children with impetigo. Am J Dis Child 1973; 124:800–806.

54. Taplin D, Lansdell L, Allen AM, Rodriguez R, Cortes A. Prevalence of streptococcalpyoderma in relation to climate and hygience. Lancet 1973; 1:501–503.

55. Margolis HS, Lum MKW, Bender TR, Elliott SL, Fitzgerald MA Harpster AP. Acute glomerulonephritis and streptococcal skin lesions in Eskimo children. Am J Dis Child 1980; 134:681–685.

56. Cruickshank JG, Lightfoot NF, Sugars KH, Colman G, Simmons MD, Tolliday J, Oakley EHN. A large outbreak of streptococcal pyoderma in a military training establishment. J Hyg 1982; 89:9–21.

57. Glezen WP, DeWalt JI, Lindsay RL, Dillon HC Jr. Epidemic pyoderma caused by nephritogenic streptococci in college athletes Lancet 1972; 1:301–303.

58. Ludlam H, Bookson B. Scrum kidney: epidemic pyoderma caused by a nephritogenic streptococcus pyogenes in a rugby team. Lancet 1986; 2:331–333.

59. Dillon HC Jr. Post-streptococcal glomerulonephritis following pyoderma. Rev Infect Dis 1979; 1:935–943.

60. Anthony BF, Yamauchi T, Penso, JS, Kamei I, Chapman SS. Classroom outbreak of scarlet fever and acute glomerulonephritis related to type 2 (M-2,T-2) group A streptococcus. J Infect Dis 1974; 129:336–340.

61. Stetson CA, Rammelkamp CH, Krause RM, Kohen RN, Perry WD. Epidemic acute nephritis: studies on etiology, natural history and prevention. Medicine 1955; 34:431–450.

62. Anthony BF, Kaplan EL, Wannamaker LW, Briese FW, Chapman SS. Attack rates of acute nephritis after type 49 streptococcal infection of the skin and of the respiratory tract. J Clin Invest 1969; 48:1697–1704.

63. Kaplan EL, Anthony BF, Chapman SS, Wannamaker LW. Epidemic acute glomerulonephritis associated with type 49 streptococcal pyoderma. Am J Med 1970; 48:9–27.

64. Derrick CW, Reeves MS, Dillon HC Jr. Complement in overt and asymptomatic nephritis after skin infection. J Clin Invest 1970; 49:1178–1187.

65. Sadick NS. Current aspects of bacterial infections of the skin. Dermatol Clin 1997; 15:341–349.

66. Ferrieri P, Dajani AS, Wannamaker LW. A controlled study of pencillin prophylaxis against streptococcal impetigo. J Infect Dis 1974; 129: 429–438.

Acute Poststreptococcal Glomerulonephritis

STIG E. HOLM, ANNIKA NORDSTRAND,
DENNIS L. STEVENS AND MARI NORGREN

Epidemics of acute poststreptococcal glomerulonephritis (APSGN) are well described in the literature [1–9], yet in total numbers the sporadic form accounts for more cases. The peak incidence is in children ages 2–6 years and overall, APSGN is much more common in children than adults. Spread of this disease among family members is well described. Males more frequently have clinical nephritis, whereas females are more likely to have subclinical disease [10,11]. In the tropics, skin infection (i.e., impetigo) during the summer is usually the initiating event [9] whereas in more temperate zones APSGN occurs more commonly in the winter months, associated with pharyngotonsillitis. Epidemics of APSGN may also occur with a cyclical variation in frequency [7]. Acute poststreptococcal glomerulonephritis mainly follows infection with certain M types of group A streptococci; these types have been designated *nephritogenic* [10,12,13], although their nephritogenic capacity is variable and seems instead to be strain-specific. Furthermore, cases have been associated with streptococcal types beyond these "nephritogenic" types as well as with streptococci belonging to groups C and G [15,16]. The identification of nephritic strains has led to the hypothesis that factors unique to these strains initiate immune responses leading to nephritis.

CLINICAL MANIFESTATIONS

The latent period between streptococcal infection and onset of nephritis depends on the site of infection: following pharyngitis, it is usually 1 to 3 weeks, whereas after skin infection, it is more prolonged at 3 to 6 weeks [10]. The preceding infection may be accompanied by severe symptoms (i.e., fever, pharyngitis), or patients may be relatively asymptomatic. For many patients, it is not possible to identify an antecedent streptococcal infection with certainty. Regional lymphadenopathy, when present, may persist even after other symptoms and signs of the primary infection have resolved. Typically, the acute nephritic syndrome lasts 4 to 7 days; however, it may be more prolonged in adults, especially in those presenting with rapidly progressive glomerulonephritis and crescentic glomerulonephritis [17].

The clinical presentation of patients with APSGN can be quite variable. As illustrated in Table 9.1, the most common symptoms are edema, gross hematuria, and back pain [17]. Generalized symptoms, including anorexia, malaise, nausea, and vomiting, are also common at initial presentation but are not particularly helpful in establishing a diagnosis. Anasarca is more common among young children [12]. Oc-

Table 9.1 Clinical and Laboratory Manifestations of Acute Poststreptococcal Glomerulonephritis

Manifestation	Patients (%)	
Clinical		
Edema	85	
Gross hematuria	30	
Back pain	5–10	
Oliguria (transient)	50	
Hypertension	60–85	
Nephrotic syndrome	5	
Laboratory		
Urinalysis: proteinuria, hematuria, casts	100	
Edema	>50	
Nephrotic range proteinuria	10	
Serum creatinine >2 mg/dl	25	
Streptococcal antibody profile (streptozyme)	>95	positive in patients with pharyngitis
	80	positive in patients with skin infection
	5	false-positive rate; early treatment prevents antibody response
C3, C4, and/or CH_{50} depressed	>90	
Hypergammaglobulinemia	90	
Cryoglobulinemia	75	

casionally, patients with gross hematuria complain of dysuria. Transient oliguria is present in approximately one-half of the patients, but anuria is rare [12].

On physical examination, hypertension is the most common finding and is present in about 60% to 85% of patients at initial presentation. Severe hypertension may result in encephalopathy and seizures in <1% of patients with APSGN [11,12]. Rarely, encephalopathy may occur in the absence of significant hypertension. Congestive heart failure may also be evident during the course of acute illness, likely due to sodium retention. Both hypertension and heart failure usually resolve after diuresis. If arthralgias or skin rash are present, other causes of glomerulonephritis should also be considered (i.e., lupus, vasculitis). Backache in the lumbar region results from intrarenal edema and stretching of the renal capsule.

LABORATORY FINDINGS AND DIAGNOSIS

The occurrence of red blood cells in urine, sometimes as red blood cell cylinders, is the hallmark of glomerular injury; these cells are best evaluated in a freshly voided specimen. White blood cell casts, granular and pigmented casts, and renal cell casts are also found during the acute stage. Proteinuria is always found and quantitation has revealed levels in the nephrotic range of 5% at initial presentation [13,18,19]. Laboratory findings vary with stage and severity of the disease. Occasionally, proteinuria increases subsequent to initial presentations to the nephrotic range, despite improvement in glomerular filtration.

The serum creatinine level is usually elevated but may remain within the upper limits of normal values. Only 25% of patients will have a serum creatinine level higher than 2 mg/dl [12]. The glomerular filtration rate is almost always depressed during the initial stages of the disease and should return toward normal values with disease resolution. Serum complement levels are very useful in establishing a diagnosis of APSGN. Still, in patients with mild disease or those presenting late in the course of disease, complement levels may have returned to normal by the time of initial presentation. Nonetheless, during the early stage of APSGN (the first 2 weeks) the serum C3 and total hemolytic complement (CH_{50}) levels are depressed in more than 90% of patients [12,20–23]. C2 and C4 levels are usually normal or slightly depressed. Elevation of plasma levels of the terminal complement components (C5b-9) has also been described [24]. Serum complement levels return to normal by 4 weeks in most patients, and the level or rate of decline of complement levels has neither positive nor negative predictive value in terms of prognosis. Persistent hypocomplementemia, however, is unusual and suggests another diagnosis [23]. C3 nephritic factor may be present in low amounts. Marked or persistent elevations are more typical of membranoproliferative glomerulonephritis [13]. Increased serum concentrations of gamma globulin are present in 90% of patients, and this may be detected as cryoglobulins in 75% of individuals [12,25] or as a positive rheumatoid factor in 30% of patients, particularly early in the course of disease [12].

Although glomerulonephritis related to group A streptococcal infection may be suspected because of demographic factors and clinical presentation, proof rests upon positive cultures or appropriate titers for antibodies to extracellular products of streptococci.

The first signs of APSGN usually appear when the primary infection is already cured. Thus the etiology is often based on the case history combined with information from serologic analyses. Because group A streptococci release an array of biologically active immunogenic substances, several serologic tests have been developed to cover the immune response in various streptococcal infections and at various stages of infection. In one of them, a crude streptococcal culture filtrate was used as an antigen pool that allowed analysis of several antibodies in a single test (the streptozyme test). This test is still used in many countries, while in others, clinicians prefer to use individual tests, as the antibody response against the various streptococcal antigens differs in relation to the site of infection and stage of disease. Thus, e.g., the antibody level to streptolysin O will usually increase within the first weeks and then decline after several months [15], whereas antibody titers toward DNAse B start to increase somewhat later but will persist several months longer [28–30]. Individuals with skin infection may not develop antistreptolysin O antibodies, as streptolysin binds to lipids in the skin. In this situation, determination of DNAse B antibodies is helpful, since DNAse B is not bound to the skin. In this way it is possible to establish the etiology of a glomerulonephritis when the primary infection has already healed. The serologic diagnosis should be

based on repeated antibody determinations. Antibodies against M protein [31] or cationic protein may also be useful; however, there are no routine assays available [12,26]. It should be noted that early treatment with antibiotic therapy may prevent the antibody response.

PATHOLOGY

Histologically a diffuse glomerulonephritis is commonly present, although the severity of involvement may vary among individual glomeruli and also within segments of a glomerulus [1,2,18,32]. During the first 2 weeks of APSGN, microscopy of kidney biopsy specimens reveals cellular infiltration by neutrophils, eosinophils, and monocytes in both the mesangium and capillary lumen of virtually all glomerular tufts [13,33]. Proliferation of endothelial and mesangial cells occurs early during the exudative stage. The lumens of capillaries may become occluded with cells or fibrin thrombi, resulting in tissue necrosis. Segmental subepithelial humps and crescent formation may also be present at this stage [13]. Early in the course of disease, the number of CD4 cells usually exceeds the number of CD8 cells, whereas CD8 cells predominate in the glomeruli at later stages [33]. Still later, intermittent thickening of capillary walls, corresponding to large subepithelial humps, may be observed by trichrome staining. After 4 to 6 weeks, hypercellularity with mononuclear cells (mesangial cells or monocytes) predominates and neutrophils are no longer present. Glomerular hypercellularity gradually resolves and capillary lumens become patent.

Immunofluorescence microscopy of renal biopsy specimens at various stages of illness have greatly improved our understanding of the pathophysiology of APSGN while providing excellent diagnostic criteria. For example, deposits of immunoglobulin G (IgG) and C3 are distributed in a diffuse granular pattern within the mesangium and capillary walls [32,34]. C3 is invariably present, whereas the presence of IgG depends on the timing of the biopsy, and it is not uncommon to see only C3 deposits very early or late in the disease. Immunoglobulin M may be present in small amounts, and fibrin deposits are occasionally detected in patients with more severe disease. Significant amounts of IgA suggest an alternative diagnosis, whereas anti-Ig antibody may be present within the mesangium [12]. C1q and C4 are not usually detected; however, properdin and terminal complement components (C5b-9) are frequently present and distributed in a granular pattern [24]. C3 may be present in the absence of detectable immunoglobulin, either very early in the disease (<2 weeks) or with disease resolution. Early in the disease, the granular appearance of immune deposits often gives a "starry sky" appearance [32,34,35]. With resolution of disease (i.e., 4–6 weeks after onset), the immune deposits take on a more mesangial pattern and may appear as "rope" or "garland" associated with persistent mesangial hypercellularity. These patterns may be apparent for months and are associated with heavy proteinuria and the subsequent development of glomerulosclerosis [34]. By contrast, transition to a more mesangial pattern is usually associated with clinical and pathologic resolution.

Electron microscopy also provides useful diagnostic information to distinguish APSGN from other causes of acute glomerulonephritis. Dome-shaped subepithelial electron-dense deposits that resemble camel "humps" are likely due to IgG, are associated with heavy proteinuria during the first months of illness, and are the most characteristic feature on electron microscopy [35]. Proliferation of cells and infiltration by leukocytes is apparent by electron microscopy, but the types of cells seen are dependent upon the stage of disease. The basement membrane itself is usually of normal diameter, although thickening has occasionally been observed [36].

PATHOGENESIS

After many decades of research into the pathogenesis of APSGN, it is clear that only certain strains of streptococci are nephritogenic, and that only certain hosts develop disease. A popular theory that originated in the 1960s is that deposition of streptococcal antigens occurs within glomeruli [37,38]. One possible pathogenic scenario is as follows: Proteins with unique antigenic determinants are produced only by nephritogenic strains of streptococci. These proteins have a particular affinity for sites within the normal glomerulus. Following release into the circulation from skin or pharyngeal infection, they lodge within the glomerulus, binding to sites for which they have intrinsic affinity. Once glomerulus-bound, they activate complement directly by attracting properdin, leading to stimulation of the alternative pathway. These glomerulus-bound streptococcal proteins interact with circulating antistreptococcal antibodies to form immune complexes, resulting in additional complement fixation and further influx of cells into the glomerulus.

The M Protein and M-like Proteins

An association between APSGN and certain M types of group A streptococcus (GAS) has been seen, including M1, 4, 12, 49, 55, 57, and 60 [39]. A common characteristic of M proteins is the presence of a repeating heptad periodicity in the distribution of nonpolar and charged residues, a characteristic of α-helical coiled-coil proteins [40]. It was demonstrated that the patterns of heptad periodicity in the N-terminal half of the nephritis-associated M49 and M57 proteins are similar to each other, but they are distinct from the patterns of ARF-associated M5 and M6 proteins [41]. The functional significance of these differences is unknown. Immunoglobulin G titers against the C-terminal, but not the N-terminal region of the M12 protein were reported to be markedly higher among APSGN patients than patients with pharyngitis, chronic glomerulonephritis, and healthy controls [42]. M proteins in complexes with fibrinogen in the circulation have been reported to localize in glomeruli [43], and injection of M protein–M protein/fibrinogen complexes was observed to induce signs of glomerulonephritis in mice [44] (Fig. 9.1). In addition, M proteins may be antigenically cross-reactive with the glomerular basement membrane (GBM) [45]. Binding of IgG and IgG aggregates was commonly demonstrated among nephritis GAS isolates, as well as strains of M types associated with APSGN [46–49]. Fc-receptor (Fc-R)–positive rather than FcR-negative GAS strains gave rise to circulating anti-IgG, as well as renal deposition of IgG and C3 in rabbits immunized with GAS [50]. The authors suggested that the FcRs might in some way induce

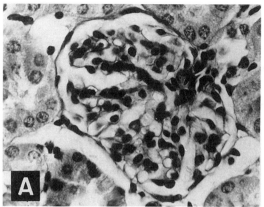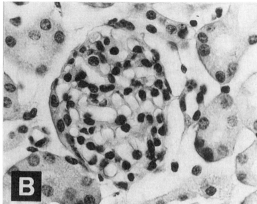

Figure 9.1 Kidney sections of glomeruli stained with hematoxylin and periodic acid–Schiff. (A) Glomerulus from mouse infected with a nephritis GAS isolate. The glomerulus was regarded positive for hypercellularity, occlusion of capillaries, and lobulation. (B) Glomerulus regarded negitive for morphological signs of APSGN. Magnification × 1000.

immune complex formation or enhance precipitation of complexes. However, morphological changes in the glomeruli of the rabbits did not correspond to those seen in APSGN in humans. In addition, if deposition of antibodies were the initiating mechanism of APSGN in humans, IgG would be detected before C3 in the glomeruli, which is usually not the case.

Streptokinase

Streptokinase is a 46 kDa, 414 amino acid extracellular protein believed to be involved in the spread of streptococci through tissue because of its ability to activate plasminogen to plasmin. Although the streptokinase gene (*ska* in GAS, *skc* in GCS, etc.) is present in virtually all group A, C, and G streptococci, not all strains that harbor the gene were observed to produce the protein in vitro [51]. The streptokinase gene is highly conserved. The nucleotide sequence identity between the nephritis GAS isolate NZ131 (M type 49) and the non-nephritis–associated group C strain *Streptococcus equisimilis* H46A is 90%, and 85% at the amino acid level [52]. The nonidentical amino acids are located in two major regions—variable regions 1 (V1) and 2 (V2)—corresponding to amino acid residues 174–244 and 270–290, respectively [51]. The V1 regions of nephritis-associated *ska* alleles show more than 95% homology with each other at the nucleotide level, but less than 60% homology with

the non-nephritis–associated *ska* alleles [53]. By endonuclease digestion of polymerase chain reaction (PCR)-amplified V1 regions, nine different variants of *ska* were identified, of which *ska*1, *ska*2, *ska*6, and *ska*9 were exclusively identified in APSGN isolates [53,54]. The V1 region was reported to appear more hydrophobic as well as to have a higher content of ordered secondary structures in nephritis-associated streptokinase molecules compared to non-nephritis–associated ones [55]. It was hypothesized that amino acid differences in V1 might lead to different affinity of streptokinases to glomerular epitopes and thereby be related to the nephritogenic capacity of a strain [56]. Formation of the complement activator plasmin by a streptokinase-plasmin(ogen) complex in situ was suggested to be a possible explanation for the initial glomerular C3 deposition. The predicted amino acid sequences of highly divergent *ska* alleles were observed to give strikingly similar hydrophilicity and hydrophobicity profiles, distribution of amphiphatic and flexible regions, surface probability plots, and antigenic indices, which taken together indicate that despite extensive nucleotide polymorphism in V1 and V2, selective pressure has constrained overall structural divergence [57]. Despite this finding, streptokinase of a nephritis-associated variant (*ska*2) was observed to contain three energetic folding units, whereas the non–nephritis-associated streptokinase from H46A contains two units, as well as has higher sensitivity to trypsin digestion of the C-terminal region [58]. Nephritis-associated streptokinase was observed to bind more tightly to glomeruli in vitro than the streptokinase from H46A [59]. However, it was also reported that no unique reactivity to streptokinase could be demonstrated in sera of APSGN patients and that streptokinase could not be detected in renal biopsies early in the course of 10 APSGN patients [60]. An animal model for APSGN has been established in mice where the GAS infection is initiated from a subcutaneously implanted tissue cage [61] (Fig. 9.2). Morphological and immunohistological changes in the kidneys resembling those of APSGN in humans, including urinary findings such as proteinuria and hematuria and deposition of C3, were noted in the mice after 7 and 16 days of infection with the APSGN isolates, but not with a non-APSGN isolate. Streptokinase was demonstrated in the kidneys of mice infected with two nephritis strains (NZ131 and EF514). Detection of streptokinase increased with the degree of glomerular hypercellularity. It was speculated that the severity of the pathological process may be a reflection of the degree of streptokinase bound in the kidney. Infection with isogenic strains of the APSGN isolate NZ131 (*ska*1), differing in the ability to produce streptokinase, showed no sign of APSGN. Thus, in strain NZ131, streptokinase production was required for induction of APSGN in the model [62]. To investigate the role of allelic variants in the pathogenesis of APSGN, the streptokinase allele (*ska*1) of strain NZ131 was exchanged to a non-nephritis–associated allele *ska*5 from strain H46A (Nordstrand A., McShan W.M., Ferretti J.J., Holm S.E., and Norgren M., unpublished results). Infection with this strain resulted in signs of APSGN after 7 days of infection, and only C3 deposition after 16 days. The results strongly support the hypothesis that certain isotypes of streptokinase can initiate the nephritis process by binding to the glomeruli. This will facilitate streptokinase-mediated plasminogen activation with and local activation of the complement cascade as a possible pathogenic mechanism (Fig. 9.3). One of four strains that produced a nephritis-associated streptokinase isotype did not induce nephritis in the model, a finding that indicates involvement of additional factors in the disease process.

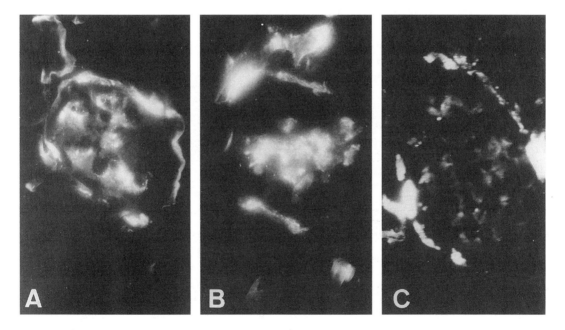

Figure 9.2 Kidney sections of glomeruli with immunofluorescent staining for the complement factor C3. (Λ) and (B) Glomeruli from mice infected with a nephritis GAS isolate. The glomeruli were regarded positive for C3 deposition, with granular deposits along capillary walls and partially blurred boundaries in the mesangium. (C) Glomerulus regarded negative for C3 deposition. Magnification × 1000.

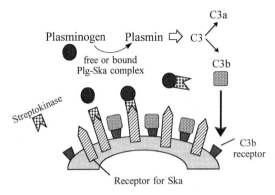

Figure 9.3 Proposed mechanism for the induction of acute poststreptococcal glomerulonephritis. Ska, streptokinase; Plg, plasminogen.

Endostreptosin and Preabsorbing Antigen

Endostreptosin, a 40–50 kDa protein obtained after disruption of GAS nephritis isolates, was suggested to be involved in the pathogenesis of APSGN [63]. It was detected in glomeruli of APSGN patients during the early phase but could not be demonstrated during the late phase of the disease. Antibody titers to endostreptosin were reported to be higher in APSGN patients than in the normal population as well as in most acute rheumatic fever (ARF) patients [65]. It was suggested that elevated levels of antibody to endostreptosin may be diagnostic for APSGN [65]. Endostreptosin may be identical to the 43 kDa preabsorbing antigen (PA-Ag) [66,67]. Antibody reactivity against PA-Ag was demonstrated in sera from 30 of 31 patients with APSGN, but rarely in control groups. In addition, PA-Ag was reported to be an activator of the alternative pathway of the complement system [67]. Slight to moderate proliferation as well as C3 deposition in glomeruli was reported after subcutaneous administration of PA-Ag to rabbits [68]. The authors argued that PA-Ag is present in glomeruli of APSGN patients at the early stage of the disease and that it may be involved in the pathogenesis of the disease via in situ complex formation and complement activation [67,68].

Cationic Antigens

Because cationic moieties are known to have affinity for the polyanionic GBM, cationic anti-gens have been considered to be factors that might be involved in the pathogenesis of APSGN [69]. Antibodies raised against a number of different cationic proteins from GAS nephritis isolates were reported to stain almost half the examined renal biopsies from APSGN patients, whereas staining was not detected in renal biopsies from patients with immune complex glomerulonephritis without streptococcal association. In addition, antibodies to these cationic antigens were noted in the APSGN patients studied. The authors suggested that such an antigen(s) could possibly initiate acute glomerulonephritis by means of in situ immune complex formation [69]. It may be hypothesized that, through such a mechanism of involvement, they may be more likely to be involved in the later phase of the disease, since C3 deposition precedes that of IgG in APSGN.

NATURAL HISTORY AND PROGNOSIS

The overall prognosis for patients with APSGN is very good: less than 0.5% die of the initial disease and fewer than 2% of patients die or progress to end-stage renal disease [3,6,8,18, 34,54]. Both the natural history of this disease and the modern clinical management of its complications contribute to the excellent outcome. Children have a better prognosis than adults, and patients older than 40 years with rapidly progressive renal failure and crescentic glomerulonephritis have a worse prognosis [6,10,12]. There appears to be no difference in outcome with either epidemic or sporadic forms, although conclusions regarding prognosis derive largely from well-documented epidemics in children. By contrast, opinion for less favorable outcomes comes from smaller series of sporadic cases in adults [12]. Persistent urinary and histologic abnormalities are common in both adults and children and may last for years [6,72]. In most large series of well-documented cases, these abnormalities eventually resolve, and the incidence of chronic renal failure is low. Patients with prolonged nephrotic syndrome or persistence of heavy proteinuria have a worse prognosis, and this is often associated with evolution to a garland-like pattern of immune deposits with disease progression [34]. In one series of adults with APSGN, a larger percentage of patients developed persistent hypertension or end-state renal disease or both, years after the initial episode of acute glomerulonephritis [16,73]. Among such patients, it is unclear whether progressive renal failure is due to nephrosclerosis associated with poorly controlled hypertension or progressive glomerular scarring. Regardless of the course of disease, it seems clear that a small group of patients will develop progressive renal insufficiency.

TREATMENT AND PREVENTION

The major aims of therapy of acute nephritis are control of blood pressure and treatment of volume overload. During the acute phase of the disease, salt and water intake should be restricted. The acute phase of the illness usually resolves within a week, and most patients undergo spontaneous diuresis within the first week. However, if significant edema or hypertension develops, diuretics should be administered. Furosemide usually provides a prompt diuresis, with reduction of blood pressure. For hypertension uncontrolled by diuretics, vasodilators (i.e., calcium channel blockers or angiotensin-converting enzyme [ACE] inhibitors) are usually effective. Intravenous nitroprusside or other parenteral agents are rarely required for the management of severe or malignant hypertension. The serum potassium level should be monitored and treated appropriately. Dialysis may be necessary to treat uremia. Restriction of physical activity is appropriate during the first few days of the illness but is unnecessary once the patient feels well.

Steroids, immunosuppressive agents, and plasmapheresis are generally not indicated. In patients with rapidly progressive renal failure, however, a renal biopsy may be useful for diagnostic reasons. If crescents are present in more than 30% of glomeruli, some practitioners recommend treatment with a short course of intravenous pulse steroid therapy (500 mg–1 g/1.73 m^2 of intravenous methylprednisolone daily, for 3–5 successive days) [74]. Although there are no controlled trials of this therapy in patients with APSGN, it has been beneficial in patients with rapidly progressive glomerulonephritis associated with other diseases. Prolonged treatment

with steroids or other immunosuppressive therapy is not indicated [74]. Long-term antihypertensive therapy in patients with hypertension and chronic renal insufficiency is essential to prevent the development of renal failure, and ACE inhibitors are the drug of choice for this purpose [74].

Specific therapy for streptococcal infections is an essential part of the therapeutic regimen. This includes treatment of both the patient and the infected family members or persons with close personal contact [74]. Throat cultures should be performed on all these individuals, and treatment with penicillin, or erythromycin for patients allergic to penicillin, administered. Whether early treatment of infected patients prevents nephritis is debated. For patients with skin infections, attention to personal hygiene is also essential. In endemics, empirical prophylactic treatment of patients at risk, including persons with close contact, and family members, is recommended.

REFERENCES

1. Dodge WF, Spargo BH, Travis LB, Srivastava RN, Carjaval HF, DeBeukeaer MM, Longley MP, Menchaca JA. Poststreptococcal glomerulonephritis. N Engl J Med 1972; 286:273–278.
2. Fish AJ, Herdman RC, Michael AF, Pickering RJ, Good RA. Epidemic acute glomerulonephritis associated with type 49 streptococcal pyoderma I. Am J Med 1970; 48:28–38.
3. Garcia R, Rubio L, Rodriguez-Iturbe B. Long term prognosis of epidemic poststreptococcal glomerulonephritis in Maracaibo: follow-up studies 11–12 years after the acute episode. Clin Nephrol 1981; 15:291–298.
4. Kaplan EL, Anthony BF, Chapman SS, Wannamaker LW. Epidemic acute glomerulonephritis associated with type 49 streptococcal pyoderma II. Clinical and laboratory findings. Am J Med 1970; 48:9–27.
5. Lewy JE, Salinas-Madrigal L, Herdson PB, Metcoff J. Clinico-pathologic correlations in acute poststreptococcal glomerulonephritis. Medicine 1971; 50:453–501.
6. Lien JWK, Matthew TH, Meadows R. Acute poststreptococcal glomerulonephritis in adults: a long-term study. Q J Med 1979; 48:99–111.
7. Rodriguez-Iturbe B. Epidemic poststreptococcal glomerulonephritis. Kidney Int 1984; 25:129 136.
8. Vogl W, Renke M, Mayer-Eichberger D, Schmitt H, Bohle A. Long-term prognosis for endocapil-

lary glomerulonephritis of poststreptococcal type in children and adults. Nephron 1986; 44:58–65.

9. Anthony BF, Kaplan EL, Wannamaker LW, Briese FW, Chapman SS. Attack rates of acute nephritis after type 49 streptococcal infection of the skin and respiratory tract. J Clin Invest 1969; 48:1697–1704.

10. Nissenson AR, Baraft LJ, Fine RN, Knutson MD. Poststreptococcal acute glomerulonephritis: Fact and controversy. Ann Intern Med 1979; 91:76–86.

11. Rodriguez-Iturbe B, Rubio L, Garcia R. Attack rate of poststreptococcal nephritis in families. Lancet 1981; 1:401–403.

12. Rodriguez-Iturbe B. Acute poststreptococcal glomerulonephritis. In: Schrier RW, Gottschalk CW (ed). Diseases of the Kidney, 5th ed. Boston: Little, Brown, 1993; 1715–1730.

13. Glassock RJ. Primary glomerular diseases. In: Brenner BM, Rector F (eds). The Kidney, 5th ed. Philadelphia: W.B. Saunders 1996; 1393–1497, Volume II.

14. Barnham M, Thornton TJ, Lange K. Nephritis caused by *Streptococcus zooepidermicus* (Lancefield group C). Lancet 1983; 1:945–948.

15. Barnham M, Ljunggren Å, McIntyre M. Human infections with *Streptococcus zooepidemicus* (Lancefield group C): three case reports. Epidemiol Infect 1987; 98:183–190.

16. Grann JW, Gray BM, Griffin FM, Dismunke WE. Acute glomerulonephritis following group G streptococcal infection. J Infect Dis 1987; 156:411–412.

17. Washio M, Okuda S, Yanase T, Miishima C, Fujimi S, Ohchi N, Nanichi F, Onoyama K, Fujishama M. Clinicopathological study of post-streptococcal glomerulonephritis in the elderly. Clin Nephrol 1994; 41:265–270.

18. Baldwin DS, Gluck MD, Schacht RG, Gallo GR, Feiner HD. The long-term course of poststreptococcal glomerulonephritis. Ann Intern Med 1974; 80:342–358.

19. Hinglis N, Garcia-Torres R, Kleinknecht D. Long-term prognosis in acute glomerulonephritis: the predictive value of early clinical and pathological features. Am J Med 1974; 56:52–60.

20. Madaio MP, Harrington JT. The diagnosis of acute glomerulonephritis. N Engl J Med 1983; 309:1299–1302.

21. Sjoholm AG. Complement components and complement activation in acute poststreptococcal glomerulonephritis. Arch Allerg Appl Immunol 1979; 58:274–284.

22. Lewis EJ, Carpenter CB, Shur PH. Serum complement levels in human glomerulonephritis. Ann Intern Med 1971; 75:555–560.

23. Cameron JS. Plasma C3 and C4 concentration in the management of human glomerulonephritis. BMJ 1973; 3:688–672.

24. Matsell D, Roy S, Tamerius JD, Morrow PR, Kolb W, Wyatt RJ. Plasma terminal complement complexes in acute poststreptococcal glomerulonephritis. Am J Kidney Dis 1991; 27:311–316.

25. McIntosh RM, Kulvinskas C, Kaufman DB. Cryoglobulins: III. Further studies on the nature, incidence, diagnostic, prognostic and immunopathologic significance of cryoproteins in renal disease. Q J Med 1975; 44:285–307.

26. Zaum R, Vogt A, Rodriguez-Iturbe B. Analysis of the immune response to streptococcal proteinase in poststreptococcal disease. Abstract from Xth Lancefield International Symposium on Streptococci and Streptococcal Disease. 1987; Abstract p 63, Cologne, Germany, Sept 1–4 1987.

27. Stollerman GH, Lewis AJ, Schultz I, Taranta A. Relationship of immune response to group A streptococci to the course of acute and chronic recurrent rheumatic fever. Am J Med 1956; 20:163–169.

28. Wannamaker LW. Differences between streptococcal infections in the throat and of the skin. N Engl J Med 1970; 282:78–85.

29. Bisno AL, Nelson KE, Waytz P, Brunt J. Factors influencing serum antibody response in streptococcal pyoderma. J Lab Clin Med 1973; 81:410–420.

30. Dillon H, Reeves M. Streptococcal immune responses in nephritis after skin infection. Am J Med 1974; 56:333–346.

31. Stollerman GH. Streptococcal immunology: protection versus injury. Ann Intern Med 1978; 88:422–423.

32. Feldman JD, Mardiney MR, Shuler SE. Immunology and morphology of acute poststreptococcal glomerulonephritis. Lab Invest 1965; 15:283–301.

33. Parra G, Platt JL, Falk RJ, Rodriguez-Jturbe B, Michael AF. Cell populations and membrane attack complex in glomeruli of patients with post-streptococcal glomerulonephritis: identification using monoclonal antibodies by indirect immunofluorescence. Clin Immunol Immunopathol 1984; 33:324–332.

34. Sorger K, Gessler M, Hubner FK, Kohler H, Olbing H, Schulz W, Thoenes GH, Thoenes W. Follow-up studies of three subtypes of acute postinfectious glomerulonephritis ascertained by renal biopsy. Clin Nephrol 1987; 27:111–124.

35. Kimmelstiel P. The hump a lesion of acute glomerulonephritis. Bull Pathol 1965; 6:187.

36. Earle DP, Jennings RB. Studies of poststreptococcal nephritis and other glomerular diseases. Ann Intern Med 1959; 51:851–

37. Zabriskie JB. The role of streptococci in human glomerulonephritis. J Exp Med 1971; 134:180S.

38. Treser G, Seman M, McVicar M, Franklin M, Ty A, Sagel J, Lange K. Antigenic streptococcal components in acute glomerulonephritis. Science 1969; 163:676–677.

39. Wannamaker LW. Differences between streptococcal infections of the throat and of the skin. N Engl J Med 1970; 282:78–85.

40. Manjula BN, Acharya AS, Mische SM, Fairwell T, Fischetti VA. The complete amino acid acid sequence of a biologically active 197-residue fragment of M protein from type 5 group A streptococci. J Biol Chem 1984; 259:3686–3693.

41. Khandke KM, Fairwell T, Manjula BN. Difference in the structural features of streptococcal M proteins from nephritogenic and rheumatogenic serotypes. J Exp Med 1987; 166:151–162.

42. Mori K, Ito Y, Kamikawaji N, Sasazuki T. Elevated titer against the C region of streptococcal M protein and its immunodeterminants in patients with poststreptococcal acute glomerulonephritis. J Pediatr 1997; 131:293–299.

43. Kantor FS. Fibrinogen precipitation by streptococcal M protein: I. Identity of the reactants and stoichiometry of the reaction. J Exp Med 1965; 121:849–879.

44. Humair L, Kwaan HC, Potter EV. The role of fibrinogen in renal disease II. Effect of anticoagulants and urokinase on experimental lesions in mice. J Lab Clin Med 1969; 74:72–78.

45. Markowitz M. Changing epidemiology of group A streptococcal infections. Pediatr Infect Dis J 1964; 92:565.

46. Burova LA, Koroleva IV, Ogurtzov RP, Murashov SV, Svensson ML, Schalén C. Role of streptococcal IgG receptor in tissue deposition of IgG in rabbits immunized with Streptococcus pyogenes. APMIS 1992; 100:567–574.

47. Christensen P, Sjöholm AG, Holm S, Hovelius B, Mårdh PA. Binding of aggregated IgG in the presence of fresh serum by group A streptococci producing pharyngeal infection: possible connection with types frequently involved in acute nephritis. Acta Pathol Microbiol Scand Sect B 1978; 86:29–33.

48. Schalén C, Christensen P, Kurl D, Sramek J, Svensson M-L. Interaction of nephritis-associated group A streptococci with aggregated human IgG. In: Kimura Y, Kotami S, Shiokawa S (eds.). Recent Advances in Streptococci and Streptococcal Diseases. Chertsey, Surrey: Reedbooks, 1985; 81–83.

49. Tewodros W, Kronvall G. Distribution of presumptive pathogenicity factors among beta-hemolytic streptococci isolated from Ethiopia. APMIS 1993; 101:295–305.

50. Burova LA, Naornev VA, Pigarevsky PV, Gladilina MM, Selivstova G, Schalén C, Totolian AA. Triggering of renal tissue damage in the rabbit by IgG Fc-receptor–positive group A streptococci. APMIS 1998; 106:277–287.

51. Huang TT, Malke H, Ferretti JJ. Heterogeneity of the streptokinase gene in group A streptococci. Infect Immun 1989; 57:502–506.

52. Huang TT, Malke H, Ferretti. The streptokinase gene of group A streptococci: cloning, expression in Escherichia coli, and sequence analysis. Mol Microbiol 1989; 3:197–205.

53. Johnston KH, Chaiban JE, Wheeler RC. Analysis of the variable domain of the streptokinase gene from streptococci associated with poststreptococcal glomerulonephritis. In: Orefici G (ed). New Perspectives on Streptococci and Streptococcal Infections. Stuttgart: Gustav Fischer Verlag, 1992; 339–341.

54. Wheeler RC, Chaiban JE, Johnston KH. Analysis of the streptokinase gene from group C streptococci S. equisimilis and S. zooeidemicus by the polymerase chain reaction and possible relation to poststreptococcal glomerulonephritis. In: Orefici G (ed). New Perspectives on Streptococci and Streptococcal Infections. Stuttgart: Gustav Fischer Verlag, 1992; 343–345.

55. Malke H. Polymorphism of the streptokinase gene: implications for the pathogenesis of poststreptococcal glomerulonephritis. Int J Med Microbiol Virol Parasitol Infect Dis 1993; 278:246–257.

56. Holm SE. The pathogenesis of acute poststreptococcal glomerulonephritis in new lights. APMIS 1988; 96:189–193.

57. Kapur V, Kanjilal S, Hamrick MR, Li L-L, Whittam TS, Saqyer SA, Musser JM. Molecular population genetic analysis of the streptokinase gene of Streptococcus pyogenes; mosaic alleles generated by recombination. Mol Microbiol 1995; 16:509–519.

58. Wefle K, Misselwitz R, Schaup A, Gerlach D, Wefle H. Conformation and stability of strepto-kinases from nephritogenic and nonnephritogenic strains of streptococci. Proteins 1997; 26–35.

59. Peake PW, Pussell BA, Karplus TE, Riley EH, Charlesworth JA. Poststreptococcal glomerulonephritis: studies on the interaction between nephritos strain–associated protein (NSAP), complement and the glomerulus. APMIS 1991; 99:460–466.

60. Mezzano S, Burgos E, Mahabir R, Kemeney E, Zabriskie JB. Failure to detect unique reactivity to streptococcal streptokinase in either the sera or renal biopsy specimens of patients with acute poststreptococcal glomerulonephritis. Clin Nephrol 1992; 38:305–310.

61. Nordstrand A, Norgren M, Holm SE. An experimental model for acute poststreptococcal glomerulonephritis in mice. APMIS 1996; 104:805–816.

62. Nordstrand A, Norgren M, Ferretti J, Holm SE. Streptokinase as a mediator of acute poststreptococcal glomerulonephritis in an experimental mouse model. Infect Immun 1998; 66:315–321.

63. Lange K, Ahmed U, Kleinberger H, Treser G. A hitherto unknown antigen and its probable relation to acute poststreptococcal glomerulonephritis. Clin Nephrol 1976; 5:206–207.

64. Lange K, Seligson G, Cronin W. Evidence for the in situ origin of poststreptococcal GN: glomerular localization of endostreptosin and the clinical

significance of the subsequent antibody response. Clin Nephrol 1983; 19:3–10.

65. Seligson G, Lange K, Majeed HA, Deol HL, Cronin W, Boyle R. Significance of endostreptosin antibody titers in poststreptococcal glomerulonephritis. Clin Nephrol 1985; 24:69–75.

66. Yoshizawa N, Treser G, Sagel I, Ty A, Ahmed U, Lange K. Demonstration of antigenic sites in glomeruli of patients with acute poststreptococcal glomerulonephritis by immunofluorescein and immunoferritin techniques. Am J Pathol 1973; 70:131–150.

67. Yoshizawa N, Oshima S, Sagel I, Shimizu J, Treser G. Role of a streptococcal antigen in the pathogenesis of acute poststreptococcal glomerulonephritis. Characterization of the antigen and a proposed mechanism for the disease. J Immunol 1992; 148:3110–3116.

68. Yoshizawa N, Oshima S, Takeuchi A, Kondo S, Oda T, Shimizu J, Nishiyama J, Ishida A, Nakabayashi I, Tazawa K, Sakuria Y. Experimental acute glomerulonephritis induced in the rabbit with a specific streptococcal antigen. Clin Exp Immunol 1996; 107:61–67.

69. Oite T, Batsford SR, Miatsch MJ, Takamiya H, Vogt A. Quantitative studies of in situ immune complex formation glomerulonephritis in the rat induced by planted, cationized antigen. J Exp Med 1982; 155:460–474.

70. Vogt A, Batsford S, Rodriguez-Iturbe B, Garcia R. Cationic antigen in poststreptococcal glomerulonephritis. Clin Nephrol 1983; 20:271–279.

71. Drachman R, Aladjem M, Vardy PA. Natural history of an acute glomerulonephritis epidemic in children: an 11 to 12 year follow up. J Med Sci 1986; 18:603–607.

72. Buzio C, Allegri L, Mutti A, Perazzoli F, Bergamaschi E. Significance of albuminuria in the follow-up of acute poststreptococcal glomerulonephritis. Clin Nephrol 1994; 41:259–264.

73. Baldwin DS. Chronic glomerulonephritis: nonimmunologic mechanisms of progressive glomerular damage. Kidney Int 1982; 21:109–120.

74. Kobrin S, Madaio MP. Acute poststreptococcal glomerulonephritis and other bacterial infection-related glomerulonephritides. In: Schrier RW (ed). Diseases of the Kidney, 6th ed. Philadelphia: Lippincott-Raven, 1997; 1579–1594.

10

Life-Threatening Streptococcal Infections: Scarlet Fever, Necrotizing Fasciitis, Myositis, Bacteremia, and Streptococcal Toxic Shock Syndrome

DENNIS L. STEVENS

Invasive streptococcal infections have been observed for several centuries and include the following unique clinical illnesses: puerperal sepsis, scarlatina maligna, septic scarlet fever, bacteremia, erysipelas, necrotizing fasciitis, streptococcal gangrene, and myositis. Marked attenuation in the incidence and severity of all forms of streptococcal infections have been apparent since before the turn of the century. Some would attribute the decline of serious streptococcal infection to improved socioeconomic conditions. Similarly, modern medicine has had a major impact on the prevention of rheumatic fever and puerperal sepsis. However, the mortality of certain group A streptococcal (GAS) infections such as scarlet fever declined in this continent and Europe well before antibiotics were available. Thus, the milder streptococcal infections since the turn of the century are more likely a result of reduced virulence of the streptococcus itself.

Recently, more aggressive GAS infections have been described in virtually every country of the world. The course of infection is rapid and cannot be matched by any other infectious disease. Acquisition of novel virulence factors by GAS could explain this newfound aggressiveness. Still, if the explanations were this simple, why have we not witnessed major epidemics of GAS infections due to common-source exposure? Instead we are experiencing an increased incidence of sporadic cases. Thus, if the presence of a new virulence factor alone were sufficient to induce infection, then major epidemics should have occurred. The susceptibility of the human host must vary even within regional domains and is dependent upon the presence or absence of humoral or cellular immunity against putative streptococcal virulence factors. Alternatively, predisposing factors might affect the susceptibility of the human host.

The interactions between GAS and the human host are intimate, complex, and sophisticated. For example, evidence is mounting that the organism has the ability to neutralize a variety of host defense mechanisms (see Chapter 2). Alternatively, GAS cell constituents and toxins can induce exaggerated host responses in terms of cytokine production or T cell activation (see Chapter 2). Clinically, these unique interactions lead to several presentations of invasive strepto-coccal disease, such as bacteremia, necrotizing fasciitis, myositis, and streptococcal toxic shock syndrome (TSS) [1]. The features of each of these entities will be discussed separately.

SCARLET FEVER

The mortality and morbidity of scarlet fever have declined dramatically since before the turn of the century and well before the availability of penicillin. The best descriptions of scarlet fever, therefore, are those of the 19th century physician Osler. He described three types of malignant scarlet fever: atactic, hemorrhagic, and anginose [2]. The anginose form was basically membranous exudation of the throat, with necrosis of the soft tissues of the pharynx and soft palate. Exudation could continue into the trachea, bronchi, eustachian tubes, and middle ear. He noted that in some cases, necrosis and sloughing of tissue about the tonsils was so severe that necrosis of the carotid artery occurred with fatal hemorrhage. Osler did not specify the time course of this form; Holt [3] subsequently stated that "the duration of the symptoms in fatal cases is from six to fourteen days." In the second variety, hemorrhages into the skin, hematuria, and epistaxis occurred. "Enfeebled children" were the most common group associated with this form, and death, when it occurred, was usually within the first 2–3 days of illness [2,3]. In the third form, atactic scarlet fever, children presented with the characteristics of an acute intoxication [2]. The disease began with great severity, high fever, extreme restlessness, headache, and delirium [2]. Temperatures were frequently 107°–108°F and, Osler observed, "rare cases have been observed in which the thermometer has registered even higher" [2]. Convulsions, coma, severe dyspnea, and rapid feeble pulses were the most common presentation [2]. Patients died within 24–48 h [2].

Weaver [4] combined all these definitions into the following groups: mild, moderate, toxic, and septic. Thus, benign scarlet fever could be either mild or moderate, and the fatal or malignant form of scarlet fever could be either septic or toxic. The toxic cases invariably began with a severe sore throat, marked fever (107°–108°F),

delirium, skin rash, and painful cervical lymph nodes [2]. In severe cases (similar to the malignant scarlet fever described by Osler [2] and Rotch [5]), fulminating fevers to 107°–108°F, pulses of 130–160, severe headache, delirium, convulsions, little if any skin rash, and death within 24 h were the usual findings. These cases occurred before the advent of antibiotics, antipyretics, and anticonvulsants. The septic cases were similar to those described by Wood [6] as scarlatina anginosa, and by Osler [2] as the anginose form of scarlet fever. Here, local invasion of the soft tissues of the neck were the prominent features with subsequent upper airway obstruction, otitis media with perforation, profuse mucopurulent drainage from the nose, bronchopneumonia, and death. Note that necrotizing fasciitis and myositis were not described in association with scarlet fever, the only exception being locally invasive infection of the soft tissues of the neck as a complication of pharyngitis. In modern times, scarlet fever has been of the benign form and could be described as streptococcal pharyngitis with skin rash.

NECROTIZING FASCIITIS

Necrotizing fasciitis is a deep-seated infection of the subcutaneous tissue that results in progressive destruction of fascia and fat but spares the skin itself. Historically, Pfanner [7] is credited with the first description of what he called necrotizing erysipelas. Several years later, Meleney [8] described 20 patients with hemolytic streptococcal gangrene in China, and he argued that this entity was different from erysipelas and should have a different name. These cases were probably due to group A streptococci as we now know them, though at that time they only characterized the organism as hemolytic streptococci. Still, in Meleney's series [8], 7 of 17 patients who had blood cultures had bacteremia due to the hemolytic streptococcus and the only organism grown from the site (or reported) was hemolytic streptococci. Interestingly, all age groups were affected and the mortality was 20%. Subsequently, necrotizing fasciitis has become the preferred term, since bacteria other than streptococci such as *Clostridium perfringens*, *C. septicum*, *Staphylococcus aureus*, and mixed aerobic-anaerobic bacteria can produce a similar pathologic process. Characteristically streptococcal gangrene begins at the site of trivial or inapparent trauma. Within 24 h of the initial lesion, which frequently is only mild erythema, there is aggressive development of swelling, heat, erythema, and tenderness with rapid spreading proximally and distally from the original focus [8]. During the next 24–48 h, the erythema darkens, changing from red to purple and then to blue, and blisters and bullae containing clear yellow fluid form [8]. On the fourth or fifth day the purple areas become frankly gangrenous [8]. From the seventh to tenth day, the line of demarcation of infection becomes sharply defined and the dead skin begins to separate at the margins or break in the center, revealing an extensive necrosis of the subcutaneous tissue [8]. Up until this time the patient continues to be febrile, prostration increases, and the patient becomes more emaciated [8]. In more severe cases, the process advances rapidly until several large areas of skin have become gangrenous, and the intoxication renders the patient dull, unresponsive, mentally cloudy, or even delirious. Subsequently, the patient may develop metastatic abscesses, bronchopneumonia, or lung abscess. It should be remembered that this description of hemolytic streptococcal gangrene by Meleney was in 1924, well before the advent of antibiotics [8]. In fact, he was the first to advocate aggressive "bear scratch" fasciotomy and debridement [8]. Using this approach as well as Dakan's solution irrigation, mortality rates of as low as 20% were observed [8]. In contrast, subsequent series written between the 1950 and 1980 suggest that mortality rates of greater than 50% are common, even with antibiotics and aggressive surgical debridement. The term necrotizing fasciitis encompasses a variety of etiologies including hemolytic streptococcus, *Staphylococcus aureus*, and enteric organisms, including clostridia either singly or in combination. For example, in the study by Rea and Wyrick [9], of 44 patients 19 had positive cultures for *Staphylococcus aureus*, 19 had positive cultures for hemolytic streptococcus, and 14 had cultures positive for both *Staphylococcus aureus* and hemolytic streptococcus. In that study, 80% of patients had sustained minor trauma and 20% developed infection following surgical procedures. In addi-

tion, most patients had either diabetes or peripheral vascular disease. The age was not suggested, although 18 of the 44 patients were greater than 50 years of age, and of those over age 50, the mortality rate was 63% despite antibiotics and surgery. Similarly, an additional study of necrotizing fasciitis isolated *Staphylococcus aureus* in 88% of patients, but in that series, the mortality rate was only 8.7%. Interestingly, all patients under age 30 had experienced either stab wounds, gunshot wounds, or appendectomy. Similarly, Quintiliani and Engh's study [10] of overwhelming GAS bacteremia involved seven patients undergoing orthopedic procedures who developed severe streptococcal soft tissue infections and overall, 57% died. The mean age of patients was 41 years, although this is misleading since one of the seven patients was only 2 years of age. Several patients had either peripheral vascular disease or diabetes. In Aitken et al.'s 1982 study [11], the mean age was 61 and infection developed following minor trauma. The mortality rate despite antibiotics and surgery, was 55%, although most patients had diabetes, cachexia, peripheral vascular disease, or cirrhosis or were receiving corticosteroids. If one compares these reports [8–12] with descriptions of cases of streptococcal TSS [1], several differences are apparent. Older series describe elderly patients with multiple medical problems [8–12]. Perhaps the higher mortality in subsequent series (1950–1970) despite antibiotics could be related to the presence of underlying diseases in many patients, the older age, and the association with major trauma—i.e., orthopedic procedures, gunshot wounds, stab wounds, and major intra-abdominal surgery. Recent cases have occurred in all age-groups. The unique epidemiology of streptococcal TSS is that it may attack young, healthy individuals with no underlying disease. Usually some other nonimmunologic predisposing factor may be present, such as antecedent viral illness, minor trauma, or use of nonsteroidal anti-inflammatory agents. Meleney's patients (reported from China) were also probably young, healthy individuals who sustained some minor trauma; however, the major difference between this study and later ones is the lower mortality rate in his series (20%) [8] than in recently described cases (30%–60%) [9–11]. Meleney's lower mortality rate was at a time when antibiotics were not yet available [8]. In addition, in Meleney's series, there are descriptions of necrotizing fasciitis evolving over the course of 7–10 days. Modern cases generally run their course in 3–4 days, despite appropriate antibiotic use. Another reason for the increased mortality and morbidity of necrotizing fasciitis could be the emergence of increased virulence of the streptococcus itself [1] (see Pathogenic Mechanisms and Molecular Epidemiology, below).

STREPTOCOCCAL MYOSITIS

Streptococcal myositis has been an extremely uncommon GAS infection. Adams et al. [13] documented only 21 cases that had been reported from 1900 to 1985 and Svane [14] found only 4 cases among over 20,000 autopsies. In our series of 20 patients with invasive GAS infection [1], one had myositis alone, three had myositis as well as necrotizing fasciitis, and five had necrotizing fasciitis alone. Recently, deep soft tissue infections such as necrotizing fasciitis and myositis have also been described in reports from Norway [15], Sweden [16], and Canada [17]. Although GAS can infect viable muscle via a direct penetrating injury or surgical incision, usually there is no history of such an event. Most cases develop spontaneously, or secondary to very minor blunt trauma or muscle strain, and most patients have not experienced symptomatic pharyngitis or tonsillitis [1,13–16,18,19]. Translocation of GAS must occur from the pharynx to the site of muscle injury via hematogenous spread. Severe pain may be the only presenting symptom, and early physical findings may only demonstrate swelling and erythema, although patients may rapidly develop muscle compartment syndromes [1,13–16,18–20]. In most cases, a single muscle group may be involved, however, because patients are frequently bacteremic, multiple sites of myositis can occur [1,13]. Distinguishing streptococcal myositis from spontaneous gas gangrene due to *C. perfringens* or *C. septicum* [21] may be difficult; the presence of crepitus or gas in the tissue would favor clostridial infection [19]. Distinguishing necrotizing fasciitis from myositis is easily done anatomically through surgical exploration or in-

cisional biopsy. In streptococcal cases, most patients may have evidence of both necrotizing fasciitis and myositis [1,13]. In published series, the case-fatality rate for necrotizing fasciitis is between 20% and 50%, whereas GAS myositis has a fatality rate of between 80% and 100% [1,13,14,16,18,19,21]. Aggressive surgical debridement is of extreme importance because the poor efficacy of penicillin described in human cases [1,13,14,18,19] as well as in experimental streptococcal models of myositis [22,23] (see discussion of antibiotic efficacy under Treatment, below). The term "myositis" connotes inflammation of muscle; however, in most cases of streptococcal myositis, frank necrosis is present. Thus a better term would be "myonecrosis."

BACTEREMIA

Bacteremia associated with GAS pharyngitis is uncommon and even during the course of scarlet fever occurs in only 0.3% of febrile patients [24]. Streptococcal bacteremia has been most common in the very young and elderly [25–34]. Among children, predisposing factors other than scarlet fever include burns, varicella, malignant neoplasm, immunosuppression, and age less than 2 years [25–34]. In patients with scarlet fever, the pharynx is the most common source of GAS and frequently such patients have complications such as extension of infection into the sinuses, peritonsillar tissue, or mastoids (septic scarlet fever or scarlet fever anginosa) [4,5]. In patients with burns and varicella the integument is the most common source and in the latter case bacteremia occurs later as the vesicles are crusting and drying up [24]. The least common source of bacteremia in children has been the lower respiratory tract and when it occurs, is usually associated with prior viral infections. For example, secondary bacterial pneumonia has occurred in approximately 3.0% of patients with varicella and invariably occurs in children less than 7 years of age [24]; GAS pneumonia complicating varicella in adults is rarely found, even though primary varicella pneumonia occurs commonly. Among all children with varicella, GAS bacteremia occurred in approximately 0.5% of patients [24].

In elderly patients, GAS bacteremia is invariably secondary to infections of the skin, such as cellulitis or erysipelas [25–34]. Predisposing factors for GAS sepsis in the elderly include diabetes, peripheral vascular disease, malignancy, and corticosteroid use [25–34]. Epidemics of GAS bacteremia associated with soft tissue infection among the institutionalized elderly have been reported for over 50 years [35,36]. In most series, the mean age of patients with bacteremia has been between the 5th and 6th decades of life. Not surprising, mortality rates of 35%–80% have been described in this patient population [25–34].

Group A streptococcal bacteremia in the age-group from 14 to 40 years of age has been rare in the past, with two notable exceptions [25–34]. In the mid-1900s, puerperal sepsis accounted for most bacteremia in this age-group [25]. Currently, such cases are uncommon, largely because of the epidemiologic and "infection control policies" put forth by Semmelweiss in Europe [37] and Oliver Wendell Holmes in the United States [38]. The other exception is due to modern cultural changes. Specifically, intravenous drug abuse has emerged as a leading cause of GAS bacteremia in this age group in the modern era [31,34]. In contrast, in our study of invasive GAS infection in the Rocky Mountain area there was a marked increase in the prevalence of GAS bacteremia in younger adults, yet only 10% of patients had a history of intravenous (IV) drug abuse. This finding has also been substantiated by public health officials in England [39], Norway [15], the United States [40], and Sweden [16]. Martin and Hoiby [15] have convincingly demonstrated that the prevalence of GAS bacteremia in Norway has increased in all age-groups, but the greatest increase (600%–800%) has been among adolescents and young adults [15]. Thus, the demographics of bacteremia have changed dramatically since the mid-1980s [1,15,39–41].

STREPTOCOCCAL TOXIC SHOCK SYNDROME

Recently, severe invasive GAS infections have been reported with increasing frequency predominantly from North America and Europe [1,15,16,39,40,42–48]. Such cases are particularly dramatic, because for the previous years, the frequency, severity, and complications of GAS infections had declined. In the late 1980s, reports of invasive GAS infections began to appear associated with bacteremia, deep soft-tissue infection, shock, and multiorgan failure. Since 1985 over 100 publications or abstracts have documented the appearance of aggressive streptococcal infections associated with bacteremia and shock in all age groups [1,16,42, 48–50]. Several studies suggest that the elderly are most commonly affected, but patients between the ages of 20 and 50 are also afflicted and many patients (>50%) do not have predisposing underlying diseases (reviewed in ref. [50]). This is in sharp contrast to the previous reports of GAS bacteremia in which patients were either less than 10 years of age or greater than 60 years of age and most had underlying diseases such as cancer, renal failure, leukemia, or severe burns or were receiving corticosteroids or other immunosuppressing drugs [25–34]. Regardless of age, bacteremia, severe soft tissue infection, shock, acute respiratory distress syndrome (ARDS), and renal failure are common complications of this infection and overall, 30% of patients have died despite aggressive modern treatments [1]. It is these clinical manifestations that have shaped the case definition of Streptococcal TSS depicted in Table 10.1.

Table 10.1 Streptococcal Toxic Shock Syndrome: Case Definition

1. *Isolation of group A streptococcus*
   A. From a sterile body site
   B. From a nonsterile body site

2. *Clinical signs of severity*
   A. Hypotension *and*
   B. Clinical and laboratory abnormalities (requires two or more of the following):
   Renal impairment
   Coagulopathy
   Liver abnormalities
   Acute respiratory distress syndrome
   Extensive tissue necrosis, i.e., necrotizing fasciitis
   Erythematous rash

Definite case = 1A + 2(A + B)
Probable case = 1B + 2(A + B)[a]

[a]Data from the Working Group on Severe Streptococcal Infections [21].

Acquisition of Group A Streptococcus: Portal of Entry, Colonization, and Transmission

In general, transmission of GAS from person to person is well documented and epidemics of streptococcal pharyngitis, rheumatic fever, scarlet fever, and impetigo are well described. Open wounds, burns, and lacerations may be easily contaminated from endogenous sources or exogenously from contact with others; this type of infection resulted in epidemics in the mid-1800s. In contrast, most cases of streptococcal TSS have occurred sporadically, and this likely accounts for the relatively low attack rate of severe infections, i.e., between 1 and 5 cases per 100,000 population. Why is this so? First, although the skin is both the portal of entry and the source of GAS in approximately 25% of cases of streptococcal TSS [1,51], skin carriage in normal individuals (reviewed in ref. [52]) or in patients with GAS bacteremia due to IV drug abuse [31] occurs in far less than 1% of the population. High rates of skin colonization have occurred in only unique settings, such as umbilical colonization with GAS among infants on maternity wards [53–55] and among impoverished children during epidemics of impetigo [56,57]. Asymptomatic colonization of certain mucous membranes is much more common; 5% of adult patients [58] and 20%–40% of children may have pharyngeal colonization during the winter months and particularly under crowded conditions [59]. Other mucous membrane sites are much less commonly colonized with GAS. For example, Finegold et al. [60] demonstrated that GAS could be isolated from stool samples in only 2 of 141 normal subjects. Among patients with GAS pharyngitis or rheumatic fever, the percentage of patients with positive GAS cultures increased to 20% [61]. Similarly, vaginal colonization with GAS was found in less than 1% of normal females [62], in less than 0.3% of pregnant females [63,64], and rarely in premenarcheal females [65] unless they also had GAS pharyngitis [66]. In 50% of patients with streptococcal TSS, a definite portal of entry cannot be established (Table 10.2). Based upon the information above, directly or indirectly, the source of GAS in most cases of streptococcal TSS is from indigenous flora of the pharynx.

Table 10.2 Acquisition of Group A Streptococci in Cases of Streptococcal Toxic Shock Syndrome

Portal of Entry	Cases (%)
Skin	35
Minor trauma	
Surgical procedures	
IV drug abuse	
Mucous membrane	20
Pharynx	
Vagina	
Unknown	45

Table adapted from Stevens et al. [1], with permission.

The risk of secondary cases of streptococcal TSS must be low, given the low prevalence of this disease despite a high prevalence of "virulent strains of GAS" in the population at large [66a]. Yet, clusters of GAS-invasive infections have been described in nursing homes [36,35,67], in health-care workers [68,69], and among family members [67,69]. Finally, patients may acquire GAS from hospital personnel. This was best demonstrated by Semmelwise [37] in Vienna and Holmes [38] in the United States, and even in contemporary settings such transmission is well documented [68–70].

Symptoms of Streptococcal Toxic Shock Syndrome

Pain—the most common initial symptom of streptococcal TSS—is abrupt in onset, severe [1,51], and frequently of a crescendoing nature and usually precedes tenderness or physical findings. The pain most commonly involves an extremity but may also mimic peritonitis, pelvic inflammatory disease, acute myocardial infarction, or pericarditis [1,51]. Prior to the onset of pain, 20% of patients experience an influenza-like syndrome characterized by fever, chills, myalgia, and diarrhea (Table 10.3; [1,51]). Recently, nausea and vomiting associated with fever have been observed in patients who subsequently develop streptococcal TSS (D.L. Stevens, unpublished observations).

Physical Findings of Streptococcal Toxic Shock Syndrome

Fever is the most common presenting sign, although 10% of patients may present with pro-

Table 10.3 Defining Streptococcal Toxic Shock Syndrome[a]

Symptoms

Early symptoms are vague
  Viral-like prodrome
  Severe pain and erythema of an extremity
  Mental confusion

Signs

Hypotension, systolic
  Fever >38°C
  Soft tissue swelling
  Tenderness
  Respiratory failure, rales, cyanosis, tachypnea

Laboratory features

Hematologic
  Marked left shift
  Decline in hematocrit
  Thrombocytopenia
Renal azotemia (2.5 times normal on admission) and
  hematuria
Hypocalcemia
Hypoalbuminemia
Creatinine phosphokinase elevation
Pulmonary abnormalities
  Pulmonary infiltrate on chest X-ray
  Hypoxia

---

[a]An acute, febrile illness that begins with a mild, viral-like prodrome of minor soft-tissue infection and may progress to shock, multiorgan failure, and death.

Table adapted from Stevens 1992 [1], with permission.

found hypothermia secondary to shock [1,51]. Confusion is present in 55% of patients and in some patients coma or combativeness are manifest [1,51]. Signs of soft tissue infection such as localized swelling, tenderness, pain, and erythema are often present at the time of admission, particularly when there is a cutaneous portal of entry. The appearance of violaceous bullae [71] in patients with fever and toxicity suggests deeper soft-tissue infection such as necrotizing fasciitis or myositis. In one series [51], 70% of patients required surgical debridement, fasciotomy, or amputation [51]. The remainder of these cases displayed a variety of clinical presentations such as endopthalmitis, myositis, perihepatitis, peritonitis, myocarditis, puerperal sepsis, septic arthritis, pharyngitis, and overwhelming sepsis [1,51]. Nearly 50% of patients with normal blood pressure (systolic pressure >110 mm Hg) on admission rapidly develop hypotension within the subsequent 4 h [1,51]. Massive local swelling develops rapidly at the site of necrotizing fasciitis and myositis; however, a dif-

fuse capillary leak commonly occurs in patients with streptococcal TSS, resulting in swelling of noninfected sites, such as digits and face, and in pleural and peritoneal effusions, particularly following IV fluid resuscitation.

Laboratory Test Results in Patients with Streptococcal Toxic Shock Syndrome

In the series discussed above [1,51], renal involvement was apparent in 80% of patients at the time of admission, as evidenced by the presence of hemoglobinuria and by serum creatinine values that were on average >2.5 times normal values [1,51]. Hypoalbuminemia was associated with hypocalcemia on admission and throughout the hospital course. The serum creatinine phosphokinase level was useful in detecting the presence of deeper soft-tissue infections, and when the level was elevated or rising, there was a good correlation with necrotizing fasciitis or myositis [1,51]. Although the initial complete blood count (CBC) demonstrates only mild leukocytosis, the mean percentage of immature neutrophils (including band forms, metamyelocytes, and myelocytes) can be striking and in our series reached 43% [1,51].

Clinical Course

Hypotension is apparent at the time of admission or within 4–8 h in virtually all patients (Table 10.4). In our series, 10% of patients presenting with hypotension attained normal systolic blood pressure 4–8 h after administration of antibiotics, albumin, and electrolyte solutions containing salts or dopamine. In most patients, however, shock persisted. Similarly, renal dysfunction progressed or persisted in all patients

Table 10.4 Complications of Group A Streptococcal Soft Tissue Infection

Complication	Patients (%)
Shock	95
Acute respiratory distress syndrome	55
Renal impairment	80
Irreversible	10
Reversible	70
Bacteremia	60
Mortality	30

Table adapted from [1], with permission.

for 48–72 h in spite of treatment, and several patients required dialysis for 10–20 days [1,51]. Among survivors, renal function returned to normal within 4 to 6 weeks. Renal dysfunction precedes hypotension in many cases and is apparent early in the course of shock in all others. Acute respiratory distress syndrome (ARDS) occurred in 55% of patients and generally after the onset of hypotension [1,51]. Supplemental oxygen, intubation, and mechanical ventilation was necessary in the 90% of patients who developed this syndrome [1,51]. Bacteremia occurred in 60%–70% of patients with streptococcal TSS [1,51]. Mortality rates of 30% to 60%–70% have been documented. Morbidity is also high; in our series, 13 of 20 patients required major surgical procedures, which included fasciotomy, surgical debridement, exploratory laparotomy, intraocular aspiration, amputation, or hysterectomy [1,51]. Surgical exploration documented concomitant myonecrosis in over one-half the patients with necrotizing fasciitis.

Factors Affecting Development and Progression of Streptococcal Toxic Shock Syndrome

Strains of GAS associated with streptococcal TSS are found widely in communities, yet epidemics have not materialized, suggesting that simple contact with a virulent strain is not sufficient to cause streptococcal TSS. This implies that predisposing factors or host factors may be necessary for streptococcal TSS to occur. Certain viral infections such as chicken pox can disrupt cutaneous and mucosal anatomical barriers. Similarly, influenza virus infection alters respiratory epithelium sufficiently to provide a portal of entry. These viral infections may also have significant effects on the immune system, although these have not been adequately studied. Disruption of anatomical barriers from other causes such as lacerations, burns, slivers, surgical procedures, decubitus ulcers, IV drug abuse, and bites (insects, dogs, cats, etc.) provides cutaneous portals of entry. Childbirth, another risk factor, compromises the integrity of the uterine mucosal barrier, allowing entry of GAS into this normally sterile site. The source of bacteria in this setting is usually GAS colonizing the vagina (rare); introduction of GAS into the birth canal

from hospital sources [70] has been well described for nearly 150 years.

In nearly 50% of patients with documented GAS bacteremia, a portal of entry such as one described above cannot be ascertained [1,51,52], and in some series, 50% of patients have cryptogenic bacteremia [52]. Since the 1980s these cases have frequently been associated with deep-seated infection such as necrotizing fasciitis and myositis [1,51,13]. In these instances, a clinical diagnosis may be difficult to establish until late in the course of the disease. In fact, a diagnosis of GAS bacteremia or necrotizing fasciitis may not be entertained until shock and organ failure develop. In these cases, other predisposing factors are probably required. For example, these deep soft-tissue infections invariably occur at the exact site of blunt trauma, muscle strain, hematoma, or joint effusion. These observations raise two important questions. First, how does nonpenetrating local trauma predispose an area to development of infection at that exact site? Second, in the absence of a penetrating injury, how does GAS arrive at the site of infection? The most plausible hypothesis is that GAS translocates to the site of injury, probably through a transient bacteremia from a mucous membrane, i.e., a pharyngeal source, and the site of injury somehow favors bacterial growth at the expense of clearance by professional phagocytes. Increasingly severe pain develops within the tissue and precedes any of the other cardinal manifestations of inflammation. At this point in time, many patients subject themselves to an additional risk factor: the patient begins to take pain killers such as nonsteroidal anti-inflammatory agents (NSAIDs). These agents adversely affect chemotaxis, phagocytosis, and bacterial killing. Although symptoms improve transiently, and fever (if any) is suppressed, the GAS infection progresses. A diagnosis may be difficult at this time because the infection is deep in muscle or fascia and there may not be evidence of cellulitis, lymphangitis, or erysipelas. In fact, there may be no redness or swelling, even though tenderness is generally present. The physician is frequently quite puzzled and concludes that musculoskeletal pain or perhaps deep vein thrombophlebitis is causative. The NSAIDs may again be given for treatment of symptoms. Invariably, within 24 h the patient returns with fever, rigors, hypotension, massive swelling of the affected area, and evidence of cellulitis with or without the tell-tale sign of necrotizing fasciitis—purple bullae. The NSAIDs may directly contribute to shock by augmenting tumor necrosis factor (TNF) production [72]. The diagnosis is quite obvious at that point; however, the mortality and morbidity, despite modern medicine, is severe. Thus, in situations where there is not an obvious portal of entry, it is difficult to have a high index of suspicion of GAS infection since nonpenetrating trauma to an extremity is very common, particularly in young, healthy individuals who are physically active.

Clinical Clues, Differential Diagnosis, and Diagnostic Considerations

Patients with streptococcal TSS most commonly present with community-acquired deep-seated infection such as necrotizing fasciitis or shock. Thus, this section will discuss the differential diagnosis of each of these entities.

The abrupt onset of shock in a previously healthy individual has a limited number of causes. In addition to streptococcal TSS, staphylococcal TSS must be considered, particularly in a female during menstruation, or in either sex in association with recent surgery or any localized staphylococcal abscess. Gram-negative sepsis can mimic streptococcal TSS, yet it is uncommon in nonhospitalized, non-neutropenic patients. The exception is typhoid fever, which certainly attacks normal individuals. Sporadic cases of bacteremia due to salmonella do occur in association with food-borne illnesses, but typhoid fever is usually related to natural disasters such as hurricanes, floods, and earthquakes. Renal impairment frequently precedes hypotension in streptococcal TSS, whereas in gram-negative shock, renal failure (acute tubular necrosis) develops only after hypotension. Similarly, the white blood count is generally normal or elevated with a marked left shift in streptococcal TSS, whereas in gram-negative shock, typhoid fever in particular, the white blood count is usually low. Rocky Mountain spotted fever (RMSF) must be distinguished from streptococcal TSS because both cause shock in otherwise healthy individuals. In RMSF, the rash is most commonly petechial, whereas in streptococcal TSS

it is diffusely erythematous. Rash is present in most patients with RMSF, whereas in streptococcal TSS rash is present in only 10%. If rash is not present, distinguishing between these two etiologies is difficult. Meningococcemia could be confused with streptococcal TSS, although the rash resembles RMSF. Meningitis, though common in meningococcemia, is uncommon in streptococcal TSS. Some cases of streptococcal TSS have respiratory symptoms and on presentation to the hospital have lobar consolidation and empyema. When such patients present with shock, it may be difficult to distinguish them from those with overwhelming *Streptococcus pneumoniae* sepsis. Heat stroke has been confused with some cases of streptococcal TSS largely because of the presence of elevated temperature, dehydration with evidence of renal impairment, confusion, and hypotension.

The differential diagnosis of deep soft-tissue infection with or without shock includes the following clinical entities. Acute hemorrhage in the form of a retroperitoneal, intra-abdominal, or deep soft-tissue bleed can result in increasing pain at the site of previous injury or surgery, and if blood loss is massive, hypotension can result. The absence of fever and a normal white blood count and differential would weigh against a diagnosis of streptococcal TSS. In cases where necrotizing fasciitis develops following a penetrating injury, progression of the cutaneous infection to necrotizing fasciitis is more obvious. In situations where necrotizing fasciitis develops in the deep tissue following nonpenetrating trauma, there may be no cutaneous signs of infection until late in the course of disease when violaceous bullae may appear. Thus, in these cases, increasing pain at the site of injury, fever, marked left shift, and elevated creatine phosphokinase (CPK) may be clues to the diagnosis of streptococcal TSS. At this stage the symptoms are frequently attributed to a putative thrombophlebitis secondary to prior trauma. Venograms are invariably normal and soft tissue radiograms and computed tomography (CT) scan results usually demonstrate diffuse soft-tissue swelling, moderate fluid accumulation in the muscle compartments, no abscess formation, and no gas. Frequently, the interpretation is "results compatible with prior muscle injury, hematoma or deep vein thrombophlebitis." In the setting of chills, fever, and marked left shift, such an interpretation is inappropriate and frequently delays surgical exploration. In contrast, necrotizing fasciitis and myonecrosis caused by mixed aerobic-anaerobic bacteria or *Clostridium* species are associated with gas in the tissues, and thus soft tissue radiograms are of more value. Magnetic resonance imaging (MRI) and CT scans may be useful to localize the site of infection, but they do not provide the specificity that is clinically useful.

Once the site of deep soft-tissue infection has been localized either by clinical clues or radiographic techniques, surgical intervention is not only useful for diagnostic purposes but of major therapeutic importance. The decision to surgically explore a patient is easy when there is cutaneous evidence of an infectious process, severe localized pain, and the patient is either not responding to medical management or is clinically deteriorating. It is more difficult to suspect necrotizing fasciitis in a patient with only increasing pain and fever and no cutaneous evidence of infection. Since about 50% of patients with streptococcal TSS have deep-seated soft tissue infections and only about 50% have obvious portals of entry, the aforementioned presentation is quite common. The physician's job gets even more difficult when patients are taking NSAIDs, aspirin, or Tylenol, since these agents reduce pain and suppress fever. In some cases, the rapid onset of shock and organ failure may preclude surgical intervention.

Pathogenic Mechanisms and Molecular Epidemiology

Pyrogenic exotoxins induce fever in humans and animals and also participate in shock by lowering the threshold to exogenous endotoxin [51] (see also Chapter 4). Streptococcal pyrogenic exotoxin A (SPE A) and SPE B induce human mononuclear cells to synthesize not only tumor necrosis factor α (TNF-α) [73] but also interleukin-1β (IL-1β) [74] and IL-6 [74–76], which suggests that TNF could mediate the fever, shock, and tissue injury observed in patients with streptococcal TSS [1]. Pyrogenic exotoxin C has been associated with mild cases of scarlet fever in the United States (D.L. Stevens, unpublished observations) and in England [77]. The roles of two newly described pyrogenic exotoxins, strep-

tococcal superantigen (SSA) [78] and mitogenic factor (MF) [79] (See Chapters 2 and 4) in streptococcal TSS have not been elucidated.

M protein contributes to invasiveness through its ability to impede phagocytosis of streptococci by human polymorphonuclear leukocytes (PMNL) [80]. Conversely, type-specific antibody against the M protein enhances phagocytosis [80]. Following infection with a particular M type, specific antibody confers resistance to challenge to viable GAS of that M type [80]. While M type 1 and 3 strains have accounted for the vast majority of strains isolated from cases of streptococcal TSS, many other M types, including some nontypeable strains, have also been isolated from such cases. M types 1 and 3 are also commonly isolated from asymptomatic carriers, patients with pharyngitis, and mild scarlet fever [81,82].

Could streptococcal TSS be related to the ability of SPE A or M protein type 1 or 3 to act as "super antigens?" [83] There are data to suggest that SPE A and a number of staphylococcal toxins (TSST-1 and staphylococcal enterotoxins A, B, and C) can stimulate T cell responses through their ability to bind to both the class II MHC complex of antigen-presenting cells and the Vβ region of the T cell receptor [83]. The net effect would be to induce T cell stimulation with production of cytokines capable of mediating shock and tissue injury. Hackett and Stevens demonstrated that SPE A induced both TNF-α and TNF-β from mixed cultures of monocytes and lymphocytes [84], supporting the role of lymphokines (TNF-β) in shock associated with strains producing SPE A. Kotb et al. [85] have shown that a digest of M protein type 6 can also stimulate T cell responses by this mechanism; however, the role of specific superantigens in this or any other infectious disease has not been proven. Proof would require demonstration of massive expansion of T cell subsets bearing Vβ repertoire specific for the putative superantigen. However, quantitation of such T cell subsets in patients with acute streptococcal TSS demonstrated deletion rather than expansion, suggesting that perhaps the life span of the expanded subset was shortened by a process of apoptosis [86]. In addition, the subsets deleted were not specific for SPE A, SPE B, SPE C, or MF, suggesting that perhaps an as-yet undefined superantigen may play a role [86].

Cytokine production by less exotic mechanisms may also contribute to the genesis of shock and organ failure. Peptidoglycan, lipoteichoic acid [87], and killed organisms [88,89] are capable of inducing TNF-α production by mononuclear cells in vitro [51,89,90]. Exotoxins such as streptolysin O (SLO) are also potent inducers of TNF-α and IL-1β. SPE B, a proteinase precursor, has the ability to cleave pre-IL-1β to release IL-1β [91]. Finally, SLO and SPE A together have additive effects in the induction of IL-1β by human mononuclear cells [84]. Whatever the mechanisms, induction of cytokines in vivo is likely the cause of shock, and SLO, SPE A, SPE B, and SPE C as well as cell-wall components, etc. are potent inducers of TNF and IL-1 [92]. Finally, a cysteine protease formed from cleavage of SPE B may play an important role in pathogenesis by the release of bradykinin from endogenous kininogen and by activating metalloproteases involved in coagulation [93]. Boyle and Raeder have shown that GAS protease cleaves the terminal portion of the M protein, rendering the organism more susceptible to phagocytosis by normal serum but resistant to phagocytosis in the presence of type-specific antibody [94].

The mere presence of virulence factors, such as M protein or pyrogenic exotoxins, may be less important in streptococcal TSS than the dynamics of their production in vivo. For example, Chaussee et al. [92] have demonstrated that among strains from patients with necrotizing fasciitis and streptococcal TSS, ~40% and ~75% produced SPE A or SPE B, respectively. In addition, the quantity of SPE A but not SPE B was higher for strains from streptococcal TSS patients than from noninvasive cases [92]. Cleary et al. have proposed a regulon in GAS that controls the expression of a group of genes coding for virulence factors such as M protein and C5-peptidase [95] (see Chapter 3). Using DNA fingerprinting, differences were shown in M-1 strains isolated from patients with invasive disease compared to M-1 strains from patients with noninvasive GAS infections [96]. Finally, strains of GAS may acquire genetic information coding for SPE A or SPE C via specific bacteriophage, and following lysogenic conversion, pyrogenic exotoxins are synthesized synchronously with growth of the streptococcus [97–99]. Multilocus enzyme electrophoresis demonstrates two patterns that correspond to M-1 and M-3 type organisms that produce pyrogenic exotoxin A, a finding that fits epidemiologic studies implicating these strains in invasive GAS infections [100] in the United States. There are currently little data that quantify the dynamics of pyrogenic exotoxin production in vivo.

The interaction between these microbial virulence factors and an immune or nonimmune host determines the epidemiology, clinical syndrome, and outcome. Since horizontal transmission of invasive strains of GAS in general is well documented, a major explanation for the low attack rate of invasive infection in the population is the presence of significant herd immunity against one or more of the virulence factors responsible for streptococcal TSS. This model explains (1) why epidemics have not materialized and (2) why a particular strain of GAS can cause different clinical manifestations in the same community [101].

TREATMENT

Antibiotic Therapy: Importance of the Mechanism of Action

Streptococcus pyogenes remains exquisitely susceptible to β-lactam antibiotics, and numerous studies have demonstrated the clinical efficacy of penicillin preparations for treating erysipelas, impetigo, and cellulitis. In addition, Wannamaker et al. [102] demonstrated that penicillin therapy prevented the development of rheumatic fever following streptococcal pharyngitis if therapy was begun within 8 to 10 days of the onset of sore throat. Nonetheless, clinical failures of penicillin treatment of streptococcal infection do occur. In addition, penicillin fails to eradicate bacteria from the pharynx of patients with documented streptococcal pharyngitis in 5%–20% of patients [41,103,104]. Finally, more aggressive GAS infections (such as necrotizing fasciitis, empyema, burn wound sepsis, subcutaneous gangrene, and myositis) respond less well to penicillin and continue to be associated with high mortality and extensive morbidity [1,13,15,45,49,51,105]. For example, a recent report of 25 cases of streptococcal myositis reported an overall mortality of 85% despite penicillin therapy [13]. Studies in experimental infection have demonstrated that penicillin fails when large numbers of organisms are present [22,23]. For example, in a mouse model of myositis due to *Streptococcus pyogenes*, penicillin was ineffective when treatment was delayed ≥2 h after initiation of infection [23]. Survival of erythromycin-treated mice was greater than that of both penicillin-treated mice and untreated controls, but only if treatment was begun within 2 h. Mice receiving clindamycin, however, had survival rates of 100%, 100%, 80%, and 70% when treatment was delayed 0, 2, 6, and 16.5 h, respectively [23,106].

Eagle suggested that penicillin failed in this type of infection because of the "physiologic state of the organism" [22]. This phenomenon has recently been attributed to both in vitro and in vivo inoculum effects [107,108]. It has also been observed that penicillin and other β-lactam antibodies are most efficacious against rapidly growing bacteria. In vivo, early in the stages of infection or in mild infections, organisms are growing rapidly but are present in rather small numbers. With delays in treatment, higher concentrations of GAS accumulate and growth begins to slow to a stationary phase. That high concentration of *Streptococcus pyogenes* accumulate in deep-seated infection is supported by data from Eagle et al. [22]. Why should penicillin lose its efficacy when large numbers of group A streptococci are present or when they are making the transition from logarithmic growth to stationary? Since penicillin mediates its antibacterial action against GAS by intimately interacting with the expressed penicillin binding proteins, we compared the penicillin-binding protein (PBP) patterns from membrane proteins of group A streptococci isolated from different stages of growth, i.e., mid-log phase and stationary phase. Binding of radiolabeled penicillin by all PBPs was decreased in stationary cells. In fact, PBPs 1 and 4 were undetectable at 36 h [107]. Thus, the loss of certain PBPs during stationary-phase growth in vitro may be responsible for the inoculum effect observed *in vivo* and may account for the failure of penicillin in both experimental and human cases of severe streptococcal infection.

The greater efficacy of clindamycin in severe GAS infections is due to many factors. First, its efficacy is not affected by inoculum size or stage of growth [107,109]. Secondly, clindamycin suppresses bacterial toxin synthesis [110,111]. Third, clindamycin facilitates phagocytosis of *Streptococcus pyogenes* by inhibiting M protein synthesis [111]. Fourth, clindamycin suppresses synthesis of PBPs which, in addition to being targets for penicillin, are also enzymes involved in cell-wall synthesis and degradation [109]. Fifth, clindamycin has a longer postantibiotic effect than β-lactams such as penicillin. Lastly, we have recently shown that clindamycin suppresses liposaccharide (LPS)-induced monocyte synthesis of TNF-α [112]. Thus, clindamycin's efficacy may also be related to its ability to modulate the immune response to GAS infection.

Other Treatment Measures

Although antibiotic selection is critically important, other measures such as prompt and aggressive exploration and debridement of suspected deep-seated *Streptococcus pyogenes* infection is mandatory. It is critically important that our surgical colleagues be involved early in such cases, since later in the course of treatment surgical intervention may be impossible due to toxicity or because infection has extended to vital areas that are impossible to debride (i.e., the head and neck, thorax, or abdomen). Frequently patients have fever, excruciating pain, and systemic toxicity. Yet definite cutaneous evidence of necrotizing fasciitis and myositis may appear quite late. Therefore, prompt surgical exploration through a small incision with visualization of muscle and fascia, and timely Gram stain of surgically obtained material may provide an early and definitive etiologic diagnosis [20]. Anecdotal reports suggest that hyperbaric oxygen may be helpful; however, no controlled studies are underway, nor is it clear if this treatment is useful.

Because of intractable hypotension and diffuse capillary leak, massive amounts of intravenous fluids (10–20 liters/day) are often necessary and about 10% of patients have significant clinical improvement. Pressors such as dopamine are used frequently, although no controlled trials have been performed for streptococcal TSS. In patients with intractable hypotension, vasoconstrictors such as epinephrine have been used, but symmetrical gangrene of digits seems to result frequently (D.L. Stevens, unpublished observations), often with loss of limb. In these cases it is difficult to determine if symmetrical gangrene is due to pressors or infection or both.

Neutralization of circulating toxins would be a desirable therapeutic modality, yet appropriate antibodies are not commercially available in the United States or Europe. Commercial intravenous gamma globulin has been reported to be useful for treating streptococcal TSS in two case reports and one nonrandomized clinical trial [113–115] (see also Chapter 2 for further discussion of IVIG). Because numerous streptococcal factors induce cytokines, strategies to inhibit their effects may provide useful treatments. Recently, a monoclonal antibody against TNF-α showed promising efficacy in a baboon model of streptococcal TSS [116].

In summary, if a wild, "flesh-eating strain" has recently emerged, then a major epidemic with a high attack rate would be expected. Clearly, epidemics of streptococcal infections, including impetigo, pharyngitis, scarlet fever, and rheumatic fever, have occurred in the past. In the last decade subsequent to early reports of streptococcal TSS, we can conclude that the incidence has remained relatively low. Large outbreaks of streptococcal TSS have not occurred because (1) the vast majority of the population probably has immunity to one or more streptococcal virulence factors [51,117]; (2) predisposing conditions (varicella, use of NSAIDs, etc.) are required in a given patient [72]; and (3) there may be only a small percentage of the population having an inherent predisposition to severe streptococcal infection by virtue of constitutional factors such as HLA class II antigen type [118,119], B cell allogantigens [120], or specific Vβ regions on lymphocytes. This hypothesis is further supported by the observation that secondary cases of streptococcal TSS, though reported [67], have been rare.

REFERENCES

1. Stevens DL, Tanner MH, Winship J, Swarts R, Reis KM, Schlievert PM, Kaplan E. Reappearance of scarlet fever toxin A among streptococci in the Rocky Mountain West: severe group A streptococcal infections associated with a toxic shock–like syndrome. N Engl J Med 1989; 321(1):1–7.

2. Osler W. Practice of Medicine, 2nd ed. New York: Appleton, 1895.

3. Holt LE. Scarlet fever. In: Holt LE (ed). The Diseases of Infancy and Childhood. New York: Appleton, 1897; 888–910.

4. Weaver GH. Scarlet fever. In: Abt IA (ed). Pediatrics. Philadelphia: W.B. Saunders, 1925; 298–362.

5. Rotch TM. Pediatrics: The Hygienic and Medical Treatment of Children. Philadelphia: J.B. Lippincott, 1896.

6. Wood GB. A Treatise on the Practice of Medicine, 5th ed. Philadelphia: J.B. Lippincott, 1858.

7. Pfanner W. Zur Kenntnis und Behandlung des nekrotisierenden Erysipels. Dtsch Z Chir 1918; 144:108.

8. Meleney FL. Hemolytic streptococcus gangrene. Arch Surg 1924; 9:317–364.

9. Rea WJ, Wyrick WJ Jr. Necrotizing fasciitis. Ann Surg 1970; 172:957–964.

10. Quintiliani R, Engh GA. Overwhelming sepsis associated with group A beta hemolytic streptococci. J Bone Joint Surg Am 1971; 53:1391–1399.

11. Aitken DR, Mackett MCT, Smith LL. The changing pattern of hemolytic streptococcal gangrene. Arch Surg 1982; 117:561–567.

12. Wilson B. Necrotizing fasciitis. Am Surg 1952; 18:416–431.

13. Adams EM, Gudmundsson S, Yocum DE, Haselby RC, Craig WA, Sundstrom WR. Streptococcal myositis. Arch Intern Med 1985; 145:1020–1023.

14. Svane S. Peracute spontaneous streptococcal myositis. A report on 2 fatal cases with review of literature. Acta Chir Scand 1971; 137:155–163.

15. Martin PR, Hoiby EA. Streptococcal serogroup A epidemic in Norway 1987–1988. Scand J Infect Dis 1990; 22:421–429.

16. Holm SE, Norrby A, Bergholm AM, Norgren M. Aspects of pathogenesis of serious group A streptococcal infections in Sweden, 1988–1989. J Infect Dis 1992; 166:31–37.

17. Demers B, Simor AE, Vellend H, Schlievert PM, Byrne S, Jamieson F, Walmsley S, Low DE. Severe invasive group A streptococcal infections in Ontario, Canada: 1987–1991. Clin Infect Dis 1993; 16:792–800.

18. Nather A, Wong FY, Balasubramaniam P, Pang M. Streptococcal necrotizing myositis—a rare entity: a report of two cases. Clin Orthop 1987; 215:206–211.

19. Yoder EL, Mendez J, Khatib R. Spontaneous gangrenous myositis induced by Streptococcus pyogenes: case report and review of the literature. Rev Infect Dis 1987; 9:382–385.

20. Bisno AL, Stevens DL. Streptococcal infections in skin and soft tissues. N Engl J Med 1996; 334:240–245.

21. Stevens DL, Musher DM, Watson DA, Eddy H, Hamill RJ, Gyorkey F, Rosen H, Mader J. Spontaneous, nontraumatic gangrene due to *Clostridium septicum*. Rev Infect Dis 1990; 12:286–296.
22. Eagle H. Experimental approach to the problem of treatment failure with penicillin. I. group A streptococcal infection in mice. Am J Med 1952; 13:389–399.
23. Stevens DL, Bryant-Gibbons AE, Bergstrom R, Winn V. The Eagle effect revisited: efficacy of clindamycin, erythromycin, and penicillin in the treatment of streptococcal myositis. J Infect Dis 1988; 158:23–28.
24. Bullowa JGM, Wishik SM. Complications of varicella I. Their occurrence among 2,534 patients. Am J Dis Child 1935; 49:923–926.
25. Keefer CS, Ingelfinger FJ, Spink WW. Significance of hemolytic streptococcic bacteremia; a study of two hundred and forty-six patients. Arch Intern Med 1937; 60:1084–1097.
26. Duma RJ, Weinberg AN, Medrek TF, Kunz LJ. A bacteriologic and clinical study of streptococcal bacteremia. In: Anonymous Streptococcal Infections, 48th ed. Baltimore: Williams & Wilkins, 1969; 87–127.
27. Ispahani P, Donald FE, Aveline AJ. *Streptococcus pyogenes* bacteremia: an old enemy subdued, but not defeated. J Infect 1988; 16:37–46.
28. Henkel JS, Armstrong D, Blevins A, Moody MD. Group A beta-hemolytic streptococcus bacteremia in a cancer hospital. JAMA 1970; 211:983–986.
29. Hable KA, Horstmeier C, Wold AD, Washington JA. Group A beta-hemolytic streptococcemia. Bacteriological and clinical study of 44 cases. Mayo Clin Proc 1973; 48:336–339.
30. Trence DL, Khan MY, Gerding DN. Beta hemolytic streptococcal bacteremia in adults: association with cold weather in Minnesota. Minn Med 1981; 64:657–679.
31. Barg NL, Kish MA, Kauffman CA, Supena RB. Group A streptococcal bacteremia in intravenous drug abusers. Am J Med 1985; 78:569–574.
32. Francis J, Warren RE. *Streptococcus pyogenes* bacteraemia in Cambridge—A review of 67 episodes. Q J Med 1988; 256:603–613.
33. Barnham M. Invasive streptococcal infections in the era before the acquired immune deficiency syndrome: a 10 years' compilation of patients with streptococcal bacteraemia in North Yorkshire. J Infect 1989; 18:231–248.
34. Braunstein H. Characteristics of group A streptococcal bacteremia in patients at the San Bernardino County Medical Center. Rev Infect Dis 1991; 13:8–11.
35. Auerbach SB, Schwartz B, Facklam RR, Breiman R, Jarvis WR. Outbreak of invasive group A streptococcal (GAS) disease in a nursing home. In: Programs & Abstracts of the Interscience Conference on Antimicrobial Agents and Chemotherapy, Atlanta, GA. Washington, D.C.: American Society for Microbiology, Abstract #508.1990.
36. Hohenboken JJ, Anderson F, Kaplan EL. Invasive group A streptococcal (GAS) serotype M-1 outbreak in a long-term care facility (LTCF) with mortality. In: Program & Abstracts of the Interscience Conference on Antimicrobial Agents and Chemotherapy, Orlando, FL. Abstract# J189.1994.
37. Carter KC, Carter BR. Childbed Fever: A Scientific Biography of Ignaz Semmelweis. Westport, CT: Greenwood Press, 1994.
38. Holmes OW. In: Holmes OW (ed). Medical Essays 1842–1882: The writings of Oliver Wendell Holmes. Boston: Houghton, Mifflin, 1891.
39. Gaworzewska E, Colman G. Changes in the patterns of infection caused by *Streptococcus pyogenes*. Epidemiol Infect 1988; 100:257–269.
40. Schwartz B, Facklam RR, Brieman RF. Changing epidemiology of group A streptococcal infection in the USA. Lancet 1990; 336:1167–1171.
41. Gatanaduy AS, Kaplan EL, Huwe BB, McKay C, Wannamaker LW. Failure of penicillin to eradicate group A streptococci during an outbreak of pharyngitis. Lancet 1980; 2:498–502.
42. Wheeler MC, Roe MH, Kaplan EL, Schlievert PM, Todd JK. Outbreak of group A streptococcus septicemia in children. Clinical, epidemiologic, and microbiological correlates. JAMA 1991; 266:533–537.
43. Bartter T, Dascal A, Carroll K, Curley FJ. "Toxic strep syndrome": manifestation of group A streptococcal infection. Arch Intern Med 1988; 148:1421–1424.
44. Cone LA, Woodard DR, Schlievert PM, Tomory GS. Clinical and bacteriologic observations of a toxic shock-like syndrome due to *Streptococcus pyogenes*. N Engl J Med 1987; 317:146–149.
45. Hribalova V. *Streptococcus pyogenes* and the toxic shock syndrome. Ann Intern Med 1988; 108:772.
46. Greenberg RN, Willoughby BG, Kennedy DJ, Otto TJ, McMillian R, Bloomster TG. Hypocalcemia and "toxic" syndrome associated with streptococcal fasciitis. South Med J 1983; 76:916–918.
47. Jackson H, Cooper J, Mellinger WJ, Olsen AR. Group A β-hemolytic streptococcal pharyngitis—results of treatment with lincomycin. JAMA 1965; 194:1189–1192.
48. Thomas JC, Carr SJ, Fujioka K, Waterman SH. Community-acquired group A streptococcal deaths in Los Angeles county. J Infect Dis 1989; 160:1086–1087.
49. Kohler W. Streptococcal toxic shock syndrome. Zentralbl Bakteriol 1990; 272:257–264.
50. Stevens DL. Streptococcal toxic shock syn-

drome: spectrum of disease, pathogenesis and new concepts in treatment. Emerg Infect Dis 1995; 1:69–78.

51. Stevens DL. Invasive group A streptococcus infections. Clin Infect Dis 1992; 14:2–13.

52. Bibler MR, Rouan GW. Cryptogenic group A streptococcal bacteremia: experience at an urban general hospital and review of the literature. Rev Infect Dis 1986; 8:941–951.

53. Boissard JM, Eton B. Neonatal umbilicus as a source of streptococcal infections in a maternity unit. BMJ 1956; 2:574–576.

54. Kwantes W, James JRE. Haemolytic streptococci on the neonatal umbilicus. BMJ 1956; 2:576–578.

55. Berg U, Bygdeman S, Henningsson A, Nystrom B, Tunnell R. An outbreak of group A streptococcal infection in a maternity unit. J Hosp Infect 1982; 3:333–339.

56. Dudding BA, Burnett JW, Chapman SS, Wannamaker LW. The role of normal skin in the spread of streptococcal pyoderma. J Hyg (Camb) 1970; 68:19–28.

57. Ferrieri P, Dajani AS, Wannamaker LW, Chapman SS. Natural history of impetigo. 1. Site sequence of acquisition and familial patterns of spread of cutaneous streptococci. J Clin Invest 1972; 51:2851–2862.

58. Commission on Acute Respiratory Diseases. The role of Lancefield groups of beta-hemolytic streptococci in respiratory infections. N Engl J Med 1947; 236:157–166.

59. Cornfield D, Hubbard JP. A four-year study of the occurrence of beta-hemolytic streptococci in 64 school children. N Engl J Med 1961; 264:211–215.

60. Finegold SM, Sutter VL, Mathisen GE. Normal indigenous intestinal flora. In: Hentges DJ (ed). Human Intestinal Microflora in Health and Disease. New York: Academic Press, 1983; 3–31.

61. Hare R, Maxted WR. The classification of hemolytic streptococci from the stools of normal pregnant women and of cases of scarlet fever by means of precipitin and biochemical tests. J Pathol Bacteriol 1935; 41:513–520.

62. Sweet RL, Gibbs RS. Clinical microbiology of the female genital tract. In: Sweet RL, Gibbs RS (eds). Infectious Diseases of the Female Genital Tract, 2nd ed. Baltimore: Williams & Wilkins, 1990; 2–10.

63. Beargie R, Lynd P, Tucker E, Duhring J. Perinatal infection and vaginal flora. Am J Obstet Gynecol 1975; 122:31–33.

64. Lancefield RC, Hare R. The serological differentiation of pathogenic and non-pathogenic strains of hemolytic streptococci from parturient women. J Exp Med 1935; 61:335–349.

65. Heller RH, Joseph JM, Davis HJ. Vulvovaginitis in the premenarcheal child. J Pediatr 1969; 74:370–377.

66. Hedlund P. Acute vulvovaginitis in streptococcal infections. Acta Paediatr Scand 1953; 42:388–389.

66a. Cockerill FR, MacDonald KL, Thompson RL, Roberson F, Kohner PC, Besser-Wiek J, Manahan JM, Musser JM, Schlievert PM, Talbot J, Frankfort B, Steckelberg JM, Wilson WR, Osterholm MT. An outbreak of invasive Group A streptococcal disease associated with high carriage rates of the invasive clone among school-aged children. JAMA 1997; 277:38–43.

67. Schwartz B, Elliot JA, Butler JC, Simon PA, Jameson BL, Welch GE, Facklam RR. Clusters of invasive group A streptococcal infections in family, hospital, and nursing home settings. Clin Infect Dis 1992; 15:277–284.

68. Valenzuela TD, Hooton TM, Kaplan EL, Schlievert PM. Transmission of 'toxic strep' syndrome from an infected child to a firefighter during CPR. Ann Emerg Med 1991; 20:1:123–125.

69. Dipersio JR, Define LA, Gardner W, Stevens DL, Kaplan EL, File TM. Use of pulsed field gel electrophoresis to investigate the clonal spread of severe Gp A streptococcal disease. In: Program & Abstracts of the American Society for Microbiology, Washington, DC. Washington, DC: American Society for Microbiology, 1995, Abstract C189.

70. Stamm WE, Feeley JC, Facklam RR. Wound infections due to group A streptococcus traced to a vaginal carrier. J Infect Dis 1978; 138:287–292.

71. Stevens DL. Streptococcal infections of skin and soft tissues. In: Stevens DL, Mandell GL (eds). Atlas of Infectious Diseases. New York: Churchill Livingstone, 1995; 3.1–3.11.

72. Stevens DL. Could nonsteroidal anti-inflammatory drugs (NSAIDs) enhance the progression of bacterial infections to toxic shock syndrome? Clin Infect Dis 1995; 21:977–980.

73. Fast DJ, Schlievert PM, Nelson RD. Toxic shock syndrome–associated staphylococcal and streptococcal pyrogenic toxins are potent inducers of tumor necrosis factor production. Infect Immun 1989; 57:291–294.

74. Hackett SP, Schlievert PM, Stevens DL. Cytokine production by human mononuclear cells in response to streptococcal exotoxins. Clin Res 1991; 39:189A.

75. Norrby-Teglund A, Norgren M, Holm SE, Andersson U, Andersson J. Similar cytokine induction profiles of a novel streptococcal exotoxin, MF, and pyrogenic exotoxins A and B. Infect Immun 1994; 62:3731–3738.

76. Muller-Alouf H, Alouf JE, Gerlach D, Fitting C, Cavaillon JM. Cytokine production by murine cells activated by erythrogenic toxin type A superantigen of *Streptococcus pyogenes*. Immunobiology 1992; 186:435–448.

77. Hallas G. The production of pyrogenic exotox-

ins by group A streptococci. J Hyg (Camb) 1985; 95:47–57.

78. Mollick JA, Miller GG, Musser JM, Cook RG, Grossman D, Rich RR. A novel superantigen isolated from pathogenic strains of *Streptococcus pyogenes* with aminoterminal homology to staphylococcal enterotoxins B and C. J Clin Invest 1993; 92:710–719.

79. Norrby-Teglund A, Newton D, Kotb M, Holm SE, Norgren M. Superantigenic properties of the group A streptococcal exotoxin SpeF (MF). Infect Immun 1994; 62:5227–5233.

80. Lancefield RC. Current knowledge of type specific M antigens of group A streptococci. J Immunol 1962; 89:307–313.

81. Johnson DR, Stevens DL, Kaplan EL. Epidemiologic analysis of group A streptococcal serotypes associated with severe systemic infections, rheumatic fever, or uncomplicated pharyngitis. J Infect Dis 1992; 166:374–382.

82. Kohler W, Gerlach D, Knoll H. Streptococcal outbreaks and erythrogenic toxin type A. Zentralbl Bakteriol Mikrobiol Hyg 1987; 266:104–115.

83. Mollick JA, Rich RR. Characterization of a superantigen from a pathogenic strain of *Streptococcus pyogenes*. Clin Res 1991; 39:213A.

84. Hackett SP, Stevens DL. Streptococcal toxic shock syndrome: synthesis of tumor necrosis factor and interleukin-1 by monocytes stimulated with pyrogenic exotoxin A and streptolysin O. J Infect Dis 1992; 165:879–885.

85. Kotb M, Ohnishi H, Majumdar G, Hackett S, Bryant A, Higgins G, Stevens D. Temporal relationship of cytokine release by peripheral blood mononuclear cells stimulated by the streptococcal superantigen pep M5. Infect Immun 1993; 61:1194–1201.

86. Watanabe-Ohnishi R, Low DE, McGeer A, Stevens DL, Schlievert D, Newton B, Schwartz B, Kreiswirth B. Selective depletion of Vβ-bearing T cells in patients with severe invasive group A streptococcal infections and streptococcal toxic shock syndrome. J Infect Dis 1995; 171:74–84.

87. Stevens DL, Bryant AE, Hackett SP. Gram-positive shock. Curr Opin Infect Dis 1992; 5:355–363.

88. Hackett S, Ferretti J, Stevens D. Cytokine induction by viable group A streptococci: suppression by streptolysin O. In: Program & Abstracts of the American Society for Microbiology, Las Vegas, NV. Washington, DC: American Society for Microbiology, 1994; Abstract B-249.

89. Muller-Alouf H, Alouf JE, Gerlach D, Ozegowski JH, Fitting C, Cavaillon JM. Comparative study of cytokine release by human peripheral blood mononuclear cells stimulated with *Streptococcus pyogenes* superantigenic erythrogenic toxins, heat-killed streptococci and lipopolysaccharide. Infect Immun 1994; 62:4915–4921.

90. Hackett SP, Stevens DL. Superantigens associated with staphylococcal and streptococcal toxic shock syndromes are potent inducers of tumor necrosis factor beta synthesis. J Infect Dis 1993; 168:232–235.

91. Kappur V, Majesky MW, Li LL, Black RA, Musser JM. Cleavage of Interleukin 1β (IL-1β) precursor to produce active IL-1β by a conserved extracellular cysteine protease from *Streptococcus pyogenes*. Proc Natl Acad Sci USA 1993; 90:7676–7680.

92. Chaussee MS, Liu J, Stevens DL, Ferretti JJ. Genetic and phenotypic diversity among isolates of *Streptococcus pyogenes* from invasive infections. J Infect Dis 1996; 173:901–908.

93. Burns EH, Marciel AM, Musser JM. Activation of a 66-kilodalton human endothelial cell matrix metalloprotease by *Streptococcus pyogenes* extracellular cysteine protease. Infect Immun 1996; 64:4744–4750.

94. Raeder RH, Boyle MDP. A secreted streptococcal cysteine protease can cleave a surface expressed M1 protein and alters its immunoglobulin-binding properties. In: Program & Abstracts of the ASM Conference on Microbes, Haemostasis, and Vascular Biology. American Society for Microbiology, Washington, D.C. Galveston: 1998.

95. Cleary P, Chen C, Lapenta D, Bormann N, Heath D, Haanes E. A virulence regulon in *Streptococcus pyogenes*. In: Program & Abstracts of the Third International ASM Conference on Streptococcal Genetics, Minneapolis, MN. Washington, DC: American Society for Microbiology, 1990; Abstract #19.

96. Cleary PP, Kaplan EL, Handley JP, Wlazlo A, Kim MH, Hauser AR, Schlievert PM. Clonal basis for resurgence of serious *Streptococcus pyogenes* disease in the 1980s. Lancet 1992; 339:518–521.

97. Nida SK, Ferretti JJ. Phage influence on the synthesis of extracellular toxins in group A streptococci. Infect Immun 1982; 36:745–750.

98. Hauser AR, Goshorn SC, Kaplan E, Stevens DL, Schlievert PM. Molecular analysis of the streptococcal pyrogenic exotoxins. In: Program & Abstracts of the Third International ASM conference on Streptococcal Genetics, Minneapolis, MN. Washington, DC: American Society for Microbiology, 1990.

99. Johnson LP, Tomai MA, Schlievert PM. Bacteriophage involvement in group A streptococcal pyrogenic exotoxin A production. J Bacteriol 1986; 166:623–627.

100. Musser JM, Hauser AR, Kim MH, Schlievert PM, Nelson K, Selander RK. *Streptococcus pyogenes* causing toxic-shock-like syndrome and other invasive diseases: clonal diversity and pyrogenic exotoxin expression. Proc Natl Acad Sci USA 1991; 88:2668–2672.

101. Stevens DL. Invasive group A streptococcal infections: the past, present and future. Pediatr Infect Dis J 1994; 13:561–566.

102. Wannamaker LW, Rammelkamp CH Jr, Denny FW, Brink WR, Houser HB, Hahn EO, Dingle JH. Prophylaxis of acute rheumatic fever by treatment of the preceding streptococcal infection with various amounts of depot penicillin. Am J Med 1951; 10:673–695.

103. Kim KS, Kaplan EL. Association of penicillin tolerance with failure to eradicate group A streptococci from patients with pharyngitis. J Pediatr 1985; 107:681–684.

104. Brook I. Role of beta-lactamase-producing bacteria in the failure of penicillin to eradicate group A streptococci. Pediatr Infect Dis 1985; 4:491–495.

105. Gaworzewska ET, Coleman G. Correspondence: group A streptococcal infections and a toxic shock–like syndrome. N Engl J Med 1989; 321:1546.

106. Stevens DL, Bryant AE, Yan S. Invasive group A streptococcal infection: new concepts in antibiotic treatment. Int J Antimicrobial Agents 1994; 4:297–301.

107. Stevens DL, Yan S, Bryant AE. Penicillin binding protein expression at different growth stages determines penicillin efficacy in vitro and in vivo: an explanation for the inoculum effect. J Infect Dis 1993; 167:1401–1405.

108. Yan S, Mendelman PM, Stevens DL. The in vitro antibacterial activity of ceftriaxone against *Streptococcus pyogenes* is unrelated to penicillin-binding protein 4. FEMS Microbiol Lett 1993; 110:313–318.

109. Yan S, Bohach GA, Stevens DL. Persistent acylation of high-molecular-weight penicillin binding proteins by penicillin induces the post antibiotic effect in *Streptococcus pyogenes*. J Infect Dis 1994; 170:609–614.

110. Stevens DL, Maier KA, Mitten JE. Effect of antibiotics on toxin production and viability of *Clostridium perfringens*. Antimicrob Agents Chemother 1987; 31:213–218.

111. Gemmell CG, Peterson PK, Schmeling D, Kim Y, Mathews J, Wannamaker L, Quie PG. Potentiation of opsonization and phagocytosis of *Streptococcus pyogenes* following growth in the presence of clindamycin. J Clin Invest 1981; 67:1249–1256.

112. Stevens DL, Bryant AE, Hackett SP. Antibiotic effects on bacterial viability, toxin production, and host response. Clin Infect Dis 1995; 20:S154–S157.

113. Barry W, Hudgins L, Donta S, Pesanti E. Intravenous immunoglobulin therapy for toxic shock syndrome. JAMA 1992; 267:3315–3316.

114. Yong JM. Letter. Lancet 1994; 343:1427.

115. Kaul R, McGeer A, Norrby-Teglund A, Kotb M, Schwartz B, O'Rourke K, Talbot J, Low DE and the Canadian Streptococcal Study Group. Intravenous immunoglobulin therapy in streptococcal toxic shock syndrome: A comparative observational study. Clin Infect Dis 1999; 28(4):800–807.

116. Stevens DL, Bryant AE, Hackett SP, Chung A, Peer G, Kosanke S, Emerson T, Hinshaw L. Group A streptococcal bacteremia: the role of tumor necrosis factor in shock and organ failure. J Infect Dis 1996; 173:619–626.

117. Stegmayr B, Bjorck S, Holm S, Nisell J, Rydvall A, Settergren B. Septic shock induced by group A streptococcal infections: clinical and therapeutic aspects. Scand J Infect Dis 1992; 24:589–597.

118. Greenberg LJ, Gray ED, Yunis E. Association of HL-A5 and immune responsiveness in vitro to streptococcal antigens. J Exp Med 1975; 141:934–943.

119. Weinstein L, Barza M. Gas gangrene. N Engl J Med 1972; 289:1129.

120. Zabriskie JB, Lavenchy D, Williams RC Jr, et al. Rheumatic-fever associated B-cell alloantigens as identified by monoclonal antibodies. Arthritis Rheum 1985; 28:1047–1051.

121. The Working Group on Severe Streptococcal Infections. Defining the group A streptococcal toxic shock syndrome: rationale and consensus definition. JAMA 1993; 269:390–391.

11

Molecular Pathogenesis of Group B Streptococcal Disease in Newborns

VICTOR NIZET
PATRICIA FERRIERI
CRAIG E. RUBENS

In the last two decades group B streptococci (GBS) have emerged as the leading cause of invasive bacterial infections in human neonates, with an incidence of 2–3 cases per 1000 live births. The early-onset form of GBS disease typically presents in the first 24 h of life, with fulminant pneumonia, septicemia, and high mortality (10%–15%) despite intensive supportive care. The less common late-onset (>7 days of age) form of GBS disease can present more indolently, with meningitis, occult bacteremia, or osteoarthritis. Whereas prematurity and maternal obstetric complications are important risk factors for early-onset disease, late-onset infections most commonly affect term newborns with unremarkable perinatal histories. The GBS isolates from neonates with early-onset infection are well distributed among the various capsular serotypes, while most isolates from infants with late-onset disease (and infants with meningitis regardless of age of onset) are of serotype III.

Recognition of the prevalence and severity of human neonatal disease has fueled intensive investigation toward elucidating the pathogenesis of GBS infection. Epidemiologic data and clinical experience frame the questions that must be addressed by basic microbiologic studies: How do GBS colonize pregnant women? How are GBS transmitted to the infant prior to or at delivery? What allows GBS to evade host defenses such as phagocytes, antibodies, and the complement system? How do GBS gain entry to the bloodstream and cross the blood-brain barrier? Do GBS elaborate specific factors that injure host tissues or induce sepsis syndrome? Why are newborns, in particular those born prematurely, uniquely susceptible to GBS infection? What explains the different clinical features and serotype distribution of the early- and late-onset forms of GBS disease?

Advances in our knowledge of GBS pathogenesis have been achieved through development of (1) in vitro model systems in which strains of the organism are allowed to interact with host tissues or components of the host immune system, and (2) animal models where the physiology and pathology of infection with GBS are examined directly. Application of modern molecular genetic techniques to GBS has begun to yield isogenic mutant strains varying solely in production of a particular component (e.g., capsular polysaccharide). Such mutants are critical reagents in establishing the biological relevance of a given trait and its requirement for virulence in vivo. As a byproduct, several GBS genes have now been identified and sequenced. This chapter will review our current understanding of the pathogenesis of GBS infection in newborns from a bacteriologic and immunologic standpoint, with special reference to recent molecular genetic discoveries.

PATHOGENESIS OF GROUP B STREPTOCOCCAL NEONATAL INFECTION: AN OVERVIEW

The process of human infection by GBS is complex and multifactorial. The marked increase in available experimental data has clarified many aspects of the pathogenic process, provided conflicting information in a few instances, and highlighted important gaps in our knowledge. The pathogenesis of GBS is perhaps best understood in the framework of an evolutionary relationship between the bacterium and its host. Selective pressure exists for GBS to establish transient or long-term colonization of the human, and to ensure successful transmission to new susceptible individuals. Therefore, those traits are favored which allow GBS to interact with human epithelial surfaces, or to penetrate to deeper tissues if a suitable survival niche can be found. Also favored are phenotypic features that permit GBS to resist, avoid, or counteract components of the host immune system directed at containing or eliminating bacteria.

Production of serious disease in the human is, from an evolutionary standpoint, an inadvertent and undesired outcome of GBS infection. Clearly, since the great majority of invasive disease is restricted to a small subset of the population (i.e., newborn infants), host factors play a central role in determining the pathogenic potential of GBS. Bacterial traits that have evolved to allow colonization or stable infection of the adult host may in turn represent significant virulence determinants for the neonate. Mode of acquisition, inadequate epithelial barrier function, and deficiencies in immune clearance undoubtedly contribute to the unique susceptibility of newborns to invasive GBS disease. Subsequent tissue injury is both a byproduct of

bacterial factors and the host inflammatory response they elicit.

Stages in the pathogenesis of GBS newborn infection are summarized schematically in Figure 11.1. The organism must first establish vaginal colonization in the pregnant mother, a process which comprises adherence to vaginal epithelial cells and resistance to mucosal immune defenses, such as secreted immunoglobulin A (IgA). To gain access to the fetus, GBS may next ascend into the amniotic cavity by penetration of placental membranes. Chorioamnionitis and bacterial proliferation allow the organism to enter the fetal lung through aspiration of infected amniotic fluid. Alternatively, the infant may acquire the organism on passage through the birth canal. After delivery, the GBS must successfully replicate within the alveoli of the neonate, adhere to respiratory epithelium, and avoid clearance by pulmonary macrophages. Pneumonia with lung epithelial and endothelial cell injury are characteristic of early-onset disease, and may be mediated in part by the cytotoxic properties of GBS beta-hemolysin and the influx of host neutrophils.

Group B streptococci are capable of "invading" alveolar epithelial and pulmonary endothelial cells within membrane-bound vacuoles. This process may allow the organism to gain stepwise entry into the bloodstream. Host phagocytic defenses are subsequently called upon to clear the pathogenic bacteria. Newborn infants, and particularly premature infants, have fewer alveolar macrophages than adults and exhibit poor neutrophil chemotaxis. Furthermore, GBS are inefficiently phagocytosed in the absence of opsonization by specific antibody or complement, both of which may be present in diminished amounts in neonatal serum. The polysaccharide capsule of GBS has a marked inhibitory effect on phagocytic clearance by preventing complement deposition on the bacterial surface. The GBS also produce a specific protease that inactivates the human complement component C5a, an important recruiter of human neutrophils to the site of infection. The alpha and beta components of GBS surface protein C may both retard opsonization and decrease intracellular killing of GBS taken up by neutrophils.

Cell wall–associated components of circulating GBS induce a sepsis syndrome characterized

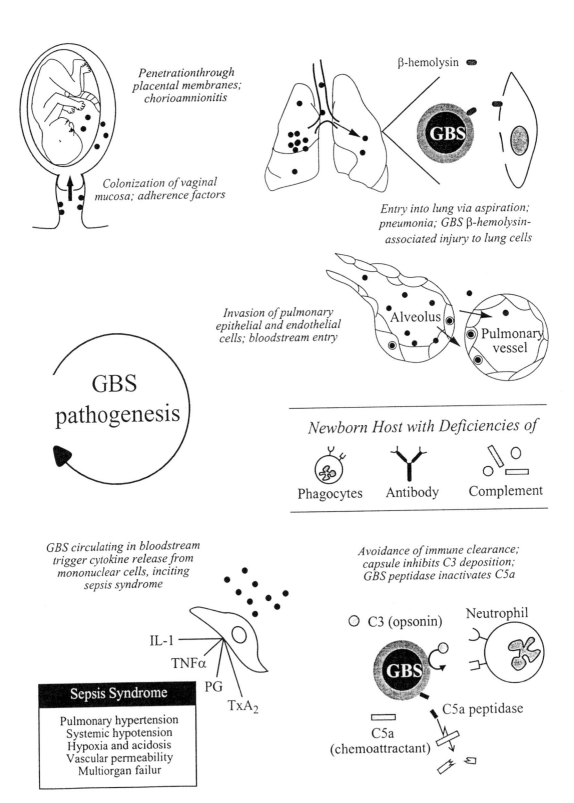

Penetration through
placental membranes;
chorioamnionitis

Colonization of vaginal
mucosa; adherence factors

β-hemolysin

GBS

Entry into lung via aspiration;
pneumonia; GBS β-hemolysin-
associated injury to lung cells

Invasion of pulmonary
epithelial and endothelial
cells; bloodstream entry

Alveolus

Pulmonary
vessel

GBS
pathogenesis

Newborn Host with Deficiencies of

Phagocytes   Antibody   Complement

GBS circulating in bloodstream
trigger cytokine release from
mononuclear cells, inciting
sepsis syndrome

Avoidance of immune clearance;
capsule inhibits C3 deposition;
GBS peptidase inactivates C5a

IL-1

TNFα

PG

TxA₂

C3 (opsonin)   Neutrophil

GBS

Sepsis Syndrome

Pulmonary hypertension
Systemic hypotension
Hypoxia and acidosis
Vascular permeability
Multiorgan failur

C5a peptidase

C5a
(chemoattractant)

Figure 11.1 Stages in the pathogenesis of group B streptococcal infection of the newborn.

by severe systemic hypotension, pulmonary hypertension, hypoxemia, and acidosis. This syndrome reflects the injurious effects of a host inflammatory response mediated by release of tumor necrosis factor (TNF), interleukins, prostaglandins, and thromboxane. Bloodstream dissemination allows GBS to reach multiple body sites, where subsequent tissue penetration results in end-organ disease manifestations (e.g., meningitis). Extracellular GBS products such as hyaluronidase, protease, and collagenase are postulated by certain investigators to facilitate spread of the organism through tissue barriers.

The pathogen–host interaction between GBS and human newborns becomes increasingly complex when one considers that bacterial attributes which promote virulence at a given stage in pathogenesis may attenuate virulence at other stages. For example, presence of the antiphagocytic polysaccharide capsule has an inhibitory effect on GBS invasion of host epithelial and endothelial cells. Furthermore, by cloaking proinflammatory cell wall components, encapsulated GBS strains are associated with less pulmonary hypertension and meningeal irritation than unencapsulated mutants. Whether GBS are capable of up- or down-regulating expression of capsular polysaccharide and other potential virulence factors at specific stages of the infectious process is unknown.

Finally, the pathogenesis of GBS disease in its late-onset form (>1 week of age) appears to be substantially different from the early-onset form. A less fulminant clinical course and frequent localization of infection (e.g., meningitis, osteomyelitis) likely reflect the progressive maturation of the host immune response. The GBS must establish carriage in the upper respiratory tract of the infant, whereupon mucosal disruption by an intercurrent viral infection might facilitate access to the bloodstream. The predominance of serotype III GBS isolates in late-onset disease indicates a unique role of the sialylated type III polysaccharide capsule in resisting subsequent immune clearance. In contrast, early-onset disease is evenly distributed among the various GBS capsular serotypes. A strong association with maternal peripartum fever and membrane rupture suggest that GBS replication in the amniotic fluid may deliver an overwhelming bacterial inoculum to the neonatal

lung, irrespective of the GBS serotype involved. Non-serotype-restricted virulence properties such as bacterial toxin release, lung cell invasion, and cell-wall activation of host cytokines may play a more prominent role, such that lung injury, entry of GBS into the bloodstream, and sepsis syndrome develop before an effective phagocytic response is recruited. Surfactant deficiency and underdeveloped local and systemic immune responses render the premature neonate particularly vulnerable to early-onset GBS pneumonia and invasive disease.

STAGES IN THE PATHOGENESIS OF NEONATAL GROUP B STREPTOCOCCAL INFECTIONS

Colonization of Pregnant Mothers

The presence of GBS in the genital tract of the mother at delivery substantially determines whether or not the newborn will acquire the organism and be at risk of invasive disease. Group B streptococci frequently inhabit the genital tract and lower gastrointestinal tract of healthy adult females. Approximately 20%–30% of mothers have positive rectovaginal cultures at delivery, and comparison of maternal culture status with surface culture of the newborn indicates a vertical transmission rate of approximately 50%–70% [1–3]. Infants born to women identified prenatally as GBS carriers have a 29-fold greater risk of early-onset disease than infants born to women with negative prenatal cultures [4]. A direct relationship also exists between the magnitude of GBS vaginal carriage, the risk of vertical transmission [5], and the likelihood of serious disease in the newborn [6]. Consequently, a critical step in the pathogenesis of GBS invasive disease in the newborn is, in fact, the asymptomatic colonization of pregnant women.

To establish colonization of the female genital tract, GBS must successfully adhere to epithelial cells of the vagina. In comparison to other microorganisms, GBS bind very efficiently to exfoliated human vaginal cells or vaginal tissue culture cells [7]. The ability to adhere to vaginal epithelial cells varies among GBS isolates, but these differences are not dependent on capsular serotype [8]. Binding is maximal at the acidic pH characteristic of vaginal mucosa [9,10]. Attachment itself does not depend on bacterial viability, as it is unaffected by UV irradiation of the GBS [9,11].

The specific molecular interactions that mediate GBS attachment to vaginal epithelial cells are not known. Importantly, GBS adherence is not restricted to the vaginal mucosa; indeed, lower gastrointestinal tract colonization may play a principal role in carriage by healthy adults [12]. In vitro, GBS bind effectively to human cells from a variety of fetal, infant, and adult tissues, including placental membranes [13], buccal or pharyngeal mucosa [8,14], alveolar epithelium [10], and endothelium [15], each relevant to vertical transmission and production of invasive disease in the infant. These findings suggest two possibilities: (1) the specific component of the host cell surface to which GBS attaches is widely distributed among human tissues, or (2) GBS can adhere to multiple cell surface components. Experimental evidence exists to suggest that both ionic and hydrophobic interactions contribute significantly to GBS host cell adherence. Increasing osmolality by addition of sodium chloride decreases GBS adherence, although calcium and magnesium do not effect binding at physiologic concentrations [10]. Treatment of epithelial cells with sialidase increases surface hydrophobicity and GBS attachment [11]. Binding is inhibited by preincubating the cells with hydrophobic GBS surface proteins or preincubating the GBS with antibodies to these proteins [16].

Isogenic mutants deficient in polysaccharide capsule production bind more efficiently to epithelial cells than the parent strain [10], and attachment of small-capsule GBS-phase variants to endothelial cells is more than 10-fold greater than attachment of large-capsule variants [15]. Thus the GBS capsule appears to attenuate the adherence potential of organism. Potential mechanisms include steric hindrance of a high-affinity adhesin-receptor interaction, or a decrease in repulsive forces generated between negatively charged sialic acid residues on the GBS capsule and the surface of host cells [10]. The presence of specific GBS protein adhesins is supported by the fact that epithelial cell binding is inhibited by pretreatment of the GBS with

a variety of proteases [10,11,17]. Alternatively, the principal GBS surface ligand may be lipoteichoic acid (LTA), as suggested by competitive inhibition experiments in which soluble LTA inhibited epithelial cell adherence [18,19]. However, others have shown no effect of exogenous LTA on epithelial cell binding [10,20], and any such experiments are complicated by potential cytotoxic effects of LTA on tissue culture monolayers [17]. Interestingly, topical administration of LTA or glycerol phosphate, a subunit component of LTA putatively involved in binding, may decrease GBS vaginal colonization of pregnant mice [21].

Pathogenic bacteria may bind to mammalian tissues by adhering to extracellular matrix (ECM) proteins such as fibronectin, fibrinogen, laminin, collagen, or integrins [22]. Recent data presented by Tamura and Rubens [23] indicate that GBS bind to fibronectin immobilized on polystyrene, but not to several other ECM proteins tested (laminin, type I collagen, vitronectin, and tenascin). Clinical isolates bind fibronectin with varying efficiency (4%–60% of the input inoculum), but differences are not correlated to capsule serotype or C protein expression [23,24]. Protein blot analysis reveals that GBS are binding to a high-molecular-weight form of nonreduced fibronectin monomers and dimers. It is intriguing to note that GBS do not bind fibronectin in its soluble form [23,25]. This suggests that GBS adherence to fibronectin is a low-avidity interaction, requiring the close proximity of multiple fibronectin molecules and GBS adhesins favored by a solid phase model.

Analysis of a random plasmid integrational mutant library of GBS has identified a genetic locus involved in human fibrinogen binding. One open reading frame encodes a putative response regulator of 218 amino acids, another, a putative histidine kinase of 444 amino acids [26]. These genes share significant homology with several gram-positive two-component regulator systems. The association of this locus with the fibrinogen-binding properties of GBS was confirmed by targeted knockout of the putative response regulator. Adherence of GBS to laminin involves the gene *lmb*, which encodes a homologue of the streptococcal Lra1 adhesin family [27]. Targeted mutagenesis of the *lmb* locus results in diminished adherence of GBS to immobilized laminin. The contributions of fibrinogen or laminin binding to GBS pathogenesis have not yet been elucidated.

Acquisition of GBS by the Infant

Newborns may be exposed to GBS in utero following ascending infection of the placental membranes and amniotic fluid. Alternatively, they may become contaminated with GBS upon passage through the birth canal. The GBS proliferate readily in amniotic fluid, and several lines of evidence suggest that infection by the ascending route plays a more pivotal role in the pathogenesis of early-onset disease. For example, the risk of GBS acquisition by the neonate is clearly increased by prolonged rupture of placental membranes and by the presence of maternal peripartum fever or chorioamnionitis [28]. A direct relation exists between the duration of placental membrane rupture prior to delivery and attack rate [29], while an inverse relation exists between the duration of membrane rupture and the age at which symptoms of early-onset pneumonia and sepsis first appear [30]. In the rhesus monkey model of intra-amniotic infection, neither maternal GBS immune status nor pre-pregnancy immunization influenced intra-amniotic bacterial proliferation or infection of the fetus, emphasizing the importance of magnitude and duration of in utero bacterial exposure in disease pathogenesis [31].

The GBS bacterium may not be a simple opportunist dependent upon mechanical rupture of placental membranes for ascent into the amniotic cavity. Histologic examination of placentae from women with chorioamniotis show bacterial infiltration along a choriodecidual course, implying that ascending infection may be a primary trigger event in many instances of premature rupture [32]. Experiments in which GBS are inoculated endocervically in pregnant ewes support this proposed route of ascending infection [33]. One epidemiologic study found that women with GBS in their urine during pregnancy had a greater than twofold increased risk of primary rupture of placental membranes and premature delivery [34]. This finding would suggest that heavy maternal colonization with GBS (for which bacteruria is a marker) favors placental infection and membrane rupture.

Mechanisms by which GBS may promote membrane rupture and premature delivery are being examined. Isolated chorioamniotic membranes exposed to GBS have decreased tensile strength, elasticity, and work to rupture [35]. Peptide fragments released from these membranes suggest that the organism is producing one or more proteases that degrade the placental tissue. Group B streptococci are known to exhibit a cell wall–associated collagenolytic activity that could disrupt the collagen fibrils of the amniotic membrane [36]. Alternatively, GBS may induce placental membrane rupture indirectly by alteration of host cell processes. For example, the presence of GBS within the lower uterine cavity or cervix activates the maternal decidua cell peroxidase-H_2O_2-halide system, which could promote oxygen radical–induced damage to adjacent fetal membranes [37]. Filtered extracts of GBS modify the arachidonic acid metabolism of cultured human amnion cells, favoring production of prostaglandin E_2 [38,39]. High local concentrations of this compound are known to stimulate the onset of normal labor, and may also be a mechanism for initiation of premature labor [40]. Group B streptococci stimulate macrophage inflammatory protein-1α and interleukin-8 (IL-8) production from human chorion cells; these chemokines are important mediators signaling migration of inflammatory cells and may also contribute to the pathogenesis of infection-associated preterm labor [41].

It appears that on occasion, GBS can penetrate into the amniotic cavity through intact placental membranes, as fulminant early-onset disease develops in some infants delivered by cesarean section with no identifiable obstetric risk factors [1,42]. Rapid death and advanced lung inflammatory changes on autopsy of such patients strongly imply that the onset of infection occurred in utero [43]. Migration of GBS through freshly isolated chorioamnionotic membranes has been documented by scanning and transmission electron microscopy [13]. The organisms bound to the maternal surface by 2 h and appeared on the fetal surface within 8 h of inoculation. The ability of GBS to interact with placental membranes may exhibit strain variation, as isolates from septic neonates adhere more avidly to chorionic epithelial cells than isolates from asymptomatic carriers [44].

When GBS gain access to the uterine cavity and proliferate over time in the amniotic fluid, an overwhelming inoculum may be delivered to the fetal lung. In utero infection likely accounts for the 40%–60% of newborns with early-onset disease who have poor Apgar scores and develop pulmonary symptoms within a few hours of birth [29,45]. Such infants almost invariably display clinical and/or histologic evidence of congenital pneumonia. Conversely, when GBS are encountered in the immediate peripartum or upon passage through the birth canal, a lesser inoculum is transmitted to the infant. Specific properties must then allow the organism to establish and sustain itself on mucosal surfaces of the newborn host. For example, certain GBS strains adhere better to buccal epithelial cells from neonates than from adults [14]. Although a small but meaningful risk of subsequent invasive disease exists, the great majority of newborns who are contaminated with GBS through swallowing of infected vaginal secretions will have asymptomatic colonization limited to mucosal surfaces [46].

Although prolonged rupture of placental membranes is frequently encountered in association with premature delivery, it is clear that the latter is a significant independent risk factor for acquisition of GBS infection. An inverse relation exists between gestational age and the incidence of early-onset GBS disease, such that the very lowest–birth-weight infants have an infection rate 10–25 times higher than term newborns [46,47]. Immaturity of pulmonary and systemic host defense mechanisms provide considerable rationale for this epidemiologic association, as discussed in later sections. Also of potential importance is the observation that GBS show increased adherence to buccal epithelial cells from premature neonates compared to term neonates [48].

Group B Streptococcal Pneumonia and Lung Injury

Consistent with the proposed route of acquisition, early-onset GBS disease is heralded by respiratory symptoms including tachypnea, retractions, and cyanosis. Marked hypoxia and pulmonary hypertension are common associated

features [49]. Autopsies of fatal early-onset cases reveal that 80% have histologic evidence of lobar or multilobar pneumonia [50,51]. The GBS pneumonia mimics severe surfactant-deficient respiratory distress syndrome clinically, radiologically, and morphologically. Dense bacterial infiltration, epithelial cell damage, alveolar hemorrhage, interstitial inflammatory exudate, and hyaline membrane formation are present in most pulmonary lesions [43,52]. Immunofluorescence studies show deposition of immunoglobluin, complement, and fibrin in the lungs of infants with fatal early-onset GBS disease [53]. The pattern is similar to that seen in premature infants with respiratory distress syndrome. It is possible the two disease processes induce a common inflammatory response, including immune complex–mediated injury to lung tissue.

Establishment of GBS pneumonia is a consequence of the size of the bacterial inoculum and the failure of local alveolar clearance mechanisms in the newborn host. An inverse relation appears to exist between the age of experimental animals and their ability to clear GBS from the lung following aerosol challenge. Compared to the adult, infant rats show diminished alveolar macrophage phagocytosis of GBS and a delayed rate of neutrophil accumulation in the lungs [54]. Enhanced susceptibility of rabbits to GBS in the immediate postnatal period is due in part to ineffective intracellular killing by alveolar macrophages [55,56]. The poorer resolution of GBS pneumonia in preterm versus term rabbits may result from a quantitative deficiency of pulmonary alveolar macrophages, mandating the recruitment of neutrophils as a secondary phagocytic defense mechanism [57]. Inhibition of prostaglandin synthesis by indomethecin fails to impair pulmonary clearance of GBS, indicating that prostaglandin H synthase–derived oxygen radicals do not contribute to pulmonary microbicidal activity [58]. Deficient clearance by the host allows multiplying GBS to attain very high concentrations within the alveolar spaces [43]. Indeed, when GBS pneumonia develops in newborn primates exposed by intra-amniotic injection, bacterial density reaches 10^9 to 10^{11} organisms per gram of lung tissue [59].

Morphologic findings of alveolar exudate and hemorrhage in autopsy studies of GBS pneumonia attest to significant pulmonary epithelial and endothelial cell injury [52,60]. Because cases of early-onset pneumonia are relatively evenly distributed among the common GBS capsular serotypes, certain constant noncapsular phenotypic traits of GBS are likely to have an important role in the pathogenesis of lung injury. In particular, a beta-hemolysin produced by the overwhelming majority of GBS clinical isolates appears to possess significant toxicity to pulmonary tissue. A direct, quantitative correlation exists between the degree to which GBS strains express beta-hemolytic activity and their ability to injure human alveolar epithelial or pulmonary endothelial cells in tissue culture [61,62]. Isogenic GBS transposon mutants with a non-hemolytic phenotype are noninjurious, and those with a hyperhemolytic phenotype are hyperinjurious, to the cell monolayers. Transposon mutant strains of GBS devoid of beta-hemolysin expression demonstrate diminished virulence upon intrathoracic inoculation of infant rats [63], but are equally virulent compared to the parent strain following subcutaneous injection in rats [64]. These animal data suggest a unique role for GBS beta-hemolysin in the preliminary respiratory tract stages of early-onset disease.

Group B streptococcal beta-hemolysin-associated epithelial cell injury is inhibited by the major phospholipid component of human surfactant, DPPC, providing additional rationale for the unusual susceptibility of premature, surfactant-deficient newborns to severe GBS pneumonia [61]. Treatment with exogenous surfactant reduces histolgocal evidence of lung inflammation, improves lung compliance, and mitigates bacterial growth in preterm rabbits infected with GBS [65,66]. Several small clinical studies exploring the effect of surfactant administration on human infants with GBS sepsis also suggest a beneficial effect [67–69]. Mice deficient in surfactant protein A, a pulmonary collectin that facilitates opsonophagocytosis, were more susceptible to bloodstream dissemination of GBS [70]. However, treatment with a monoclonal antibody against surfactant protein A did not increase bacterial proliferation in GBS-infected newborn rabbits [71].

Early-onset GBS pneumonia is associated with a marked inflammatory and hemodynamic response of the pulmonary vasculature. Characteristic features include increased pulmonary vascular permeability, neutrophil trapping in lung vessels, and pulmonary hypertension [72]. Group B streptococcal beta-hemolysin expression is associated with dose-dependent increases in albumin transit across polar endothelial cell monolayers, suggesting it may contribute to pulmonary vascular leakage [62]. Protein efflux from pulmonary vessels into the terminal air spaces is consistent with the clinical pattern of alveolar congestion and hyaline membrane formation seen in early-onset pneumonia. Pre-exposure to the type III GBS polysaccharide capsule antigen promotes attachment of neutrophils to human endothelial cells, while inhibiting chemotactic properties that may be required for neutrophils to reach the site of infection in the alveolar spaces [73].

Infusion of GBS increases pulmonary vascular resistance in isolated piglet lung preparations [74]. This finding implies that pulmonary hypertension in GBS pneumonia results from a direct interaction of the organism with target cells in lung microvasculature, independent of other organ system participation. Studies employing isogenic GBS transposon mutants demonstrate that neither the polysaccharide capsule nor beta-hemolysin are essential for GBS to cause acute pulmonary hypertension in piglets [75]. In fact, nonencapsulated GBS mutants can produce significantly higher changes in pulmonary artery pressure and resistance than encapsulated strains [76], suggesting that capsule may partially cloak the hemodynamically active GBS component. Pulmonary hypertension in the animal model can be correlated to efficiency of bacterial killing, and each is inhibited by the oxygen radical scavenger dimethylthiourea [77]. Thus activation of an oxygen-radical dependent bactericidal mechanism may contribute to acute lung injury and pulmonary hemodynamic abnormalities. Live but not heat-killed GBS induce release of the vasoactive eiconasoids prostacyclin and prostaglandin E_2 from cultured lung microvascular cells [78]. Animal experiments using specific antagonists have further implicated the host inflammatory mediators leukotriene D_4 [79] and thromboxane A_2 [80] as components of the pulmonary vascular response in GBS pneumonia.

Invasion of Pulmonary Epithelium and Endothelium

To gain access to the systemic circulation from a primary focus of infection in the lung, GBS must traverse three host barriers: the alveolar epithelium, the pulmonary interstitium, and the pulmonary endothelium. Lung epithelial and endothelial cell injury secondary to beta-hemolysin or the host inflammatory response could produce focal lesions in these barriers, thus allowing GBS to reach the bloodstream. However, wholesale barrier disruption does not appear to be a fundamental prerequisite for GBS bacteremia, since the organism is capable of penetration into the very host cells that comprise the intact lung–bloodstream interface. The first evidence of GBS entry into host cells came from a primate model in which early-onset pneumonia and septicemia was established following intra-amniotic inoculation of the organism [59]. Electron microscopy of lung tissue from the infant macaque demonstrated GBS within membrane-bound vacuoles of type I and II alveolar epithelial cells and interstitial fibroblasts (Fig. 11.2). These findings suggest that GBS can enter alveolar epithelial cells by stimulating their own endocytosis. Such "cellular invasion" may be an important mechanism through which GBS transit epithelial barriers and disseminate from the alveolar space [59]. This virulence attribute of GBS is reminiscent of certain enteric bacterial pathogens for which invasion of gut epithelial cells is a primary step in establishment of systemic infection [81,82].

The phenomenon of cellular invasion by GBS has been further elucidated by development of a tissue culture model [83]. This in vitro system represents an adaptation of the gentamicin protection assay developed for studying *Yersinia* entry into epithelial cells [84]. The GBS are allowed to interact with the eukaryotic cell monolayer for a period of time, after which nonadherent bacteria are washed away, and medium containing the antibiotics penicillin and gentamicin is added. Because gentamicin penetrates the eukaryotic cell membrane very poorly, only extracellular bacteria are killed. Subsequent lysis of the tissue culture cells releases internalized bacteria, which are plated to determine viable counts. As assessed by this model, GBS readily enter and survive within cultured A549 human alveolar epithelial cells [83]. Electron microscopic analysis confirms the presence of intracellular organisms within membrane-bound vacuoles. Time-course studies indicate the bacteria do not replicate appreciably after entering the host cell. Addition of specific inhibitors demonstrates that active bacterial DNA, RNA, and protein synthesis are necessary for invasion, and that the host endocytotic mechanism involves actin microfilaments but not microtubular cytoskeletal elements [83]. Uptake of GBS appears to require induction of protein-kinase signal transduction pathways in the epithelial cell [85]. These pathways may be dependent upon calmodulin, as entry of GBS into epithelial cells is inhibited in a dose-dependent manner when the extracellular calcium concentration is reduced [85].

The GBS isolates of capsular serotypes Ia, Ib, Ia/c, II, and III all invade alveolar epithelial cells in tissue culture, but some strain variation exists in the magnitude of invasion [86]. The polysaccharide capsule itself does not appear to be essential for invasion of alveolar epithelial cells. Rather, an isogenic nonencapsulated mutant invades more efficiently than the type III clinical isolate from which it was derived [86]. Preincubation of the epithelial cell monolayer with purified type III GBS capsular polysaccharide has no effect on invasion. As discussed above, the GBS capsule decreases adherence of the organism to alveolar epithelium [10], presumably through steric interference of certain receptor–ligand interactions. Should initial adherence to the epithelial cell be a requirement for subsequent invasion, inhibition of invasion by the presence of capsule would be anticipated. Likewise, capsule may mask other "invasin" molecules on the GBS surface that promote epithelial cell uptake independent of adherence. Finally, one must consider the fact that the polysaccharide capsule confers an important survival advantage to GBS through inhibition of macrophage and neutrophil phagocytosis. Should alveolar epithelial cells share rudimentary aspects of their endocytotic uptake mechanism with these "professional" phagocytes, capsule inhibition of invasion may be a byproduct of the stronger selective pressure placed on GBS to avoid immunologic clearance.

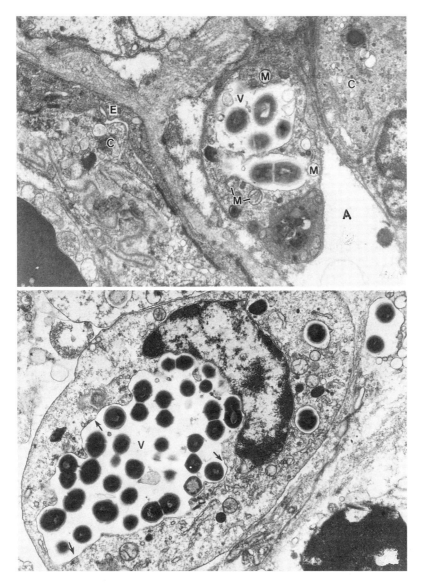

Figure 11.2 Group B streptococcal invasion of alveolar epithelial cells in neonatal primates following intramniotic exposure. Multiple intracellular organisms are seen within membrane-bound vacuoles. v, vacuole; M, mitochondria; E, endothelial cell; c, pulmonary capillary. (From Rubens et al. [59], with permission.)

If cellular invasion allows GBS to transit the alveolar epithelium into the pulmonary interstitial space, an additional barrier separates the organism from the circulation. The GBS must encounter and penetrate the pulmonary endothelium. Electron microscopy of lung tissue from newborn primates with GBS pneumonia demonstrates GBS inside capillary endothelial cells [87]. In vitro antibiotic protection assays confirm the ability of GBS to invade primary cultures of human umbilical vein or piglet lung endothelial cells [78,87]. The GBS invade more efficiently into pulmonary microvascular endothelial cells than into endothelial cells of pulmonary artery origin [78], suggesting a tropism for particular endothelial surfaces. As with epithelial monolayers, polysaccharide capsule retards the efficiency of GBS endothelial cell invasion [87].

Direct experimental evidence is accumulating to indicate that cellular invasion is a crucial component in the pathogenesis of neonatal GBS disease. When tested in the tissue culture model,

GBS isolates from the blood of infected neonates are significantly more invasive for respiratory epithelia than isolates from vaginal carriers or colonized neonates without clinical symptoms [88]. These results indicate that in vitro invasion of human epithelial cell monolayers is a marker for the ability of a GBS to produce invasive disease in vivo. Furthermore, a GBS transposon mutant has been created that is deficient in the ability to invade alveolar epithelial cells in tissue culture [89]. In contrast to the parent strain, this mutant fails to produce bacteremia when administered by aerosolization to newborn rats. This finding is consistent with the hypothesis that cellular invasion is required for GBS to bypass the pulmonary epithelial barrier.

Evasion of Host Defense Mechanisms

Upon penetration of GBS into the lung tissue or bloodstream of the newborn infant, an immunologic response is recruited to clear the organism. The central elements of this response are host phagocytic cells of the neutrophil, and to a lesser extent, monocyte–macrophage cell lines. However, as is the case with most other pathogenic bacteria, effective phagocytosis of GBS by neutrophils and macrophages requires opsonization. Without the participation of specific antibodies and serum complement, phagocytosis of GBS is dramatically reduced [90–92]. The predilection of certain neonates to suffer invasive GBS disease may thus reflect quantitative or qualitative deficits in (1) phagocytic cell function, (2) specific anti-GBS immunoglobulin, or (3) the classic and alternate complement pathways. In addition to these host factors, GBS possess a number of unique virulence attributes that interfere with effective opsonophagocytosis, chief among them, the type-specific polysaccharide capsule.

Some investigators have hypothesized that neonatal neutrophils are inherently defective in phagocytosis of GBS. Experiments designed to address this question have yielded conflicting results. Infusion of adult rather than neonatal neutrophils increases survival of newborn rats challenged with GBS [93]. However, the in vitro bactericidal kinetics of human newborn neutrophils are comparable to adult neutrophils under appropriate opsonic conditions [83]. Meta-bolic demands of fighting infection in the in vivo model could explain these differences, since impaired respiratory burst activity is present in neutrophils from severely "stressed" infants when compared to those from healthy newborns [84]. Ineffective respiratory burst function may be an especially significant risk factor for infection with GBS, which is surprisingly 10-fold more resistant to killing by oxygen metabolites than the catalase-producing *Staphylococcus aureus* [96]. The protection of GBS against oxidative damage is correlated in part with a greater endogenous content of the oxygen-metabolite scavenger glutathione. Group B streptococci can persist intracellularly in macrophages for 24–48 h, in part because of the ability of the organism to impair host cell protein kinase C–dependent signal transduction required for microbicidal activity [97].

Insufficient magnitude of the neutrophil response to GBS infection may compound specific defects in neonatal neutrophil function. Neutropenia and depletion of the marrow neutrophil storage pool is a frequent finding in human newborns with septicemia [98]. Whereas adult rats infected with GBS develop neutrophilia and an increase in granulocytic stem cells, infected neonatal rats develop severe neutropenia without a change in stem cells counts [99]. Fatal GBS infection in neonatal rats is associated with failure of depleted myeloid storage pools to recover [100]. An explanation for this may lie in the observation that the proliferative rate of neutrophils in noninfected neonatal animals is already maximal or near maximal, and cannot further increase in response to bacterial challenge [101]. Following exposure to GBS, the neutrophil chemiluminescent response of premature neonates is further impaired when compared to term infants [102].

Preliminary indications that specific antibody was important in the immunologic clearance of GBS came from Lancefield's work in the mouse and rabbit models. She found that multiple specific antibodies directed to either polysaccharide or protein antigens of a single strain were protective against lethal challenge with GBS displaying these antigens [103]. Abundant clinical data have been accumulated to support these observations. A strong correlation exists between low levels of maternal specific anticapsular antibody to type III GBS and the risk of invasive disease in the infant [104,105]. These data suggest that transplacental transfer of maternal antibody protects infants from invasive type III GBS infection. Similar clinical correlations have been reported for type Ia [106], Ib [107], and II [108] strains. Because transfer of IgG across the placenta is inefficient until after the 34th week of gestation, infants born prematurely have proportionately lower passive antibody titers [109]. The opsonic capacity of serum from premature neonates is reduced compared to term neonates [102]. Deficiency in maternally acquired specific antibodies against GBS no doubt contributes to the well-documented increased risk of invasive GBS disease in premature neonates.

When examined in vitro using adult neutrophils, sera from septic neonates with low maternal-acquired IgG antibody levels invariably lack opsonic activity for the infecting GBS strain [50]. Conversely, sera from healthy infants with high passive anticapsular antibody titers promote bacterial killing [105]. In vivo studies corroborate the importance of type-specific antibody in resistance to GBS infection. Maternally acquired type-specific antibody is protective for GBS-exposed newborn rhesus monkeys [110]. Administration of human sera from adults vaccinated with type III capsular polysaccharide also protects mice challenged with a type III GBS strain [111]. Finally, pregnant adult mice given a single inoculation of serum raised in rabbits against conjugate type III GBS polysaccharide vaccine passively protect 100% of their offspring to a type III GBS challenge [112].

Both IgG and IgM are opsonic for type III GBS [113], however, 100-fold higher concentrations of IgG than IgM antibody are required for optimal opsonization [114]. The marked protective activity of the IgM human antibody is due to its enhanced avidity and ability to trigger the complement system [114]. Moreover, hybridoma anticapsular IgM antibody appears to stimulate the release of neutrophil reserves into the bloodstream and improve neutrophil migration to infected tissues [101]. In contrast to maternal IgG antibodies, IgM antibodies are not transported effectively across the placenta, even at term. IgM deficiency in newborn infants may therefore increase their susceptibility to invasive GBS disease [113].

The interaction between GBS, specific antibody, and components of the complement system is uniquely complex and varies significantly among GBS capsule serotypes. The classical pathway of complement activation is a cascade of proteolytic cleavage and protein-binding reactions, traditionally in response to antigen–antibody complex formation, which promotes complement fixation, immune adherence, and release of proinflammatory and chemoattractant mediators. As expected, participation of the classic complement pathway maximizes specific anticapsular antibody opsonization of type I, II, and many type III strains of GBS [115]. However, certain type Ia and type II strains appear to be capable of activating C1 and the classic pathway in the absence of immunoglobulin [116,117]. The alternative pathway of complement activation was first described as an antibody-independent response to endotoxins of Gram-negative bacteria; nevertheless, alternative complement pathway-mediated opsonization and phagocytosis is facilitated by specific antibody to type III or type V GBS [118]. Quantitative deficiencies of proteins from both the classical [119] and alternative [120] complement pathways are seen in newborn sera when compared to older infants and adults, suggesting that each may play a key role in the age-dependent susceptibility to GBS infection.

Situated at the convergence of the classical and alternative pathways, deposition of C3 on the bacterial surface, with subsequent cleavage and degradation to opsonically active fragments C3b and iC3b, is a pivotal element in host defense against invasive infections. C3 deposition and degradation occurs on the surface of GBS representing a variety of serotypes [121]. However, the extent of C3 deposition by the alternative pathway is inversely related to the size and density of the polysaccharide capsule present on the surface of type Ib and type III GBS strains [122,123]. Isogenic mutant type III strains expressing a sialic acid–deficient capsule, or lacking capsular polysaccharide altogether, bind 8- to 16-fold greater amounts of C3 and are more efficiently phagocytosed than the parent strain [123]. Asialo- and acapsular type III GBS mutants exhibit a 100-fold increase in LD50 in a neonatal rat model [124]. Thus, interference of effective C3 deposition by sialylated polysaccharide capsule appears to be an important virulence mechanism of GBS. Some data suggest that antibody against type III capsular polysaccharide can overcome this interference, allowing activation of C3 and conferring protection against lethal infection [125].

The opsonic requirements of type II GBS strains are variable and correlate in part with surface protein antigen phenotype. Type II strains displaying both components of the c protein antigen are more resistant to phagocytic killing than Type II strains lacking c protein [126]. Presence or absence of c protein does not appear to affect internalization of the type II GBS into human neutrophils; however, intracellular killing of strains possessing c protein is apparently diminished [127]. A potential mechanism for this finding relates to the observation that strains bearing the c protein antigen displayed increased nonimmune binding to serum IgA and decreased C3 deposition on their surface [127]. The beta antigen of c protein is known to bind human IgA [128], and IgA deposited nonspecifically on the surface of GBS could conceivably inhibit interactions with opsonically-active complement or IgG [127].

Evidence indicates that specific neutrophil receptors recognize opsonizing complement or antibody on the surface of GBS and initiate phagocytosis. Blockade of the neutrophil complement receptors CR1 or CR3 inhibits phagocytosis of GBS by adult or neonatal neutrophils [129]. Of particular interest is CR3, the surface membrane expression of which is impaired in neonatal neutrophils [130]. The lectin-binding site of CR3 plays a greater role in opsonophagocytic killing of type III GBS, while the iC3b binding epitope of CR3 participates to a larger extent in killing of type Ia GBS [129]. Whether differential CR3 utilization contributes to strain variations in GBS virulence is unknown. Blockade of neutrophil receptors FcRII and FcRIII, both of which bind multimeric IgG, also decreases killing of type III GBS [131]. FcRIII, which is involved in initial binding of the neutrophil to the antibody–GBS complex, is invariably required. FcRII, which is involved in internalization and activation of the respiratory burst, may not be required in GBS opsonized with complement in addition to specific antibody [131]. The

dominant roles of neutrophil complement receptor CR3 and neutrophil IgG-receptor FcRIII have been corroborated in phagocytic assays using GBS serotypes IV and V [132,133].

In addition to opsonization, the serum complement system contributes to host defense through generation of soluble chemotactic factors that promote neutrophil mobilization, in particular, C5a. In response to type III GBS, neonatal sera is inherently impaired in C5a production and neutrophil chemotaxigenesis compared to adult sera [91]. Group B streptococci further contribute to poor neutrophil mobilization by production of an enzyme that specifically cleaves and inactivates human C5a [134]. Additional neutrophil chemoattractants are produced cells of monocyte lineage (e.g., alveolar macrophages), including interleukin-8 and leukotriene B4. Adult monocytes release IL-8 and leukotriene B4 in greater quantities than neonatal monocytes when exposed to GBS [135]. Insufficient production of these two chemotactic factors may contribute to the neonate's poor phagocytic response to GBS.

Optimal immune clearance of GBS may involve the soluble form of the plasma glycoprotein fibronectin. Addition of fibronectin increases uptake of antibody-coated GBS by adult neutrophils [136] and neonatal monocytes [137], while coadministration of fibronectin and type-specific antibody improves survival in infected neonatal rats [136]. Fibronectin enhancement of opsonophagocytosis appears to involve direct stimulation of the phagocytic cell, since soluble fibronectin does not bind detectably to a large panel of GBS strains [25]. A potential link between fibronectin and the age-limited susceptibility to GBS infections has been suggested, inasmuch as serum fibronectin levels are lowest at birth and rise significantly in the first few months of life [138], and decreased fibronectin levels are noted in the serum of septic neonates when compared to noninfected controls [139]. Interestingly, some opsonic and protective activity of human cord serum can be demonstrated that is independent of type-specific antibody, complement, or fibronectin [140]. Moreover, type III GBS possess a 21-kDa surface protein that directly binds to macrophages [141]. These data may explain in part why some infants born to GBS-colonized mothers with low type-specific antibody levels do not develop invasive infection [142].

Bacteremia and Induction of the Sepsis Syndrome

If failures in epithelial barrier function and immunologic clearance allow GBS to establish bacteremia in the neonate, development of the sepsis syndrome, and in many cases profound septic shock, may be the consequence. Severe early-onset GBS disease is clinically indistinguishable from septic shock associated with Gram-negative endotoxemia. Findings include systemic hypotension, persistent pulmonary hypertension, tissue hypoxemia and acidosis, temperature instability, disseminated intravascular coagulation, neutropenia, and ultimately, multiple-organ system failure. Because infusion of GBS produces similar pathophysiologic changes in neonatal animal models of sepsis, several investigations have begun to elucidate the patterns in which GBS activate host inflammatory mediators to induce sepsis syndrome and circulatory shock.

Animal models in which GBS are infused intravenously demonstrate a biphasic host inflammatory response [72,143,144]. The acute phase (<1 h) is manifest by increased pulmonary artery pressure and decreased arterial oxygenation, and is associated with a rise in serum levels of thromboxane B_2 (TxB_2), a stable metabolite marker of the pulmonary vasoconstrictor thromboxane A_2 (TxA_2). Pulmonary hypertension and hypoxemia persist through the late phase (2 to 4 h), in which a progressive pattern of systemic hypotension, decreased cardiac output, and metabolic acidosis develops together with hematologic abnormalities and organ system dysfunction. Inflammatory markers of the late phase include increases in serum TxB_2, TNF-α, and 6-keto-prostaglandin $F_{1\alpha}$ (6-keto-$PGF_{1\alpha}$, a stable metabolite of prostacyclin). Experiments employing specific antagonists confirm the importance of these compounds in producing the hemodynamic alterations of GBS sepsis, and demonstrate the involvement of still additional mediators in the host inflammatory cascade.

Thromboxanes and prostacyclin are byproducts of the cyclooxygenase pathway of arachidonic acid metabolism. Inhibition of the cyclooxygenase pathway by indomethacin is associated with decreased serum TxB_2 and 6-keto-$PGF_{1\alpha}$, less myocardial dysfunction, and a significant rise in systemic blood pressure in rabbits infused with GBS [145,146]. Venous infusions of GBS extracts produce significant pulmonary and systemic arterial vascular perturbations in neonatal lambs, all of which could be ameliorated by inhibition of the cyclooxygenase pathway [147]. Indomethicin therapy does not, however, protect against sepsis-induced hematologic abnormalities including neutropenia and thrombocytopenia [146]. Thromboxane may be particularly important in the pulmonary hemodynamic manifestations of GBS septicemia, as treatment of GBS-infected piglets with the specific thromboxane synthesis inhibitor, dazmegrel, rapidly normalizes pulmonary artery pressures and resistance [148]. Lipooxygenase products of arachidonic acid metabolism may also participate in the early inflammatory response. Treatment with the leukotriene antagonist FPL 57231 attenuated pulmonary hypertension without altering TxB_2 and 6-keto-$PGF_{1\alpha}$ levels [149].

As a known stimulator of both the cyclooxygenase and lipooxygenase pathways, IL-1 may occupy a proximal position in the cytokine cascade of septic shock [150]. Treatment with an IL-1 receptor antagonist improves cardiac output and mean arterial pressure and increases the length of survival in piglets receiving a continuous infusion of GBS [151]. In mice, GBS induce a "Th1-like" cytokine response (IL-2, interferon-γ [IFN-γ], IL-12) in the absence of cytokines important in B-cell help (IL-4, IL-5, IL-10) [152]. This pattern of response may allow GBS to evade antibody production important for clearance. The cytokine IL-12 may also play a particularly important role in systemic GBS infection. IL-12 elevation is seen 12–72 h after GBS challenge in the neonatal rat. Pretreatment with a monoclonal antibody against IL-12 results in greater mortality and levels of bacteremia, whereas therapeutic administration of IL-12 results in lower mortality and bloodstream cfu [153].

Incubation of piglet mesenteric arteries with heat-killed GBS produces a marked hyporesponsiveness to noradrenaline, the endothelial cell–derived vasoconstrictor ET-1, and the synthetic TxA_2 analog U46619. This hyporesponsiveness appears to result from enhanced release of nitric oxide (NO), suggesting a role for nitric oxide synthetase (iNOS) induction in the systemic hypotension in GBS sepsis [154]. The GBS-treated pulmonary arteries also exhibited NO-mediated hyporesponsiveness to noradrenaline and ET-1, but responded normally to U46619 [154]. Absence of the TxA_2-induced component of NO-mediated pulmonary hyporesponsiveness might help explain the coexistence of pulmonary hypertension with systemic hypotension during GBS sepsis syndrome.

Some ambiguity exists as to the precise role played by TNF-α in GBS septicemia of the newborn. One can frequently detect TNF-α in the blood, urine, or cerebrospinal fluid of infants with invasive GBS disease [155]. Human mixed mononuclear cell cultures exposed to GBS release TNF-α in a dose- and time-dependent manner; moreover, neonatal monocytes exhibit a larger TNF-α response than adult cells [155]. Infusion of GBS in piglets is associated with TNF-α release during the late phase of hemodynamic response, but the TNF-α inhibitor pentoxiphylline has only modest effects on the ongoing pulmonary hypertension, hypoxemia, and systemic hypotension [156]. Marked improvement in these hemodynamic parameters is seen when pentoxyphilline treatment is combined with indomethicin inhibition of TxB_2 and prostacyclin synthesis [157]. Serum TNF-α levels in the mouse and rat also rise after challenge with GBS, however, administration of polyclonal or monoclonal anti-TNF-α antibody does not affect overall mortality in these models [157,158].

In contrast to Gram-negative pathogens and endotoxin, the specific nature of the GBS component(s) that trigger the host cytokine cascade are less well understood. Cell wall preparations of GBS cause TNF-α release from human monocytes in a manner requiring CD14 and complement receptor types 3 and 4 [159]. The group B polysaccharide and peptidoglycan appear to be significantly greater stimulators of TNF-α release from monocytes than lipotechoic acid or type-specific capsular polysaccharide [160]. Release of IL-1 and IL-6 is also stimulated by soluble GBS cell-wall antigens [161].

Studies using isogenic type III GBS mutants lacking polysaccharide capsule have shown that the presence of capsule has no effect on pro-

duction of TNF-α by human mononuclear cells in vitro [155], and does not change the degree of pulmonary hypertension observed in vivo [75]. In contrast, capsule-deficient mutants of a type Ib GBS strain actually produce a greater degree of pulmonary hypertension than the parent strain in the piglet model [76]. The latter finding implies that the type-specific Ib capsular polysaccharide may actually cloak the GBS cell-wall component responsible for triggering the early phase of the host inflammatory response. This property of GBS capsule may be an important virulence attribute, allowing the organism to multiply and spread beyond a pulmonary focus before adequate host clearance mechanisms are recruited.

Meningitis

Group B streptococcus is the most common cause of neonatal meningitis, and 20% to 30% of surviving infants will be left with major neurological sequelae, including mental retardation, spastic quadriplegia, cortical blindness, deafness, seizures, hydrocephalus, or hypothalamic dysfunction [162,163]. These sequelae may be seen in infants suffering meningitis as a complication of either early or late-onset GBS infection. However, autopsy studies of nonsurvivors show the histopathologic appearance of the central nervous system (CNS) inflammation to vary significantly with infant age. In early-onset meningitis, most cases demonstrate little or no evidence of leptomeningeal inflammation, despite the presence of abundant bacteria, vascular thrombosis, and parenchymal hemorrhage [60,164]. In contrast, infants with late-onset disease usually have diffuse purulent arachnoiditis with prominent involvement of the base of the brain [165]. These histopathologic differences may be attributable to underdevelopment of the host immunologic response in the immediate neonatal period, and the consequent rapid course to death in the setting of overwhelming early-onset septicemia. Similar age-dependent differences in central nervous system pathology are evident in the infant rat model of invasive GBS disease. Older infected animals (11–15 days old) show thickened meninges infiltrated with neutrophils, macrophages, and bacteria. Younger infected animals (5–10 days old) demonstrate numerous GBS distributed in a perivascular pattern within the subarachnoid space, but almost invariably lack an accompanying leukocytic infiltrate [166].

To produce meningitis, GBS must penetrate human brain microvascular endothelial cells (BMEC), the single-cell layer that constitutes the blood-brain barrier. The GBS invasion of tissue culture monolayers of human BMEC was recently demonstrated [167]. Intracellular GBS were found within membrane-bound vacuoles, suggesting that the organism induced its own endocytic uptake. Furthermore, GBS demonstrated transcytosis across intact, polar BMEC monolayers grown on Transwell membranes. Serotype III strains, which account for the majority of CNS isolates, invaded BMEC more efficiently than strains from other common GBS serotypes. At high bacterial densities, GBS invasion of BMEC was accompanied by evidence of cellular injury; this cytotoxicity was correlated to beta-hemolysin production by the organism. It is hypothesized that GBS invasion of BMEC is a primary step in the pathogenesis of meningitis, allowing bacteria access to the CNS by transcytosis or by injury and disruption of the endothelial blood-brain barrier [167].

Some information on the pathogenesis of brain injury in GBS meningitis has emerged from recent animal studies. When GBS meningitis is established by intracisternal injection of the organism in neonatal rats, a vascular distribution of cortical lesions indicates that disturbances of cerebral blood flow are likely to contribute significantly to neural damage [168]. Direct application of GBS to the surface of the brain in adult rats leads to progressive dilation of pial arterioles [169], which is consistent with the intensely hyperemic appearance of the postmortem surface of the brain in human infants [165]. This arteriolar dilation cannot be attributed to cerebrospinal fluid acidosis, but instead is associated with the presence of oxygen free radicals, perhaps a byproduct of the phagocytic killing mechanism of infiltrating leukocytes [169]. Inflammation of individual CNS vessels could lead to focal brain lesions, while diffuse alterations of cerebral blood flow could cause generalized hypoxic/ischemic injury and cerebral edema [168,170]. Ischemic tissue damage in GBS meningitis appears to induce release of the

excitatory amino acid glutamate, which may reach neurotoxic levels in the cerebrospinal fluid and propagate further neuronal injury [171]. Finally, intraventricular injection of GBS in piglets leads to impaired retinal blood flow regulation, indicating that retinal damage and blindness seen in meningitis survivors may also have vasopathogenic origin [172].

In the neonatal rat, simultaneous intracisternal administration of dexamethasone with GBS leads to a marked reduction in subarachnoid inflammation, vasculopathy, and neuronal injury [168]. Dexamethasone may alter the release of proinflammatory cytokines or granulocyte–endothelial cell interactions, thereby attenuating meningeal inflammation [173]. Induction of TNF-α in particular appears to contribute to apoptosis of hippocampal neurons [174] and increases in blood-brain barrier permeability [175] during GBS meningitis in the neonatal rat model. Intraventricular inoculation of newborn piglets with GBS results in an early sharp rise in cerebrospinal fluid TNF-α levels, followed shortly by prostaglandin release and neutrophil influx [176]. The magnitude of the observed TNF-α response and inflammatory cascade is markedly increased when an isogenic nonencapsulated mutant is tested in place of the type III parent strain [176]. These findings suggest that a component of the underlying GBS cell wall and not capsule is responsible for inducing the inflammatory response. A corollary may exist in the Gram-positive meningeal pathogen *Streptococcus pneumoniae*, where studies have shown that intracisternal injection of the purified techoic acid–containing cell wall produces inflammatory changes equivalent to that of live organisms [177,178].

PARADIGM FOR GROUP B STREPTOCOCCAL VIRULENCE STUDIES: TYPE III CAPSULAR POLYSACCHARIDE

Capsule Biochemistry and Host Antibody Response

Group B streptococci associated with human disease are almost invariably encapsulated, belonging to one of the nine recognized capsule serotypes: Ia, Ib, or II–VIII. With minor exceptions, the various GBS capsular polysaccharide antigens are composed of the same four component monosaccharides: glucose, galactose, N-acetylglucosamine, and sialic acid. However, serotype-specific epitopes of each polysaccharide are created by differing arrangement of component sugars into a unique repeating unit [179]. As described earlier, hyperimmune rabbit antisera directed against a given type-specific polysaccharide antigen provide passive protection to mice from lethal challenge with virulent strains from the homologous but not heterologous serotypes. The importance of anticapsular antibody in the host response to GBS infection is further supported by serotype-specific opsonizing activity in phagocytic assays using human neutrophils and macrophages. Finally, seroepidemiologic studies show that a low level of human maternal anticapsular IgG is a major risk factor for development of invasive GBS infections in the neonate [104].

The biochemistry and immunology of GBS capsular polysaccharide has been studied most thoroughly in serotype III organisms, which account for a disproportionate share of neonatal infections. The native type III capsular polysaccharide is a high-molecular-weight polymer composed of more than 100 repeating pentasaccharide units. Each pentasaccharide unit contains a trisaccharide backbone of galactose, glucose, and N-acetylglucosamine with a side chain of galactose and a terminal sialic acid moiety [179,180]. Except for the terminal sialic acid residues, this core polysaccharide is identical to that of pneumococcal type 14 capsule [179]. Sialic acid is known to be a critical element in the epitope of type III GBS polysaccharide capsule that confers protective immunity. After treatment with sialidase, the altered capsular polysaccharide fails to elicit protective antibodies against GBS infection. Moreover, protective antibodies derived from native type III capsule do not bind to the altered (asialo) capsule backbone structure [181]. Human infants who possess antibodies that react only to the desialylated capsule remain at high risk for invasive disease [181].

Proof that Sialylated Type III GBS Capsule Is a Virulence Factor

A correlation between the sialic acid component of type III GBS capsule and animal virulence was first noted in studies employing chemical modification or spontaneous but genetically uncharacterized mutants. Organisms treated with sialidase are opsonized more effectively by complement through the alternative pathway, and are consequently more readily phagocytosed by human neutrophils in vitro [118]. Sialidase treatment of type III GBS results in diminished lethality of the organism upon intravenous administration to neonatal rats [182]. Serial subculture of a wild-type GBS strain in the presence of type III specific antiserum allows identification of mutants that lacked the terminal sialic acid component of the polysaccharide capsule. These mutants possess a 1000-fold greater LD_{50} following tail-vein injection in mice [183].

More direct evidence for the role of type III GBS capsule in virulence is provided by the construction of isogenic capsule-deficient mutants, i.e., mutants differing from the parent strain by only a single trait. This feat has been achieved by means of transposon Tn916 (or Tn916ΔE) mutagenesis [124,184]. Tn916 is a mobile genetic element that can be introduced into GBS via conjugation with a high-frequency donor strain of Enterococcus faecalis, whereupon it inserts itself into (more or less) random locations throughout the recipient chromosome. Tn916 carries an antibiotic resistance marker that allows for selection of GBS possessing one or more chromosomal transposon insertions. Libraries of GBS:Tn916 transconjugates may be screened by immunoblot analysis for alterations in capsule expression. Two major types of type III GBS capsule mutants have been identified by this method. The first mutant phenotype completely lacks evidence of capsular material and fails to react with antisera to type III GBS or to type 14 pneumococcus (which recognizes the asialo core structure of type III capsule) [184,185]. The absence of extracellular capsular polysaccharide in these mutants is confirmed by immune electron microscopy (Fig. 11.3). The second mutant phenotype reacts only with pneumococcal type 14 antisera, and has been shown by structural carbohydrate chemistry to lack specifically the terminal sialic acid residues of the native type III capsule [186].

Southern blot analysis allows enumeration of Tn916 insertions in each capsule mutant, and

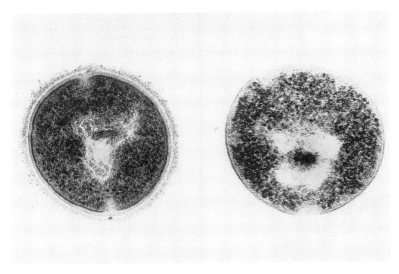

Figure 11.3 Immune electron microscopy of type III GBS wild-type strain (left) and an isogenic nonencapsulated transposon mutant (right). Each bacterium was exposed to IgG against type III capsular polysaccharide, followed by a ferritin-labeled secondary anti-IgG antibody. The transposon mutant lacks detectable extracellular capsule polysaccharide. (From Wessels et al. [85], with permission.)

those possessing a single insertion have been chosen to test the specific role of the sialylated type III capsular polysaccharide using in vitro and in vivo model systems [187]. In comparison to the parent strains, isogenic capsule mutants are susceptible to opsonophagocytosis in the presence of complement and peripheral blood neutrophils [123]. The acapsular mutant binds significantly more complement factor C3 fragments than the parent strain. Moreover, C3 fragments bound to the acapsular mutant are predominantly in the active form, C3b, whereas the inactive form, C3bi, is predominantly bound to the surface of the parent strain. The asialo capsule mutant binds less C3b than the acapsular mutant, and less C3bi than the wild-type strain [123]. These studies demonstrate that type III capsular polysaccharide, and in particular, the sialic acid residues, inhibit the alternative complement pathway by blocking binding of C3 to the organism and promoting inactivation of C3b.

The type III GBS capsule mutants are also significantly less virulent in animal models of GBS infection. In a model of neonatal GBS pneumonia and bacteremia, neonatal rats have been inoculated with either the parent strain or an acapsular mutant by intratracheal injection. In animals who receive the acapsular mutant, fewer GBS are recovered per gram of lung, more

bacteria are associated with resident alveolar macrophages, and the animals become significantly less bacteremic than animals that receive the parent strain [188]. Subcutaneous injection of the acapsular or asialo mutants in neonatal rats results in similar LD_{50} values that are at least 100-fold greater than those obtained with the parent strain [184,185]. Taken together, these data provide compelling evidence that the capsule protects the organism from phagocytic clearance during the initial pulmonary phase and the later bacteremic phase of early-onset GBS infection.

Molecular Genetic Basis of Group B Streptococcal Capsule Expression

The Type III Capsule Gene Locus

In addition to providing capsule-deficient strains for virulence testing, transposon insertional mutagenesis has provided a tool by which several genes responsible for GBS capsule biosynthesis have been identified. DNA sequences flanking the unique transposon insertion sites from the acapsular and asialo mutants have been cloned and used to probe a cosmid library of type III GBS chromosomal DNA in *E. coli* [184,189]. The transposon insertion sites for both types of mutants map to the same 30 kb region of type III chromosome [189,190]. Southern analyses with genomic DNA samples from other clinical isolates indicate that the entire capsule gene region is highly conserved among several GBS strains representing a variety of serotypes [189]. Nucleotide sequence analysis of DNA corresponding to the transposon insertion sites in the acapsular and asialo mutants reveals several open reading frames that share significant homology to polysaccharide capsule synthesis genes of other organisms. It appears these GBS capsule genes are clustered according to specific functions important for the various steps in biosynthesis of the capsule [191], akin to the capsule gene loci of *E. coli* [192] or *Haemophilus influenzae* [193].

Our current understanding of the molecular genetic basis of type III capsule expression in GBS is summarized in Figure 11.4. Several open reading frames have been identified within the capsule gene cluster, including 11 that appear to encode gene products involved in biosynthesis and transport of complex polysaccharides (*cpsA-cpsJ*, *cpsR*) and a twelfth that encodes a transcriptional regulatory element (*lysR*). In the prototype GBS strain COH1, the type III capsule genes are situated in close proximity to a 1442 bp insertion sequence, IS861, which is present in multiple copies throughout the COH1 chromosome [195]. However, at least one other type III GBS strain with an intact capsule gene locus does not possess any copies of IS861 [194]. The GBS capsule genes can be divided into three groups corresponding to different stages in the biosynthesis of capsular polysaccharide [191]. Genes in the first group (*cspE* and *cspF*) participate in monosaccharide synthesis and activation, genes in the second group (*cspD*, *cpsG*, *cpsH*, *cpsI*, and *cpsJ*) appear to be responsible for synthesis of the oligosaccharide repeating unit, and genes in the final group (*cpsR*, *cspA*, *cpsB*, and *cpsC*) are likely involved with polymerization of the oligosaccharide repeating unit and export of the mature capsular polysaccharide to the cell surface.

Monosaccharide Synthesis and Activation

In the first step of microbial capsule biosynthesis, monosaccharides must be endogenously synthesized or scavenged from the environment, then activated with a nucleotide by a condensation reaction before incorporation into the oligonucleotide subunit [195]. Tn916 insertion into open reading frame *cpsF* results in a mutant that produces asialo capsular polysaccharide on its surface [196]. Although this mutant fails to sialylate its capsule, accumulation of free sialic acid is noted intracellularly. This observation suggests a defect, not in synthesis of sialic acid but rather in its subsequent activation to CMP-sialic acid, a reaction catalyzed by CMP-sialic acid synthetase: CTP + sialic acid → CMP-sialic acid + PPi. Indeed, CMP-sialic acid synthetase activity is detectable in the parent strain and all type III isolates [197] but not in the asialo mutant [196]. The interrupted *cpsF* open reading frame shares significant homology with the CMP-sialic acid synthetase gene of *E. coli* K1, *NeuA*. When a recombinant plasmid containing GBS *cpsF* is transformed into an *E. coli* K1 *neuA* mutant, production of the sialylated form of the K1 polysaccharide on the surface of the organism is restored [198]. The 45 kDa *cpsF* gene product has been expressed and catalyses the condensation of CTP with sialic acid to form CMP-sialic acid [198].

Immediately upstream from *cpsF*, but in a different reading frame, is an open reading frame designated *cpsE*. The predicted gene product of *cpsE* is a 20-kDa protein that shares homology with another *E. coli* K1 capsule gene, *neuD* [199]. Mutations in *neuD* abolish capsule polysaccharide in *E. coli* K1; specific GBS *cpsE* mutants have yet to be created. Sequence similarities between *cpsE*, *neuD*, and acetyltransferase enzymes from other bacterial species suggest that the *cpsE* gene product may be involved in transfer of an acetyl group during monosaccharide synthesis—for example, acetylation of N-acetylglucosamine or sialic acid, the two acetylated sugars in the type III polysaccharide [191].

Formation of the Pentasaccharide Repeating Unit

Once the component monosaccharides are synthesized and activated they must be linked by specific glycosidic bonds to form the pentasaccharide repeating unit (Fig. 11.4). Association

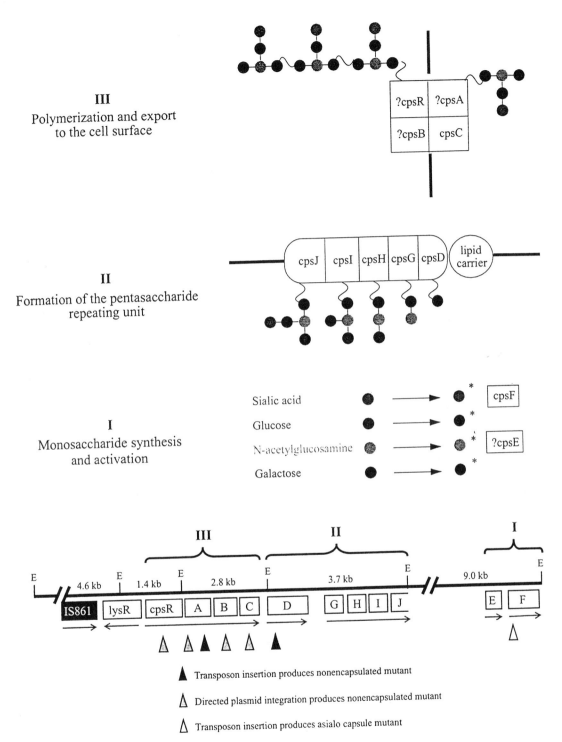

Figure 11.4 The group B streptococcal capsule gene locus and proposed mechanism of polysaccharide capsule biosynthesis.

with a lipid phosphate intermediate is necessary for oligosaccharide subunit synthesis in a number of encapsulated bacteria, including *Salmonella* [200], *E. coli* [201], and *Rhizobium* [202], but is not required for the production of hyaluronic acid capsule in group A streptococcus [203]. Tn916 insertion in the open reading frame *cpsD* abolishes type III capsule production in GBS, and no evidence of oligosaccharide precursors can be found in the cytoplasm, on the surface of the organism, or in supernatant fractions [204]. GBS *cpsD* shows homology to several galactosyl transferase genes, e.g., *rfbP* of *Salmonella* [205], and *exoY* of *Rhizobium* [206], each of which is involved in glycolipid biosynthesis. Using an assay that measures the transfer of galactose from UDP-galactose to a lipid acceptor, the acapsular GBS *cpsD* mutant exhibits decreased galactosyl transferase activity relative to the parent strain [204]. These data suggest that synthesis of type III GBS capsule requires a lipid intermediate, and that mutation of *cpsD* likely prevents transfer of one or both galactose residues into the nascent pentasaccharide subunit [204].

Sequence analysis downstream of *cpsD* identifies four additional open reading frames *cpsG–J*, which share homology with other glycosyl transferases from several organisms (Yim, H.H. and Rubens, C.E., unpublished observations). Glycosyl transferases are often involved in synthesis through lipid intermediates of both prokaryotic and eukaryotic oligo- and polysaccharides. Therefore, the arrangement of these genes may represent an operon reflective of the synthesis order for polymerization of the pentasaccharide repeating unit.

Polymerization of the Oligosaccharide Repeating Unit and Export to the Cell Surface

Once synthesized, the pentasaccharide repeating units must be polymerized into high-molecular-weight capsular polysaccharide and exported to the cell surface (Fig. 11.4). Components of this complex bacterial transport process are only beginning to be understood. In several gram-negative species, ATP-binding cassette (ABC) transporters are a central component of membrane-spanning protein complexes that concurrently polymerize and translocate capsular polysaccharides through sites of inner and outer membrane fusion [207]. Upstream of *cpsD* in the type III GBS capsule locus is an open reading frame designated *cpsC*. Sequence analysis of *cpsC* reveals substantial homology with the gene *exoP* from *Rhizobium meliloti*. *ExoP* belongs to a cluster of genes encoding membrane-spanning proteins important in the polymerization, export, and processing of succinoglycan by *Rhizobium* [208]; in strains expressing a mutated ExoP protein, only low-molecular-weight succinoglycan can be detected [209]. It is possible that *cpsC* and contiguous genes serve a similar function in polymerization and export of the type III GBS capsular polysaccharide [191].

Northern blot and primer extension analysis have shown that *cpsC* is transcribed coordinately with the upstream open reading frames *cpsB*, *cpsA*, and *cpsR* [210]. The nature of the gene products encoded by these genes is unknown, but operon structures identical to *cpsRABC* have recently been identified in the capsule gene clusters of types 19F and 14 pneumococci [211,212] and *Streptococcus thermophilus* [213]. A Tn916 insertion in *cpsA* is associated with a nonencapsulated phenotype [191]. Recently, plasmid integrational mutagenesis has been employed to create targeted knockouts of the *cpsR*, *cpsA*, *cpsB*, and *cpsC* open reading frames. In each case, the resultant GBS mutant fails to produce any immunologically detectable capsular polysaccharide [210].

Regulation of Group B Streptococcal Capsule Expression

Group B streptococci are known to regulate the degree of capsular polysaccharide expression with cell growth rate [214]. Organisms passed on solid growth media become less encapsulated (phase shifting) than when they are passed in animals [215]. Mouse passage of various serotypes of GBS is followed by increases in sialylated capsule content that correlate with increased virulence [216]. Subpopulations of heavily or poorly encapsulated GBS can be subcultured from strains isolated from infected infants [217].

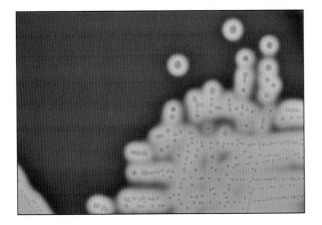

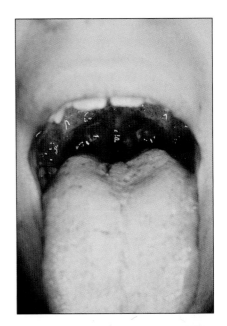

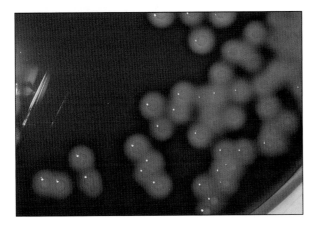

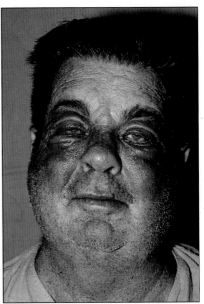

Plate 1. Beta-hemolysis is apparent on a sheep blood-agar plate after overnight incubation. Hemolysis is due to the extracellular toxins streptolysins O and S.

Plate 2. Mucoid colony of *Streptococcus pyogenes*. The larger size of the colony is related to increased hyaluronic acid production and may occur with many M types, although mucoidity recently has been associated mainly with M-type 18 strains. Mucoid colony type may be associated with rheumatic fever.

Plate 3. Pharyngitis. The most common of the group A streptoccal infections, streptococcal pharyngitis typically affects school-aged children, although adults are still highly susceptible. Transmission is through close personal contact, or via saliva droplets produced during sneezing or coughing, with infection rates peaking in the winter months. This slide demonstrates the cardinal manifestations of erythema, pharyngeal exudate, and palatial petechiae. *Courtesy of John Tobin.*

Plate 4. Erysipelas. Characteristic appearance of a salmon red, painful, confluent erythema in a "butterfly" distribution involving the nasal eminence, cheeks, and nose, with abrupt borders along the nasolabial fold. Erythema increases over a course of 3-6 days, and usually resolves in 7-10 days. Erysipelas is associated with high fevers, bacteremia, and possible death, even in modern times. The fluctuation in severity may reflect cyclical changes in the virulence of group A beta-hemolytic streptococci.

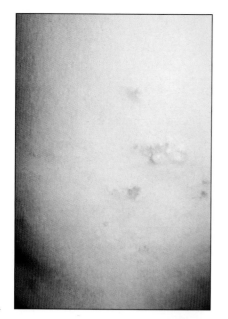

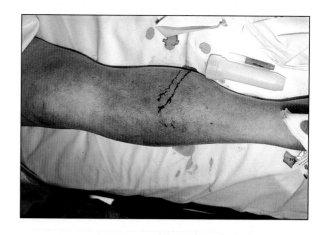

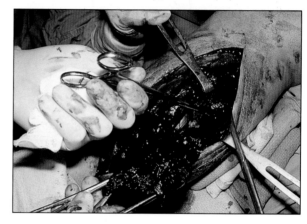

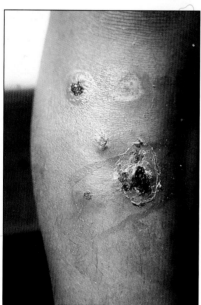

A

B

Plate 5. Streptococcal pyoderma (impetigo). (A) Early vesicular lesions in a toddler from Red Lake, Minnesota. Vesicles like these are infrequently observed by medical personnel. A pure culture of group A streptococci was obtained. (B) More typical purulent, crusted, and healing lesions in a child from Red Lake. The crusted lesions contained a mixed culture of group A streptococcus and *Staphlococcus aureus*.

Plate 6. Necrotizing fasciitis and myositis. The patient had sudden onset of excruciating pain and signs of systemic toxicity. Note the swelling of the leg and two small purple or violaceous bullae on the anterior shin, whereas the adjacent skin appears healthy. The pressures in the anterior and lateral compartments were measured by placing a needle in the deep tissue (hence the blood at the sampling site). Pressures were elevated and surgical exploration was performed. The fascia overlying the deep musculature was friable and brown to dishwater-gray in appearance, establishing a diagnosis of necrotizing fasciitis. Deeper exploration of muscle compartments is warranted in such cases.

Plate 7. Musculature in streptococcal myositis is deep red, reddish-blue, or black. Necrotic muscle must be aggressively debrided.

It is interesting to speculate that GBS may regulate capsule expression in response to the host environment at different stages in the pathogenic process. Nonencapsulated mutants are more adherent and significantly more invasive for respiratory epithelium than the parent strain [10,86]. These findings suggest that the capsule hinders interaction with the epithelial cell surface and/or partially masks important bacterial surface ligands that recognize receptors on the epithelial surface [218]. In mucosal colonization and the early stages of newborn infection, a dynamic balance may exist between producing enough capsule to avoid immune clearance but not so much as to prevent bacterial–epithelial cell interaction [187]. Once the organism invades tissues or circulates in the bloodstream, an up-regulation of GBS capsule expression may then be favored as a means of preventing rapid opsonophagocytic clearance. In vitro, it appears that only brief periods of fast growth are required for up-regulation of *cps* gene-specific mRNAs and expression of high levels of cell-associated capsule [219].

Recent DNA sequence analysis has identified an open reading frame in GBS with homology to the LysR family of transcriptional regulators. The GBS *lysR* gene is situated immediately upstream, but in the opposite orientation to the *cpsRABC* operon [210] (Fig. 11.4). Genes of the LysR family are known to autoregulate their own expression as well as regulate the expression of divergently transcribed genes [220]. Of particular note is the finding that the LysR-family gene *phcA* of the phytopathogen *Pseudomonas sonacearum* regulates transcription of genes encoding for its primary virulence factor, the exopolysaccharide EPS I [221]. In addition, the LysR-related *spvR* regulatory locus of nontyphoidal *Salmonellae* responds to environmental signals to control transcription of several virulence plasmid genes required for production of sustained bacteremia in the mouse model [222]. It remains to be proven whether *lysR* may respond to certain signals in the host environment to regulate nearby genes (*cpsRABC*) involved in expression of surface capsular polysaccharide [210].

OTHER POTENTIAL VIRULENCE FACTORS OF GROUP B STREPTOCOCCUS

C5a Peptidase

A hallmark feature of severe early-onset GBS disease is the poor influx of host neutrophils into sites of tissue infection [50]. The principal compound responsible for attracting neutrophils in humans is C5a, a 74 amino acid cleavage product of C5 that is released when the complement cascade is activated [223]. C5 is synthesized by alveolar epithelial cells and plays an active role in pulmonary inflammation [224]. Hill et al. [134] were the first to report that a majority of GBS strains of diverse serotypes directly inactivate the chemotactic properties of complement-activated human serum. Furthermore, this GBS activity was shown to involve partial degradation of the C5a peptide, as demonstrated by an increase in its mobility on SDS-PAGE [134]. Subsequent availability of recombinant human C5a has allowed more elaborate studies, in which GBS are shown to inactivate C5a by proteolytic cleavage between histidine-67 and lysine-68 near the C-terminus [225]. This finding is consistent with the known critical role of the C-terminus of C5a in activation of human neutrophils as demonstrated by site-directed mutagenesis [226]. Specific interference by GBS with C5a-mediated neutrophil chemotaxis may be an important virulence determinant, serving to delay recruitment of host phagocytic defenses to sites of mucosal colonization or tissue invasion.

The peptidase activity from GBS that inactivates human C5a is normally cell associated, but can be released into the media by treatment of the organism with mutanolysin, a muramidase that solubilizes the cell wall [227,228]. The soluble C5a peptidase activity has been purified to apparent homogeneity by chromatographic methods, revealing an enzyme with a molecular weight of approximately 120,000 Daltons on SDS-PAGE [226]. The GBS C5a peptidase appears to be a serine esterase based on sensitivity to the inhibitor di-isopropyl fluorophosphate [226]. The enzymatic activity of soluble C5a peptidase is completely neutralized by serum from normal human adults, in large part because of naturally occurring IgG antibodies [134]. IgG also neutralizes C5a peptidase on the surface of a capsule-deficient GBS mutant, but fails to neutralize the enzyme on the surface of the intact encapsulated type III parent strain [134]. This suggests that the GBS capsular polysaccharide serves to protect the cell-associated C5a-peptidase from inactivation by naturally occurring antibodies. Finally, the GBS C5a-peptidase is restricted in its ability to inactivate C5a prepared from different mammalian species. While cleaving human and bovine C5a, it fails to abolish the chemoattractant activity of mouse, rat, rabbit, pig, and sheep C5a preparations [229]. Therefore, the most frequently employed animal models of human GBS infection may underestimate the virulence of the organism by omitting the contribution of C5a-peptidase. Recently, an in vivo model employing a C5-deficient mouse strain has been developed to overcome this problem [230]. In this model, GBS expression of C5a-peptidase reduces neutrophil recruitment to the lungs of C5-deficient mice reconstituted with human C5a.

C5a peptidase activity is also associated with group A streptococci (GAS) [231] and group G streptococci [209]. The GAS enzyme is surface bound, cleaves human C5a at histidine-67, and enhances clearance of streptococci from tissue foci of infection in the mouse model [233,234]. Biochemically, the GBS C5a peptidase is distinct from the GAS enzyme, since they migrate differently on SDS-PAGE [228]. However, the complete nucleotide and deduced amino acid sequence of the GBS C5a-peptidase gene (scpB) was recently obtained [235] and found to be highly homologous (97%–98% similarity) to the C5a peptidase genes (scpA) of two GAS species [236,237]. This high degree of similarity between scpA and scpB suggests that either (a) group A and group B streptococci evolved from a common ancestor possessing a peptidase gene, or (b) horizontal transmission of DNA has occurred between these two species of streptococci. Because all of a large panel of GBS clinical strains, representing a variety of serotypes, contained a copy of scpB, horizontal transfer of the gene must be presumed to have preceded evolution of capsular serotypes in GBS [235]. The recombinant gene product of scpB has now been expressed in E. coli and is identical in size

to the enzyme extracted from the parental GBS strain [236]. A C5a-peptidase-deficient mutant strain of GBS has been created by Tn916ΔE mutagenesis, possessing three chromosomal insertions of the transposon, including one in or near the scpB gene [230].

Beta Hemolysin

The vast majority (>98%) of GBS clinical isolates demonstrate beta hemolysis when plated on sheep blood agar [238]. Hemolysin activity is constitutively expressed, requires an energy source, and peaks in the exponential or early stationary phase of growth [239,240]. Some evidence exists to suggest the hemolysin is normally associated with the bacterial surface membrane [241]. The degree of beta-hemolytic activity correlates with the amount of an orange carotenoid like–pigment produced by the organism, suggesting a genetic linkage of the two phenotypes [242]. The GBS hemolysin(s) itself has never been isolated, owing largely to the fact that its activity is unstable. High-molecular-weight carrier molecules such as starch, albumin, Tween 80, or lipotechoic acid are required to preserve hemolysin activity in GBS culture supernatants [239,240,243]. Because the hemolysin does not alter the gel column elution behavior of various carrier molecules, it appears to be a small molecule [243]. Sensitivity to the protease subtilisin suggests that it is a protein [239], but attempts to raise antibody against crude preparations have been unsuccessful [244].

A potential role for beta-hemolysin in lung epithelial injury has been demonstrated by the development of GBS transposon mutants expressing either a nonhemolytic (NH) or hyperhemolytic (HH) phenotype [61]. When monolayers of human alveolar epithelial cells are exposed to log-phase GBS or stabilized hemolysin extracts of GBS cultures, cellular injury can be assessed by release of the cytoplasmic enzyme, lactate dehydrogenase (LDH). Whereas NH strains produce no detectable injury beyond baseline (media alone), hemolysin-producing strains induce LDH release from lung epithelial cells in direct correlation to their ability to lyse sheep erythrocytes [61]. The extent of LDH release produced by HH strains is reduced in a stepwise fashion when dipalmitoyl phosphatidylcholine (DPPC), the major component of human surfactant [245], is added in concentrations corresponding to the physiologic increase in alveolar fluid DPPC during the third trimester of pregnancy [61]. This finding provides a theoretical rationale for the increased incidence of severe GBS pneumonia in premature, surfactant-deficient neonates [61,246]. The DPPC inhibition of hemolysin-associated injury may also help explain why mechanically ventilated, preterm rabbits administered GBS intratracheally have less pronounced inflammatory changes on histologic examination of lung tissue when treated with exogenous surfactant [247].

Beta hemolysin also appears to play a role in GBS-induced injury of pulmonary endothelium. Hyperhemolytic mutants produce a greater degree, and NH mutants a lesser degree, of LDH release from lung endothelial cells in tissue culture [62]. Disruption of the integrity of an entire polar endothelial cell monolayer is demonstrated by increased directional passage of albumin upon exposure to the HH GBS mutant [62]. The GBS injury to cultured lung epithelial and endothelial cells can be documented at bacterial concentrations of 10^6 (most hemolytic clinical isolate) to 10^8 (least hemolytic clinical isolate) GBS per milliliter [61,62]. When GBS pneumonia is induced in newborn primates, bacterial density reaches 10^9 to 10^{11} per gram of lung tissue [59], indicating that an ample local reservoir exists for beta-hemolysin production and host cell injury.

Electron microscopic studies of A549 cell monolayers exposed to HH GBS mutants reveal global loss of microvillus architecture, disruption of cytoplasmic and nuclear membranes, and marked swelling of the cytoplasm and organelles (Fig. 11.5; [61]). These findings suggest that the beta hemolysin acts as a pore-forming cytolysin, similar to the alpha toxin of Staph. aureus [248] or the terminal membrane attack complex (C5b-9) of human complement [249]. Earlier studies have shown that radiolabeled rubidium ($^{86}Rb^+$) and hemoglobin exhibit identical efflux kinetics from sheep red blood cells exposed to GBS beta-hemolysin, an indication that the toxin produces membrane lesions of large size [250].

The requirement of GBS beta-hemolysin expression for animal virulence is being investigated. A NH transposon mutant of GBS demon-strates equal virulence to the type III parent strain following subcutaneous injection in neonatal rats [64]. The parent and NH mutant also elicit comparable degrees of thromboxane-associated pulmonary hypertension following intravenous infusion in neonatal piglets [75]. It is important to note that each of these modes of administration bypasses the initial pulmonary alveolar stage of neonatal infection. If instead the bacterial inoculum is delivered directly into the rat lung by transthoracic puncture, a different NH GBS transposon mutant exhibits a 1000-fold increased LD_{50} over that of a wild type strain [63]. Using intranasal inoculation, a comparison of chemically derived NH and HH GBS mutants shows that increased beta-hemolytic activity is associated with a decreased LD_{50} and an earlier time to death for a given inoculum [251]. Taken together, these data suggest a unique role for beta-hemolysin expression in GBS disease acquired via the respiratory tract. Potential systemic effects of GBS hemolysin, however, cannot be discounted. As an example, intravenous administration of filter-purified GBS beta-hemolysin extracts to rabbits or rats produces dose-dependent hypotensive changes and a limited number of deaths due to shock, findings not seen with streptolysin S from Streptococcus pyogenes [252].

The molecular basis of GBS beta-hemolysin expression has yet to be defined. Comparative analysis of highly concentrated, purified protein extracts from isogenic GBS hemolysin mutants permits polyacrylamide gel electrophoresis resolution of an 11-kDa candidate beta-hemolysin protein absent in NH mutants and overexpressed by HH mutants [63]. In genetic studies, a recombinant plasmid containing GBS chromosomal DNA conferred a beta-hemolytic phenotype on host E. coli, and allowed identification of a putative GBS beta-hemolysin gene encoding a protein of 230 amino acids [253]. However, when an intragenic fragment of this gene sequence is used to create targeted knockouts in two wild-type GBS strains through homologous recombination and plasmid integrational mutagenesis, hemolytic activity is unaffected, indicating that the gene does not encode the major GBS beta-hemolysin determinant [63]. Analysis of a random plasmid integrational mutant library of GBS for non-

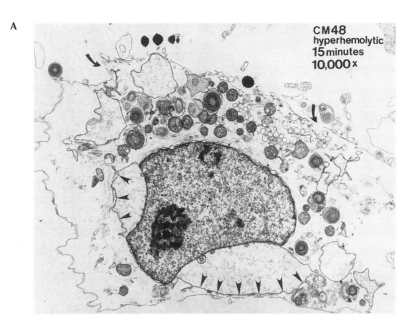

A   CM48
hyperhemolytic
15 minutes
10,000 ×

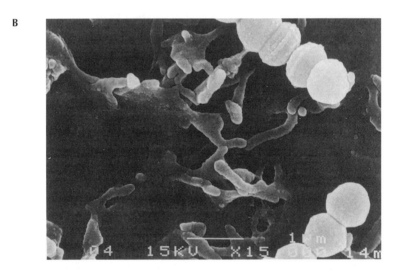

B

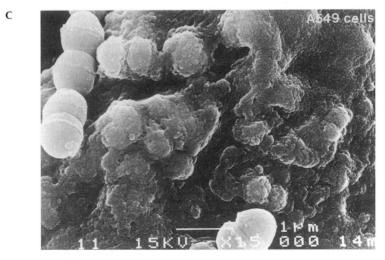

C   A549 cells

hemolytic isolates has identified a genetic locus involved in beta-hemolysin expression [254]. Three open reading frames encoding proteins with significant homologies to prokaryotic multidrug-resistance ABC transporters were sequenced. Targeted knockout of two of these open reading frames reproduced the NH phenotype, confirming that an ABC transporter-type function is required for the hemolytic activity of GBS.

Lipotechoic Acid

The amphiphilic molecule lipotechoic acid (LTA) is a component of most Gram-positive bacteria. A glycerol-phosphate (GP) polymer that extends through the peptidoglycan layer of the cell wall, LTA is attached to the cytoplasmic membrane via hydrophobic interactions between its glycolipid anchor and the cytoplasmic membrane [255]. The LTA of GBS averages about 22 GP units in length and contains complex lipids and short-chain fatty acid [20]. Inhibition of GBS peptidoglycan synthesis with penicillin enhances LTA synthesis and release into the culture media, whereas inhibition of protein synthesis with chloramphenicol inhibits synthesis of LTA and results in its depletion from the cell surface [256]. Clinical isolates of GBS from infants with early- or late-onset invasive disease possess significantly higher levels of cell-associated LTA than strains from asymptomatically colonized infants, suggesting that LTA may participate somehow in disease pathogenesis [257]. The LTA purified from GBS is cytotoxic for a variety of human cell monolayers in tissue culture, including human embryonic brain and human embryonic amnion cells [17,20]. The potential contribution of soluble LTA to GBS-induced tissue injury is uncertain, however, since little LTA is released from the cytoplasmic membrane under normal growth conditions [258].

Lipotechoic acid is known to mediate host cell attachment by other Gram-positive pathogens, including GAS [259,260]. Certain experimental evidence seems to suggest that LTA also participates in GBS adherence to host tissues. Topical administration of LTA or GP decreases GBS vaginal colonization of pregnant mice [21]. Binding of GBS to human buccal epithelial cells is significantly inhibited by preincubation with purified LTA, but not by preincubation with the group B or type III polysaccharide antigens [18]. Moreover, GBS with high levels of LTA bind more efficiently to buccal cells of fetal rather than adult origin, suggesting a potential link to the age-restricted susceptibility to GBS disease [18]. Studies with ^{3}H-labeled purified LTA indicate that binding to adult cells involves only hydrophobic interactions with the lipid portion of the polymer, while binding to fetal cells involves hydrophobic as well as specific interactions due to the glycerolphosphate backbone [261]. Strain differences in fetal buccal cell binding appear to be attributable to longer LTA chains (30–35 GP units) in strains isolated from infants with invasive disease than LTA chains (10–12 GP units) from asymptomatically colonized infants [261]. Mild enzymatic treatment of the fetal buccal epithelial cells with trypsin or periodate abolishes LTA binding, suggesting the presence of a glycoprotein receptor(s) not present on human adult buccal epithelial cells [261].

In contrast, purified LTA does not competitively inhibit binding of GBS to cultured human amnion cells [20] or alveolar epithelial cells [10]. In these studies, the human cells are present in a solid-phase monolayer, which allows more vigorous washing and results in lower levels of adherence (0.01% to 0.2%) than calculated in the liquid-phase buccal cell assays (4% to 95%). It is possible, therefore, that LTA mediates a relatively low-affinity interaction with human cells not detected in solid-phase assays [10]. Alternatively, one may consider that cultured cell lines

Figure 11.5 Group B streptococcal beta-hemolysin-associated injury to alveolar epithelial cells. (*A*) Transmission electron micrograph of epithelial cell exposed to hyperhemolytic GBS mutant demonstrates discrete cytoplasmic membrane disruptions, splitting of the nuclear membrane, loss of cytoplasmic density and clumping of nuclear chromatin. Scanning electron microscopic comparison of weakly hemolytic parent strain (*B*) with hyperhemolytic mutant (*C*) reveals loss of microvillus architecture and bleb formation on the cell surface. Pattern of injury suggests the beta-hemolysin acts as a pore-forming cytolysin. (From Nizet et al. [61], with permission.)

are known to differ widely in their expression of the extracellular matrix glycoprotein fibronectin [262], which acts as an LTA receptor for GAS on oropharyngeal cells [263]. As GBS are likewise capable of adhering to fibronectin attached to a solid phase [23], it is possible that experimental differences in the contribution of LTA to binding are related to variations in the amount of cell-associated fibronectin [19]. Finally, exfoliated buccal cells may not express the same array of potential surface receptors as epithelial cells of the chorioamnion and/or lower respiratory tract.

Surface Protein Antigens

Group B streptococci express three major surface protein antigens, c, R, and Rib, which can be purified following HCl extraction or mutanolysin digestion of the cell wall [264,265]. The surface localization of proteins C and R is confirmed by the use of ferritin-labeled polyclonal rabbit antisera, which reveal filamentous projections external to the cell wall upon electron microscopic examination [266]. The precise role of surface protein antigens in GBS pathogenesis and protective immunity to GBS disease has yet to be defined. It is important to note that (1) expression of these surface proteins varies significantly among the different GBS capsular serotypes, and (2) no single protein antigen is expressed by all strains within a given serotype [267].

The C antigen of GBS is a protein complex consisting of two distinct components: alpha, which is sensitive to the protease trypsin, and beta, which is trypsin-resistant [268,269]. The alpha component is expressed as a series of proteins that demonstrate a laddering pattern on immunoblots and vary greatly in molecular weight (14 kDa to 145 kDa) among GBS strains [264,270,271]. Large, identical, tandem repeat units make up 74% of the DNA sequence in the alpha-antigen gene and are likely to play a role in generating the size diversity observed in alpha-antigen expression [272]. The beta component of C protein is typically expressed as a single 130 kDa protein capable of binding human IgA, although smaller non-IgA-binding variants are seen in some strains [128,273]. Determination of the nucleotide sequence of the complete

beta antigen gene shows that it encodes a polypeptide typical of other Gram-positive cell-wall proteins [274]. There is a long signal sequence of 37 amino acids at the N-terminus. Four of the five C-terminal amino acid residues are basic and are preceded by a hydrophobic stretch that appears to anchor the C-terminus in the cell membrane. The IgA-binding activity can be localized to two distinct regions of the beta antigen by analysis of subfragments expressed as fusion proteins [274].

Overall, one or both components of the c protein are found in approximately 60% of GBS clinical isolates [269,275]. More specifically, all Ib strains possess at least one of the C protein components, with 84% exhibiting both of them. All Ic strains contain C protein, but 96% possess only the alpha component. Of the 59% of type II strains with C protein, 81% lack the beta component. In marked contrast, C protein components are found in less than 1% of type III strains [275].

Mounting evidence suggests that C protein may contribute to GBS virulence. Type II strains possessing both the alpha and beta components of C protein produce significantly higher mortality in the infant rat model than type II strains lacking C protein [264]. In vitro studies showed that type II strains without C protein were more easily killed than C protein–positive strains in an opsonophagocytic bactericidal assay [126]. This limitation in phagocytosis of alpha and beta containing type II strains is not due to differential uptake by the neutrophils, since the organisms are efficiently internalized, but rather to an apparent defect in intracellular killing [127]. Protection against phagocytosis may reflect nonimmune binding of IgA by the beta component [128], which appears to interfere sterically with deposition of opsonically active complement protein C3 on the GBS surface [127]. Inactivation of the alpha antigen gene (bca) by allelic replacement resulted in a five- to seven-fold attenuation in lethality in the mouse model compared with the isogenic wild-type strain [276].

The C protein also appears to represent an important target of the host humoral immune response to GBS. Hyperimmune rabbit antisera against the purified alpha and beta components of C protein are highly protective against lethal type II/C protein–positive GBS infection in neonatal rats [264]. Antisera raised in rabbits against *E. coli* containing plasmid clones of the alpha and beta C protein antigens provides protective immunity to mice challenged by GBS strains carrying the C proteins, but not to those mice challenged by non–C-protein-bearing strains [270]. A mouse monoclonal antibody identifies a protective epitope on the alpha antigen that is encoded within the tandem repeats of its genetic sequence [270,272]. Active immunization of adult female mice with the C protein beta antigen prior to mating subsequently confers protection against lethal infection with beta-positive GBS to their offspring [277]. Finally, antibodies to the alpha component of C protein did not passively protect neonatal mice from lethal challenge with the *bca* gene knockout mutant, suggesting that the antigen is a target for protective immunity [276].

The R protein antigens of GBS resemble the alpha component of C protein in a number of respects: the presence of multiple molecular-weight forms, resistance to trypsin, lack of binding of human IgA, and immunogenicity in a variety of animal species [270,271,278]. R proteins are also found in GAS and other streptococci, and can be classified into four species (R1, R2, R3, and R4) based on immunoprecipitin reaction patterns in agarose [279]. Overall, more than one-third of GBS isolates express R antigen, predominantly species R4 [280]. Production of the R protein and the alpha component of C protein appear to be mutually exclusive. For example, 80% of type II strains without alpha antigen contain R protein, compared to 0% of the type II/alpha antigen–positive strains. R protein is also common in type III strains (71%), which characteristically lack C protein components [280]. R proteins from GBS are immunogenic in rabbits and antibodies to them can be detected in adult and newborn infant human sera [281,282]. Administration of R protein antibodies to mice protects them against challenge with type II but not type III GBS bearing the R protein [283]. However, seroepidemiologic data suggest that adequate levels of anti-R protein IgG may be crucial in preventing invasive infection in human neonates with type II or type III GBS that bear the R antigen [281].

Protein Rib is a recently described trypsin-resistant, size-variable surface antigen of GBS found in a large proportion of type III strains [265]. Rabbit antiserum against Rib passively protects mice against lethal infection with Rib-expressing strains [265], as does active immunization of the mice with highly purified preparations of Rib [284]. The GBS Rib protein, R proteins, and alpha component of C protein are structurally related and define a family of streptococcal surface proteins with extremely repetitive structures [285]. Still another surface protein antigen of analogous structure and protective immunogenicity has now been identified in 63% of type V GBS [286]. It is possible that with further biochemical characterization, this protein and the Rib protein may actually prove to be R proteins or other repetitive alpha-like molecules.

Hyaluronate Lyase

Group B streptococci secrete a protein that degrades hyaluronic acid, an important component of the extracellular matrix in higher organisms. This enzyme had been misidentified as a neuraminidase in the earlier literature [287–289], but its true substrate specificity was confirmed when the cleavage product was shown to be an α,β-unsaturated disaccharide derivative of hyaluronic acid by anion-exchange chromatography and electron impact mass spectrometry [290]. Characterization of the purified enzyme reveals that it degrades hyaluronic acid by a novel mechanism compared to that of other known hyaluronidases, making an initial random cut in the hyaluronan chain and then progressively moving along the chain, releasing disaccharide units [291]. The GBS hyaluronate lyase gene has been cloned and expressed in *E. coli*, and shares 50.7% amino acid identity with the pneumococcal hyaluronidase [292].

Hyaluronate lyase is expressed in increased levels by type III GBS isolates [288], and strains obtained from neonates with bloodstream infections produced higher levels of the enzyme than strains from asymptomatically colonized infants [287] or adults with noninvasive disease [293]. In strains lacking hyaluronate lyase activity, a novel insertional element, IS1548 may be found within the structural gene [295]. The biological role of the hyaluronate lyase in GBS pathogenesis remains uncertain. Theoretically, breakdown of hyaluronic acid in the extracellular matrix could facilitate tissue spread by the organism [291]. High concentrations of hyaluronic acid in term placentas and preterm amniotic fluid may represent important targets for hyaluronate lyase during the course of infection, in which case it could act as a scavenger enzyme. Interference of normal immune system function by hyaluronate lyase is also possible, since human macrophages, neutrophils, and lymphocytes express the CD44 receptor that binds specifically to hyaluronan [294]. Lymphocyte adherence to endothelial cells is inhibited by bovine testicular and fungal hyaluronidases [296], and presumably would also be sensitive to the GBS hyaluronate lyase [291].

CAMP Factor

The CAMP phenomenon, named after the original investigators Christie, Atkins, and Munch-Peterson [297], refers to synergistic hemolysis zones produced by colonies of GBS streaked adjacent to colonies of *Staph. aureus* on sheep blood agar. Group B streptococcal CAMP factor is an extracellular protein of 23.5 Kda that further unstabilizes and lyses erythrocyte membranes pretreated with beta toxin, a staphylococcal sphingomyelinase [298]. CAMP factor is released from log-phase GBS cultures into the media, and is capable of binding weakly to the Fc region of human IgG and IgM [299]. The complete amino acid sequence of CAMP factor has been determined, and partial sequence homology exists with the Fc-binding regions of *Staph. aureus* protein A [300]. The CAMP factor gene (*cfb*) has been cloned and expressed in *E. coli* [301], and the recombinant protein elicits antibodies that inhibit the CAMP phenomenon [302].

It has been postulated that CAMP factor protein could contribute to GBS virulence, either by toxic activity against cell membranes or through nonimmune binding to circulating antibodies. Human erythrocytes, like sheep erythrocytes, have not been observed to undergo hemolysis with CAMP factor alone. The limited evidence for direct toxicity comes from experiments in which partially purified CAMP factor preparation produces mortality in rabbits

when injected intravenously [303]. In the mouse model, however, data favor a role for CAMP factor in resistance to immune clearance. Mice treated with a sublethal dose of GBS but then injected with purified CAMP factor develop septicemia and die [304]. However, neither CAMP factor alone nor various peptide fragments of the CAMP factor coadministered with the bacteria result in similar mortality.

Proteases

Group B streptococcal proteolytic activity has been identified in culture supernatants, but no correlation exists between the proteolytic activity of a given strain and its virulence in a mouse model [305]. Recently, a cell-associated collagenase activity of GBS was postulated [36]. Antibodies raised against collagenase from *Clostridium histolyticum* cross-reacted with cell-associated proteins produced by GBS and inhibited GBS hydrolysis of a synthetic peptide collagen analogue [36]. Disruption of collagen fibrils could theoretically play a role in GBS penetration of the chorioamnion and premature rupture of membranes. However, when the gene for this enzyme (*pep*B) was cloned, sequenced, and expressed, it was found incapable of solubilizing a film of reconstituted rat tail collagen [306]. Rather, it appears to be a zinc metallopeptidase capable of degrading a variety of small bioactive peptides (e.g., bradykinin, neurotensin).

Nucleases

In agar diffusion studies, 74 of 75 GBS strains tested exhibited deoxyribonuclease activity [307]. Three nucleases of differing molecular weight and electrophoretic mobility have been isolated and purified, each of which is capable of digesting RNA as well as DNA substrates. The GBS nucleases differ immunologically from nucleases of GAS. Neutralizing antibodies against the GBS nucleases are found in human sera and are more prevalent in pregnant women colonized with GBS and in their infants [307]. The role of these enzymes in disease pathogenesis has not been studied.

Platelet Aggregation Factor

Certain type III strains of GBS promote platelet aggregation [308,309]. The GBS platelet aggregating activity is trypsin-sensitive, which suggests the participation of specific bacterial proteins [310]. Whole-cell fractionation allows partial purification of a fibrinogen-binding activity that has been termed clumping factor [311]. The clumping factor fraction appears to be capable of inducing fatal disseminated intravascular coagulation in mice [312], but the results must be viewed cautiously since such preparations contain multiple cell components including the type III polysaccharide antigen.

Opacity Variants

Group B streptococci exhibit high-frequency variation in the colonial opacity, and the transition from transparent to opaque correlates with an increase in bacterial chain length [313]. Transparent and opaque variants differ in several ways, including capsular architecture, buoyant density, and cell-surface protein profile and growth in Todd-Hewitt media [313]. Compared to transparent forms, opaque GBS are less immunogenic, more susceptible to neutrophil killing, and less virulent in newborn mice [314]. Transparent, opaque, or mixed cultures of GBS can be directly isolated from humans [314], but the significance of opacity phase-shifting in the pathogenesis of GBS disease is not known.

Group B Streptococcal "Toxin"

Extensive fractionation from large volumes of GBS culture supernatant has led to identification of a noncapsular, high-molecular-weight polysaccharide that induces certain features of GBS sepsis symptomatology when injected into animals, including pulmonary hypertension, increased vascular permeability, and neutrophil trapping [72,315]. Analysis of this putative GBS "toxin" reveals it to be a mannan with a repeating unit of nine mannose residues and phosphodiester-linked mannosyl moiety essential for biologic activity [316]. The potential cellular location or mode of production of this substance is not known. As mannans have not previously been described in streptococcal capsules or cell walls, further studies must be done to rigorously prove that the toxin originates from GBS and is not a component present in the complex growth media.

SUMMARY

Group B streptococcal infection represents a complex interaction between the bacterial pathogen and the susceptible newborn. Human infants exhibit several well-documented deficiencies in host defense mechanisms, creating an environment in which a variety of potential GBS virulence factors are revealed. Chief among these is the polysaccharide surface capsule, whose role in pathogenesis has been established by the creation of specific isogenic mutants defective in capsule expression. These mutants are more susceptible to opsonophagocytosis and exhibit decreased virulence in animal models. The transposon insertion sites identified show a specific chromosomal locus containing numerous genes involved in capsule biosynthesis. The alpha component of the C protein antigen has been cloned and sequenced, and targeted mutagenesis demonstrates that the gene product contributes to virulence and is also a target of protective immunity. Another virulence attribute, the C5a-peptidase, has been characterized genetically and biochemically, and demonstrated to impair neutrophil recruitment both in vitro and in vivo; final confirmation of its role in GBS pathogenesis awaits construction and thorough testing of isogenic mutants lacking C5a-peptidase activity. Studies using isogenic mutants with altered beta-hemolysin expression indicate that it may contribute to lung injury in GBS pneumonia, but to date, neither the hemolysin molecule nor its structural gene have been identified. Recent advances in molecular genetic techniques applicable to Gram-positive bacteria should allow (1) more in-depth molecular analyses of these and other potential GBS virulence factors (e.g., hyaluronate lyase), (2) identification of novel virulence factors involved in complex pathogenic processes such as host cell adherence and invasion, and (3) construction of specific GBS mutants for virulence testing in relevant animal models of GBS disease. A fundamental understanding of GBS pathogenesis at the molecular level will provide invaluable information toward rational design of therapeutic and immunoprophylactic strategies to combat this foremost of neonatal infections.

REFERENCES

1. Ferrieri P, Cleary PP, Seeds AE. Epidemiology of group-B streptococcal carriage in pregnant women and newborn infants. J Med Microbiol 1977; 10:103–114.
2. Siegel JD, McCracken GH, Threlkeld N, Milvenan B, Rosenfeld CR. Single-dose penicillin prophylaxis against neonatal group B streptococcal infections. A controlled trial in 18,738 newborn infants. N Engl J Med 1980; 303:769–775.
3. Lewin E, Amstey MS. Natural history of group B streptococcus colonization and its therapy during pregnancy. Am J Obstet Gynecol 1981; 139:512–515.
4. Boyer KM, Gotoff SP. Strategies for chemoprophylaxis of GBS early-onset infections. Antibiot Chemother 1985; 35:267–280.
5. Ancona RJ, Ferrieri P, Williams PP. Maternal factors that enhance the acquisition of group B streptococci by newborn infants. J Med Microbiol 1980; 13:273–280.
6. Pass MA, Gray BM, Khare S, Dillon HC. Prospective studies of group B streptococcal infections in infants. J Pediatr 1979; 95:437–443.
7. Sobel JD, Myers P, Levison ME, Kaye D. Comparison of bacterial and fungal adherence to vaginal exfoliated epithelial cells and human vaginal epithelial tissue culture cells. Infect Immun 1982; 35:697–701.
8. Jelinkova J, Grabovskaya KB, Ryc M, Bulgakova TN, Totolian AA. Adherence of vaginal and pharyngeal strains of group B streptococci to human vaginal and pharyngeal epithelial cells. Zentralbl Bakteriol Mikrobiol Hyg A 1986; 262:492–499.
9. Zawaneh SM, Ayoub EM, Baer H, Cruz AC, Spellacy WN. Factors influencing adherence of group B streptococci to human vaginal epithelial cells. Infect Immun 1979; 26:441–447.
10. Tamura GS, Kuypers JM, Smith S, Raff H, Rubens CE. Adherence of group B streptococci to cultured epithelal cells: roles of environmental factors and bacterial surface components. Infect Immun 1994; 62:2450–2458.
11. Bulgakova TN, Grabovskaya KB, Ryc M, Jelinkova J. The adhesin structures involved in the adherence of group B streptococci to human vaginal cells. Folia Microbiol Praha 1986; 31:394–401.
12. Badri MS, Zawaneh S, Cruz AC, Mantilla G, Baer H, Spellacy WN, Ayoub EM. Rectal colonization with group B streptococcus: relation to vaginal colonization of pregnant women. J Infect Dis 1977; 135:308–312.
13. Galask RP, Varner MW, Petzold CR, Wilbur SL. Bacterial attachment to the chorioamniotic membranes. Am J Obstet Gynecol 1984; 148:915–928.
14. Broughton RA, Baker CJ. Role of adherence in the pathogenesis of neonatal group B streptococcal infection. Infect Immun 1983; 39:837–843.
15. Kallman J, Schollin J, Hakansson S, Andersson A, Kihlstrom E. Adherence of group B streptococci to human endothelial cells in vitro. APMIS 1993; 101:403–408.
16. Wibiwan IWT, Lammler C, Pasaribu FH. Role of hydrophobic surface proteins in mediating adherence of group B streptococci to epithelial cells. J Gen Microbiol 1992; 138:1237–1242.
17. Miyazaki S, Leon O, Panos C. Adherence of Stretococcus agalactiae to synchronously growing human cell monolayers without lipotechoic acid involvement. Infect Immun 1988; 56:505–512.
18. Nealon TJ, Mattingly SJ. Role of cellular lipoteichoic acids in mediating adherence of serotype III strains of group B streptococci to human embryonic, fetal, and adult epithelial cells. Infect Immun 1984; 43:523–530.
19. Teti G, Tomasello F, Chiofalo MS, Orefici G, Mastroeni P. Adherence of group B streptococci to adult and neonatal epithelial cells mediated by lipotechoic acid. Infect Immun 1987; 55:3057–3064.
20. Goldschmidt JC, Panos C. Techoic acids of Streptococcus agalactiae: chemistry, cytotoxicity, and effect on bacterial adherence to human cells in tissue culture. Infect Immun 1984; 43:670–677.
21. Cox F, Taylor L, Eskew EK, Mattingly SJ. Prevention of group B streptococcal colonization and bacteremia in neonatal mice with topical vaginal inhibitors. J Infect Dis 1993; 167:1118–1122.
22. Westerlund B, Korhonen TK. Bacterial proteins binding to the mammalian extracellular matrix. Mol Microbiol 1993; 9:687–694.
23. Tamura GS, Rubens CE. Group B streptococci adhere to a variant of fibronectin attached to a solid phase. Mol Microbiol 1995; 15:581–589.
24. Zabel LT, Neuer A, Manncke B. Fibronectin binding and cell surface hydrophobicity contribute to adherence properties of group B streptococci. Zentralbl Bakteriol 1996; 285:35–43.
25. Butler KM, Baker CJ, Edwards MS. Interaction of soluble fibronectin with group B streptococci. Infect Immun 1987; 55:2404–2408.
26. Spellerberg B, Rozdzinski E, Martin S, Lutticken R. Two-component regulatory system

controls fibrinogen binding of group B streptococci. ASM Conference on Streptococcal Genetics, Vichy, France. Washington, DC: American Society for Microbiology 1998; Abstract 2C-14.

27. Spellerberg B, Rozdzinski E, Martin S, Weber-Heynemann J, Schnitzler N, Lutticken R, Dodbielski A. Lmb, a protein with similarities to the LraI adhesin family, mediates attachment of streptococcus agalactiae to human laminin. Infect Immun 1999; 67:871–878.

28. Centers for Disease Control. Prevention of perinatal group B streptococcal disease: a public health perspective. MMWR Morb Mortal Wkly Rep 1996; 45:1–24.

29. Stewardson-Krieger PB, Gotoff SP. Risk factors in early-onset neonatal group B streptococcal infections. Infection 1978; 6:50–53.

30. Tseng PI, Kandall SR. Group B streptococcal disease in neonates and infants. N Y State J Med 1974; 74:2169–2173.

31. Hemming VG, London WT, Curfman BL, Patrick DF, Fischer GW. Maternal humoral immunity and neonatal GBS infection: studies in a primate model. Antibiot Chemother 1985; 35:194–200.

32. Evaldson GR, Malmborg AS, Nord CE. Premature rupture of the membranes and ascending infection. Br J Obstet Gynaecol 1982; 89:793–801.

33. Evaldson GR, Malmborg AS, Nord CE, Ostensson K. *Bacteroides fragilis, Streptococcus intermedius* and group B streptococci in ascending infections of pregnancy. An animal experimental study. Gynecol Obstet Invest 1983; 15:230–241.

34. Moller M, Thomsen AC, Borch K, Dinesen K, Zdravkovic M. Rupture of fetal membranes and premature delivery associated with group B streptococci in urine of pregnant women. Lancet 1984; 2(8394):69–70.

35. Schoonmaker J, Lawellin DW, Lunt B, McGregor JA. Bacteria and inflammatory cells reduce chorioamniotic membrane integrity and tensile strength. Obstet Gynecol 1989; 74:590–596.

36. Jackson RJ, Dao ML, Lim DV. Cell-associated collagenolytic activity by group B streptococci. Infect Immun 1994; 62:5647–5651.

37. Sbarra AJ, Thomas GB, Cetrulo CL, Shakr C, Chaudhury A, Paul B. Effect of bacterial growth on the bursting pressure of fetal membranes in vitro. Obstet Gynecol 1987; 70:107–110.

38. Lamont RF, Rose MP, Elder MG. Effect of bacterial products on prostaglandin E production by amnion cells. Lancet 1985; 2(8468):131–1333.

39. Bennett PR, Rose MP, Myatt L, Elder MG. Preterm labor: stimulation of arachidonic acid metabolism in human amnion cells by bacterial products. Am J Obstet Gynecol 1987; 156:649–655.

40. Gomez R, Ghezzi F, Romero R, Munoz H, Tolosa JE, Rojas I. Premature labor and intraamniotic infection. Clinical aspects and role of the cytokines in diagnosis and pathophysiology. Clin Perinatol 1995; 22:281–342.

41. Dudley DJ, Edwin SS, Van Wagoner J, Augustine NH, Hill HR, Mitchell MD. Regulation of decidual cell chemokine production by group B streptococci and purified bacterial cell wall components. Am J Obstet Gynecol 1997; 177:666–672.

42. Eickhoff TC, Klein JO, Daly AK, Ingal P, Finland M. Neonatal sepsis and other infections due to group B beta-hemolytic streptococci. N Engl J Med 1964; 271:1221–1228.

43. Katzenstein AL, Davis C, Braude A. Pulmonary changes in neonatal sepsis to group B beta-hemolytic *Streptococcus:* relation of hyaline membrane disease. J Infect Dis 1976; 133:430–435.

44. Helmig R, Halaburt JT, Uldbjert N, Thomsen AC, Stenderup A. Increased cell adherence of group B streptococci from preterm infants with neonatal sepsis. Obstet Gynecol 1990; 76:825–827.

45. Baker CJ. Early onset group B streptococcal disease. J Pediatr 1978; 93:124–125.

46. Baker CJ, Edwards MS. Group B streptococcal infections. Perinatal impact and prevention methods. Ann N Y Acad Sci 1998; 549:193–202.

47. Cochi SL, Feldman RA. Estimating national incidence of group B streptococcal disease: the effect of adjusting for birth weight [letter]. Pediatr Infect Dis 1983; 2:414–415.

48. Cox F, Taylor L. Adherence of group B streptococci to buccal epithelial cells in neonates with different gestational ages. J Perinat Med 1990; 18:455–458.

49. Payne NR, Burke BA, Day DL, Christensen PD, Thompson TR, Ferrieri P. Correlation of clinical and pathologic findings in early onset neonatal group B streptococcal infection with disease severity and prediction of outcome. Pediatr Infect Dis J 1988; 7:836–847.

50. Hemming VG, McCloskey DW, Hill HR. Pneumonia in the neonate associated with group B streptococcal septicemia. Am J Dis Child 1976; 130:1231–1233.

51. Vollman JH, Smith WL, Ballard ET, Light IJ. Early onset group B streptococcal disease: clinical, roentgenographic, and pathologic features. J Pediatr 1976; 89:199–203.

52. Ablow RC, Driscoll SG, Effmann EL, Effman EL, Gross I, Jolles CJ, Uauy R, Warshaw JB. A comparison of early-onset group B streptococcal neonatal infection and the respiratory-distress syndrome of the newborn. N Engl J Med 1976; 294:65–70.

53. Pinnas JL, Strunk RC, Fenton LJ. Immunofluorescence in group B streptococcal infection and idiopathic respiratory distress syndrome. Pediatrics 1979; 63:557–561.

54. Martin TR, Rubens CE, Wilson CB. Lung antibacterial defense mechanisms in infant and adult rats: implications for the pathogenesis of group B streptococcal infections in the neonatal lung. J Infect Dis 1988; 157:91–100.

55. Sherman M, Goldstein E, Lippert W, Wennberg R. Group B streptococcal lung infection in neonatal rabbits. Pediatr Res 1982; 16:209–212.

56. Sherman MP, Lehrer RI. Oxidative metabolism of neonatal and adult rabbit lung macrophages stimulated with opsonized group B streptococci. Infect Immun 1985; 47:26–30.

57. Sherman MP, Johnson JT, Rothlein R, Hughes BJ, Smith CW, Anderson DC. Role of pulmonary phagocytes in host defense against group B streptococci in preterm versus term rabbit lung. J Infect Dis 1992; 166:818–826.

58. Pauly TH, Aziz SM, Horstman SJ, Gillespie MN. Impact of prostaglandin and thromboxane synthesis blockade on disposition of group B streptococcus in lung and liver of intact piglet. Pediatr Res 1992; 31:14–17.

59. Rubens CE, Raff HV, Jackson JC, Chi EY, Bielitzki JT, Hillier SL. Pathophysiology and histopathology of group B streptococcal sepsis in *Macaca nemestrina* primates induced after intraamniotic inoculation: evidence for bacterial cellular invasion. J Infect Dis 1991; 164:320–330.

60. Quirante J, Ceballos R, Cassady-G. Group B beta-hemolytic streptococcal infection in the newborn. I. Early onset infection. Am J Dis Child 1974; 128:659–665.

61. Nizet V, Gibson RL, Chi EY, Framson PE, Hulse M, Rubens CE. Group B streptococcal hemolysin expression is associated with injury of lung epithelial cells. Infect Immun 1996; 64:3818–3826.

62. Gibson RL, Nizet V, Rubens CE. Group B streptococcal β-hemolysin promotes injury of lung microvascular endothelial cells. Pediatr Res 1999; 45:626–634.

63. Nizet V, Gibson RL, Rubens CE. The role of GBS β-hemolysin expression in newborn lung injury. Adv Exp Med 1997; 418:627–630.

64. Weiser JN, Rubens CE. Transposon mutagenesis of group B streptococcus beta-hemolysin biosynthesis. Infect Immun 1987; 55:2314–2316.

65. Herting E, Jarstrand C, Rasool O, Curstedt T, Sun B, Robertson B. Experimental neonatal group B streptococcal pneumonia: effect of a modified porcine surfactant on bacterial proliferation in ventilated near-term rabbits. Pediatr Res 1994; 35:784–791.

66. Herting E, Sun B, Jarstrand C, Curstedt T, Robertson B. Surfactant improves lung function and mitigates bacterial growth in immature ventilated rabbits with experimentally induced neonatal group B streptococcal pneumonia. Arch Dis Child Fetal Neonatal Edit 1997; 76:F3–8.

67. Khammash H, Perlman M, Wojtulewicz MB, Dunn M. Surfactant therapy in full-term neonates with severe respiratory failure. Pediatrics 1993; 92:135–139.

68. Auten RL, Notter RH, Kendig JW, Davis JM, Shapiro DL. Surfactant treatment of full-term newborns with respiratory failure. Pediatrics 1991; 87:101–107.

69. Gortner L, Pohlandt F, Bartmann P. Bovine surfactant in full-term neonates with adult respiratory distress syndrome-like disorders. Pediatrics 1994; 93:538.

70. LeVine AM, Bruno MD, Huelsman KM, Ross GF, Whitsett JA, Korfhagen TR. Surfactant protein A–deficient mice are susceptible to group B streptococcal infection. J Immunol 1997; 158:4336–4340.

71. Hertig E, Strayer DS, Jarstrand C, Sun B, Robertson B. Lung function and bacterial proliferation in experimental neonatal pneumonia in ventilated rabbits exposed to monoclonal antibody to surfactant protein B. Lung 1998; 176:123–131.

72. Rojas J, Larsson LE, Hellerqvist CG, Brigham KL, Gray ME, Stahlman MT. Pulmonary hemodynamic and ultrastructural changes associated with group B streptococcal toxemia in adult sheep and newborn lambs. Pediatr Res 1983; 17:1002–1008.

73. McFall TL, Zimmerman GA, Augustine NH, Hill HR. Effect of group B streptococcal type-specific antigen on polymorphonuclear leukocyte function and polymorphonuclear leukocyte–endothelial cell interaction. Pediatr Res 1987; 21:517–523.

74. Bowdy BD, Aziz SM, Marple SL, Yoneda K, Pauly TH, Coonrod JD, Gillespie MN. Organ-specific disposition of group B streptococci in piglets: evidence for a direct interaction with target cells in the pulmonary circulation. Pediatr Res 1990; 27:344–348.

75. Gibson RL, Redding GJ, Truog WE, Henderson WR, Rubens CE. Isogenic group B streptococci devoid of capsular polysaccharide or beta-hemolysin: pulmonary hemodynamic and gas exchange effects during bacteremia in piglets. Pediatr Res 1989; 26:241–245.

76. Philips JB, Li JX, Gray BM, Pritchard DG, Oliver JR. Role of capsule in pulmonary hypertension induced by group B streptococcus. Pediatr Res 1992; 31:386–390.

77. Bowdy BD, Marple SL, Pauly TH, Coonrod JD, Gillespie MN. Oxygen radical-dependent bacterial killing and pulmonary hypertension in piglets infected with group B streptococci. Am Rev Respir Dis 1990; 141:648–653.

78. Gibson RL, Soderland C, Henderson WR, Chi EY, Rubens CE. Group B streptococci (GBS) injure lung endothelium in vitro: GBS invasion and GBS-induced eicosanoid production is greater with microvascular than with pulmonary artery cells. Infect Immun 1995; 63:271–279.

79. Schreiber MD, Covert RF, Torgerson LJ. Hemodynamic effects of heat-killed group B beta-hemolytic streptococcus in newborn lambs: role of leukotriene D4. Pediatr Res 1992; 31:121–126.

80. Pinheiro JM, Pitt BR, Gillis CN. Roles of platelet-activating factor and thromboxane in group B streptococcus-induced pulmonary hypertension in piglets. Pediatr Res 1989; 26:420–424.

81. Isberg RR, Falkow S. A single genetic locus encoded by *Yersinia pseudotuberculosis* permits invasion of cultured animal cells by *Escherichia coli* K-12. Nature 1985; 317:262–264.

82. Finlay BB, Heffron F, Falkow S. Epithelial cell surfaces induce *Salmonella* proteins required for bacterial adherence and invasion. Science 1989; 243:940–943.

83. Rubens CE, Smith S, Hulse M, Chi EY, van Belle G. Respiratory epithelial cell invasion by group B streptococci. Infect Immun 1992; 60:5157–5163.

84. Devenish JA, Schiemann DA. HeLa cell infection by *Yersinia enterocolitica:* evidence for lack of intracellular multiplication and development of a new procedure for quantitative expression of infectivity. Infect Immun 1981; 32:48–55.

85. Valentin-Weigand P, Jungnitz H, Zock A, Rohde M, Chhatwal GS. Characterization of group B streptococcal invasion in HEp-2 epithelial cells. FEMS Microbiol Lett 1997; 147:69–74.

86. Hulse ML, Smith S, Chi EY, Pham A, Rubens CE. Effect of type III group B streptococcal capsular polysaccharide on invasion of respiratory epithelial cells. Infect Immun 1993; 61:4835–4841.

87. Gibson RL, Lee MK, Soderland C, Chi EY, Rubens CE. Group B streptococci invade endothelial cells: type III capsular polysaccharide attenuates invasion. Infect Immun 1993; 61:478–485.

88. Valentin-Weigand P, Chhatwal GS. Correlation of epithelial cell invasiveness of group B streptococci with clinical source of isolation. Microb Pathog 1995; 19:83–91.

89. Lapenta D, Framson P, Nizet V, Rubens CE. Epithelial cell invasion by GBS is important for virulence. Adv Exp Med 1997; 418:631–634.

90. Shigeoka AO, Hall RT, Hemming VG, Allred CD, Hill HR. Role of antibody and complement in opsonization of group B streptococci. Infect Immun 1978; 21:34–40.

91. Anderson DC, Hughes BJ, Edwards MS, Buffone GJ, Baker CJ. Impaired chemotaxigenesis by type III group B streptococci in neonatal sera: relationship to diminished concentration of specific anticapsular antibody and abnormalities of serum complement. Pediatr Res 1983; 17:496–502.

92. Edwards MS, Nicholson-Weller A, Baker CJ, Kasper DL. The role of specific antibody in alternative complement pathway-mediated opsonophagocytosis of type III, group B streptococcus. J Exp Med 1980; 151:1275–1287.

93. Santos JI, Shigeoka AO, Hill HR. Functional leukocyte administration in protection against experimental neonatal infection. Pediatr Res 1980; 14:1408–1410.

94. Lopez-Osuna M, Kretschmer RR. Bactericidal kinetics of newborn polymorphonuclear leukocytes against group B streptococci type III. Infection 1984; 12:367–368.

95. Shigeoka AO, Charette RP, Wyman ML, Hill HR. Defective oxidative metabolic responses of neutrophils from stressed neonates. J Pediatr 1981; 98:392–398.

96. Wilson CB, Weaver WM. Comparative susceptibility of group B streptococci and *Staphylococcus aureus* to killing by oxygen metabolites. J Infect Dis 1985; 152:323–329.

97. Cornacchione P, Scaringi L, Fettucciari K, Rosati E, Sabatini R, Orefici G, von Hunolstein C, Modesti A, Modica A, Mincelli F, Marconi P. Group B streptococci persist inside macrophages. Immunology 1998; 93:86–95.

98. Wheeler JG, Chauvenet AR, Johnson CA, Dillard R, Block SM, Boyle R, Abramson JS. Neutrophil storage pool depletion in septic, neutropenic neonates. Pediatr Infect Dis 1984; 3:407–409.

99. Christensen RD, MacFarlane JL, Taylor NL, Hill HR, Rothstein G. Blood and marrow neutrophils during experimental group B streptococcal infection: quantification of the stem cell, proliferative, storage and circulating pools. Pediatr Res 1982; 16:549–553.

100. Zeligs BJ, Armstrong CD, Walser JB, Bellanti JA. Age-dependent susceptibility of neonatal rats to group B streptococcal type III infection: correlation of severity of infection and response of myeloid pools. Infect Immun 1982; 37:255:263.

101. Christensen RD, Hill HR, Rothstein G. Granulocytic stem cell (CFUc) proliferation in experimental group B streptococcal sepsis. Pediatr Res 1983; 17:278–280.

102. Kallman J, Schollin J, Schalen C, Erlandsson A, Kihlstrom E. Impaired phagocytosis and opsonisation towards group B streptococci in preterm neonates. Arch Dis Child Fetal Neonat Edit 1998; 78:F46–50.

103. Lancefield RC, McCarty M, Everly WN. Multiple mouse-protective antibodies directed against group B streptococci. Special reference to antibodies effective against protein antigens. J Exp Med 1975; 142:165–179.

104. Baker CJ, Kasper DL. Correlation of maternal antibody deficiency with susceptibility to neonatal group B streptococcal infection. N Engl J Med 1976; 294:753–756.

105. Baker CJ, Edwards MS, Kasper DL. Role of an-

tibody to native type III polysaccharide of group B streptococcus in infant infection. Pediatrics 1981; 68:544–549.

106. Boyer KM, Papierniak CK, Gadzala CA, Parvin JD, Gotoff SP. Transplacental passage of IgG antibody to group B streptococcus serotype Ia. J Pediatr 1984; 104:618–620.

107. Gotoff SP, Papierniak CK, Klegerman ME, Boyer KM. Quantitation of IgG antibody to the type-specific polysaccharide of group B streptococcus type Ib in pregnant women and infected infants. J Pediatr 1984; 105:628–630.

108. Gray BM, Pritchard DG, Dillon HC. Seroepidemiological studies of group B streptococcus type II. J Infect Dis 1985; 151:1073–1080.

109. Morell A, Sidiropoulos D, Herrmann U, Sidiropoulos D, Herrmann U, Christenson KK, Christensen P, Prellner K, Fey H, Skvaril F. IgG subclasses and antibodies to group B streptococci, pneumococci, and tetanus toxoid in preterm neonates after intravenous infusion of immunoglobulin to the mothers. Pediatr Res 1986; 20:933–936.

110. Larsen JW, Harper JS, London WT. Antibody to type III group B streptococcus in the rhesus monkey. Am J Obstet Gynecol 1983; 146:958–962.

111. Baltimore RS, Baker CJ, Kasper DL. Antibody to group B streptococcus type III in human sera measured by a mouse protection test. Infect Immun 1981; 32:56–61.

112. Rodewald AK, Onderdonk AB, Warren HB, Kasper DL. Neonatal mouse model of group B streptococcal infection. J Infect Dis 1992; 166:635–639.

113. Anthony BF, Concepcion NF, Opsonic activity of human IgG and IgM antibody for type III group B streptococci. Pediatr Res 1989; 26:383–387.

114. Shyur SD, Raff HV, Bohnsack JF, Kelsey DK, Hill HR. Comparison of the opsonic and complement triggering activity of human monoclonal IgG1 and IgM antibody against group B streptococci. J Immunol 1992; 148:1879–1884.

115. Hill HR, Shigeoka AO, Hall RT, Hemming VG. Neonatal cellular and humoral immunity to group B streptococci. Pediatrics 1979; 64:787.

116. Levy NJ, Kasper DL. Antibody-independent and -dependent opsonization of group B *Streptococcus* requires the first component of complement C1. Infect Immun 1985; 49:19–24.

117. Baker CJ, Webb BJ, Kasper DL, Edwards MS. The role of complement and antibody in opsonophagocytosis of type II group B streptococci. J Infect Dis 1986; 154:47–54.

118. Edwards MS, Kasper DL, Jennings HJ, Baker CJ, Nicholson-Weller A. Capsular sialic acid prevents activation of the alternative complement pathway by type III, group B streptococci. J Immunol 1982; 128:1278–1283.

119. Edwards MS, Buffone GJ, Fuselier PA, Weeks JL, Baker CJ. Deficient classical complement pathway activity in newborn sera. Pediatr Res 1983; 17:685–688.

120. Davis AE, Zalut C, Rosen FS. Human factor D of the alternative complement pathway. Physicochemical characteristics and N-terminal amino acid sequence. Biochemistry 1979; 18:5082–5087.

121. Campbell JR, Baker CJ, Edwards MS. Influence of serotype of group B streptococci on C3 degradation. Infect Immun 1992; 60:4558–4562.

122. Smith CL, Pritchard DG, Gray BM. Role of polysaccharide capsule in C3 deposition by type Ib group B streptococci (GBS) In: Program and Abstracts of the 31st Interscience Conference on Antimicrobial Agents and Chemotherapy. Washington, DC: American Society for Microbiology, 1991; Abstract 450.

123. Marques MB, Kasper DL, Pangburn MK, Wessels MR. Prevention of C3 deposition by capsular polysaccharide is a virulence mechanism of type III group B streptococci. Infect Immun 1992; 60:3986–3993.

124. Rubens CE, Wessels MR, Kuypers JM, Kasper DL, Weiser JN. Molecular analysis of two group B streptococcal virulence factors. Semin Perinatol 1990; 14:22–29.

125. Campbell JR, Baker CJ, Edwards MS. Deposition and degradation of C3 on type III group B streptococci. Infect Immun 1991; 59:1978–1983.

126. Payne NR, Ferrieri P. The relation of the Ibc protein antigen to the opsonization differences between strains of type II group B streptococci. J Infect Dis 1985; 151:672–681.

127. Payne NR, Kim YK, Ferrieri P. Effect of differences in antibody and complement requirements on phagocytic uptake and intracellular killing of "C" protein–positive and –negative strains of type II group B streptococci. Infect Immun 1987; 55:1243–1251.

128. Russell-Jones GJ, Gotschlich EC, Blaker MS. A surface receptor specific for human IgA on group B streptococci possessing the Ibc protein antigen. J Exp Med 1984; 160:1467–1475.

129. Smith CL, Baker CJ, Anderson DC, Edwards MS. Role of complement receptors in opsonophagocytosis of group B streptococci by adult and neonatal neutrophils. J Infect Dis 1990; 162:489–495.

130. Bruce MC, Baley JE, Medvik KA, Berger M. Impaired surface membrane expression of C3bi but not C3b receptors on neonatal neutrophils. Pediatr Res 1987; 21:306–311.

131. Noya FJ, Baker CJ, Edwards MS. Neutrophil Fc receptor participation in phagocytosis of type III group B streptococci. Infect Immun 1993; 61:1415–1420.

132. Hall MA, Edwards MS, Baker CJ. Complement and antibody participation in opsonophagocyto-

sis of type IV and V group B streptococci. Infect Immun 1992; 60:5030–5035.

133. Hall MA, Hickman ME, Baker CJ, Edwards MS. Complement and antibody in neutrophil-mediated killing of type V group B streptococcus. J Infect Dis 1994; 170:88–93.

134. Hill HR, Bohnsack JF, Morris EZ, Augustine NH, Parker CJ, Cleary PP, Wu JT. Group B streptococci inhibit the chemotactic activity of the fifth component of complement. J Immunol 1988; 141:3551–3556.

135. Rowen JL, Smith CW, Edwards MS. Group B streptococci elicit leukotriene B4 and interleukin-8 from human monocytes: neonates exhibit a diminished response. J Infect Dis 1995; 172:420–426.

136. Hill HR, Shigeoka AO, Augustine NH, Pritchard D, Lundblad JL, Schwartz RS. Fibronectin enhances the opsonic and protective activity of monoclonal and polyclonal antibody against group B streptococci. J Exp Med 1984; 159:1618–1628.

137. Jacobs RF, Kiel DP, Sanders ML, Steele RW. Phagocytosis of type III group B streptococci by neonatal monocytes: enhancement by fibronectin and gammaglobulin. J Infect Dis 1985; 152:695–700.

138. Patterson LE, Baker CJ, Rench MA, Edwards MS. Fibronectin and age-limited susceptibility to type III, group B streptococcus. J Infect Dis 1988; 158:471–474.

139. Domula M, Bykowska K, Wegrzynowicz Z, Lopaciuk S, Weissbach G, Kopec M. Plasma fibronectin concentrations in healthy and septic infants. Eur J Pediatr 1985; 144:49–52.

140. Kim KS, Wass CA, Hong JK, Concepcion NF, Anthony BF. Relative functional activity of purified human immunoglobulin G against a type III group B streptococcal strain. Infect Immun 1986; 52:908–910.

141. Smith LM, Laganas V, Pistole TG. Attachment of group B streptococci to macrophages is mediated by a 21-kDa protein. FEMS Immunol Med Microbiol 1998; 20:89–97.

142. Baker CJ, Webb BJ, Kasper DL, Yon MD, Beachler CW. The natural history of group B streptococcal colonization in the pregnant woman and her offspring. II. Determination of serum antibody to capsular polysaccharide from type III, group B streptococcus. Am J Obstet Gynecol 1980; 137:39–42.

143. Hemming VG, O'Brien WF, Fischer GW, Golden SM, Noble SF. Studies of short-term pulmonary and peripheral vascular responses induced in oophorectomized sheep by the infusion of a group B streptococcal extract. Pediatr Res 1984; 18:266–269.

144. Gibson RL, Truog WE, Henderson WR, Redding GJ. Group B streptococcal sepsis in piglets: effect of combined pentoxifylline and indomethacin pretreatment. Pediatr Res 1992; 31:222–227.

145. Peevy KJ, Chartrand SA, Wiseman HJ, Boerth RC, Olson RD. Myocardial dysfunction in group B streptococcal shock. Pediatr Res 1985; 19:511–513.

146. Peevy KJ, Panus P, Longenecker GL. Prostaglandin synthetase inhibition in group B streptococcal shock: hematologic and hemodynamic effects. Pediatr Res 1986; 20:864–866.

147. O'Brien WF, Golden SM, Bibro MC, Charkobardi PK, Davis SE, Hemming VG. Short-term responses in neonatal lambs after infusion of group B streptococcal extract. Obstet Gynecol 1985; 65:802–806.

148. Tarpey MN, Graybar GB, Lyrene RK, Godoy G, Oliver J, Gray BM, Phillips JB. Thromboxane synthesis inhibition reverses group B streptococcus-induced pulmonary hypertension. Crit Care Med 1987; 15:644–647.

149. Goldberg RN, Suguihara C, Streitfeld MM, Bancalari A, Clark MR, Bancalari E. Effects of a leukotriene antagonist on the early hemodynamic manifestations of group B streptococcal sepsis in piglets. Pediatr Res 1986; 20:1004–1008.

150. Dinarello CA. The role of interleukin-1 in host responses to infectious diseases. Infect Agents Dis 1992; 1:227–236.

151. Vallette JD, Goldberg RN, Suguihara C, Del Moral T, Martinez O, Lin J, Thompson RC, Bancalori E. Effect of an interleukin-1 receptor antagonist on the hemodynamic manifestations of group B streptococcal sepsis. Pediatr Res 1995; 38:704–708.

152. Rosati E, Fettucciari K, Scaringi L, Cornacchione P, Sabatini R, Mezzasoma L, Rossi R, Marconi P. Cytokine response to group B streptococcus infection in mice. Scand J Immunol 1998; 47:314–323.

153. Mancuso G, Cusumano V, Genovese F, Gambuzza M, Beninati C, Teti G. Role of interleukin-12 in experimental neonatal sepsis caused by group B streptococci. Infect Immun 1997; 65:3731–3735.

154. Villamor E, Perez-Vizcaino F, Tamargo J, Moro M. Effects of group B streptococcus on responses to U46619, endothelin-1, and noradrenaline in isolated pulmonary and mesenteric arteries of piglets. Pediatr Res 1996; 40:827–333.

155. Williams PA, Bohnsack JF. Augustine NH, Drummond WK, Rubens CE, Hill HR. Production of tumor necrosis factor by human cells in vitro and in vivo, induced by group B streptococci. J Pediatr 1993; 123:292–300.

156. Gibson RL, Redding GJ, Henderson WR, Truog WE. Group B streptococcus induces tumor necrosis factor in neonatal piglets. Effect of the tumor necrosis factor inhibitor pentoxifylline on hemodynamics and gas exchange. Am Rev Respir Dis 1991; 143:598–604.

157. Teti G, Mancuso G, Tomasello F, Chiofalo MS.

Production of tumor necrosis factor-alpha and interleukin-6 in mice infected with group B streptococci. Circ Shock 1992; 38:138–144.

158. Teti G, Mancuso G, Tomasello F. Cytokine appearance and effects of anti-tumor necrosis factor alpha antibodies in a neonatal rat model of group B streptococcal infection. Infect Immun 1993; 61:227–235.

159. Medvedev AE, Flo T, Ingalls RR, Golenbock DT, Teti G, Vogel SN, Espevik T. Involvement of CD14 and complement receptors CR3 and CR4 in nuclear factor-kappa B activation and TNF production induced by lipopolysaccharide and group B streptococcal cell walls. J Immunol 1998; 160:4535–4542.

160. Vallejo JG, Baker CJ, Edwards MS. Roles of the bacterial cell wall and capsule in induction of tumor necrosis factor alpha by type III group B streptococci. Infect Immun 1996; 64:5042–5046.

161. von Hunolstein C, Totolian A, Alfarone G, Mancuso G, Cusumano V, Teti G, Orefici G. Soluble antigens from group B streptococci induce cytokine production in human blood cultures. Infect Immun 1997; 65:4017–4021.

162. Chin KC, Fitzhardinge PM. Sequelae of early-onset group B hemolytic streptococcal neonatal meningitis. J Pediatr 1985; 106:819–822.

163. Edwards MS, Rench MA, Haffar AA, Murphy MA, Desmond MM, Baker CJ. Long-term sequelae of group B streptococcal meningitis in infants. J Pediatr 1985; 106:717–722.

164. Franciosi RA, Knostman JD, Zimmerman RA. Group B streptococcal neonatal and infant infections. J Pediatr 1973; 82:707–718.

165. Berman PH, Banker BQ. Neonatal meningitis. A clinical and pathological study of 29 cases. Pediatrics 1966; 38:6–24.

166. Ferrieri P, Burke B, Nelson J. Production of bacteremia and meningitis in infant rats with group B streptococcal serotypes. Infect Immun 1980; 27:1023–1032.

167. Nizet V, Kim KS, Stins M, Jonas M, Chi EY, Nguyen D, Rubens CE. Invasion of brain microvascular endothelial cells by group B streptococci. Infect Immun 1997; 65:5074–5081.

168. Kim YS, Sheldon RA, Elliott BR, Liu Q, Ferriero DM, Tauber MG. Brain injury in experimental neonatal meningitis due to group B streptococci. J Neuropathol Exp Neurol 1995; 54:531–539.

169. McKnight AA, Keyes WG, Hudak ML, Jones MD. Oxygen free radicals and the cerebral arteriolar response to group B streptococci. Pediatr Res 1992; 31:640–644.

170. Wahl M, Unterberg A, Baethmann A, Schilling L. Mediators of blood-brain barrier dysfunction and formation of vasogenic brain edema. J Cereb Blood Flow Metab 1988; 8:621–634.

171. Leib SL, Kim YS, Ferriero DM, Tauber MG. Neuroprotective effect of excitatory amino acid antagonist kynurenic acid in experimental bacterial meningitis. J Infect Dis 1996; 173: 166–171.

172. Bottoli I, Beharry K, Modanlou HD, Norris K, Ling E, Noya F, Amato MM, Aranda JV. Effect of group B streptococcal meningitis on retinal and choroidal blood flow in newborn pigs. Invest Ophthalmol Vis Sci 1995; 36:1231–1239.

173. Saez-Llorens X, Jafari HS, Severien C, Parras F, Olsen KD, Hansen EJ, Singer II, McCracken GH. Enhanced attenuation of meningeal inflammation and brain edema by concomitant administration of anti-CD18 monoclonal antibodies and dexamethasone in experimental Haemophilus meningitis. J Clin Invest 1991; 88:2003–2011.

174. Bogdan I, Leib SL, Bergeron M, Chow L, Tauber MG. Tumor necrosis factor-alpha contributes to apoptosis in hippocampal neurons during experimental group B streptococcal meningitis. J Infect Dis 1997; 176:693–697.

175. Kim KS, Wass CA, Cross AS. Blood-brain barrier permeability during the development of experimental bacterial meningitis in the rat. Exp Neurol 1997; 145:253–257.

176. Ling EW, Noya FJ, Ricard G, Beharry K, Mills EL, Aranda JV. Biochemical mediators of meningeal inflammatory response to group B streptococcus in the newborn piglet model. Pediatr Res 1995; 38:981–987.

177. Tuomanen E, Liu H, Hengstler B, Zak O, Tomasz A. The induction of meningeal inflammation by components of the pneumococcal cell wall. J Infect Dis 1985; 151:859–868.

178. Tauber MG, Burroughs M, Niemoller UM, Kuster H, Borschberg U, Tuomanen E. Differences of pathophysiology in experimental meningitis caused by three strains of Streptococcus pneumoniae. J Infect Dis 1991; 163:806–811.

179. Wessels MR, Pozsgay V, Kasper DL, Jennings HJ. Structure and immunochemistry of an oligosaccharide repeating unit of the capsular polysaccharide of type III group B streptococcus. A revised structure for the type III group B streptococcal polysaccharide antigen. J Biol Chem 1987; 262:8262–8267.

180. Jennings HJ, Lugowski C, Kasper DL. Conformational aspects critical to the immunospecificity of the type III group B streptococcal polysaccharide. Biochemistry 1981; 20:4511–4518.

181. Kasper DL, Baker CJ, Baltimore RS, Crabb JH, Schiffman G, Jennings HJ. Immunodeterminant specificity of human immunity to type III group B streptococcus. J Exp Med 1979; 149:327–339.

182. Shigeoka AO, Rote NS, Santos JI, Hill HR. Assessment of the virulence factors of group B streptococci: correlation with sialic acid content. J Infect Dis 1983; 147:857–863.

183. Yeung MK, Mattingly SJ. Isolation and characterization of type III group B streptococcal mu-

tants defective in biosynthesis of the type-specific antigen. Infect Immun 1983; 42:141–151.

184. Rubens CE, Wessels MR, Heggen LM, Kasper DL. Transposon mutagenesis of type III group B streptococcus: correlation of capsule expression with virulence. Proc Natl Acad Sci USA 1987; 84:7208–7212.

185. Wessels MR, Rubens CE, Benedi VJ, Kasper DL. Definition of a bacterial virulence factor: sialylation of the group B streptococcal capsule. Proc Natl Acad Sci USA 1989; 86:8983–8987.

186. Wessels MR, Benedi VJ, Kasper DL, Heggen LM, Rubens CE. The type II capsule and virulence of group B streptococcus. In: Dunny GM, Cleary PP, McKay LL (eds). Genetics and Molecular Biology of Streptococci, Lactococci, and Enterococci. Washington, DC: American Society for Microbiology, 1991; 219–223.

187. Rubens CE. Type III capsular polysaccharide of group B streptococci: role in virulence and the molecular basis of capsule expression. In: Miller VL, Kaper JB, Portnoy DA, Isberg RR (eds). Molecular Genetics of Bacterial Pathogenesis. Washington, DC: American Society for Microbiology, 1994; 327–339.

188. Martin TR, Ruzinski JT, Rubens CE, Chi EY, Wilson CB. The effect of type-specific polysaccharide capsule on the clearance of group B streptococci from the lungs of infant and adult rats. J Infect Dis 1992; 165:306–314.

189. Kuypers JM, Heggen LM, Rubens CE. Molecular analysis of a region of the group B streptococcus chromosome involved in type III capsule expression. Infect Immun 1989; 57:3058–3065.

190. Rubens CE, Kuypers JM, Heggen LM, Kasper DL, Wessels MR. 1991. Molecular analysis of the group B streptococcal capsule genes. In: Dunny GM, Cleary PP, McKay LL (eds). Genetics and Molecular Biology of Streptococci, Lactococci, and Enterococci. Washington, DC: American Society for Microbiology, 1991; 179–183.

191. Rubens CE, Haft RF, Wessels MR. Characterization of the capsular polysaccharide genes of group B streptococci. In: Ferretti JJ, Gilmore MS, Klaenhammer TR, Brown F, (eds). Genetics of Streptococci, Enterococci and Lactococci. Dev Biol Stand. 1995; 85:237–244.

192. Boulnois GJ, Roberts IS, Hodge R, Hardy KR, Jann KB, Timmis KN. Analysis of the K1 capsule biosynthesis genes of Escherichia coli: definition of three functional regions for capsule production. Mol Gen Genet 1987; 208:242–246.

193. Kroll JS, Loynds BM, Moxon ER. The Haemophilus influenzae capsulation gene cluster: a compound transposon. Mol Microbiol 1991; 5:1549–1560.

194. Rubens CE, Heggen LM, Kuypers JM. IS861, a group B streptococcal insertion sequence related to IS150 and IS3 of Escherichia coli. J Bacteriol 1989; 171:5531–5553.

195. Sutherland IW. Biosynthesis of microbial exopolysaccharides. Adv Microb Physiol 1982; 23:79–150.

196. Wessels MR, Haft RF, Heggen LM, Rubens CE. Identification of a genetic locus essential for capsule sialylation in type III group B streptococci. Infect Immun 1992; 60:392–400.

197. Haft RF, Wessels MR. Characterization of CMP-N-acetylneuraminic acid synthetase of group B streptococci. J Bacteriol 1994; 176:7372–7374.

198. Haft RF, Wessels MR, Mebane MF, Conaty N, Rubens CE. Characterization of cpsF and its product CMP-N-acetylneuraminic acid synthetase, a group B streptococcal enzyme that can function in K1 capsular polysaccharide biosynthesis in Escherichia coli. Mol Microbiol 1996; 19:555–563.

199. Annunziato PW, Wright LF, Vann WF, Silver RP. Nucleotide sequence and genetic analysis of the neuD and neuB genes in region 2 of the polysialic acid gene cluster of Escherichia coli K1. J Bacteriol 1995; 177:312–319.

200. Wright A. Mechanism of conversion of the Salmonella O antigen by bacteriophage e34. J Bacteriol 1971; 105:927–936.

201. Troy FA, McCloskey MA. Role of a membranous sialyltransferase complex in the synthesis of surface polymers containing polysialic acid in Escherichia coli. Temperature-induced alteration in the assembly process. J Biol Chem 1979; 254:7377–7387.

202. Reuber TL, Walker GC. Biosynthesis of succinoglycan, a symbiotically important exopolysaccharide of Rhizobium meliloti. Cell 1993; 74:269–280.

203. Stoolmiller AC, Dorfman A. The biosynthesis of hyaluronic acid by Streptococcus. J Biol Chem 1969; 244:236–246.

204. Rubens CE, Heggen LM, Haft R, Wessels MR. Identification of cpsD, a gene essential for type III capsule expression in group B streptococci. Mol Microbiol 1993; 8:843–855.

205. Jiang XM, Neal B, Santiago F, Lee SJ, Romana LK, Reeves PR. Structure and sequence of the rfb (O antigen) gene cluster of Salmonella serovar typhimurium (strain LT2). Mol Microbiol 1991; 5:695–713.

206. Muller P, Keller M, Weng WM, Quandt J, Arnold W, Puhler A. Genetic analysis of the Rhizobium meliloti exoYFQ operon: ExoY is homologous to sugar transferases and ExoQ represents a transmembrane protein. Mol Plant Microbe Interact 1993; 6:55–65.

207. Bliss JM, Silver RP. Coating the surface: a model for expression of capsular polysialic acid in Escherichia coli K1. Mol Microbiol 1996; 21:221–231.

208. Glucksmann MA, Reuber TL, Walker GC. Family of glycosyl transferases needed for the synthesis of succinoglycan by Rhizobium meliloti. J Bacteriol 1993; 175:7033–7044.

209. Becker A, Niehaus K, Puhler A. Low-molecular-weight succinoglycan is predominantly produced by *Rhizobium meliloti* strains carrying a mutated ExoP protein characterized by a periplasmic N-terminal domain and a missing C-terminal domain. Mol Microbiol 1995; 16:191–203.

210. Yim HH, Nittayajarn A, Rubens CE. Analysis of the capsule synthesis locus, a virulence factor in group B streptococci. Adv Exp Med 1997; 418:995–997.

211. Guidolin A, Morona JK, Morona R, Hansman D, Paton JC. Nucleotide sequence analysis of genes essential for capsular polysaccharide biosynthesis in *Streptococcus pneumoniae* type 19F. Infect Immun 1994; 62:5384–5396.

212. Kolkman MA, Morrison DA, Van Der Zeijst BA, Nuijten PJ. The capsule polysaccharide synthesis locus of *Streptococcus pneumoniae* serotype 14: identification of the glycosyl transferase gene cps14E. J Bacteriol 1996; 178:3736–3741.

213. Stingele F, Neeser JR, Mollet B. Identification and characterization of the *eps* (exopolysaccharide) gene cluster from *Streptococcus thermophilus* Sfi6. J Bacteriol 1996; 178:1680–1690.

214. Paoletti LC, Ross RA, Johnson KD. Cell growth rate regulates expression of group B streptococcus type III capsular polysaccharide. Infect Immun 1996; 64:1220–1226.

215. Gray BM, Pritchard DG. Phase variation in the pathogenesis of group B streptococcal infections. In: Orefici G (ed). New Perspectives on Streptococci and Streptococcal Infections. Proceedings of the XI Lancefield International Symposium. New York: Gustav Fisher Verlag, 1992; 452–454.

216. Orefici G, Recchia S, Galante L. Possible virulence marker for *Streptococcus agalactiae* (Lancefield group B). Eur J Clin Microbiol Infect Dis 1988; 7:302–305.

217. Hakansson S, Holm SE, Wagner M. Density profile of group B streptococci, type III, and its possible relation to enhanced virulence. J Clin Microbiol 1987; 25:714–718.

218. Tamura G, Rubens CE. Host-bacterial interactions in the pathogenesis of group B streptococcal infections. Curr Opin Infect Dis 1994; 7:317–322.

219. Ross RA, Yim JJ, Rubens CE, Paoletti LC. Expression of type III polysaccharide by group B streptococcus during adaptation to changing growth rate environments. (manuscript submitted).

220. Schell MA. Molecular biology of the LysR family of transcriptional regulators. Annu Rev Microbiol 1993; 47:597–626.

221. Huang J, Carney BF, Denny TP, Weissinger AK, Schell MA. A complex network regulates expression of *eps* and other virulence genes of *Pseudomonas solanacearum*. J Bacteriol 1995; 177:1259–1267.

222. Guiney DG, Fang FC, Krause M, Libby S. Plasmid-mediated virulence genes in non-typhoid *Salmonella* serovars. FEMS Microbiol Lett 1994; 124:1–9.

223. Fernandez HN, Hugli TE. Primary structural analysis of the polypeptide portion of human C5a anaphylatoxin. Polypeptide sequence determination and assignment of the oligosaccharide attachment site in C5a. J Biol Chem 1978; 253:6955–6964.

224. Strunk RC, Eidlen DM, Mason RJ. Pulmonary alveolar type II epithelial cells synthesize and secrete proteins of the classical and alternative complement pathways. J Clin Invest 1988; 81:1419–1426.

225. Bohnsack JF, Mollison KW, Buko AM, Ashworth JC, Hill HR. Group B streptococci inactivate complement component C5a by enzymic cleavage at the C-terminus. Biochem J 1991; 273:635–640.

226. Mollison KW, Mandecki W, Zuiderweg ER, Fayer L, Feyt A, Krause RA, Conway RG, Miller L, Edalji RP, Shalleross MA. Identification of receptor-binding residues in the inflammatory complement protein C5a by site-directed mutagenesis. Proc Natl Acad Sci USA 1989; 86:292–296.

227. De Cueninck BJ, Shockman GD, Swenson RM. Group B, type III streptococcal cell wall: composition and structural aspects revealed through endo-N-acetylmuramidase-catalyzed hydrolysis. Infect Immun 1982; 35:572–581.

228. Bohnsack JF, Zhou XN, Williams PA, Cleary PP, Parker CJ, Hill HR. Purification of the proteinase from group B streptococci that inactivates human C5a. Biochim Biophys Acta 1991; 1079:222–228.

229. Bohnsack JF, Chang JK, Hill HR. Restricted ability of group B streptococcal C5a-ase to inactivate C5a prepared from different animal species. Infect Immun 1993; 61:1421–1426.

230. Bohnsack JF, Widjaja K, Ghazizadeh S, Rubens CE, Hillyard DR, Parker CJ, Albertine KH, Hill HH. A role for C5 and C5a-ase in the acute neutrophil response to group B streptococcal infections. J Infect Dis 1997; 175:847–855.

231. Wexler DE, Nelson RD, Cleary PP. Human neutrophil chemotactic response to group A streptococci: bacteria-mediated interference with complement-derived chemotactic factors. Infect Immun 1983; 39:239–246.

232. Cleary PP, Peterson J, Chen C, Nelson C. Virulent human strains of group G streptococci express a C5a peptidase enzyme similar to that produced by group A streptococci. Infect Immun 1991; 59:2305–2310.

233. Cleary PP, Prahbu U, Dale JB, Wexler DE, Handley J. Streptococcal C5a peptidase is a highly specific endopeptidase Infect Immun 1992; 60:5219–5223.

234. Ji Y, McLandsborough L, Kondagunta A, Cleary

PP. C5a peptidase alters clearance and trafficking of group A streptococci by infected mice. Infect Immun 1996; 64:503–510.

235. Chmouryguina I, Suvorov A, Ferrieri P, Cleary PP. Conservation of the C5a peptidase genes in group A and B streptococci. Infect Immun 1996; 64:2387–2390.

236. Chen CC, Cleary PP. Cloning and expression of the streptococcal C5a peptidase gene in *Escherichia coli:* linkage to the type 12 M protein gene. Infect Immun 1989; 57:1740–1745.

237. Podbielski A, Flosdorff A, Weber-Heynemann J. The group A streptococcal *vir*R49 gene controls expression of four structural *vir* regulon genes. Infect Immun 1995; 63:9–20.

238. Facklam RR, Padula JF, Wortham EC, Cooksey RC, Rountree HA. Presumptive identification of group A, B, and D streptococci on agar plate media. J Clin Microbiol 1979; 9:665–672.

239. Marchlewicz BA, Duncan JL. Properties of a hemolysin produced by group B streptococci. Infect Immun 1980; 30:805–813.

240. Ferrieri P. Characterization of a hemolysin isolated from gruop-B streptococci. In: Holm SE, Christensen P (eds). Basic Concepts of Streptococci and Streptococcal Diseases. Proceedings of the VIIIth International Lancefield Symposium. Surrey, UK: Reedbooks, 1982; 142–143.

241. Platt MW. In vivo hemolytic activity of group B streptococcus is dependent on erythrocyte-bacteria contact and independent of a carrier molecule Curr Microbiol 1995; 31:5–9.

242. Tapsall JW. Relationship between pigment production and haemolysin formation by Lancefield group B streptococci. J Med Microbiol 1987; 24:83–87.

243. Tsaihong JC, Wennerstrom DE. Effect of carrier molecules on production and properties of extracelluluar hemolysin produced by *Streptococcus agalactiae.* Curr Microbiol 1983; 9:333–338.

244. Dal M-C, Monteil H. Hemolysin produced by group B streptococcus agalactiae. FEMS Microbiol Lett 1983; 16:89–94.

245. Rooney SA. The surfactant system and lung phospholipid biochemistry. Am Rev Respir Dis 1985; 131:439–460.

246. Tapsall JW, Phillips EA. The hemolytic and cytolytic activity of group B streptococcal hemolysin and its possible role in early onset group B streptococcal disease. Pathology 1991; 23:139–144.

247. Herting E, Jarstrand C, Rasool O, Curstedt T, Sun B, Robertson B. Experimental neonatal group B streptococcal pneumonia: effect of a modified porcine surfactant on bacterial proliferation in ventilated near-term rabbits. Pediatr Res 1994; 36:784–791.

248. Thelestam M, Blomqvist L. Staphylococcal alpha toxin—recent advances. Toxicon 1988; 26:51–65.

249. Papadimitrious JC, Drachenburg ML, Shin ML, Trump BF. Ultrastructural studies of complement mediated cell death: a biological reaction model to plasma membrane injury. Virchows Arch 1994; 424:677–685.

250. Marchlewicz BA, Duncan JL. Lysis of erythrocytes by a hemolysin produced by a group B *Streptococcus* sp. Infect Immun 1981; 34:787–794.

251. Wennerstrom DE, Tsaihong JC, Crawford JT. Evaluation of the role of hemolysin and pigment in the pathogenesis of early onset group B streptococcal infection. In: Kimura Y, Kotami S, Shiokowa Y (eds). Recent Advances in Streptococci and Streptococcal Diseases. Bracknell, UK: Reedbooks, 1985; 155–156.

252. Griffiths BB, Rhee H. Effects of haemolysins of groups A and B streptococci on the cardiovascular system. Microbios 1992; 69:17–27.

253. Conrads G, Podbielski A, Lutticken R. Molecular cloning and nucleotide sequence of the group B streptococcal hemolysin. Zentralbl Bakteriol 1991; 275:179–194.

254. Spellerberg B, Pohl B, Haase G, Martin S, Weber-Heynemann J, Lütticken R. Identification of genetic determinants for the hemolytic activity of streptococcus agalactiae by ISS1 transposition. J Bacteriol 1999; 181:3212–3219.

255. Fischer W. Physiology of lipotechoic acids in bacteria. Adv Microb Physiol 1988; 29:233–302.

256. Maurer JJ, Mattingly SJ. Molecular analysis of lipoteichoic acid from *Streptococcus agalactiae.* J Bacteriol 1991; 73:487–494.

257. Nealon TJ, Mattingly SJ. Association of elevated levels of cellular lipoteichoic acids of group B streptococci with human neonatal disease. Infect Immun 1983; 39:1243–1251.

258. Mattingly SJ, Johnston BP. Comparative analysis of the localization of lipoteichoic acid in *Streptococcus agalactiae* and *Streptococcus pyogenes.* Infect Immun 1987; 55:2383–2386.

259. Wicken AJ, Knox KW. Lipoteichoic acids: a new class of bacterial antigen. Science 1975; 187:1161–1167.

260. Beachey EH. Binding of group A streptococci to human oral mucosal cells by lipotechnoic acid. Trans Assoc Am Physicians 1975; 88:285–292.

261. Nealon TJ, Mattingly SJ. Kinetic and chemical analyses of the biologic significance of lipotechoic acids in mediating adherence of serotype III group B streptococci. Infect Immun 1985; 50:107–115.

262. Stanislawski L, Simpson WA, Hasty D, Sharon N, Beachey EH, Ofek I. Role of fibronectin in attachment of *Streptococcus pyogenes* and *Escherichia coli* to human cell lines and isolated oral epithelial cells. Infect Immun 1985; 48:257–259.

263. Beachey EH, Courtney HS. Bacterial adherence: the attachment of group A streptococci to mucosal surfaces. Rev Infect Dis 1987; 9(Suppl 5):S475–S481.

264. Ferrieri P. Surface-localized protein antigens of group B streptococci. Rev Infect Dis 1988; 10(Suppl 2):S363–S366.

265. Stalhammar-Carlemalm M, Stenberg L, Lindahl G. Protein rib: a novel group B streptococcal cell surface protein that confers protective immunity and is expressed by most strains causing invasive infections. J Exp Med 1993; 177:1593–1603.

266. Wagner B, Wagner M, Kubin V, Ryc M. Immunoelectron microscopic study of the location of group-specific and protein type-specific antigens of group B streptococci. J Gen Microbiol 1980; 118:95–105.

267. Ferrieri P, Flores AE. Surface protein expression in group B streptococcal invasive isolates. Adv Exp Med 1997; 418:635–637.

268. Wilkinson HW, Eagon RG. Type-specific antigens of group B type Ic streptococci. Infect Immun 1971; 4:596–604.

269. Bevanger L, Iversen OJ. The Ibc proteins of group B streptococci: trypsin extracted alpha antigen and detection of the alpha and beta antigens. Acta Pathol Microbiol Immunol Scand B 1983; 91:75–81.

270. Madoff LC, Hori S, Michel JL, Baker CJ, Kasper DL. Phenotypic diversity in the alpha C protein of group B streptococci. Infect Immun 1991; 59:2638–2644.

271. Flores AE, Ferrieri P. Molecular diversity among the trypsin resistant surface proteins of group B streptococci. Zentralbl Bakteriol 1996; 285:44–51.

272. Michel JL, Madoff LC, Olson K, Kling DE, Kasper Dl, Ausubel FM. Large, identical, tandem repeating units in the C protein alpha antigen gene, *bca*, of group B streptococci. Proc Natl Acad Sci USA 1992; 89:10060–10064.

273. Brady LJ, Boyle MD. Identification of non-immunoglobulin A-Fc-binding forms and low-molecular-weight secreted forms of the group B streptococcal beta antigen. Infect Immun 1989; 57:1573–1581.

274. Jerlstrom PG, Talay SR, Valentin-Weigand P, Timmis KN, Chhatwal GS. Identification of an immunoglobulin A binding motif located in the beta-antigen of the C protein complex of group B streptococci. Infect Immun 1996; 64:2787–2793.

275. Johnson DR, Ferrieri P. Group B streptococcal Ibc protein antigen: distribution of two determinants in wild-type strains of common serotypes. J Clin Microbiol 1984; 19:506–510.

276. Li J, Kasper DL, Ausubel FM, Rosner B, Michel JL. Inactivation of the alpha C protein antigen gene, *bca*, by a novel shuttle/suicide vector results in attenuation of virulence and immunity in group B streptococcus. Proc Natl Acad Sci USA 1997; 94:13251–13256.

277. Madoff LC, Michel JL, Gong EW, Rodewald AK, Kasper DL. Protection of neonatal mice from group B streptococcal infection by mater-nal immunization with beta C protein. Infect Immun 1992; 60:4989–4994.

278. Wibawan IW, Lammler C. Isolation and characterization of group B streptococcal type antigens X and R. Int J Med Microbiol 1991; 275:327–334.

279. Wilkinson HW. Comparison of streptococcal R antigens. Appl Microbiol 1972; 24:669–670.

280. Flores AE, Ferrieri P. Molecular species of R-protein antigens produced by clinical isolates of group B streptococci. J Clin Microbiol 1989; 27:1050–1054.

281. Linden V, Christensen KK, Christensen P. The occurrence of R-protein among isolates of group B streptococci from human sources. Acta Pathol Microbiol Immunol Scand 1983; 91:153–156.

282. Fasola EL, Flores AE, Ferrieri P. Immune responses to the R4 protein antigen of group B streptococci and its relationship to other streptococcal R4 proteins. Clin Diagn Lab Immunol 1996; 3:321–325.

283. Linden V. Mouse-protective effect of rabbit anti-R-protein antibodies against group B streptococci type II carrying R-protein. Acta Pathol Microbiol Immunol Scand 1983; 91:145–151.

284. Larsson C, Stalhammar-Carlemalm M, Lindahl G. Experimental vaccination against group B streptococcus, an encapsulated bacterium, with highly purified preparations of cell surface proteins Rib and alpha. Infect Immun 1996; 64:3518–3523.

285. Wastfelt M, Stalhammar-Carlemalm M, Delisse AM, Cabezon T, Lindahl G. Identification of a family of streptococcal surface proteins with extremely repetitive structure. J Biol Chem 1996; 271:18892–18897.

286. Lachenauer CS, Madoff LC. A protective surface protein from type V group B streptococci shares N-terminal sequence homology with the alpha C protein. Infect Immun 1996; 64:4255–4260.

287. Milligan TW, Baker CJ, Straus DC, Mattingly SJ. Association of elevated levels of extracellular neuraminidase with clinical isolates of type III group B streptococci. Infect Immun 1978; 21:738–746.

288. Milligan TW, Mattingly SJ, Straus DC. Purification and partial characterization of neuraminidase from type III group B streptococci. J Bacteriol 1980; 144:164–171.

289. Mattingly SJ, Milligan TW, Pierpont AA, Straus DC. Extracellular neuraminidase production by clinical isolates of group B streptococci from infected neonates. J Clin Microbiol 1980; 12:633–635.

290. Pritchard DG, Lin B. Group B streptococcal neuraminidase is actually a hyaluronidase. Infect Immun 1993; 61:3234–3239.

291. Pritchard DG, Lin B, Willingham TR, Baker JR. Characterization of the group B streptococcal hyaluronate lyase. Arch Biochem Biophys 1994; 315:431–437.

292. Lin B, Hollingshead SK, Coligan JE, Egan ML, Baker JR, Pritchard DG. Cloning and expression of the gene for group B streptococcal hyaluronate lyase. J Biol Chem 1994; 269: 30113–30116.

293. Kjems E, Perch B, Henrichsen J. Serotypes of group B streptococci and their relation to hyaluronidase production and hydrolysis of salicin. J Clin Microbiol 1980; 11:111–113.

294. Haynes BF, Telen MJ, Hale LP, Denning SM. CD44—a molecule involved in leukocyte adherence and T cell activation. Immunol today 1989; 10:423–428.

295. Granlund M, Oberg L, Sellin M, Norgren M. Identification of a novel insertion element, IS1548, in group B streptococci, predominantly in strains causing endocarditis. J Infect Dis 1998; 177:967–976.

296. Miyake K, Underhill CB, Lesley J, Kincade W. Hyaluronate can function as a cell adhesion molecule and CD44 participates in hyaluronate recognition. J Exp Med 1990; 172:69–75.

297. Christie R, Atkins NE, Munch-Peterson E. A note on a lytic phenomenon shown by group B streptococci. Aust J Exp Biol Med Sci 1944; 22:197–200.

298. Bernheimer AW, Linder R, Avigad LS. Nature and mechanism of action of the CAMP protein of group B streptococci. Infect Immun 1979; 23:838–844.

299. Jurgens D, Sterzik B, Fehrenbach FJ. Unspecific binding of group B streptococcal cocytolysin (CAMP-factor) to immunoglobulins and its possible role in pathogenicity. J Exp Med 1987; 165:720–732.

300. Ruhlmann J, Wittmann-Liebold B, Jurgens D, Fehrenbach FJ. Complete amino acid sequence of protein B. FEBS Microbiol Lett 1988; 235:262–266.

301. Schneewind O, Friedrich KH, Lutticken R. Cloning and expression of the CAMP-factor of group B streptococci in *Escherichia coli*. Infect Immun 1988; 56:2174–2179.

302. Podbielski A, Blankenstein O, Lutticken R. Molecular characterization of the *cfb* gene encoding group B streptococcal CAMP-factor. Med Microbiol Immunol 1994; 183:239–256.

303. Skalka B, Smola J. Lethal effect of CAMP-factor and UBERIS-factor—a new finding about diffusable exosubstances of *Streptococcus agalactiae* and *Streptococcus uberis*. Zentralbl Bakteriol Mikrobiol Hyg A 1981; 249:190–194.

304. Fehrenbach FJ, Jurgens D, Ruhlmann J, Sterzik B, Ozel M. Role of CAMP-factor (protein B) in virulence. 1988; 17:351–357.

305. Durham DL, Mattingly SJ, Doran TI, Milligan TW, Straus DC. Correlation between the production of extracellular substances by type III group B streptococcal strains and virulence in a mouse model. Infect Immun 1981; 34: 448–554.

306. Lin B, Averett WF, Novak J, Chatham WW, Hollingshead SK, Coligan JE, Egan ML, Pritchard DS. Characterization of PepB, a group B streptococcal oligopeptidase. Infect Immun 1996; 64:3401–3406.

307. Ferrieri P. GBS enzymes, homolysin, toxins and other products. Antibiot Chemother 1985; 35:57–80.

308. Wood EG, Gray BM. Type-specific antibody prevents platelet aggregation induced by group B streptococci type III. J Lab Clin Med 1986; 107:322–326.

309. Usui Y, Ohshima Y, Yoshida K. Platelet aggregation by group B streptococci. J Gen Microbiol 1987; 133:1593–1600.

310. Usui Y, Ichiman Y, Ohtomo T, Suganuma M, Yoshida K. Inhibition of platelet aggregation by a whole cell extract from strains of group B streptococcus. Thromb Res 1990; 58:283–291.

311. Usui Y, Yoshida K, San-Clemente CL. Characterization of partially purified group B streptococcal clumping factor. Zentralbl Bakteriol Mikrobiol Hyg A 1982; 252:299–309.

312. Usui Y, Ichiman Y, Yoshida K, Oikawa K. Possible induction of disseminated intravascular coagulation in the mouse by group B streptococcal clumping factor. Br J Exp Path 1986; 67:629–635.

313. Pincus SH, Cole RL, Wessels MR, Corwin MD, Kamango-Sollo E, Hayes SF, Cieplak W, Swanson J. Group B streptococcal opacity variants. J Bacteriol 1992; 174:3739–3749.

314. Pincus SH, Cole RL, Kamanga-Sollo E, Fischer SH. Interaction of group B streptococcal opacity variants with the host defense system. Infect Immun 1993; 61:3761–3768.

315. Hellerqvist CG, Rojas J, Green RS, Sell S, Sundell H, Stahlman MT. 1981. Studies on group B β-hemolytic streptococcus. I. Isolation and partial characterization of an extracellular toxin. Pediatr Res 1981; 15:892–898.

316. Hellerqvist CG, Sundell H, Gettins P. Molecular basis for group B beta-hemolytic streptococcal disease. Proc Natl Acad Sci USA 1987; 84:51–55.

12

Group B Streptococcal Infections

CAROL J. BAKER

Streptococcus agalactiae, or Lancefield group B streptococcus, was first isolated by Nocard and Mollereau in 1887 [1]. Lancefield not only described a serologic classification of beta-hemolytic streptococci [2] but, along with Hare, she was also first to report isolation of group B streptococci from parturient women [3]. In the same year, Congdon [4] included one fatal puerperal case of group B streptococcal septicemia and pneumonia in his summary of streptococcal infections associated with childbirth. The first case series of group B streptococcus as a cause of human disease was Fry's description of three cases of fatal puerperal sepsis [5]. Sporadic case reports appeared until the 1960s when three case series of maternal and neonatal infections were recorded [6–8]. Until the mid-1970s, however, group B streptococcus was listed in standard textbooks of medical microbiology as a cause of bovine mastitis, with no mention of its role in human disease. Reports in 1973 established its emergence as the predominant pathogen causing bacteremia, pneumonia, and meningitis in neonates and infants less than 3 months of age [9,10]. For more than two decades, the incidence of infection in neonates has remained stable, with reported attack rates ranging from 1.0 to 4.7 per 1000 live births [11,12]. Infection occasionally involves infants more than 3 months of age [13] and often in-volves pregnant women [11,14]. More recently, group B streptococci have been recognized as an increasingly occurring pathogen in nonpregnant adults with underlying medical conditions or those over 60 years of age [14,15]. Recently, implementation of recommendations for use of maternal intrapartum chemoprophylaxis has been associated with a significant decrease in the incidence of disease in neonates [16].

MEDICAL MICROBIOLOGY

Group B streptococci are facultative gram-positive diplococci that grow on a variety of bacteriologic media. Colonies are 3–4 mm in size, grayish-white, flat, and somewhat mucoid in appearance. Colonies are surrounded by a narrow zone of beta-hemolysis that for some strains is detectable only when the colony is lifted from the agar. Nonhemolytic strains account for 1%–2% of isolates, and alpha-hemolytic strains are identified rarely. Laboratory methods for presumptive identification of group B streptococci include testing for resistance to bacitracin or trimethoprim-sulfamethoxazole, hydrolysis of sodium hippurate broth, failure to hydrolyze bile esculin, production of orange pigment when cultured under certain conditions, and CAMP testing. Definitive identification relies on detection of the group B carbohydrate cell-wall antigen common to all strains. Various serologic methods employing hyperimmune group B–specific antisera or monoclonal antibodies have been developed. Latex agglutination is the most widely employed method for definitive identification (Sero STAT, Scott Laboratories; Streptex, Murex Diagnostics Limited; PathoDx, Remel Laboratories).

Group B streptococci may be further subdivided into serotypes based on type-specific capsular polysaccharides. The type-specific polysaccharides are repeating units of five to seven monosaccharides (glucose, galactose, glucosamine, and N-acetyl-neuraminic acid, or sialic acid). Each of the characterized polysaccharides includes an N-acetyl-neuraminic acid (sialic acid) residue, important in pathogenesis. Currently, eight such polysaccharides are characterized: Ia, Ib, and II–VIII [17–21]. A small proportion of strains do not react with hyperimmune sera to the characterized capsular polysaccharides, and are referred to as "nontypable." Further differentiation of type Ia strains was based on the presence of a surface protein antigen known as c, leading to the nomenclature of Ia and Ia/c serotypes. This C protein is present in other serotypes as well, but is rare in type III strains [22]. C protein has at least two distinct components, α and β, and individual strains may contain one or both. Other proteins, designated R, X, and Rib, are found in some strains but their biologic significance remains undefined.

To date, human isolates of group B streptococci have remained uniformly susceptible to penicillin G [23]. They also are susceptible to other beta-lactam antibiotics, cephalosporins, vancomycin, and imipenem. Resistance to the macrolides (erythromycin, clindamycin, clarithromycin) occurs in 3%–8% of isolates, and tetracycline resistance has risen to nearly 90% [23–25]. Resistance to bacitracin, nalidixic acid, trimethoprim-sulfamethoxazole, and metronidazole is uniform [26]. While gentamicin resistance is characteristic, when this antimicrobial is combined with either penicillin G or ampicillin, there is synergistic killing in vitro and in vivo [27,28].

Up to 5% of group B streptococcal isolates have been reported to be tolerant to penicillin [29]. The expression of this tolerance requires laboratory conditions that promote a >16-fold discrepancy between minimal inhibitory concentrations (MIC) and minimal bactericidal concentrations (MBC). Tolerant strains are characterized in vitro by delayed penicillin killing, similar rates of killing by penicillin, whether growth is exponential or stationary, an additive rather than a synergistic response to the combination of penicillin and gentamicin, and deficient autolysis. However, the clinical significance of these laboratory characteristics, if any, is unknown [29].

EPIDEMIOLOGY

Incidence

Reported attack rates for group B streptococcal disease in newborns and young infants range from 0.7 to 5.7 per 1000 live births [12,30–32]. Early-onset disease (birth to age 7 days) accounts for approximately 80% of cases [14]. Late-onset disease (8 days to 3 months) has reported attack rates from 0.3 to 1.8 per 1000 live births [31,33]. The Centers for Disease Control and Prevention conducted a multistate active surveillance program encompassing a population of 10.1 million persons in five U.S. states, and reported attack rates of 1.4 and 0.3 per 1000 live births, respectively, for early- and late-onset disease [12]. When these rates are applied to the U.S. population as a whole, a minimum of 6200 early-and 1400 late-onset cases may be expected annually. However, these rates should diminish when recommendations for use of maternal intrapartum chemoprophylaxis to prevent early-onset disease are widely implemented [16,34].

Group B streptococcal disease is also common in pregnant women. In one population-based study, the incidence of invasive disease among pregnant women was estimated at 22 cases per 100,000 births, and pregnancy-associated infections comprised 8% of all group B streptococcal disease [15]. Clinical manifestations include urinary tract infection (usually asymptomatic bacteriuria), intra-amniotic infection (chorioamnionitis), wound infections associated with cesarean delivery or episiotomy, endometritis (often with bacteremia), puerperal sepsis and occasionally meningitis, septic thrombophlebitis, or other serious complications [11,35–37]. Group B streptococci clearly cause stillbirth in some instances, and increasingly, evidence points to a causative role for these organisms in amnionitis and preterm delivery [35,38–40]. However, nonpregnant adults actually comprised the majority of cases (68%) of group B streptococcal infection from the greater Atlanta metropolitan area [15]. In these patients, underlying medical conditions are the rule.

Maternal Colonization

Infection in the neonate with group B streptococci results from exposure to the organism from the maternal genital tract following rupture of membranes [30]. In almost all cases, the mother is asymptomatically infected, or colonized. Maternal colonization rates vary widely and relate to body sites sampled, microbiologic techniques employed, and the gestation when these cultures are performed.

The site chosen for culture is critical, and sampling of more than one site improves detection [41–43]. The distal vagina more frequently yields group B streptococci than the cervix [39,44], and sampling of both vaginal and rectal sites results in optimal detection of carriers. The majority (up to two-thirds) of carriers are positive at both sites. In some patients, the rectal site is the only one that yields the organism [41,43,45,46]. Swab specimens must undergo optimal processing for greatest accuracy. These may be placed in transport media at environmental temperatures for up to 96 h. In the laboratory, they should be placed in broth media containing either gentamicin (selective broth medium) or colistin and nalidixic acid (Lim broth) rather than on solid media, since the latter will "miss" detection of up to 50% of positives [42,45,47]. After 18 to 24 h of incubation at 37°C, the broth is subcultured onto a blood agar plate and processed in the conventional manner. Finally, the proximity to delivery will affect the accuracy of predicting colonization at delivery. Cultures obtained at 35 and 37 weeks gestation predict colonization at delivery with nearly 100% accuracy [34,48]. Reported colonization rates vary, but if the above methods are employed, the overall rate is about 25% [14,49].

Much effort has been spent to define women at enhanced risk for colonization with group B streptococci. Nonpregnant women have similar colonization rates, suggesting that pregnancy does not affect colonization. Women less than 20 years of age have higher rates and multiparous (≥3 pregnancies) women have lower colonization rates [39,46,50]. Although group B streptococci are sexually transmissible, the number of partners does not influence colonization status [39,51]. However, ethnicity does affect the likelihood of colonization. In a recent survey of 2929 women from Houston and Seattle, 36.7% of African-American women were colonized, a rate significantly greater than the 23.3% in women belonging to other ethnic groups [46]. In the same study, Asian women had a significantly lower prevalence of group B streptococcal colonization (14%) than any other ethnic group. In another multicenter study, 7742 women were evaluated at 23 to 26 weeks gestation. It was noted that African-American ethnic origin, age less than 20 years, and lower educational level were independently correlated with higher group B streptococcal colonization rates [39].

Infant Colonization

Acquisition of the organism by infants born to colonized mothers (vertical transmission) occurs in 29%–72% of cases [30,31,50,52]. Detection of colonization depends on sites sampled, culture method, and timing. Acquisition is presumed to occur either by the ascending route through ruptured membranes or by contact with the organism in the genital tract during parturition. Nosocomial transmission and community acquisition occur, although infrequently [11]. Positive cultures obtained shortly after birth may indicate contamination with infected maternal secretions rather than true infant colonization. Many infant sites have been sampled, including the ear canal, axillary skin, throat, umbilicus, perineum, and rectum. However, throat and rectal swab cultures collected between 24 and 48 h of age should identify nearly 100% of colonized infants [53].

The factor most directly associated with vertical transmission and subsequent neonatal colonization is the inoculum present in the maternal genital tract. Mothers with "heavy" group B streptococcal colonization ($>10^5$ cfu/ml) are more likely to transmit the organism [50,54]. Maternal intrapartum antibiotic therapy substantially diminishes the inoculum and thereby decreases vertical transmission rates [55,56]. In a recently reported study, infant colonization was significantly diminished when intrapartum antibiotics were administered [53].

Risk Factors for Infant Disease

Vertical transmission is a prerequisite for the development of invasive, early-onset infection. There is limited evidence that most late-onset infections also follow vertical transmission [11,33]. The bacterial inoculum also influences the risk for group B streptococcal disease; women with "heavy" colonization are more likely to have symptomatically infected infants, and heavily colonized infants are more likely to develop either early- or late-onset disease [33,55,57]. Other maternal factors associated with the development of early-onset disease include labor prior to 37 weeks gestation, premature rupture of membranes or rupture of membranes 18 or more h before delivery at any gestation, and intrapartum fever [34]. Additional factors associated with significantly higher attack rates for early-onset disease are African-American ethnicity, age less than 20 years, history of previous fetal loss, history of urinary tract infection during the pregnancy, and primiparity [58]. Attack rates for late-onset infection are increased if the mother is less than 20 years of age or of African-American ethnic origin [59].

Adult Disease

An estimated 4.4/100,000 nonpregnant persons 15 years of age and older per year develop invasive group B streptococcal disease, and for those 60 years of age or older, the figure is 18/100,000 [15,60]. In nonpregnant adults, men and women are equally affected, and the incidence rises with age and is particularly high among African Americans [15,60]. The gastrointestinal tract is an important reservoir for group B streptococci in older adults, and the male genital tract is also an important source for pyelonephritis and prostatitis in older men. Case series have indicated that chronic underlying conditions are common, and population-based studies have indicated that attack rates are significantly higher in patients with diabetes mellitus [15,60], HIV infection, and cancer [61–63]. Most infections in nonpregnant adults are nosocomial. A case–control study of 219 nonpregnant adults with invasive group B streptococcal infection determined that the following conditions significantly increased risk after controlling for age: cirrhosis (odds ratio [OR], 9.7), diabetes mellitus (OR 3.0), stroke (OR 3.5), breast cancer (OR 4.0), decubitus ulcer (OR 4.0), and neurogenic bladder (OR 4.6) [64].

Serotypes of Group B Streptococci Causing Disease

Reports nearly 20 years ago indicated that the group B streptococcal serotypes colonizing pregnant women and neonates were fairly evenly divided among three types: I, II, and III [65,66]. Recently, however, a new serotype, type V, has emerged as a prominent strain [67–70]. Serotype III remains a predominant type associated with early-onset infection in infants and in pregnant women (approximately 35% each) [68,69], but the number of type Ia infections has risen in the past decade. Serotype Ia, like III, is associated with approximately one-third of early-onset and pregnancy-associated infections, and is the second-most frequent cause of disease in nonpregnant adults [67,68]. Type III continues its dominance as a cause of late-onset infant infections. Serotype V causes both early- and late-onset infections as well as serious infections in adults, but lags behind types Ia and III in prevalence. Currently, the least common serotypes causing human disease are types II and Ib/c, and types IV, VI through VIII and nontypable strains are rare.

CLINICAL FEATURES

Infant Infections

The paradigm of early- versus late-onset disease in neonates and young infants was described in 1973 by Baker and Barrett [30] when they and investigators from Colorado [10] noted the bimodal distribution of group B streptococcal infections. The syndromes of early- and late-onset disease differ in clinical presentation, prognosis, epidemiologic characteristics, and pathogenesis (Table 12.1). Early-onset disease appears during the first week of life, but nearly 90% of patients have signs of systemic infection at birth or develop these within 12 hours [11]. Infants with late-onset infection present between 8 and 90 days of age, with a median onset of about 36 days [59]. Early case series suggested that when the infant reached 3 months of age the period of risk ended, but late, late-onset infections, although rare, have been reported, usually in infants born before 32 weeks gestation who have concomitant infection with HIV or other immunodeficiency states [13,71].

Early-onset disease often (about 50% of cases) occurs in the setting of maternal complications known to increase the risk for neonatal sepsis. The three most frequent clinical presentations are septicemia without a focus, pneumonia, or meningitis [11,32]. The signs are similar for each of these presentations, and range from shock and respiratory failure at delivery to asymptomatic infection detected during evaluation of the term neonate because of maternal risk factors known to increase risk for systemic infection [72]. Respiratory signs, such as apnea, grunting respirations, tachypnea, and cyanosis, predominate. Other signs are nonspecific: lethargy, poor feeding, abdominal distention, pallor, tachycardia, and jaundice. Fever is often a feature of infection in term neonates, but premature infants usually have normal temperatures or are hypothermic. Recently reported case–fatality ratios range from 4% to 15% [32,59,71].

Late-onset disease primarily affects term infants with an unremarkable maternal and early neonatal course. More recent case series suggest that a larger number of infants born quite prematurely (less than 32 weeks gestation) develop late, late-onset infection beyond 3 months of age. Nosocomial "epidemics" of late-onset disease have also occurred in neonatal intensive care units, usually in very preterm neonates who acquire group B streptococci by horizontal spread via the hands of nursery personnel [73]. Meningitis and bacteremia without focus are the two most common manifestations of late-onset disease. Osteoarticular infections and cellulitis are less common [74,75]. Early-onset disease often presents acutely with apnea and hypotension, whereas late-onset disease typically is heralded by the occurrence of fever, irritability, and other nonspecific signs. More fulminant, rapidly progressive cases of late-onset infection, however, do occur. Recently reported case–fatality ratios for late-onset disease range from 0 to 6% [14,71].

Bacteremia without a focus is present in 27% to 87% of neonates with early-onset disease [11]. Signs of septicemia, such as respiratory distress and poor perfusion, are often present, especially in premature neonates. Asymptomatic bacteremia may occur in term infants, and in one series, this comprised 22% of cases [32], many of whom had early evaluation with institution of

Table 12.1 Characteristics of Group B Streptococcal Disease in Infants

Feature	Early-Onset	Late-Onset	Late, Late-Onset
Age at onset (median)	≤7 days (8 h)	≥7 d–90 days (36 days)	>90 days
Infants affected	Premature neonates, births after maternal obstetric complications	Term infants predominant	Premature <1500 g; immune deficiency
Presentation	Respiratory distress, apnea, and hypotension common	Fever, nonspecific signs; occasionally fulminant	Fever, nonspecific signs
Site of infection	Bacteremia (40%–55%); pneumonia (30%–45%); meningitis (6%–15%)	Bacteremia without a focus (55%); meningitis (35%); osteoarthritis (~5%); cellulitis/adenitis (~2%)	Bacteremia without a focus; focal infections as in late-onset disease
Serotypes isolated	All (Ia, III, and V most frequent)	Type III predominates	Type III predominates
Mortality	4%–15%	0–6%	<5%

empiric antimicrobial therapy. Respiratory distress is common in all forms of early-onset disease, including congenital pneumonia [9,10,76]. Radiographic findings may include infiltrates suggestive of pneumonia, small pleural effusions, a pattern similar to that of hyaline membrane disease, and increased vascular markings as seen in transient tachypnea of the newborn, or the radiographs may be normal despite pulmonary symptoms [77,78]. In preterm neonates, the presentation is often identical to that of hyaline membrane disease, and at autopsy, hyaline membranes containing bacteria and minimal inflammatory infiltrates have been described [79].

Meningitis is documented in 6% to 15% of neonates with early-onset disease [11]. As a rule, there are no signs to indicate meningeal involvement, underscoring the need to evaluate the cerebrospinal fluid (CSF) of all neonates with early-onset disease [80]. Early in the course, the CSF white blood cell count may be normal despite isolation of group B streptococci from CSF culture [81]. Respiratory distress is the most frequent clinical finding in infants with meningitis. Seizures rarely are the presenting feature, but may occur during the early course of disease in almost 50% of patients. Focal neurologic findings or a bulging fontanelle often predict poor outcome. Postmortem evaluation of infants with fatal early-onset group B streptococcal meningitis reveals hemorrhage, prominent basilar involvement, and abundant bacteria with relatively sparse inflammation [82].

Sequelae occur in 15% to 50% of survivors of early- and late-onset meningitis [81,83,84]. These sequelae include mental retardation, spastic quadriplegia, cortical blindness, deafness, uncontrolled seizures, hydrocephalus, and speech and language delay. Signs at admission that are correlated with risk for poor outcome include hypotension, coma or semicoma, status epilepticus, neutropenia, and CSF protein levels >300 mg/dl.

Osteoarthritis occurs in about 5% of late-onset infections [71]. Group B streptococci have been identified as the casual agents in 5% to 38% of cases of neonatal osteomyelitis [74,85]. The presentation of osteoarticular disease is more indolent, however, than that caused by other etiologic agents. Decreased motion of the involved extremity or pain with manipulation are common

findings. Warmth and redness are infrequent manifestations. Systemic signs are unusual. The humerus is the bone most often involved, and this is typically proximal. The femur is the second-most frequent bone involved. Unlike other forms of neonatal osteomyelitis, infection of a single rather than multiple bone sites is the rule, and blood cultures are infrequently positive. Involvement of the adjacent joint occurs frequently. A lytic lesion is often found in admission radiographs, implying that the process began weeks before. This may represent seeding of the metaphysis during an episode of asymptomatic, early-onset bacteremia [11]. In infants with septic arthritis the presentation typically is more acute, with a mean of 2 days of abnormal findings before diagnosis. The lower extremities are most often involved, especially the hip joint. Bacteremia is detected in more than 50% of cases. The diagnosis is made at a mean age of 31 days.

In one case series, 2% of late-onset group B streptococcal infections presented with cellulitis/adenitis syndrome [72]. The most frequent sites of involvement are the face or neck [75,86,87]. The mean age at presentation is estimated at 5 weeks, and there is a male predominance. The typical presentation is one of fever, irritability, poor feeding, and swelling of the affected soft-tissue area. Enlarged adjacent lymph nodes often become palpable within a few days when the submandibular area is involved. Ipsilateral otitis media was reported in four of five infants with facial or submandibular cellulitis in one case series. Other than the face or submandibular area, less commonly affected sites include the genital or inguinal region, hand, and prepatellar space [11]. Aspiration of the area of cellulitis often yields group B streptococci, and concomitant bacteremia is almost always present.

Delayed onset of late-onset infection was reported in 19% of cases of late-onset group B streptococcal disease [71], but a lesser frequency has been observed by others [87]. Immunodeficiency should be considered in children presenting beyond the usual period of risk [13]. The clinical manifestations are similar to those infants with typical late-onset infection; bacteremia without a focus and meningitis are the frequent presentations [88]. Other reported infections have included endocarditis, cellulitis, and central venous catheter infections [11].

Adult Infections

Among nonpregnant adults, skin and soft-tissue infections and bacteremia without an identifiable focus are the most common manifestations of invasive disease [14,15,61]. Many of these infections are acquired during hospitalization for another illness, and the bacteremia may be polymicrobial. The clinical spectrum also includes urosepsis, pneumonia, peritonitis, meningitis, septic arthritis, and endocarditis. Bacteremia without a focus usually occurs in patients with underlying liver or renal disease [61,62,64]. Often these patients have indwelling vascular catheters and have co-infection with staphylococci, suggesting that a significant proportion of these infections may be catheter related [15]. The skin and soft-tissue infections include cellulitis, foot ulcers, and decubitus ulcers, and more than half of these episodes occur in patients with diabetes mellitus. Osteomyelitis due to contiguous spread of infection from decubiti or foot ulcers may result, and patients with a history of mastectomy for breast cancer may present with arm or chest wall cellulitis, sometimes years postoperatively. Pneumonia usually occurs in the setting of neurological disease, such as stroke or dementia, and can be unilobar or multilobar. In older men, urinary tract infection and prostatitis are particularly common, and patients with urosepsis usually have an underlying urological abnormality (obstructive uropathy, neurogenic bladder, indwelling Foley catheter) [15,60,61]. Meningitis is uncommon, but when it occurs, at least 30% of patients have another focus of infection, often the urinary tract, soft tissue, or heart [89]. Mortality ranges from 8% to 70%, but in recent years 20% to 30% has become usual. Shock and alcoholism are associated independently with risk for death [90]. The presentation for endocarditis is usually acute, and it may occur, albeit rarely, in previously healthy adults with no underlying valvular disease [91]. Vegetations are often large and systemic embolization has been reported in 40% of patients.

Relapsing or Recurrent Infections

Second (and sometimes third) episodes of group B streptococcal infection have been reported in infants and adults [92,93]. In an infant case series from Houston, the mean age at recurrence was 44 days, with the mean duration of the interval between the first course of therapy and recurrence being 19 days [92]. Molecular epidemiologic techniques indicate that most, but not all, recurrent infections are due to the strain implicated in the first episode, suggesting that persistent mucosal colonization following treatment is the likely source. No specific risk factors are evident in these infants, but many were premature. In up to 50% of adults, second episodes often represent relapses that had unsuspected deep-seated infections. Underlying humoral immune deficiency or HIV infection should also be evaluated in patients who have no explanation for recurrence [64]. Optimal management for these patients is unknown.

DIAGNOSIS AND DIFFERENTIAL DIAGNOSIS

Isolation of group B streptococcus from a usually sterile body site, such as blood or CSF, is the only means by which a diagnosis of invasive infection can be established. Recovery of the organism from mucous membranes, surface sites, or a placenta is of no diagnostic significance. Meningitis in early-onset disease is clinically indistinguishable from bacteremia without a focus, and 10% to 38% of neonates with meningitis will have negative blood cultures [11,80]. Tracheal aspirate cultures from neonates that grow group B streptococci indicate colonization, but cannot be used to prove pulmonary invasion.

Several methods for detecting group B polysaccharide antigen in body fluid specimens from infants have been developed, but their usefulness is limited by poor sensitivity, especially for serum. Testing should be reserved for patients with meningitis who were treated with antibiotics before collection of blood or cerebrospinal cultures, and only CSF or serum should be submitted. Urine antigen testing is no longer recommended.

The presentation of early-onset group B streptococcal disease is clinically indistinguishable from neonatal infection caused by other bacterial pathogens. The prominence of respiratory signs in early-onset disease has led to confusion with noninfectious causes of respiratory distress, such as hyaline membrane disease, transient tachypnea of the newborn, and persistent fetal circulation. Clinical features that suggest group B streptococcal infection are a history of colonization in the mother, rupture of membranes more than 18 h before birth, apnea and shock in the first 24 h of life, 1 min Apgar score of 5 or less, and rapid progression of pulmonary disease [76,79,95].

The differential diagnosis for late-onset disease depends upon the focus of infection. Meningitis in infants of this age is also caused by *Listeria*, nontypable strains of *Hemophilus influenzae*, *Streptococcus pneumoniae*, *Neisseria meningitidis* or viruses, whereas soft tissue, bone or joint infections may be caused by *Staphylococcus aureus* or group A streptococci. In the absence of conclusive evidence, other potential pathogens should be considered when therapy is selected. The presentation of osteomyelitis may be subtle, with refusal to move the arm ascribed to neuromuscular disease or Erb's palsy. Careful physical examination will usually reveal point tenderness over the involved metaphyses, and radiographs often reveal a lytic defect [74]. If the organism is isolated from a bone aspirate, the diagnosis is definitive. Because infections have been reported to involve almost every body site, this organism should be included in the differential diagnosis of any focal infection occurring in infants less than three months of age.

Distinguishing between colonization and invasive infection may be difficult in adult patients. Isolation of the organism from the blood is the best indication, but since 17%–43% of group B streptococcal bacteremias are polymicrobial, sometimes clinical infection is attributed to another agent [15]. Molecular typing techniques may be useful for the evaluation of the patient with a recurrent infection [92,93] or in investigating a cluster of nosocomial infections [96].

TREATMENT

Penicillin remains the drug of choice for treatment of systemic group B streptococcal infection [23]. Empiric therapy of infants should be directed toward the agents frequently causing early- and late-onset infections, and typically include intravenous ampicillin and gentamicin, with the possible addition of cefotaxime if meningeal involvement is likely. Empiric therapy for pregnant women and nonpregnant adults include broad-spectrum agents recommended for septicemia or specific focal infections. Once group B streptococci have been identified and susceptibility verified, penicillin G can be used to complete therapy. Recommendations concerning optimal dose and duration vary and are dictated by the focus and severity of the infection (Tables 12.2 and 12.3). Several facts are pertinent when selecting the dose for penicillin or ampicillin. First, the usual minimal bactericidal concentration of penicillin for group B streptococci ranges from 0.04 to 0.8 μg/ml [23,97]. Second, only 10% to 20% of the concentration of penicillin in the serum will penetrate CSF when inflammation is present. Third, the inoculum of group B streptococci in the CSF of infants with meningitis may exceed 10^7 cfu/ml [98]. Finally, even high doses of penicillin G and ampicillin are safe in neonates, young infants, pregnant women, and elderly adults with normal renal function. To ensure rapid bacterial killing, especially in patients with meningitis, relatively high doses of penicillin are recommended [99].

In patients with meningitis, a second lumbar puncture 24 to 48 h into therapy is recommended by some experts to document CSF sterility. Patients with positive CSF cultures should be considered to have ventriculitis with obstruction, severe infection with cerebritis and vasculitis, or a very high inoculum. Since penicillin-resistant strains of group B streptococci have not been reported, patients with positive CSF cultures should have studies, including determination of penicillin susceptibility, to determine which, if any, of these circumstances accounts for the persistently positive culture. When CSF sterility and penicillin G susceptibility are verified, penicillin G is given for a minimum total

Table 12.2 Therapy for Group B Streptococcal Infections in Infants

Focus of Infection	Antibiotic Dose	Duration
Suspected sepsis[a]	Ampicillin (100–150 mg/kg/day) plus gentamicin	Until organism identified
Suspected meningitis	Ampicillin (300 mg/kg/day) plus gentamicin	Until cerebrospinal fluid sterility and penicillin G susceptibility documented (MIC ≤0.6 μg/ml)
Bacteremia	Penicillin G (200,000 units/kg/day)	10 days
Meningitis	Penicillin G (450,000–500,000 units/kg/day)	14 days minimum[b]
Osteomyelitis	Penicillin G (200,000–300,000 units/kg/day)	3–4 weeks
Endocarditis[c]	Penicillin G (200,000–300,000 units/kg/day)	4 weeks

[a]Assumes lumbar puncture has been performed and that cerebrospinal fluid has no abnormalities.

[b]This should be extended to 21 days or longer if ventriculitis, cerebritis, subdural empyema, or other suppurative complications occur.

[c]The addition of gentamicin for the first 14 days is suggested.

antimicrobial treatment of 14 days. Contrast-enhanced computer tomography scan of the head should be considered for all infants, especially for those with complications, but this should be delayed until therapy is almost completed. Infants who have shock, coma, prolonged fever (more than 5 days), cerebritis, subdural empyema or venous thrombosis may have incomplete central nervous system recovery [81,83].

Infants with bacteremia without a focus should receive intravenous therapy for a total of 10 days. A shorter duration has not been shown to be efficacious, and relapses, although rare, have been reported under these circumstances [11]. Oral therapy has no place in the manage-ment of infants with group B streptococcal disease, but these are often utilized after initial parenteral therapy in adults without underlying medical conditions. Alternative agents, such as the cephalosporins and vancomycin, are active against group B streptococci in vitro [97], but their efficacy is unknown and they are not recommended except in the patients with documented penicillin allergy (Tables 12.2 and 12.3).

Adjunctive therapies for life-threatening group B streptococcal disease in infants are under investigation. These include measures to improve developmentally impaired host defenses, such as use of intravenous immune globulin, white blood cell transfusion, and growth factors, such as granulocyte colony-stimulating factor

Table 12.3 Therapy for Group B Streptococcal Infections in Adults

Focus of Infection	Antibiotic Dose[a,b]	Duration
Bacteremia, pneumonia, soft-tissue infections	Penicillin G 9–12 MU/day	10–14 days
Meningitis	Penicillin G 30 MU/day	14 days minimum
Endocarditis	Penicillin 24 MU/day[c]	4–6 weeks
Osteomyelitis	Penicillin 10–20 MU/day	4 weeks

[a]For patients with normal renal function.

[b]In penicillin-allergic patients, vancomycin should be substituted except in those with meningitis, where cefotaxime or ceftriaxone is preferred because of superior CSF penetration.

[c]Use of gentamicin for the first 10–14 days should be considered.

and granulocyte monocyte-stimulating factor. These agents have not been adequately assessed for safety and efficacy in controlled clinical trials. Although they may be employed in the occasional patient, their use should be considered experimental.

In those very few patients who experience a recurrence, suppurative foci and humoral immune deficiency should be excluded or treated, if present. Tube dilution susceptibility testing of isolates from the first and recurrent episodes should be performed to ensure in vitro susceptibility to penicillin. If the reason for the recurrence remains unknown, it is likely that persistent mucous membrane infection with group B streptococci is the source. Beta-lactam antibiotics do not reliably eradicate group B streptococcal colonization [100]. However, successful eradication of mucosal group B streptococcal colonization following oral rifampin treatment in twins has been reported [101]. This treatment (20 mg/kg/day) after completion of parenteral therapy should be considered in infants with recurrent group B streptococcal disease, but no clinical studies have evaluated the effectiveness of this empiric therapy [92].

PREVENTION

The continuing magnitude and severity of group B streptococcal disease and its attendant mortality and morbidity underscore the desirability of prevention methods. Two approaches have been proposed: chemoprophylaxis and immunoprophylaxis.

Chemoprophylaxis

Three approaches to prevent early-onset group B streptococcal by chemoprophylaxis have been evaluated. The first was treatment of carriers during pregnancy. This temporarily suppressed colonization, but did not eradicate it at delivery nor did it interrupt vertical transmission [102,103]. The second, intramuscular penicillin given as a single dose to newborns shortly after birth, is controversial. The two controlled trials evaluating neonatal prophylaxis reached contradictory conclusions [104,105]. Since no bacterial cultures were obtained before penicillin was administered by Siegel et al. [105], it is possible that early-onset cases occurred but were not documented. In another controlled study, blood cultures were obtained before penicillin therapy, and the rates of group B streptococcal bacteremia were similar in treatment and control group [104]. The result of this latter investigation is supported by numerous observations indicating that most early-onset disease has an in utero onset [14,55].

The third approach, intrapartum chemoprophylaxis, is efficacious in the prevention of vertical transmission from colonized mothers to their neonates, of early-onset disease, and of maternal febrile morbidity. Its impact on late-onset disease, if any, is not documented. Four controlled trials involving thousands of deliveries have indicated that intrapartum penicillin G or ampicillin given intravenously to group B streptococcal carriers prevents early-onset disease in neonates [56,106–108]. The first identified group B streptococcal carriers using vaginal and rectal cultures were obtained at 26 to 28 weeks gestation [56]. Carriers who had either labor less than 37 weeks gestation, rupture of membranes >12 h before delivery, or intrapartum fever (>37.5°C) were randomized to receive intravenous ampicillin during labor or conventional care. Ampicillin reduced the rate of vertical transmission from 51% to 9% and that of early-onset disease from 6% to none ($P <$ 0.02) [56].

Intrapartum chemoprophylaxis for group B streptococcal carriers selected because of one or more risk factors for early-onset disease was supported by the American Academy of Pediatrics in 1992 [109]. These guidelines provoked controversy, and their implementation was been problematic [110]. Recently, new recommendations supported by both The American Academy of Pediatrics and The American College of Obstetricians and Gynecologists have been provided [34]. Key features of these include a choice of prevention strategies, use of penicillin G rather than ampicillin as the prophylactic agent, and an empiric algorithm for management of the infant (Table 12.4). In selected women, chemoprophylaxis is initiated at hospital admission for delivery or rupture of membranes, and consists of intravenous penicillin G (initial dose, 5 million units; subsequent doses, 2.5 million units

Table 12.4 Prevention of Early-Onset Group B Streptococcal (GBS) Disease by Intrapartum Maternal Chemoprophylaxis

Strategy	Target Population	Estimated Proportion of Cases Prevented[a]	Antibiotic/Dose
Culture-based	Women with (1) previous GBS infant; (2) GBS bacteriuria, or (3) labor <37 weeks	85–90%	Penicillin G % MU IV (initially); 2.5 MU every 4 hr until delivery
	GBS carriers with (1) membrane rupture >18 h before delivery, or (2) intrapartum fever		
	Other GBS carriers[b]		
Risk factor–Based	Women with (1) previous GBS infant, (2) GBS bacteriuria, (3) labor <37 weeks, (4) rupture of membranes >18 h before delivery, or (5) intrapartum fever (≥38°C)	68%	Same

[a]Data from Schuchat [34].

[b]Carriers without a risk factor should have the opportunity to choose chemoprophylaxis, if desired.

every 4 h) until delivery. Penicillin-allergic women are given clindamycin (900 mg) or erythromycin (500 mg) intravenously until delivery, although neither of these agents has been evaluated for efficacy. Selection of women to receive chemoprophylaxis is dictated either by group B streptococcal culture screening at 35–37 weeks of gestation or on the presence of a factor known to significantly increase the risk of early-onset disease in the neonate. These include (1) previous delivery of an infant with documented group B streptococcal disease, (2) group B streptococcal bacteriuria during the current pregnancy, (3) labor onset or membrane rupture before 37 weeks gestation, (4) rupture of membranes 18 or more h before delivery, or (5) intrapartum fever (≥38.0°C or 100.4°F). Women who have the first three risk factors need not been screened since they all should receive chemoprophylaxis. Women who are group B streptococcal carriers without one of the risk factors should receive chemoprophylaxis because up to 50% of the infants who develop early-onset dis-

ease are born to carriers without risk factors [14,111]. Group B streptococcal carriers who have either intrapartum fever or rupture of membranes more than 18 h before delivery always should receive intrapartum penicillin G prophylaxis. Women who are culture negative and have no risk factors are managed routinely (approximately 75% of obstetrical patients) [34]. Although the safety, efficacy, and cost-effectiveness of these two strategies have not been compared in clinical trials, each is estimated to be cost-beneficial [112–114].

Management of the infant born to the mother given intrapartum penicillin G prophylaxis is based on expert opinion, and depends on clinical findings at birth, gestational age, and number of doses administered to the mother [115]. If the infant is asymptomatic, has a gestational age of 35 weeks or more, and has a mother given two or more doses before delivery, neither a diagnostic evaluation nor empiric antimicrobial therapy are required. However, to assure their asymptomatic status, such infants are observed carefully for 48 h. Neonates with signs of sepsis are evaluated and empirically treated for sepsis.

Immunoprophylaxis

While efforts to implement intrapartum chemoprophylaxis are ongoing, the most promising, durable, and cost-effective method for prevention of early- and late-onset infant infections is immunoprophylaxis. This approach remains investigational, and several reviews have summarized the rationale [14,116,117]. It is based on the observation that immunity to group B streptococci is correlated with antibody directed against the type-specific capsular polysaccharides of these organisms [11]. These immunoglobulin G (IgG) class antibodies in the presence of complement and polymorphonuclear leukocytes promote opsonization, phagocytosis, and bacterial killing of group B streptococci, and protect animals against lethal challenge [118,119]. Provision of protective levels of group B streptococcal type-specific immunity to the infant could be achieved through immunization of the mother. Baker et al. [120] immunized women at a mean gestation of 31 weeks with purified type III polysaccharide vaccine. Although the immune response was not optimal (54%), placental transport of maternal antibodies (when stimulated) was excellent, and among neonates born to women who did respond to vaccination, 75% had protective levels of antibodies in their sera at 2 months of age. Additional studies immunizing nonpregnant adults with capsular polysaccharide vaccines of group B streptococcus indicated their safety, but suboptimal immunogenicity [116].

Since most pregnant women (estimated at 80% to 90%) have nonprotective levels of group B streptococcal specific antibodies in their sera at delivery, active immunization of women with improved vaccines has been proposed [117]. Initial results using candidate polysaccharide-protein conjugate vaccines in nonpregnant women suggest their safety and excellent immunogenicity [121,122]. They will require additional investigation administered as a multivalent single dose and in pregnant women to assure stimulation of class and IgG subclass of antibodies that are efficiently transported to the neonate. Furthermore, as maternal immunization is unlikely to be a strategy that will be utilized in this country, vaccine strategies that avoid pregnancy must be considered. Although immunoprophylaxis is believed to be the most cost-effective and beneficial prevention strategy for group B streptococcal infant disease [14,113], its realization will require acceptance and promotion by physicians, public health officials, parents, pharmaceutical manufacturers, and legislators.

REFERENCES

1. Nocard, M. Sur une mammite contagieuse des vaches laitières. Ann Inst Pasteur 1887; 1:109–127.
2. Lancefield RC. A serological differentiation of human and other groups of hemolytic streptococci. J Exp Med 1933; 57:571–595.
3. Lancefield RC, Hare R. The serological differentiation of pathogenic and non-pathogenic strains of hemolytic streptococci from parturient women. J Exp Med 1935; 61:335–349.
4. Congdon PM. Streptococcal infection in childbirth and septic abortion. Lancet 1935; 2:1287–1288.
5. Fry RM. Fatal infections by haemolytic streptococcus group B. Lancet 1938; 1:199–201.
6. Butter MNW, DeMoor CE. *Streptococcus agalactiae* as a cause of meningitis in the newborn, and of bacteremia in adults. Antonie van Leeuwenhoek 1967; 33:439–450.
7. Eickhoff TC, Klein JO, Daly AL, Ingall D, Finland M. Neonatal sepsis and other infections due to group B beta-hemolytic streptococci. N Engl J Med 1964; 271:1221–1228.
8. Hood M, Janney A, Dameron G. Beta hemolytic streptococcus group B associated with problems of the perinatal period. Am J Obstet Gynecol 1961; 82:809–818.
9. Baker CJ, Barrett FF, Gordon RC, Yow MD. Suppurative meningitis due to streptococci of Lancefield group B: a study of 33 infants. J Pediatr 1973; 82:724–729.
10. Franciosi RA, Knostman JD, Zimmerman RA. Group B streptococcal neonatal and infant infections. J Pediatr 1973; 82:707–718.
11. Baker CJ, Edwards MS. Group B streptococcal infections. In: Remington JS, Klein JO (eds). Infectious Diseases of the Fetus and Newborn Infant, 4th ed. Philadelphia: W.B. Saunders, 1995; 980–1054.
12. Zangwill KM, Schuchat A, Wenger JD. Group B streptococcal disease in the United States, 1990: report from a multistate active surveillance system. MMWR Morb Mortal Wkly Rep 1992; 41(Surveillance Summary-6):25–32.
13. Hussain SM, Luedtke GS, Baker CJ, Schlievert

PM, Leggiadro RJ. Invasive group B streptococcal disease in children beyond early infancy. Pediatr Infect Dis J 1995; 14:278–281.

14. Schuchat A. Epidemiology of group B streptococcal disease in the United States: shifting paradigms. Clin Microbiol Rev 1998; 11:497–513.

15. Farley MM, Harvey C, Stull T, Smith JD, Schuchat A, Wenger JD, Stephens DS. A population-based assessment of invasive disease due to group B streptococcus in nonpregnant adults. N Engl J Med 1993; 328:1807–1811.

16. Centers for Disease Control. Decreasing incidence of perinatal group B streptococcal disease—United States, 1993–1995. MMWR Morb Mortal Wkly Rep 1997; 46:473–477.

17. Henrichsen J, Ferrieri P, Jelinkova J, Kohler W, Maxted WR. Nomenclature of antigens of group B streptococci. Int J Syst Bact 1984; 34:500.

18. Jelinkova J, Motlova J. Worldwide distribution of two new serotypes of group B streptococcus: type IV and provisional type V. J Clin Microbiol 1985; 21:361–362.

19. Kogan G, Uhrín D, Brisson J-R, Paoletti LC, Kasper DL, von Hunolstein C, Oreficig, Jennings HJ. Structure of the type VI group B streptococcus capsular polysaccharide determined by high resolution NMR spectroscopy. J Carbohydr Chem 1994; 13:1071–1078.

20. Kogan G, Brisson J-R, Kasper DL, von Hunolstein C, Orefici G, Jennings HJ. Structural elucidation of the novel type VII group B streptococcus capsular polysaccharide by high resolution NMR spectroscopy. Carbohydr Res 1995; 277:1–9.

21. Kogan G, Uhrín D, Brisson J-R, Paoletti LC, Blodgett AE, Kasper DL, Jennings HJ. Structural and immunochemical characterization of the type VIII group B streptococcus capsular polysaccharide. J Biol Chem 1996; 271:8786–8790.

22. Ferrieri P. Surface-localized protein antigens of group B streptococci. Rev Infect Dis 1988; 10:S363–S366.

23. Fernandez M, Hickman ME, Baker CJ. Antimicrobial susceptibilities of group B streptococci isolated between 1992 and 1996 from patients with bacteremia or meningitis. Antimicrob Agents Chemother 1998; 42:1517–1519.

24. Berkowitz K, Regan JA, Greenberg E. Antibiotic resistance patterns of group B streptococci in pregnant women. J Clin Microbiol 1990; 28:5–7.

25. Rolston KV. I. Susceptibility of group B and group G streptococci to newer antimicrobial agents. Eur J Clin Microbiol 1986; 5:534–536.

26. Persson KM-S, Forsgren A. Antimicrobial susceptibility of group B streptococci. Eur J Clin Microbiol 1986; 5:165–167.

27. Scheld WM, Alliegro GM, Field MR, Brodeur JP. Synergy between penicillins and low concentrations of gentamicin in experimental meningitis due to group B streptococci. J Infect Dis 1982; 146:100.

28. Swingle HM, Bucciarfelli RL, Ayoub EM. Synergy between penicillins and low concentrations of gentamicin in the killing of group B streptococci. J Infect Dis 1985; 152:58–66.

29. Kim KS. Clinical perspectives on penicillin tolerance. J Pediatr 1988; 112:214–216.

30. Baker CJ, Barrett FF. Transmission of group B streptococci among parturient women and their neonates. J Pediatr 1973; 83:919–925.

31. Pass MA, Gray BM, Khare S, Dillon HC. Prospective studies of group B streptococcal infections in infants. J Pediatr 1979; 95:437–443.

32. Weisman LE, Stoll BJ, Cruess DF, Hall RT, Merenstein GB, Hemming VG, Fischer GW. Early-onset group B streptococcal sepsis: a current assessment. J Pediatr 1992; 121:428–433.

33. Dillon HC Jr, Khare S, Gray BM. Group B streptococcal carriage and disease: a 6-year prospective study. J Pediatr 1987; 110:31–36.

34. Schuchat A, Whitney C, Zangwill K. Prevention of perinatal group B streptococcal disease: a public health perspective. MMWR Morb Mortal Week Rep 1996; 45:1–24 (No. RR-7).

35. Krohn MJ, Hillier SL, Baker CJ. Maternal peripartum complications associated with vaginal group B streptococcal colonization. J Infect Dis 1999; in press.

36. Minkoff HL, Sierra MF, Pringle GF, Schwarz RH. Vaginal colonization with group B beta-hemolytic streptococcus as a risk factor for postcesarean section febrile morbidity. Am J Obstet Gynecol 1982; 142:992–995.

37. Yancey MK, Duff P, Clark P, Kurtzer T, Frentzen BH, Kubilis P. Peripartum infection associated with vaginal group B streptococcal colonization. Obstet Gynecol 1994; 84:816–819.

38. Hillier SL, Nugent RP, Eschenbach DA, Krohn MJ, Gibbs RS, Martin DH, Cotch MF, Edelman R, Pastorek JG, Vijaya Rao A, McNellis D, Regan JA, Carey JC, Klebanoff MA. Association between bacterial vaginosis and preterm delivery of a low birth weight infant. N Engl J Med 1995; 333:1737–1742.

39. Regan JA, Klebanoff MA, Nugent RP, and the Vaginal Infections and Prematurity Study Group. The epidemiology of group B streptococcal colonization in pregnancy. Obstet Gynecol 1991; 77:604–610.

40. Regan JA, Klebanoff MA, Nugent RP, Eschenbach DA, Blackwelder WC, Lou Y, Gibbs RS, Rettig PJ, Martin DH, Edelman R. Colonization with group B streptococci in pregnancy and adverse outcome. Am J Obstet Gynecol 1996; 174:1354–1360.

41. Badri MS, Zawaneh S, Cruz AC, Mantilla G, Baer H, Spellacy WN, Ayoub EM. Rectal colonization with group B streptococcus: relation to vaginal colonization of pregnant women. J Infect Dis 1977; 135:308–312.

42. Baker CJ, Goroff DK, Alpert SL, Hayes C, McCormack WM. Comparison of bacteriological

methods for the isolation of group B strepto-coccus from vaginal cultures. J Clin Microbiol 1976; 4:46–48.

43. Dillon HC Jr, Gray E, Pass MA, Gray BM. Anorectal and vaginal carriage of group B strep-tococci during pregnancy. J Infect Dis 1982; 145:794–799.

44. MacDonald SW, Manuel FR, Embil JA. Local-ization of group B beta-hemolytic streptococci in the female urogenital tract. Am J Obstet Gy-necol 1979; 133:57–59.

45. Platt MW, McLaughlin JC, Gilson GJ, Well-honer MF, Nims LJ. Increased recovery of group B streptococcus by the inclusion of rectal culturing and enrichment. Diagn Microbiol In-fect Dis 1995; 21:65–68.

46. Zaleznik DF, Krohn MA, Hillier SL, Ferrier P, Lee M-L, Platt R, Baker CJ. Group B strepto-coccal colonization in parturient women differs among racial groups. In: Abstracts of the 35th ICAAC, 1995; 322, Abstract K188.

47. Lim DV, Morales WJ, Walsh AF. Lim group B strep broth and coagglutination for rapid iden-tification of group B streptococci in preterm pregnant women. J Clin Microbiol 1987; 25:452–453.

48. Boyer KM, Gadzala CA, Kelly PD, Burd LI, Gotoff SP. Selective intrapartum chemoprophy-laxis of neonatal group B streptococcal early-onset disease. II. Predictive value of prenatal cultures. J Infect Dis 1983; 148:802–809.

49. Baker CJ. Inadequacy of rapid immunoassays for intrapartum detection of group B streptococcal carriers. Obstet Gynecol 1996; 88:51–55.

50. Anthony BF, Okada DM, Hobel CJ. Epidemi-ology of the group B streptococcus: maternal and nosocomial sources for infant acquisitions. J Pediatr 1979; 95:431–436.

51. Baker CJ, Goroff DK, Alpert S, Crockett VA, Zinner SH, Evrard JR, Rosner B, McCormack WM. Vaginal colonization with group B strep-tococcus: a study in college women. J Infect Dis 1977; 135:392–397.

52. Ferrieri P, Cleary PP, Seeds AE. Epidemiology of group B streptococcal carriage in pregnant women and newborn infants. J Med Microbiol 1976; 10:103–114.

53. Hickman ME, Rench MA, Ferrieri P, Baker CJ. Changing epidemiology of group B streptococ-cal colonization. Pediatrics 1999; in press.

54. Ancona RJ, Ferrieri P, Williams PP. Maternal factors that enhance the acquisition of group B streptococci by newborn infants. J Med Micro-biol 1980; 13:273–280.

55. Boyer KM, Gadzala CA, Kelly PD, Gotoff SP. Selective intrapartum chemoprophylaxis of neonatal group B streptococcal early-onset dis-ease. III. Interruption of mother-to-infant trans-mission. J Infect Dis 1983; 148:810–816.

56. Boyer KM, Gotoff SP. Prevention of early-onset neonatal group B streptococcal disease with se-lective intrapartum chemoprophylaxis. N Engl J Med 1986; 314:1665–1669.

57. Lim DV, Kanarek KS, Peterson ME. Magnitude of colonization and sepsis by group B strepto-cocci in newborn infants. Curr Microbiol 1982; 7:99–101.

58. Schuchat A, Deaver-Robinson K, Plikaytis BD, Zangwill KM, Mohle-Boetani J, Wenger JD. Multistate case-control study of maternal risk factors for neonatal group B streptococcal disease. Pediatr Infect Dis J 1994; 13: 623–629.

59. Schuchat A, Oxtoby M, Cochi S, Sikes RK, High-tower A, Plikaytis B, Broome CV. Population-based risk factors for neonatal group B strepto-coccal disease: results of a cohort study in metropolitan Atlanta. J Infect Dis 1990; 162: 672–677.

60. Schwartz B, Schuchat A, Oxtoby MJ, Cochi SL, Hightower A, Broome CV. Invasive group B streptococcal disease in adults. A population-based study in metropolitan Atlanta. JAMA 1991; 266:1112–1114.

61. Colford JM, Mohle-Boetani J, Vosti KL. Group B streptococcal bacteremia in adults: five years' experience and a review of the literature. Med-icine 1995; 74:176–190.

62. Gallagher PG, Watanakunakorn C. Group B streptococcal bacteremia in a community teach-ing hospital. Am J Med 1985; 78:795–800.

63. Verghese A, Mireault K, Arbeit RD. Group B streptococcal bacteremia in men. Rev Infect Dis 1986; 8:912–917.

64. Jackson LA, Hilsdon R, Farley MM, Harrison LH, Reingold AL, Plikaytis BD, Wenger JD, Schuchat A. Risk factors for group B strepto-coccal disease in adults. Ann Intern Med 1995; 123:415–420.

65. Baker CJ, Barrett FF. Group B streptococcal in-fections in infants: the importance of the vari-ous serotypes. JAMA 1974; 230:1158–1182.

66. Wilkinson HW. Analysis of group B streptococ-cal types associated with disease in human in-fants and adults. J Clin Microbiol 1978; 7:176–179.

67. Blumberg HM, Stephens DS, Modansky M, Er-win M, Elliot J, Facklam RR, Schuchat A, Baughman W, Farley MM. Invasive group B streptococcal disease: the emergence of serotype V. J Infect Dis 1996; 173:365–373.

68. Harrison LH, Elliott JA, Dwyer DM, Liborati JP, Ferrieri P, Billmann L, Schuchat A. Serotype distribution of invasive group B streptococcal isolates in Maryland: implications for vaccine formulation. J Infect Dis 1998; 177:998–1002.

69. Lin FYC, Clemens JD, Azimi PH, Regen JA, Weisman LE, Phillips JB III, Rhoads GG, Clark P, Brenner RA, Ferrieri P. Capsular polysac-charide types of group B streptococcal isolates from neonates with early-onset systemic infec-tion. J Infect Dis 1998; 177:790–792.

70. Rench MA, Baker CJ. Neonatal sepsis caused by a new group B streptococcal serotype. J Pediatr 1993; 122:638–640.

71. Yagupsky P, Menegus MA, Powell KR. The changing spectrum of group B streptococcal disease in infants: an eleven-year experience in a tertiary care hospital. Pediatr Infect Dis J 1991; 10:801–808.

72. Payne NR, Burke BA, Day DL, Christenson PD, Thompson TR, Ferrieri P. Correlation of clinical and pathologic findings in early onset neonatal group B streptococcal infection with disease severity and prediction of outcome. Pediatr Infect Dis J 1988; 7:836–847.

73. Noya FJD, Rench MA, Metzger TG, Colman G, Naidoo J, Baker CJ. Unusual occurrence of an epidemic of type Ib/c group B streptococcal sepsis in a neonatal intensive care unit. J Infect Dis 1987; 55:1135–1144.

74. Edwards MS, Baker CJ, Wagner ML, Taber LH, Barrett FF. An etiologic shift in infantile osteomyelitis: the emergence of the group B streptococcus. J Pediatr 1978; 93:578–583.

75. Baker CJ. Group B streptococcal cellulitis/adenitis in infants. Am J Dis Child 1982; 136:631–633.

76. Vollman JH, Smith WL, Ballard ET, Light IJ. Early onset group B streptococcal disease: clinical, roentgenographic, and pathologic features. J Pediatr 1976; 89:199–203.

77. Lilien LD, Harris VJ, Pildes RS. Significance of radiographic findings in early-onset group B streptococcal infection. Pediatrics 1977; 60:360–365.

78. Weller MH, Katzenstein A. Radiological findings in group B streptococcal sepsis. Radiology 1976; 118:385–387.

79. Ablow RC, Driscoll SG, Effmann EL, Gross I, Jolles CJ, Uauy R, Warshaw JB. A comparison of early-onset group B streptococcal neonatal infection and the respiratory-distress syndrome of the newborn. N Engl J Med 1976; 294:65–70.

80. Wiswell TE, Baumgart S, Gannon CM, Spitzer AR. No lumbar puncture in the evaluation for early neonatal sepsis: will meningitis be missed? Pediatrics 1995; 95:803–806.

81. Chin KC, Fitzhardinge PM. Sequelae of early-onset group B streptococcal neonatal meningitis. J Pediatr 1985; 106:819–822.

82. Quirante J, Ceballos R, Cassady G. Group B β-hemolytic streptococcal infection in the newborn. Am J Dis Child 1974; 128:659–665.

83. Edwards MS, Rench MA, Haffar AAM, Murphy M, Desmond MM, Baker CJ. Long-term sequelae of group B streptococcal meningitis in infants. J Pediatr 1985; 106:717–722.

84. Wald ER, Bergman I, Taylor HG, Chiponis D, Porter C, Kubek K. Long-term outcome of group B streptococcal meningitis. Pediatrics 1986; 77:217–221.

85. Wong M, Isaacs D, Howman-Giles R, Uren R. Clinical and diagnostic features of osteomyelitis occurring in the first three months of life. Pediatr Infect Dis J 1995; 14:1047–1053.

86. Hauger SB. Facial cellulitis: an early indicator of group B streptococcal bacteremia. Pediatrics 1981; 67:376–377.

87. Garcia-Pena BM, Harper MB, Fleisher GR. Occult bacteremia with group B streptococci in an outpatient setting. Pediatrics 1998; 102:67–72.

88. DiJohn D, Krasinski K, Lawrence R. Very late onset of group B streptococcal disease in infants infected with the human immunodeficiency virus. Pediatr Infect Dis J 1990; 9:925–928.

89. Domingo P, Barquet N, Alvarez M, Coll P, Nava J, Garau J. Group B streptococcal meningitis in adults: report of twelve cases and review. Clin Infect Dis 1997; 25:1180–1187.

90. Munoz P, Llancaqueo A, Rodriguez-Creixems M, Pelaez T, Martin L, Bouza E. Group B streptococcus bacteremia in nonpregnant adults. Arch Intern Med 1997; 157:213–216.

91. Scully BE, Spriggs D, Neu HC. Streptococcus agalactiae (group B) endocarditis—description of twelve cases and review of the literature. Infection 1987; 15:169–176.

92. Green PA, Singh KV, Murray BE, Baker CJ. Recurrent group B streptococcal infections in infants: clinical and microbiologic aspects. J Pediatr 1994; 125:931–938.

93. Harrison LH, Alia A, Dwyer DM, Libonati JP, Reeves MW, Elliott JA, Billmann L, Lashkerwala T, Johnson JA. Relapsing invasive group B streptococcal infection in adults. Ann Intern Med 1995; 123:421–427.

95. Baker CJ. Early onset group B streptococcal disease. J Pediatr 1978; 93:124–125.

96. Blumberg HM, Stephens DS, Licitra C, Pigott N, Facklam R, Swaminathan B, Wachsmuth IK. Molecular epidemiology of group B streptococcal infections: use of restriction endonuclease analysis of chromosomal DNA and DNA restriction fragment length polymorphisms of ribosomal RNA genes (ribotyping). J Infect Dis 1992; 166:574–579.

97. Kim KS. Antimicrobial susceptibility of group B streptococci. Antimicrob Agents Chemother 1985; 35:83–89.

98. Feldman WE. Concentrations of bacteria in cerebrospinal fluid of patients with bacterial meningitis. J Pediatr 1976; 88:549–552.

99. American Academy of Pediatrics. Group B streptococcal infections. In: Peter G (ed). Red Book: Report of the Committee on Infectious Diseases, 23rd ed. Elk Grove Village, IL, 1997; 495–496.

100. Paredes AB, Wong P, Yow MD. Failure of penicillin to eradicate the carrier state of group B streptococcus in infants. J Pediatr 1976; 89:191–193.

101. Millard DD, Bussey ME, Shulman ST, Yogev R. Multiple group B streptococcal infections in a

premature infant: eradication of nasal colonization with rifampin. Am J Dis Child 1985; 139:964–965.

102. Gardner SE, Yow MD, Leeds LJ, Thompson PK, Mason EO Jr, Clark DJ. Failure of penicillin to eradicate group B streptococcal colonization in the pregnant woman. Am J Obstet Gynecol 1979; 135:1062–1065.

103. Hall RT, Barnes W, Krishnan L, Harris DJ, Rhodes PG, Fayez J, Miller GL. Antibiotic treatment of parturient women colonized with group B streptococci. Am J Obstet Gynecol 1976; 124:630–634.

104. Pyati SP, Pildes RS, Jacobs NM, Ramamurthy RS, Yeh TF, Raval DS, Lilien LD, Amma P, Metzger WI. Penicillin in infants weighing two kilograms or less with early-onset group B streptococcal disease. N Engl J Med 1983; 308: 1383–1389.

105. Siegel JD, McCracken GH Jr, Threlkeld N, Milvenan B, Rosenfeld CR. Single-dose penicillin prophylaxis against neonatal group B streptococcal infections. N Engl J Med 1980; 303:769–775.

106. Garland SM, Fliegner JR. Group B streptococcus and neonatal infections: the case for intrapartum chemoprophylaxis. Aust N Z J Obstet Gynaecol 1991; 31:119–122.

107. Matorras R, Garcia-Perea A, Omenaca F, Diez-Enciso M, Madero R, Usanclizaga JA. Intrapartum chemoprophylaxis of early-onset group B streptococcal disease. Eur J Obstet Gynecol Reprod Biol 1991; 40:57–62.

108. Tuppurainen N, Hallman M. Prevention of neonatal group B streptococcal disease: intrapartum detection and chemoprophylaxis of heavily colonized parturients. Obstet Gynecol 1989; 73:583–587.

109. American Academy of Pediatrics. Guidelines for prevention of group B streptococcal infection by chemoprophylaxis. Pediatrics 1992; 90:775–778.

110. Jafari HS, Schuchat A, Hilsdon R, Whitney CG, Toomey KE, Wenger JD. Barriers to prevention of perinatal group B streptococcal disease. Pediatr Infect Dis J 1995; 14:662–665.

111. Rosenstein N, Schuchat A and Neonatal GBS Disease Study Group. Opportunities for prevention of perinatal group B streptococcal disease: a multistate surveillance analysis. Obstet Gynecol 1997; 90:901–906.

112. Allen UD, Navas L, King SM. Effectiveness of intrapartum penicillin prophylaxis in preventing early-onset group B streptococcal infection: results of a meta-analysis. Can Med Assoc J 1993; 149:1659–1665.

113. Mohle-Boetani JC, Schuchat A, Plikaytis BD, Smith JD, Broome CV. Comparison of prevention strategies for neonatal group B streptococcal infection: a population-based economic analysis. JAMA 1993; 270:1442–1448.

114. Rouse DJ, Goldenberg RL, Cliver SP, Cutter GR, Mennemeyer ST, Fargason CA Jr. Strategies for the prevention of early-onset group B streptococcal sepsis: a decision analysis. Obstet Gynecol 1994; 83:483–494.

115. American Academy of Pediatrics. Revised guidelines for prevention of early-onset group B streptococcal (GBS) infection. Pediatrics 1997; 99:489–496.

116. Baker CJ, Kasper DL. Group B streptococcal vaccines. Rev Infect Dis 1985; 7:458–467.

117. Baker CJ. Immunization to prevent group B streptococcal disease: victories and vexations. J Infect Dis 1990; 161:917–921.

118. Paoletti LC, Wessels MR, Rodewald AK, Shroff AA, Jennings HJ, Kasper DL. Neonatal mouse protection against infection with multiple group B streptococcal serotypes by maternal immunization with a tetravalent GBS polysaccharide-tetanus toxoid conjugate vaccine. Infect Immun 1994; 62:3236–3243.

119. Wessels MR, Paoletti LC, Kasper DL, DiFabio JL, Michon F, Holme K, Jennings HJ. Immunogenicity in animals of a polysaccharide-protein conjugate vaccine against type III group B streptococcus. J Clin Invest 1990; 86: 1428–1433.

120. Baker CJ, Rench MA, Edwards MS, Carpenter RJ, Hays BM, Kasper DL. Immunization of pregnant women with a polysaccharide vaccine of group B streptococcus. N Engl J Med 1988; 319:1180–1185.

121. Baker CJ, Paoletti LC, Wessels MR, Guttormsen H-K, Rench MA, Hickman ME, Kasper DL. Safety and immunogenicity of capsular polysaccharide-tetanus toxoid conjugate vaccines for group B streptococcal types Ia and Ib. J Infect Dis 1999; 179:142–150.

122. Kasper DL, Paoletti LC, Wessels MR, Guttormsen H-K, Carey VJ, Jennings HJ, Baker CJ. Immune response to type III group B streptococcal polysaccharide-tetanus toxoid conjugate vaccine. J Clin Invest 1996; 98:2308–2314.

13

Group C and G Streptococci

J. MILTON GAVIRIA
ALAN L. BISNO

Streptococci of groups C and G are frequently recovered from humans and animals. This chapter will review the taxonomy and microbiologic characteristics of these organisms as well as their role in disease.

GROUP C STREPTOCOCCI

Taxonomy

The group-specific antigen of Lancefield group C streptococci (GCS) is a polysaccharide composed of hexosamine and rhamnose. It differs from that of group A in that the terminal antigenic determinant of GCS carbohydrate is N-acetyl-galactosamine rather than N-acetylglucosamine. Streptococci possessing the group C cell-wall carbohydrate are heterogeneous with regard to biochemical reactions, hemolytic characteristics, predilection for host species, and clinical illnesses produced. These streptococci can be initially divided into two morphologic categories based on colony size. For the most part, they form large colonies ($\geq$0.5 mm in diameter) that resemble those of *Streptococcus pyogenes* when cultivated on sheep blood–agar plates. These large-colony forms can be differentiated on the basis of biochemical reactions into two species: *Streptococcus dysgalactiae* and *Streptococcus equi*. The former is alpha hemolytic and

the latter beta hemolytic. Three other GCS formerly referred to as species but now classified in *Bergey's Manual* [1] as subspecies of *Streptococcus equi* are subsp. *equi*, *equisimilis*, and *zooepidemicus*. For convenience, throughout this discussion these three subspecies will be referred to as *Streptococcus equi*, *Streptococcus equisimilis*, and *Streptococcus zooepidemicus*. The classification of small- or minute-colony types (<0.5 mm in diameter) that react with group C antisera is less straightforward. They are often designated as members of the "*Streptococcus milleri* group" [2]. Strains classified as *Streptococcus milleri* may belong to Lancefield groups A, C, G, or F or may not be groupable [1]. They may be alpha-, beta- or nonhemolytic on sheep blood agar. Small-colony forms have also been referred to as *Streptococcus anginosus*, a species designation more recently proposed on the basis of genetic and phenotypic studies to be a member of the "*Streptococcus intermedius* group," along with *Streptococcus intermedius* and *Streptococcus constellatus* [3–6]. In addition to differences in colony size, there are differences in biochemical reactions between large-colony group C and group G strains and the "minute"-colony forms carrying the group C or G carbohydrate antigens. Large-colony isolates give positive beta-glucuronidase reactions and negative Voges-Proskauer tests. The opposite is true of minute-colony forms.

Microbiology

Major features differentiating the large-colony species and subspecies of GCS are outlined in Table 13.1. Efstratiou et al. [7] proposed biochemical tests to differentiate human from animal strains of *Streptococcus equisimilis*. Nearly all animal strains fermented glycogen and produced L-prolyl-L-arginine aminopeptidase, but none of the human strains did so. Considerable homology has been found between *Streptococcus equisimilis* and the large-colony human biotype group G streptococci [8]. In addition, one-dimensional sodium dodecyl sulphate-polyacrylamide gel electrophoresis (SDS-PAGE) of the two organisms produced similar patterns, adding strength to the suggestion that these bacteria might perhaps be classified within the same species [8].

Testing for susceptibility to a low-potency bacitracin disc is a time-honored method of presumptively differentiating group A from non–group A streptococci. Although the test has high sensitivity, its specificity with regard to GCS is imperfect. Matthieu et al. [9] reported that 8 to 13 (depending on the criteria used) of 15 group C strains were inhibited by a 0.04 unit bacitracin disc. Feingold et al. [10], using a 0.02 unit bacitracin disk, found 8 of 13 GCS to be sensitive to bacitracin. The GCS are thus more appropriately differentiated from group A streptococci by techniques employing group-specific antisera. One such system (Streptex®, Wellcome Diagnostics, Dartford, England), employing latex beads coated with group-specific antisera and enzymatic extracts of the Streptococcus cell wall, has proven quite accurate in our experience. A rapid staphylococcal coagglutination technique

[9] correctly identified 500 isolates of betahemolytic streptococci, 436 group A, and 64 non–group A streptococci, when compared with the capillary precipitin test, with no false positives and no false negatives. DNA fingerprinting has also been used to identify GCS [11].

Virulence Factors

Factors contributing to virulence of GCS have been less extensively studied than those of group A streptococci. It has been demonstrated, however, that certain GCS strains possess the two major somatic virulence constituents expressed by *Streptococcus pyogenes*: M protein and hyaluronate capsule.

M proteins have been detected in GCS strains of both animal and human origin. Jean-Francois et al. [12] immunized mice with an acid-extracted M-like protein from *Streptococcus equi* and found that it conferred protective immunity. Furthermore, monoclonal antibodies to different epitopes in the M protein molecule passively protected mice from lethal challenge. Galen and Timoney [13] studied a series of *Streptococcus equi* isolates from the United States and Europe and concluded that all expressed a single M protein type. Boshwitz and Timoney [14] studied a strain of *Streptococcus equi* that resisted killing in whole equine blood. They purified M protein from this strain and raised rabbit antisera to it. The antisera promoted bacterial killing in whole equine blood, an effect due at least in part to enhanced deposition of C3 complement on the opsonized organisms. Timoney et al. [15] cloned a protective

Table 13.1 Biochemical Characteristics of Group C Streptococci

Streptococcal Species and Group	Hemolysis on Sheep Blood Agar	Lactose	Sorbitol	Trehalose	Glycogen	L-propyl-L-arginine aminopeptidase	Streptokinase	Streptolysin O
S. equi subsp. *Equisimilis* (human)	β	±	−	+	−	−	+	+
S. equi subsp. *Zooepidemicus*	β	±	−	+	+	+	+	+
S. equi subsp. *Zooepidemicus*	β	±	+	−	+	−	−	−
S. equi subsp. *Equi*	β	−	−	−	+	−	−	−
S. dysgalactiae	α or none	+	±	+	−	+	−	−

From Holt et al. [1], and Efstratiou et al. [7], with permission.

M-like gene from an equine strain of *Streptococcus zooepidemicus*. The predicted amino acid structure contained an α-helical region and showed extensive homology with the carboxy termini of M proteins of groups A and G but lacked the A-, B-, and C-repeats found in group A M proteins.

Podbielski et al. [16], utilizing polymerase chain reaction (PCR) assays and genomic fingerprinting, identified M protein (termed *emm*) genes in one-quarter of 28 human GCS isolates tested. These workers sequenced one GCS *emm* gene and found the predicted structure of the C-repeat regions to be highly homologous to those of class I M protein genes of group A and G streptococci. The N-terminal region of the molecule, however, differed from those of previously characterized group A Streptococcus M proteins.

M proteins have been demonstrated by conventional microbiologic (resistance to phagocytosis) and immunologic (type-specific opsonization and precipitation) criteria in *Streptococcus equisimilis* strains isolated from four outbreaks of human disease [17,18]. Two of these were common-source outbreaks of pharyngitis associated with contaminated foods and two were outbreaks of puerperal infections in a maternity unit. One of the pharyngitis outbreaks was associated with cases of acute glomerulonephritis. Three of these outbreaks occurred in England and were caused by a single M type. The third outbreak occurred in Romania, and strains from this outbreak exhibited a different M type. Bisno et al. [19] studied 15 strains of *Streptococcus equisimilis* isolated from the throats of college students with acute pharyngitis and 5 strains isolated from patients with noninfectious disorders. Nineteen of the 20 strains resisted phagocytic killing during incubation with normal human blood, suggesting the presence of M proteins. All these 20 strains possessed genomic DNA encoding the conserved portion of the group M protein gene *emm*24, a region that is highly conserved among M proteins of group A and G streptococci. The predicted amino acid sequences of the N-terminal (variable) portions of two pharyngitis isolates studied were identical and were 88% homologous to the amino acid sequence of a group G M protein gene. This finding is compatible with the previously suggested

hypothesis that M proteins may be acquired by horizontal transfer across serogroups [20].

Many strains of *Streptococcus zooepidemicus* and some strains of *Streptococcus equi* produce a hyaluronic acid capsule [21,22]. The hyaluronate capsule subserves an important antiphagocytic function in group A streptococci, and the same may be presumed to be true of GCS. Genes encoding fibronectin-binding proteins, cellular constituents important in binding to epithelial surfaces, have been cloned and sequenced from *Streptococcus dysgalactiae* [23] and *Streptococcus zooepidemicus* [24]. The majority of human strains of GCS express immunoglobulin binding proteins [25].

Streptococcus equisimilis produces streptolysin O [26] and *Streptococcus zooepidemicus* and *Streptococcus equi* produce hemolysins unrelated to streptolysin O [21]. Other extracellular products produced by GCS that may possibly contribute to virulence include streptokinase [27] and hyaluronidase.

Clinical Manifestations

Animal Diseases

Group C streptococci are major pathogens of animals [21]. *Streptococcus zooepidemicus* may be isolated from wound infections of horses and is a cause of mastitis in cows and of septicemia in cows, rabbits, and swine. *Streptococcus equisimilis* can be isolated from the upper respiratory tract of animals and may cause diseases similar to those associated with *Streptococcus zooepidemicus* [7]. *Streptococcus equi* is the causative agent of strangles in horses. *Streptococcus dysgalactiae* may be isolated from udders of cows with mild mastitis and from blood and tissues of lambs with polyarthritis.

Human Infections

The great majority of human GCS infections are due to organisms classified as *Streptococcus equisimilis*. Infections due to *Streptococcus zooepidemicus* are unusual and in most cases represent zoonoses transmitted to humans by ingestion of unpasteurized milk and dairy products or by contact with horses. As suggested by their epidemiologic associations, human *Streptococcus zooepi-*

demicus infections often occur in the form of common source outbreaks. The spectrum of disease processes is broad, including respiratory tract infections [28], cervical lymphadenitis [29], pneumonia [30], bacteremia [31], endocarditis [22], meningitis [32,33], septic arthritis [30,32], and cellulitis. Invasive *Streptococcus zooepidemicus* infections may be life-threatening. Of 11 patients in West Yorkshire, England who became ill after ingesting unpasteurized milk, 7 died [34]. In New Mexico 2 of 16 ill persons died after consuming contaminated cheese [35]. Yuen et al. [22] reported 11 cases of *Streptococcus zooepidemicus* septicemia in Hong Kong and reviewed 43 cases reported elsewhere. The overall mortality rate was 22%. Pigs were incriminated as a possible source of human infection in Hong Kong; the local strains formed mucoid colonies and were heavily encapsulated. Several instances of poststreptococcal acute glomerulonephritis (AGN) have been documented following *Streptococcus zooepidemicus* infection [28,30,31,36]. In the most dramatic of these episodes [36], 85 persons in a Romanian town experienced acute pharyngitis and cervical adenitis after drinking milk contaminated with *Streptococcus zooepidemicus*, and approximately one-third subsequently developed AGN. Infections of humans due to *Streptococcus dysgalactiae* [37–39] and *Streptococcus equi* [38,40,41] have been documented only very rarely.

In the following sections dealing with human infections due to both group C and G streptococci, it has frequently not been possible to ascertain from published literature whether the infections were due to large-colony or minute-colony strains. In most cases, given what is known of the pathogenicity of these organisms, it is likely that the bulk of the infections were due to beta-hemolytic, large-colony (*Streptococcus pyogenes*–like) microorganisms.

PHARYNGITIS

Streptococcus equisimilis is not infrequently isolated from the throats of normal persons, particularly adults. Fox et al. [42], for example, isolated strains of *Streptococcus equisimilis* from the throats of 2.2% of 227 persons visiting a university student health service who had noninfectious problems. The role of this organism as

a cause of endemically occurring episodes of acute pharyngitis has remained controversial, however, in part because studies have not always shown a clear-cut difference in isolation rates between symptomatic and asymptomatic individuals [43]. Recent data provide evidence for the role of these organisms in community-acquired pharyngitis. In a study of college students, Turner et al. [44] found GCS to be isolated significantly more frequently from patients with acute pharyngitis than from those with noninfectious problems (26% vs. 11%). Among patients with sore throat, those with positive cultures for GCS were significantly more likely to have fever, exudate, and anterior cervical adenopathy than those with negative cultures. Additional studies in this student population demonstrated that students from whom *Streptococcus equisimilis* was isolated had clinical features more suggestive of pyogenic infection and had higher colony counts on primary culture plates than those from whom minute-colony strains (*Streptococcus anginosus*) were recovered [45]. Cimolai et al. [46] conducted a case–control study to evaluate the association of non–group A streptococci and pharyngitis in a pediatric population. These investigators found a statistically significant relationship between isolation of large-colony strains of group C and group G streptococci (when present in moderate to heavy amounts on the culture plate) and the occurrence of pharyngitis. The GCS strains were identified biochemically as *Streptococcus equisimilis*. There was no such association between presence of small-colony strains of groups C, F, and G and pharyngitis, although the number of such isolates was quite small.

Two other studies strongly support the role of GCS as a cause of clinically significant pharyngitis. Meier et al. [47] isolated GCS more frequently from 1425 adults with sore throat than from 284 controls (6% vs. 1.4%). Moreover, the signs and symptoms of group C–associated pharyngitis were intermediate between those of group A Streptococcus and culture-negative pharyngitis. During a 3-month period Benjamin and Perriello [48] isolated GCS from the throats of 32 students at a school for boys with learning disabilities. Children with positive throat cultures had significantly higher mean serum antistreptolysin O titers than those with negative cultures, and 22 (69%) of the students with positive cultures exhibited signs and symptoms of acute pharyngitis. In neither of these two studies, however, were the organisms speciated.

INFECTIONS OF SKIN, SOFT TISSUE, AND GENITOURINARY TRACT

Group C streptococci colonize not only the throat but also in normal skin and the genitourinary tract. The organisms have thus been associated with a wide range of skin and soft-tissue infections and infections of the female genital tract. Among these infections are cellulitis [2,49,50], pyoderma [51], deep-tissue abscesses, erysipelas [2,10,52–55], necrotizing fasciitis [2] (complicated in at least one case by development of Streptococcus toxic shock syndrome [56]), and puerperal sepsis [18,53].

OTHER DEEP-TISSUE INFECTIONS

As with other Streptococcus pathogens, GCS have been associated with infection of many body sites. Clinical reports document the occurrence, for example, of septic arthritis [57–60] sinusitis [61], osteomyelitis [53], endophthalmitis [62], intraabdominal abscess [53], meningitis [33,39,41, 63,64], and pericarditis [65]. Although uncommon, GCS pneumonia is associated with significant morbidity and mortality. It is manifested by extensive pulmonary infiltration and frequent occurrence of empyema. Blood cultures are often positive, and resolution is slow despite appropriate antimicrobial therapy and drainage of the pleural space [2,30,52–55,66–70].

INFECTIVE ENDOCARDITIS

Numerous cases of GCS endocarditis have been described [52,53,55], as well as a few cases of mycotic aneurysm [53,70,71]. Bradley et al. [52] reviewed 24 cases (13 definite and 11 probable) of GCS endocarditis; 5 were due to *Streptococcus zooepidemicus*, 4 to *Streptococcus equisimilis*, and the rest unspeciated. Underlying cardiac disease was present in 7 of 12 patients in whom adequate information regarding this feature was available. The aortic and/or mitral valves were involved in 19 cases, the tricuspid in 1 case, and information was lacking in 4 cases. Most of the patients pursued a subacute course with a mean duration of symptoms of 17 days.

The course of endocarditis in these patients was complicated by heart failure and major embolic events. Eight (33%) of the patients died, but three of these received either sulfonamides alone or no antibiotics and one died within 2 days of diagnosis.

BACTEREMIA

Bacteremia due to GCS is an uncommon event. Only eight of approximately 150,000 blood cultures obtained at the Mayo Clinic between 1968 and 1977 were positive for streptococci of this serogroup [54]. This represented 1.5% of all beta-hemolytic streptococci isolated. Similarly, only 7 (3.6%) of 192 blood isolates of beta-hemolytic Streptococcus serogrouped at Massachusetts General Hospital between 1986 and 1993 were GCS [2]. Many of the patients had serious underlying diseases. Carmeli et al. [55] reported the experience in Israel from 1985 to 1992 and reviewed cases of GCS bacteremia reported in the English language between 1988 and 1993. They compared the spectrum of disease as determined in case reports (80 cases) with that found in population-based studies (59 cases) performed in Ohio; North Yorkshire, England; Madrid, Spain; Israel; and Hong Kong (the latter restricted to *Streptococcus zooepidemicus*) (Table 13.2). Compared with the case reports, underlying diseases were more prevalent (88% vs. 66%, $P < 0.01$) and animal exposure, endovascular infections, and central nervous system infections less frequent in the population-based studies. The case–fatality ratio was 22.5% in the collected case reports and 28.8% in the population-based studies. The data from both sources suggest that GCS may be opportunists in patients with malignancy, alcoholism/cirrhosis, cardiovascular disease, and diabetes mellitus.

NOSOCOMIAL INFECTIONS

Group C streptococci are at times nosocomial pathogens [53]. Clusters of infections have occurred in burn units, hospital wards, and maternity units [18,72]. An orthopedic surgeon carrying *Streptococcus equisimilis* in nares and rectum was responsible for postoperative wound infections in two patients operated upon in a 3-day period [73].

Table 13.2 Group C Streptococcal Bacteremia: Comparison of Case Reports and Cases Reported in Population-Based Studies

	Case Reports	Ohio (Salata, 1989; [53])	Hong Kong (Yuen, 1990; [22])	North Yorkshire, England (Barnham, 1989; [70])	Madrid, Spain (Berenguer, 1992; [38])	Israel (Carmeli, 1995; [55])	Population Studies (All)
Total no. patients	80	23	11	5	10	10	59
Underlying diseases	53	23	7	3	10	9	52[a]
Malignant neoplasm	14	5	2	1	2	4	14
Alcohol/cirrhosis	4	3	2	1	1	3	10[a]
Heart disease	15	6	2	1	2	3	14
Diabetes mellitis	4	3	0	0	0	2	8
Injecting drug abuse	3	1	0	0	2	0	3
Exposure to animal	23	0	0	0	0	0	0[a]
Streptococcus sps.	39	2	11	3	10	0	26
Strep. equisimilis	20	2	0	3	5	0	10
Strep. zooepidemicus	16	0	11	0	1	0	12
Strep. equi	2	0	0	0	2	0	2
Strep. dysgalactiae	1	0	0	0	2	0	2
Clinical syndromes							
Endovascular	28	3	2	1	2	0	8[a]
Primary bacteremia	19	3	1	0	4	4	12
Central nervous system infection	11	1	0	0	1	1	3
Pneumonia	4	2	2	1	2	1	8
Skin infection	4	5	4	1	1	4	15[a]
Other	16	9	2	2	0	0	13
Morbidity	17	6	1	—	—	2	9
Mortality	18	6	2	3	4	2	17

From Carmeli et al. [55], 1995; Arch Intern Med 155:1170–1176. Copyright, 1995, American Medical Association.

[a]Statistically significant difference ($P < 0.05$) between case reports and population-based studies.

Therapy

Group C streptococci are exquisitely susceptible to penicillin, which should be considered the drug of choice. Rolston et al. [74] tested 25 human isolates of GCS and 19 of group G streptococci and found the range of penicillin G minimal inhibitory concentrations (MIC) to be 0.03 to 0.06 μg/ml. Other beta lactam agents such as cephalothin (MIC_{90}, 0.06 μg/ml) and cefotaxime (0.12 μg/ml) were highly effective in vitro, as was vancomycin (0.12 μg/ml). Erythromycin MICs ranged from 0.03 to 1.0 μg/ml. Although these studies were reported well over a decade ago, there is no evidence to date of increasing resistance of GCS to penicillin or other cell wall–active agents. There has, however, been a report from England of occasional strains resistant to erythromycin [70].

Several authors have reported the occurrence of penicillin tolerance in some strains of GCS [53,75,76], raising the issue of the concomitant use of an aminoglycoside antibiotic in cases of life-threatening GCS disease. However, the clinical significance of tolerance in organisms other than enterococci remains uncertain at the present time.

GROUP G STREPTOCOCCI

Group G streptococci (GGS) were first identified by Lancefield and Hare [77] over a half-century ago. Although these organisms are part of the normal microbial flora of the skin, pharynx, vagina, and gastrointestinal tract of humans, there has been increasing recognition in recent years that GGS may cause life-threatening infections.

Taxonomy and Microbiology

The group-specific carbohydrate of GGS is a polysaccharide composed of rhamnose and galactosamine. As with streptococci belonging to serogroup C, GGS may be initially subdivided into two categories based upon colony size. Human and animal strains exhibiting large ($\geq$0.5 mm in diameter) beta-hemolytic colonies morphologically indistinguishable from those of *Streptococcus pyogenes* are designated in *Bergey's Manual of Determinative Bacteriology* as *Streptococcus canis* [1], although some authors reserve this species designation for strains isolated from animals [7]. Efstratiou et al. compared the biochemical reactions of human and animal strains of GGS. All human strains tested fermented trehalose whereas animal strains did so only occasionally. Animal strains produced α-D-galactosidase and β-D-galactosidase but human strains did not [7].

Small- or minute-colony (<0.5 mm diameter) strains of GGS display variable hemolytic reactions and have been variously categorized as *Streptococcus anginosus-milleri* or as members of the *Streptococcus intermedius* group. The taxonomic considerations are the same as those described above for the small-colony forms of GCS. In contrast to large-colony GGS, strains forming minute colonies give a positive Voges-Proskauer reaction [1]. Whereas human isolates of large-colony GGS consistently demonstrate β-D-glucuronidase activity, small colony GGS fail to do so [78].

Bacitracin susceptibility of GGS is variable. In one study [9], 10 of 18 GGS were found sensitive ($\geq$10 mm zone of inhibition) to a 0.04 unit bacitracin disc on a sheep blood–agar plate and thus would have been falsely assumed to be group A streptococci by this screening technique. Although bacitracin susceptibility testing, when properly performed, is highly sensitive in identifying group A streptococci, more specific immunologic techniques are required for differentiating group A from group G or C streptococci (see above). Random amplified polymorphic DNA (RAPD) analysis has been found to be a useful technique for distinguishing species

and strains within species of pyogenic streptococci, especially for group A and G streptococci [79].

Virulence Factors

Many large-colony GGS strains express M proteins similar in structure and function to those of group A streptococci [80–83]. These organisms resist phagocytosis in human blood [80,84] and are type-specifically opsonized by antisera raised against whole cells, purified M proteins, and synthetic peptides of M protein [85]. The GGS M protein molecules conform to the proposed class I structure of group A Streptococcus M proteins [86], a structure common to virulent rheumatogenic group A strains. All class I M proteins share a surface-exposed domain within the C-repeat (highly conserved) region of the M protein molecule located near the carboxy terminus. Although GGS strains expressing group A Streptococcus M12 protein have been identified [87], for the most part, the N-terminal (variable) portions of GGS M proteins are unique and represent a family of "new" types [81,88]. DNA–DNA hybridization studies indicate that sequences homologous to group A Streptococcus M protein genes are widely distributed in human GGS strains, but such sequences have not been identified in animal strains [89]. Studies utilizing DNA–DNA hybridization, restriction fragment length polymorphism (RFLP), and multilocus enzyme electrophoresis have provided evidence consistent with the hypothesis that horizontal transfer of *emm* genes may have occurred between group A and group G streptococci [20,88,90].

Group G streptococci possess a variety of other constituents that may be related to virulence. Among these is a C5a peptidase (similar to that produced by group A streptococci) that is capable of destroying the human chemotactin C5a [91]; the peptidase has been identified in human but not in animal isolates of GGS. The GGS also express an albumin receptor protein [92] and a fibronectin-binding protein that mediates adherence to epithelial cells [93].

As with streptococci of groups A and C, GGS express an immunoglobulin G (IgG) binding protein. The generally accepted nomenclature for such proteins recognizes five classes, with that of group A streptococci designated class II and the IgG-binding protein of groups C and G streptococci designated type III [94]. The type III IgG Fc receptor, also known as protein G [95], binds to all four classes of human IgG [96]. The IgG-binding site of protein G is located in the carboxy-terminal domain, whereas domains present on the animo-terminal portion of the molecule bind albumin and α-2 macroglobulin [95,97,98]. The presence of a type II IgG receptor in GGS has also been reported [94]. Surface proteins that bind plasminogen are expressed by both GGS and GCS [99].

Group G streptococci also elaborate extracellular products that are likely to subserve virulence functions. These include streptolysin O, streptokinase, deoxyribonuclease, and hyaluronidase. In contrast to group A streptococci and some strains of GCS, capsules have not been identified in GGS.

Clinical Manifestations

Animal Diseases

Group G streptococci may be isolated from the throats of domestic animals, including dogs [21] and cows [100]. Although *Streptococcus canis* strains usually represent commensal flora of the canine skin and mucosa, they can cause a variety of canine infections, including abscesses, dermatitis, arthritis, and mastitis. These organisms have also been documented to cause cervical lymphadenitis in laboratory rats and cats [101]. Human isolates differ from animal strains in several respects, including their expression of virulence factors such as M proteins and C5a peptidase (see above). Moreover, human and bovine isolates can be distinguished on the basis of exoenzyme production and biochemical tests [100].

Human Infections

PHARYNGITIS

Group G streptococci have been responsible for food-borne outbreaks of acute pharyngitis related to contaminated egg salad [102] and chicken salad [103]. In still another outbreak, 68 patients with acute GGS pharyngitis were treated over a 9-day period in a college student health service [104]; a common source was not identified.

As is the case with group C organisms (see above), the role of GGS in causing endemically occurring cases of acute pharyngitis remains uncertain [43,105]. Gerber et al. [106] described a community-wide outbreak of pharyngitis, during which 25% of patients with acute pharyngitis seen in a private pediatric office had positive cultures for GGS. Patients with cultures positive for group A and large-colony group G streptococci were similar with respect to clinical findings, antistreptolysin O response, and response to antimicrobial therapy. In that community outbreak, a single GGS strain characterized by a unique restriction profile predominated in isolates collected over a 6-month period [107]. This observation suggests that the propensity of GGS to cause symptomatic pharyngeal infections may relate to the virulence characteristics of strains prevalent in a particular epidemiologic setting.

SKIN AND SOFT TISSUE INFECTION

Group G streptococci colonize human skin [84,108], and infections of the integument and subcutaneous tissues are among the most common illnesses caused by this organism. Such infections include pyoderma, cellulitis, and erysipelas [109–112]. Factors predisposing to skin and soft-tissue infections include chronic leg ulcers, malignancy, vascular disease, abnormal venous or lymphatic drainage, diabetes, and intravenous drug abuse [109,113]. Group G streptococci were isolated with greater frequency than group A streptococci from the skin cultures of patients admitted to a hospital dermatology ward [109]. In that study, 21 of 34 patients with positive cultures for GGS had leg ulcers, and 28 of the 34 patients had clinically apparent infections requiring antimicrobial therapy. Of the six patients in whom antibiotics were withheld, half developed erysipelas within the succeeding few months. Nohlgard et al. [109] isolated GGS from approximately 3% of all patients admitted to a Scottish burn unit. During the latter years of the study (1987–1990), the rate of graft survival was significantly lower among patients from whom GGS were isolated than among those from whom other non–group A streptococci or *Staphylococcus aureus* was recovered. The authors speculated that disruption of fibrinous adhesions between graft and bed by GGS streptokinase might be in part responsible for this outcome [109]. Recently, a case of GGS myositis associated with Streptococcus toxic shock syndrome was reported [114]. This organism did not contain the gene for Streptococcus pyrogenic exotoxin (SPE) A, SPE B, or SPE C, but it was found to produce at least one novel SPE.

LOWER RESPIRATORY TRACT INFECTIONS

Pneumonia caused by GGS is rare. It is usually preceded by a viral respiratory tract infection in a patient with a comorbid condition such as malignancy. The disease is characterized by fever, chills, dyspnea, and chest pain, and it may be complicated by empyema [115]. One case of upper airway obstruction as a consequence of laryngeal obstruction due to vocal cord infection by GGS has also been reported.

SEPTIC ARTHRITIS AND OSTEOARTHRITIS

Numerous cases of septic arthritis due to GGS have been reported [113,116–120]. Large joints are more frequently affected, especially the knee, hip, and shoulder. Involvement of more than one joint is not uncommon and an extra-articular focus of infection is usually found, such as infected decubitus ulcer, surgical wound infection, other skin infections, or periodontal disease [72,117,118,120,121]. Predisposing factors in the joint itself are prior joint trauma, surgery on the affected knee, rheumatoid arthritis, and the presence of an articular prosthesis [72,116, 118,122,123]. Cases of septic arthritis due to GGS in parenteral drug abusers have also been reported [113,119], and these have occasionally involved the sacroiliac and sternoclavicular joints. In this setting, septic arthritis is frequently associated with endocarditis, thrombophlebitis, or cellulitis [113,119].

There have been isolated reports of osteomyelitis due to GGS, usually in patients with predisposing conditions such as malignancy, alcoholism, osteoarthritis, or the presence of a joint prosthesis. Coexisting septic arthritis may be present. Two cases of GGS osteomyelitis of the spine have also been reported [124].

BACTEREMIA

Group G streptococci account for 6%–18% of all beta-hemolytic Streptococcus bacteremias [10,69,125,126]. Underlying malignancy has been reported in 25%–83% of such patients [125,126], and many others manifest serious underlying conditions such as alcoholism, diabetes mellitus, and chronic renal failure (Table 13.3). Polymicrobial bacteremia is not uncommon, with Staph. aureus as the most frequently isolated co-pathogen. The skin is the usual portal of entry [126]. Other foci of infection associated with bacteremia include pneumonia, meningitis, puerperal infection, postoperative wound infection, septic arthritis, or cholangitis [69, 111,121,125]. In parenteral drug abusers with GGS bacteremia, there are often concurrent local signs of cellulitis and disseminated foci of infection such as infective endocarditis, septic thrombophlebitis, or septic arthritis [113]. Mortality in patients with GGS bacteremia is related to the severity of the underlying disease.

ENDOCARDITIS

Infective endocarditis caused by GGS is uncommon. The disease tends to occur in older patients with underlying conditions such as those enumerated above (see section on bacteremia) [121,125]. Although many of the patients reported had underlying cardiac conditions predisposing to endocarditis, GGS are also capable of infecting normal valves. Both native and prosthetic valves may be involved, and the left heart valves are more commonly affected. Usually the onset of symptoms is acute, and the course of the disease may be aggressive with valvular destruction and perivalvular infection. Metastatic foci are not uncommon. The usual portal of entry is the skin; other sites include the oropharynx and lower gastrointestinal and genital tracts [121,125,127]. Endocarditis due to GGS in parenteral drug abusers has been associated with tricuspid valve involvement in people with a long-standing history of parenteral drug abuse, especially when drugs are injected into the internal jugular or femoral veins because of limited venous access [113]. Concurrent manifestations are pulmonary septic emboli, cellulitis,

Table 13.3 Group G Streptococcal in Bacteremia and/or Endocarditis: Selected Series

Reference	No. Cases	Organ/Tissue Involvement (n)	Probable Portal of Entry (n)	Underlying Disease (n)	Deaths (%)
Lam, 1983 [143]	15	Bacteremia (5) Endocarditis (4) Septic arthritis (5) Meningitis (1)	Skin (3) Unknown (12)	Alcoholism (4) IVDU[a] (2) Cirrhosis (1) Malignancy (1) Prosthetic joint (2) Rheumatoid arthritis (2) Osteoarthritis (1) Prosthetic heart valve (1)	2(13.3)
Watsky, 1985 [126]	24	Septic arthritis (3) Pneumonia (3) Meningitis (2) Cellulitis (1) Skin Ulcers (16)	Skin (19) Unknown (5)	Alcoholism (8) Malignancy (6) Diabetes mellitus (5) Neurological disease (4)	4(16.7)
Packe, 1991 [111]	13	Bacteremia (2) Cellulitis (8) Bowel/biliary tree (2) Bursitis (1)	Skin (8) Bowel/biliary tree (2) Unknown (3)	Malignancy (2) Alcoholism (1) Burns (1) Diabetes mellitus (1) Chronic renal failure (1) Cardiac failure (1) None (7)	1(7.7)
Auckenthaler, 1983 [115]	38	Bacteremia (15) Cellulitis (13) Soft-tissue abscesses (5) Meningitis (1) Empyema (2) Throat (1) Urinary tract (1)	Skin (29) Gastrointestinal tract (3) Urogenital tract (2) Unknown (4)	Malignancy (24) Heart failure (2) Diabetes mellitus (2) Venous insufficiency (2) Rheumatoid arthritis (1)	9(23.7)
Duma, 1969 [125]	6	Endocarditis (2) Septicemia (2) Cellulitis (1) Cholangitis (1)	Genital tract (2) Biliary tract (1) Skin ulcer (1) Pharynx (1) Unknown (1)	Malignancy (5)	None
Vartian, 1985 [149]	24	Bacteremia (15) Endocarditis (6) Neonatal sepsis (2) Infected pacemaker wire (1)	No data	Malignancy (5) Rheumatic fever (2) Prosthetic valve (1) Bone marrow transplant (2) IVDU[a] (2) Alcoholism (2) Cirrhosis (1) Cardiac failure (4) Diabetes mellitus (1) Prematurity (2)	9(37.5)
Venezio, 1986 [121]	15	Endocarditis (7) Cellulitis (3) Septic arthritis (2) Endometritis (1) Peritonitis (1) Urinary tract infection (1)	Genital tract (2) Biliary tract (1) Unknown (7)	Malignancy (5) Cardiac disease (4) Postpartum (2) Degenerative joint disease (2) Diabetes mellitus (1) Chronic renal failure (1)	4(26.6)

[a]IVDU, intravenous drug use.

multiple skin abscesses, septic thrombophlebitis, or septic arthritis. Patients usually respond well to antimicrobial combination of a beta-lactam for at least 4 weeks in combination with an aminoglycoside for at least 2 weeks [113].

PUERPERAL INFECTION AND NEONATAL INFECTIONS

In their original paper, Lancefield and Hare [77] recovered GGS from 5 of 855 antepartum vaginal swabs and the blood of a patient with puerperal sepsis who was co-infected with *Staphylococcus aureus*. Although most cases of puerperal sepsis with GGS are described as mild, the disease may pursue an aggressive course if not treated promptly. The clinical manifestations include fever, uterine tenderness, and change in normal appearance of the lochia. Appropriate antimicrobial therapy results in rapid resolution of symptoms.

As with other forms of neonatal infection, GGS neonatal sepsis is more likely in the setting of complications such as prematurity, low birth weight, or prolonged rupture of the membranes. In most instances infection is probably acquired as the infant traverses the birth canal. In one of the reported cases the infecting organism was a "minute" (*Streptococcus anginosus*) strain. The onset of disease is usually within the first week of life. Common manifestations are hypothermia, bradypnea, irritability, hypotonic extremities, twitching, and respiratory distress. In fatal cases, progressive severe respiratory distress, shock, and disseminated intravascular coagulation may occur [128–131].

OTHER INFECTIONS

A number of other infections have been reported on rare occasion to be due to GGS. These include meningitis [132,133], brain abscess [134], epididymo-orchitis [135], ascending cholangitis [125], peritonitis [111,121], endophthalmitis [111,136], appendicitis [111,112], and Bartholin's abscess [112].

NOSOCOMIAL INFECTIONS

Nosocomial infections due to GGS often involve skin and soft tissues. These usually present as surgical wound infections or cellulitis, mostly of the lower extremities or genital regions [110,115].

Nonsuppurative Complications of Group G Streptococcus Infection

Despite the microbiologic (see section on virulence factors above) and epidemiologic similarities between streptococci of serogroups A and G, acute rheumatic fever has never been documented to follow GGS pharyngeal infection. Sterile reactive arthritis has been reported in patients with GGS bacteremia [137,138] and in one patient with acute

pharyngitis and a strongly positive throat culture for GGS [139].

There have been rare reports of GGS infection eliciting postStreptococcus acute glomerulonephritis (AGN). The cases are rather atypical in that all occurred in adults. Acute glomerulonephritis developed in a 65-year-old woman with GGS bacteremia [133], a 50-year-old woman with a GGS postoperative wound infection and bacteremia [140], and a 57-year-old man with GGS septic polyarthritis and bacteremia [141]. In each of these cases, renal biopsy confirmed the diagnosis of proliferative glomerulonephritis and demonstrated the electron-dense subepithelial "humps" characteristic of immune complex glomerulonephritis. In Trinidad [108] and Venezuela [142], GGS have frequently been isolated from impetiginous lesions of children with AGN, but the role of this organism in causing pyoderma-associated nephritis has not been definitively established.

Therapy

Group G streptococci are exquisitely susceptible to penicillin G. Minimum inhibitory concentrations are generally in the range of 0.03 to 0.06 μg/ml [76,113] or less [143]. The organisms are also highly susceptible in vitro to a variety of other antimicrobial agents, including the ureidopenicillins, most cephalosporins, and vancomycin [74]. Most GGS are inhibited by achievable blood levels of erythromycin and clindamycin, but minimum bactericidal concentrations (MBCs) of these two agents, and especially chloramphenicol, for certain GGS strains are rather high [143].

Although most GGS strains are readily killed by beta lactam antibiotics [113,121], there have been a few reports of penicillin tolerance to these agents and to vancomycin [76,144]. The biologic significance of this phenomenon is uncertain at the present time. Lam and Bayer [143], who found no evidence of classic tolerance (high MIC/MBC ratio) in their invasive GGS strains, nevertheless pointed out that bacterial killing was impaired when large GGS inocula (10^8 colony-forming units/ml) were in the stationery phase of growth. This is a common finding in group A streptococci and is most likely attributable to decreased expression of penicillin-binding proteins (i.e., the "Eagle effect") as recently reported by Stevens et al. [145,146].

Despite the susceptibility of GGS to penicillin and cell wall–active agents, several authors have noted a poor or delayed response to therapy, particularly in patients with endocarditis or septic arthritis [121,143,147]. Such suboptimal therapeutic responses are likely attributable at least in part to the underlying conditions present in patients who develop invasive GGS infection. Nevertheless, the addition of gentamicin to a cell wall–active antibiotic seems prudent in certain patients with severe and invasive GGS infections, provided there is no contraindication to use of an aminoglycoside antimicrobial agent. Such combinations have been shown to be synergistic in vitro [148]. Candidates for combined therapy, as suggested by Vartian et al. [149], might include patients with acute bacterial endocarditis or septic arthritis, especially in the presence of a prosthesis, immunosuppressive disease, or immunosuppressive therapy. Combination therapy is also appropriate for patients whose response to single-agent therapy is poor, provided such response is not due to the presence of complicating factors such as an undrained focus of infection. Such therapy must be employed, however, with the recognition that there is no acceptable clinical evidence to date of its superior efficacy.

REFERENCES

1. Holt JG, Krieg NR, Sneath PHA, Staley JT, Williams ST (eds). Gram-positive cocci. In: Bergey's Manual of Determinative Bacteriology, 9th ed. Baltimore: Williams & Wilkins, 1994; 527–558.
2. Carmeli Y, Ruoff KL. Report of cases of and taxonomic considerations for large-colony-forming Lancefield group C Streptococcus bacteremia. J Clin Microbiol 1995; 33:2114–2117.
3. Stratton CW. *Streptococcus intermedius* group. In: Mandell GL, Bennett JE, Dolin R (eds). Principles and Practice of Infectious Diseases, 4th ed. New York: Churchill Livingstone, 1995; 1861–1865.
4. Whiley RA, Hardie JM. DNA–DNA hybridization studies and phenotypic characteristics of strains within the "*Streptococcus milleri* group". J Gen Microbiol 1989; 135:2623–2633.
5. Whiley RA, Fraser HY, Hardie JM, Beighton D. Phenotypic differentiation of *Streptococcus in-*

termedius, *Streptococcus constellatus*, and *Streptococcus anginosus* strains within the "*Streptococcus milleri* group". J Clin Microbiol 1990; 28:1497–1501.
6. Whiley RA, Beighton D. Emended descriptions and recognition of *Streptococcus constellatus*, *Streptococcus intermedius*, and *Streptococcus anginosus* as distinct species. Int J Syst Bacteriol 1991; 41:1–5.
7. Efstratiou A, Colman G, Hahn G, Timoney JF, Boeufgras JM, Monget D. Biochemical differences among human and animal streptococci of Lancefield group C or group G. J Med Microbiol 1994; 41:145–148.
8. Clark S, Cimolai N, Cheong ACH. A comparison of whole cell protein profiles for sporadic human isolates of *Streptococcus equisimilis* and beta-haemolytic group G streptococci. Microbios 1994; 77:19–27.
9. Matthieu DE Jr, Wasilauskas BL, Stallings RA. A rapid staphylococcal coagglutination technic to differentiate group A from other Streptococcus groups. Am J Clin Pathol 1979; 72:463–467.
10. Feingold DS, Stagg NL, Kunz LJ. Extrarespiratory Streptococcus infections: importance of the various serologic groups. N Engl J Med 1966; 275:356–361.
11. Skjold SA, Quie PG, Fries LA, Barnham M, Cleary PP. DNA fingerprinting of *Streptococcus zooepidemicus* (Lancefield group C) as an aid to epidemiological study. J Infect Dis 1987; 155:1145–1150.
12. Jean-Francois MJ, Poskitt DC, Turnbull SJ, Macdonald LM. Protection against *Streptococcus equi* infection by monoclonal antibodies against an M-like protein. J Gen Microbiol 1991; 137:2125–2133.
13. Galan JE, Timoney JF. Immunologic and genetic comparison of *Streptococcus equi* isolates from the United States and Europe. J Clin Microbiol 1988; 26:1142–1146.
14. Boschwitz JS, Timoney JF. Inhibition of C3 deposition on *Streptococcus equi* subsp. *equi* by M protein: A mechanism for survival in equine blood. Infect Immun 1994; 62:3515–3520.
15. Timoney JF, Walker J, Zhou M, Ding J. Cloning and sequence analysis of a protective M-like protein gene from *Streptococcus equi* subsp. *zooepidemicus*. Infect Immun 1995; 63:1440–1445.
16. Podbielski A, Mignon M, Weber-Heynemann J, Schnitzler N, Lutticken R, Kaufhold A. Characterization of groups C (GCS) and G (GGS) Streptococcus M protein (*emm*) genes. In: Totolian A (ed). Pathogenic Streptococci: Present and Future. St. Petersburg, Russia: Lancer Publications, 1994; 234–236.
17. Efstratiou A, Teare EL, McGhie D, Colman G. The presence of M proteins in outbreak strains of *Streptococcus equisimilis* T-type 204. J Infect 1989; 19:105–111.
18. Galloway A, Noel I, Efstratiou A, Saint E, White

DR. An outbreak of group C Streptococcus infection in a maternity unit. J Hosp Infect 1994; 28:31–37.

19. Bisno AL, Collins CM, Turner JC. M proteins of group C streptococci isolated from patients with acute pharyngitis. J Clin Microbiol 1996; 34:2511–2515.

20. Simpson WJ, Musser JM, Cleary PP. Evidence consistent with horizontal transfer of the gene (emm12) encoding serotype M12 protein between group A and group G pathogenic streptococci. Infect Immun 1992; 60:1890–1893.

21. Deibel RH, Seeley HW Jr. Family II. Streptococcaceae. In: Buchanan RE, Gibbons NE (eds). Bergey's Manual of Determinative Bacteriology, 8th ed. Baltimore: Williams & Wilkins, 1974; 490–517.

22. Yuen KY, Seto WH, Choi CH, Ng W, Ho SW, Chau PY. Streptococcus zooepidemicus (Lancefield group C) septicaemia in Hong Kong. J Infect 1990; 21:241–250.

23. Lindgren PE, McGavin MJ, Signas C, Guss B, Gurusiddappa S, Hook M, Lindberg M. Two different genes coding for fibronectin-binding proteins from Streptococcus dysgalactiae. The complete nucleotide sequences and characterization of the binding domains. Eur J Biochem 1993; 214:819–827.

24. Lindmark H, Jacobsson K, Frykberg L, Guss B. Fibronectin-binding protein of Streptococcus equi subsp. zooepidemicus. Infect Immun 1996; 64:3993–3999.

25. Otten RA, Boyle MDP. Characterization of protein G expressed by human group C and G streptococci. J Microbiol Methods 1991; 13:185–200.

26. Gerlach D, Kohler W, Gunther E, Mann K. Purification and characterization of streptolysin O secreted by Streptococcus equisimilis (group C). Infect Immun 1993; 61:2727–2731.

27. McCoy HE, Broder CC, Lottenberg R. Streptokinases produced by pathogenic group C streptococci demonstrate species-specific plasminogen activation. J Infect Dis 1991; 164:515–521.

28. Barnham M, Thornton TJ, Lange K. Nephritis caused by Streptococcus zooepidemicus (Lancefield group C). Lancet 1983; 1(8331):945–948.

29. Kohler W, Cederberg A. Streptococcus zooepidemicus (group C streptococci) as a cause of human infection. Scand J Infect Dis 1976; 8:217–218.

30. Barnham M, Ljunggren A, McIntyre M. Human infection with Streptococcus zooepidemicus (Lancefield group C): three case reports. Epidemiol Infect 1987; 98:183–190.

31. Francis AJ, Nimmo GR, Efstratiou A, Galanis V, Nuttall N. Investigation of milk-borne Streptococcus zooepidemicus infection associated with glomerulonephritis in Australia. J Infect 1993; 27:317–323.

32. Edwards AT, Roulson M, Ironside MJ. Unpasteurised milk and Streptococcus zooepidemicus. CDR Weekly 1994; 4:241–243.

33. Low DE, Young MR, Harding GKM. Group C Streptococcus meningitis in an adult. Probable acquisition from a horse. Arch Intern Med 1980; 140:977–978.

34. Edwards AT, Roulson M, Ironside MJ. A milkborne outbreak of serious infection due to Streptococcus zooepidemicus (Lancefield group C). Epidemiol Infect 1988; 101:43–51.

35. Centers for Disease Control U. Group C Streptococcus infections associated with eating homemade cheese—New Mexico. MMWR Morb Mortal Wkly Rep 1983; 32:510, 515–516.

36. Duca E, Teodorovici GR, Radu C, Vita A, Talasman-Nicolescu P, Bernescu E, Feldi C, Rossa V. A new nephritogenic streptococcus. J Hyg 1969; 67:691–698.

37. Mollison LC, Donaldson E. Group C Streptococcus meningitis. Med J Aust 1990; 152:319–320.

38. Berenguer J, Sampedro I, Cercenado E, Baraia J, Rodriquez-Creixems M, Bouza E. Group C beta-hemolytic Streptococcus bacteremia. Diagn Microbiol Infect Dis 1992; 15:151–155.

39. Quinn RJM, Hallett AF, Appelbaum PC, Cooper RC. Meningitis caused by Streptococcus dysgalactiae in a preterm infant. Am J Clin Pathol 1978; 70:948–950.

40. Braunstein H, Tucker E, Gibson BC. Infections caused by unusual beta hemolytic streptococci. Am J Clin Pathol 1971; 55:424–430.

41. Breiman RF, Silverblatt FJ. Systemic Streptococcus equi infection in a horse handler—a case of human strangles. West J Med 1986; 145:385–386.

42. Fox K, Turner J, Fox A. Role of beta-hemolytic group C streptococci in pharyngitis: incidence and biochemical characteristics of Streptococcus equisimilis and Streptococcus anginosus in patients and healthy controls. J Clin Microbiol 1993; 31:804–807.

43. Hayden GF, Murphy TF, Hendley JO. Non–group A streptococci in the pharynx. Pathogens or innocent bystanders? Am J Dis Child 1989; 143:794–797.

44. Turner JC, Hayden GF, Kiselica D, Lohr J, Fishburne CF, Murren D. Association of group C beta-hemolytic streptococci with endemic pharyngitis among college students. JAMA 1990; 264:2644–2647.

45. Turner JC, Hayden FG, Lobo MC, Ramirez CE, Murren D. Epidemiologic evidence for Lancefield group C beta-hemolytic streptococci as a cause of exudative pharyngitis in college students. J Clin Microbiol 1997; 35:1–4.

46. Cimolai N, Morrison BJ, MacCulloch L, Smith DF, Hlady J. Beta-haemolytic non–group A streptococci and pharyngitis: a case–control study. Eur J Pediatr 1991; 150:776–779.

47. Meier FA, Centor RM, Graham L Jr, Dalton

HP. Clinical and microbiological evidence for endemic pharyngitis among adults due to group C streptococci. Arch Intern Med 1990; 150:825–829.

48. Benjamin JT, Perriello VA Jr. Pharyngitis due to group C hemolytic streptococci in children. J Pediatr 1976; 89:254–256.

49. Portnoy B, Reitler R. Cellulitis due to a haemolytic streptococcus type C. Lancet 1944; 2:597–598.

50. McKeage MJ, Humble MW, Morrison RB. *Streptococcus zooepidemicus* cellulitis and bacteremia in a renal transplant recipient. Aust N Z J Med 1990; 20:177–178.

51. Belcher DW, Afoakwa SN, Osei-Tutu E, Wurapa FK, Osei L. Non–group A streptococci in Ghanaian patients with pyoderma. Lancet 1975; 2:1032–1036.

52. Bradley SE, Gordon JJ, Baumgartner DD, Marasco WA, Kauffman CA. Group C Streptococcus bacteremia: analysis of 88 cases. Rev Infect Dis 1991; 13:270–280.

53. Salata RA, Lerner PI, Shlaes DM, Gopalakrishna KV, Wolinsky E. Infections due to Lancefield group C streptococci. Medicine 1989; 68:225–239.

54. Mohr DN, Feist DJ, Washington JA, Hermans PE. Infections due to group C streptococci in man. Am J Med 1979; 66:450–456.

55. Carmeli Y, Schapiro JM, Neeman D, Yinnon AM, Alkan M. Streptococcus group C bacteremia: survey in Israel and analytical review. Arch Intern Med 1995; 155:1170–1176.

56. Keiser P, Campbell W. "Toxic strep syndrome" associated with group C streptococcus. Arch Intern Med 1992; 152:882–883.

57. Ike RW. Septic arthritis due to group C streptococcus: report and review of the literature. J Rheumatol 1990; 17:1230–1236.

58. Ortel TL, Kallianos J, Gallis HA. Group C Streptococcus arthritis: case report and review. Rev Infect Dis 1991; 12:829–837.

59. Sobrino J, Bosch X, Wennberg P, Villalta J, Grau JM. Septic arthritis secondary to group C streptococcus typed as *Streptococcus equisimilis* [letter]. J Rheumatol 1991; 18:485–486.

60. Steinfeld S, Galle C, Struelens M, De-Gheldre Y, Farber CM, Appelboom T, Van-Voovey JP. Pyogenic arthritis caused by *Streptococcus equisimilis* (group C streptococcus) in a patient with AIDS. Clin Rheumatol 1997; 16:314–316.

61. Gallagher PG, Myer CM III, Crone K, Benzing G III. Group C Streptococcus sinusitis. Am J Otolaryngol 1990; 11:352–354.

62. Moffett DG, Edward DP. Anterior segment necrosis associated with endogenous endophthlamitis secondary to group C Streptococcus septicemia. Can J Ophthalmol 1991; 26:283–287.

63. Mohr DN, Feist DJ, Washington JA, II, Hermans PE. Meningitis due to group C streptococci in and adult. Mayo Clin Proc 1978; 53:529–532.

64. Ghoneim A. Serious infection caused by group C streptococci. J Clin Pathol 1980; 33:188–190.

65. Marsa RJ, Blomquist IK, Bansal RC, Boucek FC, Elperin LS. Acute pericarditis due to group C streptococcus: report of a medically treated case. Am J Med 1989; 86:474–476.

66. Dolinski SY, Jones PG, Zabransky RJ, Rasansky M. Group C Streptococcus pleurisy and pneumonia: a fulminant case and review of the literature. Infection 1990; 18:239–241.

67. Vartian CV. Bacteremic pneumonia due to group C streptococci. Rev Infect Dis 1991; 13:1029–1030.

68. Arditi M, Shulman ST, Davis AT, Yogev R. Group C beta-hemolytic Streptococcus infections in children: nine pediatric cases and review. Rev Infect Dis 1989; 11:34–45.

69. Nielsen SV, Kolmos HJ. Bacteraemia due to different groups of beta-haemolytic streptococci: a two-year survey and presentation of a case of recurring infection due to *Streptococcus "equisimilis"*. Infection 1993; 21:358–361.

70. Barnham M, Kerby J, Chandler RS, Millar MR. Group C streptococci in human infection: a study of 308 isolates with clinical correlations. Epidemiol Infect 1989; 102:379–390.

71. de Miguel J, Collazos J, Echeverria J, Egurbide V, Ayarza R. Group C Streptococcus pneumonia and aneurysm infection. Chest 1993; 104:1644–1645.

72. Efstratiou A. Outbreaks of human infection caused by pyogenic streptococci of Lancefield groups C and G. J Med Microbiol 1989; 29:207–219.

73. Goldman DA, Breton SJ. Group C Streptococcus surgical wound infections transmitted by an anorectal and nasal carrier. Pediatrics 1978; 61:235–237.

74. Rolston KV, LeFrock JL, Schell RF. Activity of nine antimicrobial agents against Lancefield group C and group G streptococci. Antimicrob Agents Chemother 1982; 22:930–932.

75. Portnoy D, Prentis J, Richards GK. Penicillin tolerance of human isolates of group C streptococci. Antimicrob Agents Chemother 1981; 20:235–238.

76. Rolston KVI, Chandrasekar PH, LeFrock JL. Antimicrobial tolerance in group C and group G streptococci. J Antimicrob Chemother 1984; 13:389–392.

77. Lancefield RC, Hare R. The serologic differentiation of pathogenic and non-pathogenic strains of hemolytic streptococci from parturient women. J Exp Med 1935; 61:335–349.

78. Cimolai N, Mah D. Beta-D-glucuronidase activity assay for rapid differentiation of species within beta-haemolytic group C and G streptococci. J Clin Pathol 1991; 44:824–825.

79. Bert F, Picard B, Branger C, Lambert-Ze-

chovsky N. Analysis of genetic relationships among strains of groups A, C and G streptococci by random amplified polymorphic DNA analysis. J Med Microbiol 1996; 45:278–284.

80. Bisno AL, Craven DE, McCabe WR. M proteins of group G streptococci isolated from bacteremic human infections. Infect Immun 1987; 55:753–757.

81. Collins CM, Kimura A, Bisno AL. Group G Streptococcus M protein exhibits structural features analogous to class I M protein of group A streptococci. Infect Immun 1992; 60:3689–3696.

82. Campo RE, Schultz DR, Bisno AL. M-proteins of group G streptococci: mechanisms of resistance to phagocytosis. J Infect Dis 1995; 171:601–606.

83. Jones KF, Fischetti VA. Biological and immunochemical identity of M protein on group G streptococci with M protein on group A streptococci. Infect Immun 1987; 55:502–506.

84. Lawal SF, Coker AO, Solanke EO, Ogunbi O. Serotypes among Lancefield group G streptococci isolated in Nigeria. J Med Microbiol 1982; 15:123–125.

85. Bisno AL, Campo RE, Collins CM. M proteins of group G streptococci: structural and functional studies. In: Totolian A (ed). Pathogenic Streptococci: Present and Future. St. Petersberg, Russia: Lancer Publications; 1994; 225–227.

86. Bessen DE, Fischetti VA. Differentiation between two biologically distinct classes of group A streptococci by limited substitutions of amino acids within the shared region of M protein-like molecules. J Exp Med 1990; 172:1757–1764.

87. Maxted WR, Potter EV. The presence of type 12 M-protein antigen in group G streptococci. J Gen Microbiol 1967; 49:119–125.

88. Schnitzler N, Podbielski A, Baumgarten G, Mignon M, Kaufhold A. M or M-like protein gene polymorphisms in human group G streptococci. J Clin Microbiol 1995; 33:356–363.

89. Simpson WJ, Robbins JC, Cleary PP. Evidence for group A–related M protein genes in human but not animal-associated group G Streptococcus pathogens. Microb Pathog 1987; 3:339–350.

90. Sriprakash KS, Hartas J. Lateral genetic transfers between group A and G streptococci for M-like genes are ongoing. Microb Pathog 1996; 20:275–285.

91. Cleary PP, Peterson J, Chen C, Nelson C. Virulent human strains of group G streptococci express a C5a peptidase enzyme similar to that produced by group A streptococci. Infect Immun 1991; 59:2305–2310.

92. Gupalova TV, Orlova SN, Totolian AA. Albumin receptor protein of group G streptococcus. Cloning of the gene, characterization, and usage of the protein expressed in Escherichia coli. Adv Exp Med Biol 1997; 418:753–755.

93. Kline JB, Xu S, Bisno AL, Collins CM. Identification of a fibronectin-binding protein (GfbA) in pathogenic group G streptococci. Infect Immun 1996; 64:2122–2129.

94. Smirnov OY, Denesyuk AI, Zakharov MV, Abramov VM, Zav'yalov VP. Protein V, a novel type-II IgG receptor from Streptococcus sp.: sequence, homologies and putative Fc-binding site. Gene 1992; 120:27–32.

95. Sjobring U, Bjorck L, Kastern W. Streptococcus protein G. Gene structure and protein binding properties. J Biol Chem 1991; 266:399–405.

96. Fahnestock SR, Alexander P, Nagle J, Filpula D. Gene for an immunoglobulin-binding protein from a group G streptococcus. J Bacteriol 1986; 167:870–880.

97. Raeder R, Otten RA, Boyle MD. Comparison of albumin receptors expressed on bovine and human group G streptococci. Infect Immun 1991; 59:609–616.

98. Muller HP, Rantamaki LK. Binding of native β_2-macroglobulin to human group G streptococci. Infect Immun 1995; 63:2833–2839.

99. Ben Nasr A, Wistedt A, Ringdahl U, Sjorbring U. Streptokinase activates plasminogen bound to human group C and G streptococci through M-like proteins. Eur J Biochem 1994; 222:267–276.

100. Clark RB, Berrafati JF, Janda JM, Bottone EJ. Biotyping and exoenzyme profiling as an aid in the differentiation of human from bovine group G streptococci. J Clin Microbiol 1984; 20:706–710.

101. Corning BF, Murphy JC, Fox JG. Group G Streptococcus lymphadenitis in rats. J Clin Microbiol 1991; 29:2720–2723.

102. Hill HR, Caldwell GG, Wilson E, Hager D, Zimmerman RA. Epidemic of pharyngitis due to streptococci of Lancefield group G. Lancet 1969; 2(616):371–374.

103. Stryker WS, Fraser DW, Facklam RR. Foodborne outbreak of group G Streptococcus pharyngitis. Am J Epidemiol 1982; 116:533–540.

104. McCue JD. Group G Streptococcus pharyngitis: analysis of an outbreak at a college. JAMA 1982; 248:1333–1336.

105. Cimolai N, Elford RW, Bryan L, Anand C, Berger P. Do the beta-hemolytic non–group A streptococci cause pharyngitis? Rev Infect Dis 1988; 10:587–601.

106. Gerber MA, Randolph MF, Martin NJ, Rizkallah MF, Cleary PP, Kaplan EL, Ayoub EM. Community-wide outbreak of group G Streptococcus pharyngitis. Pediatrics 1991; 87:598–603.

107. Martin NJ, Kaplan EL, Gerber MA, et al. Comparison of epidemic and endemic group G streptococci by restriction enzyme analysis. J Clin Microbiol 1990; 28:1881–1886.

108. Reid HF, Bassett DC, Poon-King T, Zabriskie JB, Read SE. Group G streptococci in healthy

school-children and in patients with glomerulonephritis in Trinidad. J Hyg 1985; 94:61–68.

109. Nohlgard C, Bjorklind A, Hammar H. Group G
Streptococcus infections on a dermatological
ward. Acta Dermatol Venereol 1992; 72:128–
130.

110. Rider MA, McGregor JC. Group G streptococcus—an emerging cause of graft loss? Br J Plast
Surg 1994; 47:346–348.

111. Packe GE, Smith DF, Reid TMS, Smith CC.
Group G Streptococcus bacteremia—a review
of thirteen cases of grampian. Scott Med J 1991;
36:42–44.

112. Brahmadathan KN, Koshi G. Epidemiology of
Streptococcus pyoderma in an orphanage community of a tropical country. J Trop Med Hyg
1988; 91:306–314.

113. Craven DE, Rixinger AI, Bisno AL, Goularte
TA, McCabe WR. Bacteremia caused by group
G streptococci in parenteral drug abusers: epidemiological and clinical aspects. J Infect Dis
1986; 153:988–992.

114. Wagner JG, Schlievert PM, Assimacopoulos AP,
Stoehr JA, Carson PJ, Komadina K. Acute group
G Streptococcus myositis associated with Streptococcus toxic shock syndrome: case report and
review. Clin Infect Dis 1996; 23:1159–1163.

115. Auckenthaler R, Hermans PE, Washington JA
II. Group G streptocococcal bacteremia: clinical study and review of the literature. Rev Infect Dis 1983; 5:196–204.

116. Ho G Jr, Su EY. Therapy for septic arthritis.
JAMA 1982; 247:797–800.

117. Fujita NK, Lam K, Bayer AS. Septic arthritis
due to group G streptococcus. JAMA 1982;
247:812–813.

118. Nakata MM, Silvers JH, George L. Group G
Streptococcus arthritis. Arch Intern Med 1983;
143:1328–1330.

119. Raucher BG, Clark R, Bottone EJ. Group G
Streptococcus sacroiliitis. Diagn Microbiol Infect Dis 1986; 4:255–257.

120. Brahmadothan KN, Koshi G. Importance of
group G streptococci in human pyrogenic infections. J Trop Med Hyg 1989; 92:35–38.

121. Venezio FR, Gullberg RM, Westenfelder GO,
Phair JP, Cook FV. Group G Streptococcus endocarditis and bacteremia. Am J Med 1986;
81:29–34.

122. Dougall HT, Laing RB, Smith CC. Opportunistic group G streptococcus infection of both prosthetic knee joints. Scott Med J 1997; 42:46.

123. Pons M, Puido A, Leal V, Viladot R. Sepsis due
to group G streptococcus after a total hip arthro-
plasty. A case report. Int Orthop 1997; 21:277–
278.

124. Hall M, Williams A. Group G Streptococcus osteomyelitis of the spine. Br J Rheumatol 1993;
32:342–345.

125. Duma RJ, Weinberg AN, Medrek TF, Kunz LJ.
Streptococcus infections: a bacteriological and

clinical study of Streptococcus bacteremia.
Medicine 1969; 48:87–127.

126. Watsky KL, Kollisch N, Densen P. Group G
Streptococcus bacteremia: the clinical experience at Boston University Medical Center and
a critical review of the literature. Arch Intern
Med 1985; 145:58–61.

127. Yap JC, Wang YT, Poh SC. Group G Streptococcus endocarditis and bacteraemia—a report
of 3 cases. Singapore Med J 1990; 31:451–453.

128. Carstensen H, Pers C, Pryds O. Group G Streptococcus neonatal septicemia: two case reports
and review of the literature. Scand J Infect Dis
1988; 20:407–410.

129. Dyson AE, Read SE. Group G Streptococcus
colonization and sepsis in neonates. J Pediatr
1981; 99:944–947.

130. Baker CJ. Unusual occurrence of neonatal septicemia due to group G streptococcus. Pediatrics
1974; 53:568–570.

131. Dylewski JS, Roy I, Libman M. Fatal postpartum infection with group G streptococcus [let-
ter]. Clin Infect Dis 1994; 19:1174–1175.

132. Raviglione MC, Tierno PM, Ottuso P, Klemes
AB, Davidson M. Group G Streptococcus
meningitis and sepsis in a patient with
AIDS. A method to biotype group G streptococcus. Diagn Microbiol Infect Dis 1990;
13:261–264.

133. Casadevall A, Freundlich LF, Pirofski L. Acute
glomerulonephritis and encephalomyelitis following group G Streptococcus bacteremia. Clin
Infect Dis 1992; 14:784–786.

134. Maniglia RJ, Roth T, Blumberg EA. Polymicrobial brain abscess in a patient infected with human immunodeficiency virus. Clin Infect Dis
1997; 24:449–451.

135. Teel LD, Shemonsky NK, Aronson N. Group G
Streptococcus bacteremia in a healthy young
man. South Med J 1989; 82:633–634.

136. Margo CE, Cole EL. Postoperative endophthalmitis and asymptomatic bacteriuria caused
by group G streptococcus. Am J Ophthalmol
1989; 107:430–431.

137. Gaunt PN, Seal DV. Group G Streptococcus infection of joints and joint prosthesis. J Infect
1986; 13:115–123.

138. Rogerson SJ, Beeching NJ. Reactive arthritis
complicating group G Streptococcus septicaemia. J Infect 1990; 20:155–158.

139. Young L, Deighton CM, Chuck AJ, Galloway A.
Reactive arthritis and group G Streptococcus
pharyngitis. Ann Rheum Dis 1992; 51:1268–
1271.

140. Gnann JW Jr, Gray BM, Griffin FM Jr, Dismukes WE. Acute glomerulonephritis following
group G Streptococcus infection. J Infect Dis
1987; 156:411–412.

141. Anonymous. Septic polyarthritis and acute renal
failure in a 57-year-old man [clinical confer-
ence]. Am J Med 1991; 91:293–299.

142. Garcia R, Rubio L, Rodriguez-Iturbe B. Long-term prognosis of epidemic postStreptococcus glomerulonephritis in Maracaibo: follow-up studies 11–12 years after the acute episode. Clin Nephrol 1981; 15:291–298.

143. Lam K, Bayer AS. Serious infections due to group G streptococci: report of 15 cases with in vitro–in vivo correlations. Am J Med 1983; 75:561–570.

144. Noble JT, Tyburski MB, Berman M, Greenspan J, Tenenbaum MJ. Antimicrobial tolerance in group G streptococci. Lancet 1980; ii:982–986.

145. Stevens DL, Gibbons AE, Bergstrom R, Winn V. The Eagle effect revisited: efficacy of clindamycin, erythromycin, and penicillin in the treatment of Streptococcus myositis. J Infect Dis 1988; 158:23–28.

146. Stevens DL, Yan S, Bryant AE. Penicillin-binding protein expression at different growth stages determines penicillin efficacy in vitro and in vivo: an explanation for the inoculum effect. J Infect Dis 1993; 167:1401–1405.

147. Bouza E, Meyer RD, Busch DF. Group G Streptococcus endocarditis. Am J Clin Pathol 1978; 70:108–111.

148. Lam K, Bayer AS. In vitro bactericidal synergy of gentamicin combined with penicillin G, vancomycin, or cefotaxime against group G streptococci. Antimicrob Agents Chemother 1984; 26:260–262.

149. Vartian C, Lerner PI, Shlaes DM, Gopalakrishna KV. Infections due to Lancefield group G streptococci. Medicine 1985; 64:75–88.

14

Nonhemolytic Streptococci

JUDY A. DALY

Nonhemolytic streptocci have routinely been associated with subacute bacterial endocarditis. However, because of the confusion with the nomenclature of this group, complete understanding of the pathogenesis of nonhemolytic streptococci is still pending [1].

The nonhemolytic species *Streptococcus bovis* is an inhabitant of the intestine and has been associated with concurrent colonic cancer [2,3]. Whether *Streptococcus bovis* is a marker for the disease or has an etiologic role in carcinoma of the colon has not been entirely determined [2–6].

The nonhemolytic species *Streptococcus milleri* group has clinical significance for purulent infections of the oral, abdominal, and thoracic cavities and the central nervous system. Using the nomenclature by Whiley et al., *Streptococcus intermedius* has been found in liver and brain abscesses while *Streptococcus anginosus* and *Streptococcus constellatus* have been isolated more frequently from alternate sites [7,8]. Again, the current confusion over taxonomy and nomenclature hinders the clarity with which definition of pathogenesis can be accomplished.

Nonhemolytic nutritionally variant streptococci can cause endocarditis [9–11]. Because of the nutritional requirements of the group and a reporting of culture-negative endocarditis, probably much more than the reported 6% of microbial endocarditis is caused by nutritionally variant streptococci [12–23]. Endocarditis due to

nonhemolytic nutritionally variant streptococci results in comparatively small vegetations, with embolization common [24]. Nonhemolytic nutritionally variant streptococci cause a variety of other infections including sepsis, cirrhosis, and pancreatic abscess [22,25]. Other wound, ear, and eye infections have also been reported [10,19,26–28].

TAXONOMY

To say that revision and expansion of the taxonomy of the streptococci and related streptococcus-like bacteria have recently occurred would be an understatement. Hyperactivity and major changes have occurred due to molecular taxonomic evaluations of the classical family *Streptococcaceae*. The most powerful approach for detailing the phylogenetic relationships among organisms has been found to be small subunit rRNA (16S RNA) sequencing [29]. The genus *Streptococcus* now includes the pyogenic and oral streptococci [29,30]. Using small subunit rRNA sequence analysis, members of the genus *Streptococcus* could be divided into six divisions (Table 14.1). Using these divisions, the oral viridans streptococci (which include nonhemolytic streptococci) can be categorized into three phylogenetic divisions (divisions III, IV, and V) because of their genetic diversity. Although classical phenotypic criteria (hemolytic reactions) for

Table 14.1 Streptococcal Species Groups Based on Small Subunit rRNA Sequence Analysis

Group	Group Name	Members
I	Pyogenic	Group A streptococci (*Streptococcus pyogenes*)
		Group B streptococci (*Streptococcus agalactiae*)
		Group C streptococci (*Streptococcus equi, Streptococcus dysgalactiae*)
II	Group D *Streptococcus*	*Streptococcus bovis*
		Streptococcus equinus
III	Pneumonococcus/viridans	*Streptococcus pneumoniae*
		Streptococcus oralis
		Streptococcus sanguis
		Streptococcus parasanguis
		"*Streptococcus milleri*" group (*Streptococcus anginosus, Streptococcus constellatus, Streptococcus intermedius*)
IV	*Streptococcus mutans*	*Streptococcus mutans*
		Streptococcus rattus
		Streptococcus cricetus
		Streptococcus sobrinus
		Streptococcus ferus
		Streptococcus macacae
		Streptococcus downei
V	*Streptococcus salivarius*	*Streptococcus salivarius*
		"*Streptococcus thermophilus*"
		Streptococcus vestibularis
VI	Unaffiliated species	*Streptococcus suis* (Lancefield groups R, S, RS, and T)

Information in this table is based on Bentley et al. [29]

LABORATORY IDENTIFICATION

Bergey's Manual of Systemic Bacteriology describes streptococci as gram-positive, catalase-negative, facultatively anaerobic bacteria that are spherical or ovoid and <2 μm in diameter [32]. Because the hemolytic reaction of the streptococcal strain may be realized early in the identification process, media with blood is desirable for primary plating purposes. Gram-positive selective media (phenylethyl alcohol or Columbia with colistin and nalidixic acid agars) and nonselective Trypticase soy agar or Columbia base with 5% sheep blood will grow streptococci. Nutritionally variant streptococci require a source of pyridoxal (0.001% of an aqueous solution) or cross-streak of *Staphylococcus aureus*. Conventionally, streptococci are incubated at 35° to 37°C in 5% CO_2 atmosphere. Although detecting the Lancefield group D antigen might be helpful in identifying *Streptococcus bovis*, detection remains a nonspecific test. Nonhemolytic streptococci are identified by physiologic tests.

Tables 14.2 and 14.3 differentiate the physiological, pathological, and clinical characteristics of nonhemolytic streptococci [33]. The ability of *Streptococcus bovis* to hydrolyze the glycoside esculin in the presence of 40% bile distinguishes it from nonhemolytic viridans isolates [34].

Nonhemolytic streptococci in the viridans group are vancomycin-susceptible and produce

classification of the streptococci remain valid for identification schemes, use should be adjusted by new taxonomic knowledge. Among nonhemolytic streptococcal isolates, part of the viridans group, part of the nutritionally variant streptococci, and *Streptococcus bovis* comprise a number of species groups [31].

Table 14.2 Differentiation of Nonhemolytic Streptococci[a]

Type or Species of Streptococcus	Bile Esculin	Satelliting Behavior
"Viridans"	–	–
Streptococcus bovis	+	–
Nutritionally variant[b]		+

[a]Strains of group B streptococci may be nonhemolytic. Serologic methods or the CAMP test should be used to rule out possible group B strains.

[b]PYR positive.

Information in this table is adapted from Ruoff [71,72].

Table 14.3 Gram-Positive Cocci—Catalase-Negative, Nonhemolytic

Organism	Gram Stain	Hemolysis	Lancefield Group	Vanco	PYR	LAP	Bile Esculin	6.5% Salt	Gas/Glucose	Natural Habitat	Clinical Significance	Comments
Nutritionally variant strep	c/cb pr, ch	γ, (α)	None	S	+	+	-	-	-	URT GIT GUT	Endocarditis	Require pyridoxal
Streptococcus bovis	c/cb pr, ch	γ, (α)	D	S	-	+	+	-	-	GIT	*Streptococcus bovis* I: endocarditis; bacteremia associated with colon cancer. *Streptococcus bovis* II: bacteremia associated with a hepatobiliary source	*Streptococcus bovis* I: mannitol+ insulin ± levans+[a]. *Streptococcus bovis* II: mannitol− inulin− levans−
Streptococcus viridans	c/cb pr, ch	γ, (α), (β)	*Streptococcus milleri* group: A, C, F, G, or none. Others: varying Lancefield groups or none	S	-	+	−[b]	-	-	URT GIT GUT	*Streptococcus milleri* group: abscesses and pyogenic infections. Others: bacteremia, endocarditis, dental caries	

Abbreviations: c, cocci; cb, coccobacilli; ch, chains; A C D F G Lancefield Groups; GIT, gastrointestinal tract; GUT, genitourinary tract; LAP, leucine aminopeptidase; pr, pairs; PYR, pyrrolidonyl arylamidase; S, susceptible; URT, upper respiratory tract.

[a]levans: detected on mitis-salivarius agar as nonadherent gummy colonies.

[b]Some "viridans" streptococci may be bile exculin+ (e.g., *Streptococcus mutans*, *Streptococcus intermedius*).

Adapted from information based on Ruoff [71,72].

Table 14.4 Differentiating Features of Gram-Positive Cocci with Negative or Weakly Positive Catalase Reactions

Genus	PYR	Vancomycin	LAP	Gas from Glucose[a]	Esculin Hydrolysis	Growth in 6.5% NaCl
Streptococcus (nonhemolytic)	V[b]	S	+	−	V	V[c]
Lactococcus	V	S	+	−	V[d]	V
Leuconostoc	−	R	−	+	V	V
Pediococcus	−	R	+	−	V[d]	V
Gemella	+	S	V[e]	−	−	−
Aerococcus[f]	+	S	−	−	V	+

Abbreviations: +, positive; −, negative; V, variable; S, susceptible; R, resistant; PYR, pyrrolidonyl arylamidase; LAP, leucine aminopeptidase.

[a]Gas production from glucose in sealed MRS broth.

[b]Nutritionally variant streptococci are PYR positive.

[c]Viridans and group D streptococci are negative; group B streptococci may be positive.

[d]Most strains are positive.

[e]G. haemolysans is usually LAP negative; G. morbillorum is usually LAP positive.

[f]A. urinase, a newly described urinary tract pathogen, is PYR negative and LAP positive.

Data are based on Ruoff [71,72].

the enzyme leucine aminopeptidase (LAP), but do not produce the enzyme pyrrolidonyl arylamidase (PYR). These tests can differentiate nonhemolytic viridans streptococci from other genera that may be misidentified as viridans group, including *Leuconostoc, Pediococcus, Aerococcus, Lactococcus,* and *Gemella* (Table 14.4, Fig. 14.1).

Classification of these streptococci (nonhemolytic viridans group) has still not been finalized. The Facklam and Washington scheme summarized by Ruoff (Table 14.5) remains what is available for a diagnostic algorithm [33].

SPECIES GROUP DESCRIPTIONS

The nonhemolytic cariogenic *Streptococcus mutans* group consists of approximately seven physiologically similar but genetically distinct species. Extracellular polysaccharides (dextrans) are produced that may contribute to pathogenicity. Human mouths host *Streptococcus sobrinus, Streptococcus rattus,* or *Streptococcus mutans.* Reports of endocarditis in addition to dental caries have occurred [35].

Another nonhemolytic viridans species group consists of *Streptococcus salivarius, Streptococcus thermophilus, Streptococcus intestinalis,* and *Streptococcus vestibularis.* These human pathogens produce the polysaccharide levan, which might con-

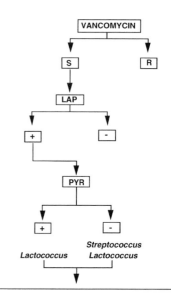

Figure 14.1 Schema showing nonhemolytic catalase-negative gram-positive cocci. Gram stains of *Gemella morbillorum* may appear streptococcal, but are distinctive in that individual cells in a given pair are often of unequal sizes. Data adapted from Ruoff [71,72].

Table 14.5 Differentiation of Commonly Isolated Nonhemolytic Viridans Streptococci

Species	VP	Arginine	Esculin	Mannitol	Sorbitol	Urease
Streptococcus mutans group	+	−[a]	+	+	+	−
Streptococcus salivarius group	+[b]	−	+	−	−	±
Streptococcus bovis	+	−	+	±[c]	−	−
"*Streptococcus milleri*" group	+	+	±	±	−	−

Abbreviations: +, positive; −, negative; ±, variable results may occur; VP,

[a]*Streptococcus rattus* is arginine positive.

[b]*Streptococcus vestibularis* is voges proskauer (VP) variable. *Streptococcus vestibularis* is also alpha-hemolytic, unlike the nonhemolytic *Streptococcus salivarius*.

[c]*Streptococcus bovis* biotype I is positive; biotype II is negative.

Information in this table is adapted from Ruoff [33] and Coykendall [35].

tribute to the gumdrop appearing colonies on sucrose-containing agar. These strains are probably also producers of urease, a characteristic that is unique among streptococcal isolates. In patients with cancer, bacteremia with *Streptococcus salivarius* has been described [1].

The nonhemolytic *Streptococcus bovis* classic description has included group D antigen and nonenterococcal streptococci identification. However, physiological tests are probably a better choice for identification purposes. Physiologically, *Streptococcus bovis* and *Streptococcus salivarius* (see Table 14.5) are similar. Two biotypes of *Streptococcus bovis* exist: biotype II is mannitol negative, inulin negative, and levan negative and biotype I is able to form large watery colonies on sucrose agar because of polysaccharide production (Table 14.3).

Nonhemolytic streptococci from oral infections were first called *Streptococcus milleri*. The nomenclatural history of the *Streptococcus milleri* group has progressed as follows: 1956, *Streptococcus milleri* [36]; 1977, *Streptococcus anginosus-constellatus*, *Streptococcus MG-intermedius* [37]; 1984, *Streptococcus anginosus*, *Streptococcus constellatus*, *Streptococcus inter-*

medius [38]; 1987 *Streptococcus anginosus* [39]; and 1991, *Streptococcus anginosus*, *Streptococcus constellatus*, *Streptococcus intermedius* [40]. In Tables 14.6 and 14.7, the discriminating reactions can be seen. Unfortunately, many of the substrates listed are not commercially available in traditional diagnostic test kits for identifying streptococci, therefore a large, current database for those organisms is not available. The isolates of the *Streptococcus milleri* group cause serious purulent infections and are normal flora of the oral cavity and upper respiratory and intestinal tracts.

The nonhemolytic nutritionally variant streptococci satellite around yeast, staphylococci, other streptococci, and family *Enterobacteriaceae* strains [14,19,22]. Exceptions to this include isolates of *Streptococcus pyogenes* and *Pseudomonas aeruginosa* [22,25]. Pyridoxal hydrochloride at a concentration of 0.001% or L-cysteine at a concentration of 0.01% will support the growth of nutritionally variant streptococci [10,14,19,20,22,25,41,42]. Overall, unsupplemented tryptic soy agar with 5% sheep blood does not support nutritionally variant streptococci, and growth on chocolate agar is variable

Table 14.6 Nonhemolytic Viridans Streptococci and Nutritionally Variant Streptococci

Organism	Cell Morphology	PYR	Pyridoxal Requirement
Nonhemolytic viridans streptococci	Coccobacilli in pairs, chains	−	−
Nutritionally variant streptococci	Like streptococci, or pleomorphic and gram-variable	+	+

Adapted from Ruoff [71,72].

Table 14.7 Current Classification of the Nonhemolytic *Streptococcus Milleri Species Group*

Enzyme	*Streptococcus anginosus*	*Streptococcus constellatus*	*Streptococcus intermedius*
Beta-*D*-fucosidase	−	−	+
Beta-*N*-acetylglucosaminidase	−	−	+
Beta-*N*-galactosaminidase	−	−	+
Sialidase	−	−	+
Beta-galactosidase	−	−	+
Beta-glucosidase	+	−	±
Hyaluronidase	−	+	+

+, positive; −, negative; ± variable.

Adapted from Ruoff [72] and Whiley [73]

[43,44]. Variable growth has been observed with brain heart infusion, Todd-Hewitt broth, and Columbia blood agar [43,45,46]. Growth of nutritionally variant streptococci occurs with thioglycolate or thiol broths [10,43,44,46,47].

Because nonhemolytic strains of nutritionally variant streptococci cause endocarditis, the support of their growth in blood culture media is relevant. If human blood (pyridoxal is contained in human erythrocytes) is added to traditional blood culture media, nutritionally variant streptococci growth [44,46,48]. Therefore, thioglycolate, thiol, and tryptic soy (supplemented with pyridoxal) will grow these strains. Subculture at 48 h enhances growth [46,48]. If the Dupont isolator system is used, horse blood agar supplemented with pyridoxal is required for plating media [49].

The nonhemolytic species of nutritionally variant streptococci include *Streptococcus defectivus* biotype I and *Streptococcus adjacens* biotypes 2 and 3. These species are resistant to optochin and susceptible to vancomycin. Both species produce pyrrolidonyl arylamidase and leucine aminopeptidase. These species do not produce alkaline phosphatase, hippurate, and arginine; no acidification of D-ribose, L-arabinose, D-mannitol, sorbitol, or glycogen occurs and polysaccharides are not produced from sucrose [9]. Table 14.8 has the distinguishing tests listed for the species.

SUSCEPTIBILITY TESTING

Nonhemolytic streptococci including *Streptococcus bovis* should be tested for susceptibility

Table 14.8 Differential Characteristics of *Streptococcus defectivus* and *Streptococcus adjacens*

Characteristics	Reaction[a]	
	Streptococcus defectivus	*Streptococcus adjacens*
Production of		
α- and β-galactosidases	+	−
β-glucuronidase	−	±
β-glucosidase	−	±
Acidification of		
Trehalose	+	−
Insulin	−	±
Lactose	±	−
D-raffinose	±	−
Starch	+	−

[a]+, positive; −, negative; ±, variable.

Information in this table is based on Ruoff [72].

to antimicrobials typically when isolated from blood culture or normally sterile body sites. Mixed culture evaluation is discouraged. Recommended therapy for strains causing endocarditis is penicillin with or without gentamicin; the level of pencillin resistance is usually used to determine the need for and duration of combination therapy with an aminoglycoside [50]. Because of the variability in resistance among nonhemolytic streptococci, minimal inhibitory concentration ([MIC] range 0.015 to >4 μg/ml) strains causing endocarditis should be tested for susceptibility [51–55]. The National Committee for Clinical Laboratory Standards [NCCLS] recommendations for testing techniques are listed in Table 14.9 [56,57]. The Bauer-Kirby technique may not be appropriate when testing nonhemolytic streptococci [57]. Troubling overlap in MICs is observed in isolates with zones of inhibition in the intermediate range and isolates with zones of inhibition in the susceptible range. Hindler et al. demonstrated potential with the E test [58]. However, data with other commercially available testing systems are lacking.

Testing nonhemolytic streptococci is recommended for susceptibility to third-generation cephalosporins [59,60]. Although nonvancomycin

resistance has been reported, vancomycin susceptibility is used as an identification tool. Genera resistant to vancomycin include *Lactobacillus*, *Leuconostoc*, or *Pediococcus* and might be confused with nonhemolytic streptococci. Not enough is known about the high-level streptomycin or gentamicin resistance for the NCCLS to make recommendations concerning nonhemolytic streptococci, although some resistance to these drugs has been reported [59,60].

The nutritionally variant streptococci species, both *Streptococcus defectivus* and *Streptococcus adjacens*, are a susceptibility testing challenge because of their requirements for pyridoxal and L-cysteine. Traditional testing techniques are listed in Table 14.9. In addition, a recent evaluation used numerous media for the E test and compared the E test to MICs done in Todd Hewitt broth supplemented with 0.001% pyridoxal HCl and Mueller Hinton agar supplemented with 5% horse blood and 0.001% pyridoxal HCl. In the 14 susceptible isolates, using the standard agar dilution medium for both E test and the reference test, the percent agreement ($\pm$1% dilution) was 93%. Most of the MIC categorical errors were due to the E test being one dilution higher than the reference MIC [61]. Endo-

Table 14.9 Considerations for Susceptibility Testing of Nonhemolytic Streptococci

Organism Group	Preferred Therapy		Routine Testing Indicated	Rationale	Testing Methods (Media)[a]
	Primary	Secondary			
Nutritionally variant	Penicillin + gentamicin	Vancomycin + gentamicin	No	Penicillin/ gentamicin combined therapy recommendation not dependent on penicillin results	AD (MHA + 5% LHB/.001% PdHCl) BD (MHB + 5% LHB/.001% PdHCl)
"Viridans" streptococci and *Streptococcus bovis*	Penicillin $\pm$ gentamicin	Vancomycin $\pm$ gentamicin	Yes	Level of penicillin resistance used to establish need for combined therapy with gentamicin; prevalence of aminoglycoside resistance unknown, probably rare	AD (MHA + 5% SB) BD (MHB + 2%–5% LHB)

[a]Testing in 5% to 7% CO_2 atmosphere enhances growth of most streptococci. Method abbreviations: AD, agar dilution; BD, broth microdilution. Media abbreviations: LHB, lysed horse blood; MHA(B), Mueller-Hinton agar (broth); PdHCl, pyridoxal-HCl; SB, sheep blood.

Information in this table is based on Sahm [74] and recommendations from the National Committee for Clinical Laboratory Standards [56,57]

carditis due to nutritionally variant streptococci should be treated with penicillin and aminoglycoside dual therapy [62,63]. Penicillin susceptibility of nutritionally variant streptococci is unpredictable (MIC range ≤0.03 to >4.0 μg/ml) [43,62]. In addition, the effectiveness of combination therapy does not correlate with penicillin resistance [62,64]. To date, resistance to vancomycin and high levels of aminoglycoside has not been observed. Therefore, because of the limited usefulness of in vitro data for guiding therapy and the difficulty of testing and interpreting that is related to specific growth requirements, susceptibility testing is rarely necessary for nutritionally variant streptococci [62,64]. Therapy should be selected according to whether the isolate was identified as a nutritionally variant streptococcus.

CLINICAL LABORATORY CONSIDERATIONS

Once a nonhemolytic streptococci isolate has been deemed significant enough to be evaluated, both identification and susceptibility testing procedures should be accomplished. Significance usually correlates with strains isolated repeatedly and in pure culture from normally sterile body fluids, such as blood, cerebrospinal fluid (CSF), and other fluids, tissue specimens, and prosthetic devices. However, nonhemolytic streptococci may be significant even when present with other isolates (for example, *Streptococcus milleri* with anaerobes or other bacteria) in the case of the immunocompromised patient.

Because of the existence of penicillin-resistant nonhemolytic streptococcal strains, susceptibility testing of significant isolates should be done [41]. In addition, as mentioned before, to distinguish strains from the vancomycin-resistant genera that could be confused with nonhemolytic streptococci, vancomycin susceptibility testing should also be done.

In addition to the identification tests listed in Table 14.5, commercially available testing systems exist [65]. In one evaluation, varying levels of agreement (50% to 74%) among five testing systems resulted [65]. It is important to note whether supplemental testing is needed for each of the kit techniques presented. Evaluations include API Rapid Strep, Baxter MicroScan Pos ID Panel, BBL Minitek Differential Identification System, IDS RapID STR System, and Vitek GPI. In another evaluation, the bioMérieux Rapid ID 32 Strep was tested, revealing good accuracy, with supplemental testing required [66]. Although different commercially available products use different nomenclature systems, perhaps we are approaching consensus as the knowledge of taxonomy and pathogenesis grows.

Nutritionally variant streptococci should be suspected when microscopic observation shows variable morphology and variable gram-stained cells but culture results are negative. To culture nutritionally variant streptococci, media can be supplemented with filter-sterilized pyridoxal hydrochloride solutions (added to produce a final concentration of 0.001%), pyridoxal-containing filter paper disks (commercially available), or cross-streaks of a suitable colony (*Staph. aureus*) to allow satelliting growth. Routine use of pyridoxal containing plating media is not recommended by Reimer and colleagues because of the apparent detrimental effects on other pathogens (for example, *Streptococcus pyogenes*) [67].

If a suspected isolate is confirmed to require pyridoxal, a positive pyrrolidonyl arylamidase test along with typical morphology fulfills the criteria for confirmatory identification of nutritionally variant streptococci. The API Rapid Strep Strip, using pyridoxal supplementation, has been used to further define nutritionally variant streptococci [11,13,68].

Susceptibility testing of nutritionally variant streptococci, either with a commercially available test or using NCCLS criteria, remains a not entirely satisfying experience [13,61,69,70]. The limited usefulness of in vitro data guiding therapy, along with the drawbacks of problems related to specific growth requirements, suggests that susceptibility tested is not often useful. It is better to select therapy on the basis of a strain's identification as nutritionally variant streptococci.

REFERENCES

1. Awada A, van der Auwera P, Meunier F, Daneau D, Klastersky J. Streptococcal and enterococcal

bacteremia patients with cancer. Clin Infect Dis 1992; 15:33–48.

2. Murray HW, Roberts RB. *Streptococcus bovis* bacteremia and undergastrointestinal disease. Arch Intern Med 1978; 138:1097–1099.

3. Burns CA, McCaughey M, Lauter CB. The association of *Streptococcus bovis* fecal carriage and colon neoplasia: possible relationship with polyps and their premalignant potential. Am J Gastroenterol 1985; 80:42–46.

4. Reynolds JG, Silva E, McCormack WM. Association of *Streptococcus* bacteremia with bowel disease. J Clin Microbiol 1983; 17:696–697.

5. Klein RS, Recco RA, Catalano MT, et al. Association of *Streptococcus* with carcinoma of the colon. N Engl J Med 1977; 297:800–802.

6. Klein RS, Catalano MT, Edberg SC, et al. *Streptococcus bovis* septic and carcinoma of the colon. Ann Intern Med 1979; 91:560–562.

7. Reed TMS, Davidson AI. *Streptococcus milleri* liver abscess. Lancet 1976; 2:648–649.

8. Koepke JA. Meningitis due to *Streptococcus anginosus* (Lancefield group F). JAMA 1965; 193:739–740.

9. Bouvet A, Grimont F, Grimont PAD. *Streptococcus defectivus* sp. nov. and *Streptococcus adjacens* sp. nov., nutritionally variant streptococci from human clinical specimens. Int J Syst Bacteriol 1989; 39:290–294.

10. George RH. The isolation of symbiotic streptococci. J Med Microbiol 1974; 7:77–83.

11. Pompei R, Caredda E, Piras V, Serra C, Pintus L. Production of bacteriolytic activity in the oral cavity by nutritionally variant streptococci. J Clin Microbiol 1990; 28:1623–1627.

12. Roberts RB, Krieger AG, Schiller NL, Gross KC. Viridans streptococcal endocarditis: the role of various species, including pyridoxal-dependent streptococci. Rev Infect Dis 1979; 1:955–965.

13. Bosley GS, Facklam RR. Biochemical and antimicrobic testing of "nutritionally variant streptococci." In: Abstracts from the 90th Annual Meeting of the American Society for Microbiology. Washington, DC: ASM Press, 1990; 395, Abstract C-307.

14. Cayeux P, Acar JF, Chabbert YA. Bacterial persistence in streptococcal endocarditis due to thiol-requiring mutants. J Infect Dis 1971; 124:247–254.

15. Coto H, Berk SL. Endocarditis caused by *Streptococcus morbillorum*. Am J Med Sci 1984; 287:54–58.

16. Dykstra MA, Polly SM, Sanders CS, Chastain DE, Sanders WE. Vitamin B$_6$-dependent streptococcus mimicking fungi in a patient with endocarditis. Am J Clin Pathol 1983; 80:107–110.

17. Eisenberg FP, Lorber B, Suh B, McDonough MT. Case report: prosthetic valve endocarditis due to a nutritionally variant streptococcus. Am J Med Sci 1985; 289:249–250.

18. Feder HM, Olsen N, McLaughtlin JC, Barlett RC, Chameides L. Bacterial endocarditis caused by vitamin B$_6$-dependent viridans group streptococcus. Pediatrics 1980; 66:309–312.

19. Frenkel A, Hirsch W. Spontaneous development of L forms of streptococci requiring secretions of other bacteria or sulphydryl compounds for normal growth. Nature 1961; 191:778–730.

20. Koshi G, Lalitha MK. Satelliting streptococci causing infective endocarditis—a short communication. Indian J Med Res 1978; 67:538–541.

21. Levine JF, Hanna BA, Pollock AA, Simberkoff MS, Rahal JJ. Case report: penicillin sensitive nutritionally variant streptococcal endocarditis: relapse after penicillin therapy. Am J Med Sci 1983; 286:31–36.

22. McCarthy LR, Bottone EJ. Bacteremia and endocarditis caused by satelliting streptococci. Am J Clin Pathol 1974; 61:585–591.

23. Narasimhan SL, Weinstein AJ. Infective endocarditis due to a nutritionally deficient streptococcus. J Pediatr 1980; 96:61–62.

24. Stein DS, Nelson KE. Endocarditis due to nutritionally deficient streptococci: therapeutic dilemma. Rev Infect Dis 1987; 9:908–916.

25. Carey RB, Gross KC, Roberts RB. Vitamin B$_6$-dependent *Streptococcus mitior* (*mitis*) isolated from patients with systemic infections. J Infect Dis 1975; 131:722–726.

26. Wofsy D. Culture-negative septic arthritis and bacterial endocarditis: diagnosis by synovial biopsy. Arthritis Rheum 1980; 23:605–607.

27. Barrios H, Bump CM. Conjunctivitis caused by a nutritionally variant streptococcus. J Clin Microbiol 1986; 23:379–380.

28. Ormerod LD, Ruoff KL, Meisler DM, Wasson PJ, Kintner JC, Dunn SP, Lass JH, van de Rijn I. Ophthalmology 1991; 98:159–169.

29. Bentley RW, Leigh JA, Collins MD. Intrageneric structure of *Streptococcus* based on comparative analysis of small-subunit rRNA sequences. Int J Syst Bacteriol 1991; 41:487–494.

30. Ludwig W, Seewaldt E, Kilpper-Balz R, Schleifer KH, Magrum L, Woese CR, Fox GE, Stackebrandt E. The phylogenetic position of *Streptococcus* and *Enterococcus*. J Gen Microbiol 1985; 131:543–551.

31. Bouvet A, Grimont F, Grimont PAD. *Streptococcus defectivus* sp. nov. and *Streptococcus adjacens* sp. nov., nutritionally variant streptococci from human clinical specimens. Int J Syst Bacteriol 1989; 39:290–294.

32. Hardie JM. Genus *Streptococcus* Rosenbach 1884, 22^{AL}. In: Sneath PHA, Mair NS, Sharpe ME, Holt JG (eds). Bergey's Manual of Systematic Bacteriology, Vol. 2. Baltimore: Williams & Wilkins 1986; 1043–1071.

33. Ruoff KL. Streptococcus, leuconostoc, pediococcus, stomatococcus, and miscellaneous gram-positive cocci that grow aerobically. In: Murray PR, Baron EJ, Pfaller MA, Yolken RH (eds).

Manual of Clinical Microbiology. Washington DC: ASM Press, 1995; 299–323.

34. Ruoff KL, Miller SI, Garner CV, Ferraro MJ, Calderwood SB. Bacteremia with *Streptococcus bovis* and *Streptococcus salivarius:* clinical correlates of more accurate identification of isolates. J Clin Microbiol 1989; 27:305–308.

35. Coykendall AL. Classification and identification of the viridans streptococci. Clin Microbiol Rev 1989; 2:315–318.

36. Guthof, O. Über pathogene "vergrunende Streptokokken." Streptokoken-Befunde bei dentogenen Abszessen und Infiltraten in Bereich der Mundhole. Zentralb Bakteriol Parasitenkd Infektionskr Hyg Abt 1 Orig Reihe A 1956; 166:553–564.

37. Facklam RR. Physiological differentiation of viridans streptococci. J Clin Microbiol 1977; 5:184–201.

38. Facklam RR. The major differences in the American and British *Streptococcus* taxonomy schemes with special reference to *Streptococcus milleri.* Eur J Clin Microbiol 1984; 3:91–93.

39. Coykendall AL, Wesbescher PM, Gustafson KB. "*Stretococcus milleri,*" *Streptococcus constellatus,* and *Streptococcus intermedius* are later synonyms of *Streptococcus anginosus.* Int J Syst Bacteriol 1987; 37:222–228.

40. Whiley RA, Beighton D. Emended descriptions and recognition of *Streptococcus constellatus,* *Streptococcus intermedius,* and *Streptococcus anginosus* as distinct species. Int J Syst Bacteriol 1991; 41:1–5.

41. Sherman SP, Washgton JA II. Pyridoxine inhibition of a symbiotic streptococcus. Am J Clin Pathol 1978; 70:689–690.

42. Schiller NL, Roberts RB. Vitamin B_6 requirements of nutritionally variant *Streptococcus mitior.* J Clin Microbiol 1982; 15:740–743.

43. Peterson CE, Cook JL, Burke UP. Media-dependent subculture of nutritionally variant streptococci. Am J Clin Pathol 1981; 75:634–636.

44. Reimer LG, Reller LB. Growth of nutritionally variant streptococci on common laboratory and 10 commercial blood culture media. J Clin Microbiol 1981; 14:329–332.

45. Cooksey RC, Thompson FS, Facklam RR. Physiological characterization of nutritionally variant streptococci. J Clin Microbiol 1979; 10:326–330.

46. Tillotson GS. Evaluation of ten commercial blood culture systems to isolate a pyridoxal-dependent streptococcus. J Clin Pathol 1981; 34:930–934.

47. Farber BF, Yee Y. High-level aminoglycoside resistance mediated by aminoglycoside-modifying enzymes among viridans streptococci: implications for the therapy for endocarditis. J Infect Dis 1987; 155:948–953.

48. Gross KC, Houghton MP, Roberts RB. Evaluation of blood culture media for isolation of pyridoxal-dependent *Streptococcus mitior* (*mitis*). J Clin Microbiol 1981; 14:266–272.

49. Gill VJ, Williams D. Usefulness of pyridoxal-containing blood agar as a primary plating medium to enhance recovery of nutritionally deficient streptococci. Diagn Microbiol Infect Dis 1988; 9:119–121.

50. Bisno AL, Dismukes WE, Durack DT, Kaplan EL, Karchmer AW, Kaye D, Rahimtoola SH, Sande MA, Sanford JP. Antimicrobial treatment of infective endocarditis due to viridans streptococci, enterococci, and staphylococci. JAMA 1989; 261:1471–1477.

51. Bourgault AM, Wilson WR, Washington JA II. Antimicrobial susceptibilities of viridans streptococci. J Infect Dis 1979; 140:315–321.

52. Etienne J, Gruer LD, Fleurette J. Antibiotic susceptibility of streptococcal strains associated with infective endocarditis. Am Heart J 1984; 5:33–37.

53. Venditti M, Baiocchi P, Santini C, Brandimarte C, Serra P, Gentile G, Girmenia C, Martino P. Antimicrobial susceptibilities of *Streptococcus* species that cause septicemia in neutropenic patients. Antimicrob. Agents Chemother 1989; 33:580–582.

54. Goldfarb J, Wormser GP, Glaser JH. Meningitis caused by multiply antibiotic-resistant viridans streptococci. J Pediatr 1984; 105:891–895.

55. Quinn JP, DiVincenzo CA, Lucks DA, Luskin RL, Shatzer KL, Lerner SA. Serious infections due to penicillin-resistant strains of viridans streptococci with altered penicillin-binding proteins. J Infect Dis 1988; 157:764–769.

56. National Committee for Clinical Laboratory Standards. Performance Standards for Antimicrobial Susceptibility Testing, 4th Informational Supplement, M100-S4. Villanova, PA: National Committee for Clinical Laboratory Standards, 1992.

57. National Committee for Clinical Laboratory Standards. Performance Standards for Antimicrobial Disk Susceptibility Tests, 4th ed., M2-A4. Villanova, PA: National Committee for Clinical Laboratory Standards, Washington DC: ASM Press, 1990.

58. Hindler JA, Bruckner DA. MIC testing of viridans streptococci using E test as compared to a reference method. In: 33rd Interscience Conference on Antimicrobial Agents and Chemotherapy, 1993; 166, Abstract 254.

59. Potgieter E, Carmichael M, Koornhof HJ, Chalkley LJ. In vitro susceptibility of viridans streptococci isolated from blood cultures. Eur J Clin Microbiol Infect Dis 1992; 11:543–546.

60. Wilcox, MH. Susceptibility of alpha-hemolytic streptococci causing endocarditis to benzylpenicillin and ten cephalosporins. J Antimicrob Chemother 1993; 32:63–69.

61. Douglas CP, Siarakas S, Gottlieb T. Evaluation of E test as a rapid method for determining MICs for nutritionally variant streptococci. J Clin Microbiol 1994; 32:2318–2320.

62. Stein DS, Nelson KE. Endocarditis due to nutritionally deficient streptococci: therapeutic dilemma. Rev Infect Dis 1987; 9:908–916.

63. Medical Letter. The choice of antibacterial agents. Med Lett 1992; 34:49–56.
64. Cooksey RC, Swenson JM. In vitro antimicrobial inhibition patterns of nutritionally variant streptococci. Antimicrob Agents Chemother 1979; 16:514–518.
65. Hinnebusch CJ, Nikolai DM, Bruckner DA. Comparison of API rapid STREP, Baxter MicroScan Rapid Pos ID Panel, BBL Minitek Differential Identification System, IDA RapID STR System, and Vitek GPI to conventional biochemical tests for identification of viridans streptococci. Am J Clin Pathol 1991; 96:459–463.
66. Freney J, Bland S, Etienne J, Desmonceaux M, Boeufgras JM, Fleurette J. Description and evaluation of the semiautomated 4-hour Rapid ID 32 Strep method for identification of streptococci and members of related genera. J Clin Microbiol 1992; 30:2657–2661.
67. Reimer LG, Reller LB. Effect of pyridoxal on growth of nutritionally variant streptococci and other bacteria on sheep blood agar. Diagn Microbiol Infect Dis 1983; 1:273–275.
68. Bouvet A, Villeroy F, Cheng F, Lamesch C, Williamson R, Gutman L. Characterization of nutritionally variant streptococci by biochemical tests and penicillin binding proteins. J Clin Microbiol 1985; 22:1030–1034.
69. Carey RB. Antimicrobial susceptibility of 22 strains of pyridoxal dependent streptococci. In: Program Abstracts of the 24th Interscience Conference on Antimicrobial Agents and Chemotherapy. Washington, DC: ASM Press, 1984; 267, Abstract 1005.
70. Thornsberry C, Swenson JM, Baker CN, McDougal LK, Stocker SA, Hill BC. Methods for determining susceptibility of fastidious and unusual pathogens to selected antimicrobial agents. Diagn Microbiol Infect Dis 1988; 9:139–153.
71. Ruoff KL. Nutritionally variant streptococci. Clin Microbiol Rev 1991; 4:184–190.
72. Ruoff KL. Dealing with viridans streptococci in the clinical laboratory. Clin Microbiol Newslett 1993; 15:73–76.
73. Whiley RA, Beighton D. Emended descriptions and recognition of Streptococcus constellatus, Streptococcus intermedius, and Streptococcus anginosus as distinct species. Int J Syst Bacteriol 1991; 41:1–5.
74. Sahm DF. Streptococci and staphylococci: laboratory considerations for in vitro susceptibility testing. Clin Microbiol Newslett 1994; 16:9–14.
75. Facklam RR, Washington II JA. Streptococcus and related catalase-negative gram-positive cocci. In: Balows A, Hausler WJ. (eds). Manual of Clinical Microbiology. Washington, DC: American Society for Microbiology, 1991; 238–257.
76. Facklam R, Hollis D, Collins MD. Identification of gram-positive coccal and coccobacillary vancomycin-resistant bacteria. J Clin Microbiol 1989; 27:724–730.
77. Janda WM. Streptococci and "Streptococcus-like" bacteria: old friends and new species. Clin Microbiol Newslett 1994; 16:161–170.
78. Oberhofer TR. Value of the L-pyrrolidonyl-B-naphthylamide hydrolysis test for identification of select gram-positive cocci. Diagn Microbiol Infect Dis 1986; 4:43–47.
79. Ruoff KL. The "new" catalase-negative, gram-positive cocci. Clin Microbiol Newslett 1994;16: 153–156.
80. Schleifer KH, Kilpper-Balz R. Molecular and chemotaxonomic approaches to the classification of streptococci, enterococci and lactococci: a review. Syst Appl Microbiol 1987; 10:1–9.
81. Bucher C, von Graevenitz A. Differentiation in throat culture of group C and G streptococci with identical antigens. Eur J Clin Microbiol 1984; 3:44–45.
82. Coykendall AL. Classification and identification of the viridans streptococci. Clin Microbiol Rev 1989; 2:315–328.
83. Gossling J. Occurrence and pathogenicity of the Streptococcus milleri group. Rev Infect Dis 1988; 10:257–285.
84. Ruoff KL. Streptococcus anginosus ("Streptococcus milleri"): the unrecognized pathogen. Clin Microbiol Rev 1988; 1:102–108.

15

Laboratory Evaluation of Streptococci

DIANA R. MARTIN

Streptococci are gram-positive, catalase-negative, facultatively anaerobic bacteria. Microscopically they appear spherical or ovoid. Chaining of cells is a common phenomenon. In recent years the classification of the species included in the genus *Streptococcus* has undergone review. Enterococci (previously classified as Lancefield group D streptococci) and lactococci (previously Lancefield group N) now reside in the genera *Enterococcus* and *Lactococcus*, respectively [1].

Streptococci form the dominant flora of the respiratory and genital tracts of humans. Some are parasites of other mammals. Broadly, streptococci can be divided into two groups. The first group, involving species identified serologically as Lancefield groups A, B, C, and G, are responsible for pyogenic infections and recognized in the laboratory by their ability to produce beta-hemolysis on blood agar. The second group, containing a number of genetically diverse species including the nutritionally variant streptococci [2], are mostly alpha-hemolytic on blood agar. Of these, the most important species medically is *Streptococcus pneumoniae* (pneumococcus). Other species, too numerous to list, are collectively referred to as the "viridans" group. These streptococci contribute significantly to the flora of the mouth and oropharynx but are capable of causing serious infections including subacute bacterial endocarditis, deep-seated abscesses,

and bacteremia particularly in immunocompromised hosts.

This chapter deals with the detection, isolation, identification, and differentiation of streptococci at the species and serogroup level and diagnostic immune responses generated by beta-hemolytic streptococci. Methods available for epidemiologic discrimination of streptococci at the subspecies and strain level are then described.

BETA-HEMOLYTIC STREPTOCOCCI

Streptococcus pyogenes (group A streptococcus), undoubtedly the most common and important of the beta-hemolytic streptococci, is responsible for pharyngitis (tonsillitis), commonly known as a strep throat. This streptococcus is highly infectious and can spread rapidly through a household, school, or community. Primary impetigo and skin infections are caused by group A streptococci. In the late stage of impetigo, and in infections following cuts, abrasions, or insect bites, other organisms such as staphylococci may also be present. Hematogenous spread from the throat or skin sites leads to suppurative complications including peritonsillar abscess, otitis media, cellulitis, septic arthritis, puerperal sepsis, deep-seated abscesses, myositis, and necrotising fasciitis. Group A streptococci are responsible for the two important nonsuppurative sequelae, acute glomerulonephritis and acute rheumatic fever, the latter leading to chronic rheumatic heart disease. Streptococci belonging to groups C and G are primarily residents of the upper respiratory tract but may cause tonsillitis, endocarditis, or bacteremia.

Group B streptococci (*Streptococcus agalactiae*) are an important cause of neonatal infection characterized by septicemic (early-onset) or meningitic (late-onset) infection. Vaginal and rectal carriage is quite common, particularly during pregnancy. Infection arises intrapartum from the maternal vaginal tract. Conditions such as malignancy often predispose group B infections in nonpregnant adults. The most common presentations in adults are bacteremia, and skin and soft tissue infections.

Detection, Isolation, Identification, and Differentiation

Specimen Types for Diagnostic Testing

Streptococcal involvement in superficial and deep-seated infections may be demonstrated by the isolation of a beta-hemolytic streptococcus from a particular focal site or specimen type. Alternatively, elevated anti-streptococcal antibodies in the serum of a patient may be demonstrated, but measurement of antibodies is generally limited to infections caused by *Streptococcus pyogenes*. However, the isolation of a streptococcus, with or without elevation of one or more streptococcal antibodies, provides supporting evidence for the diagnosis of a streptococcal infection or sequelae, only when accompanied by the appropriate clinical profile in a patient.

The most frequent specimens received in a clinical laboratory from which beta-hemolytic group A, C, and G streptococci are isolated are throat swabs, pus, serous fluids, aspirates, or blood. Pus from cuts, abrasions, and insect bites often yield a mixture of both streptococci and staphylococci. In contrast, serous fluid taken from the vesicle of a primary impetigenous lesion yields a pure culture of streptococci, providing the surrounding skin has not been touched during specimen collection. Specimens of tissue, blood, and aspirates, properly collected, should yield pure cultures of streptococci. Vaginal and anorectal swabs from pregnant women and aspirates or swabs of orifices in newborns are the most usual specimens for recovery of group B streptococci. Other bacteria will also be present at these sites.

Accurate diagnosis of streptococcal pharyngitis is important because eradication of *Streptococcus pyogenes* from the throat will prevent rheumatic fever [3]. Confirmation of streptococcal involvement depends either on a positive throat culture or a positive direct detection test. As most sore throats are caused by viruses, only 15%–30% of symptomatic patients subjected to a throat culture will test positive for *Streptococcus pyogenes*, assuming the throat swab has been properly taken [4]. Since the clinical features of streptococcal pharyngitis are nonspecific, diagnosis cannot be made on clinical grounds alone. Throat swabs from patients with streptococcal tonsillitis frequently yield a large number of *Streptococcus pyogenes* in contrast to swabs taken from the throats of carriers. However, there is no definite correlation between colony count and the presence or absence of infection [5]. Antibody responses can be detected even when numbers of streptococci are few [6].

The optimal method for establishing the presence of *Streptococcus pyogenes* in the throat has been the subject of much debate. The traditional approach and gold standard for detection of *Streptococcus pyogenes* is based on laboratory culture, whereas more recent approaches use direct detection systems or genetic probes, used either in a near-patient situation or in a laboratory. Regardless of the detection system, sensitivity is dependent on several variables including the adequacy of the swabbing technique, conditions operating for transportation of the swab, the methodology employed to detect *Streptococcus pyogenes*, and the interpretation of the results obtained [7]. Immediate processing of a swab is the best procedure but, in most situations, there will be a need for swabs to be transported to the laboratory, which can involve considerable time delays.

The type of swab (cotton or synthetic fiber) used for specimen collection is usually determined by the choice available at the point of collection. Survival of streptococci has been shown to be less than optimal on swabs that remain moist for a long time during transit, particularly in higher temperatures [8]. Transport media present in the tubes of commercial swabs provide environments suitable for retaining viability of beta-hemolytic streptococci for up to 48 h. Some commercial swab systems use a liquid medium, Modified Stuart's transport medium, contained on a pad at the base of the tube. Types that use an agarose butt of Amies semi-solid transport medium are better for the recovery of streptococci as the agar plug surrounding the swab protects streptococci from changes in humidity within the tube.

If transportation to the laboratory is prolonged, streptococci are more likely to remain viable if held in a dry state [8]. This can be achieved by replacing swabs in their tube, by placing the swab in contact with sterile desiccant (silica gel removes moisture from around the swab) [8] or, by smearing on to sterile filter paper strips housed in foil [9]. When a dry method of transportation is used, care should be taken that swabs are not left exposed to ultraviolet light or extreme temperatures.

Rapid Streptococcal Detection Tests

Rapid streptococcal detection systems for *Streptococcus pyogenes* have the advantage over throat culturing of being simple, with results available almost immediately, particularly when performed near-patient. In contrast, culturing takes 24–48 h to produce a result, with the consequent delay in implementation of antibiotic therapy.

A number of rapid streptococcal identification tests are marketed. Most rapid kits detect the group-specific polysaccharide antigen present in the cell wall of *Streptococcus pyogenes* and are based on the use of either nitrous acid or enzymes to extract group-specific antigen from streptococci collected on a throat swab. Detection of extracted antigen then relies on specific recognition by group-specific antibody and visualization of the reaction. In some systems group-specific antibody is coupled to particles and a reaction with specific antigen results in visible agglutination. Latex, liposomes, or protein A on

the surface of *Staphylococcus aureus* (co-agglutination), function as the particles for antibody attachment [10,11]. A competitive inhibition enzyme immunoassay, requiring laboratory facilities, has also been developed [12]. Results can be provided in 3–4 h. The most recently developed technique is optical immunoassay (OIA). Antigen extracted from a swab binds to group-specific antibody immobilized on a silicon wafer causing an observable change in the reflection of light [13]. This method has a high sensitivity and specificity.

Optimal culturing methods are regarded as the gold standard against which the use of rapid antigen detection tests are compared. A polymerase chain reaction (PCR)-based assay in association with optimal culturing was recently used to establish a reference standard [14]. Reported specificities for rapid kits have ranged from 85% to 100% and sensitivities varied from 31% to 95% [6,14,15]. Collective results show that rapid detection kits currently used are of insufficient sensitivity to replace the standard culture for detection of group A streptococci, particularly in populations at risk for rheumatic fever. Positive results from a rapid detection assay can be acted on, usually without question, but negative results provide no security and backup culturing is still required [16].

A nucleic acid probe assay for detecting *Streptococcus pyogenes* has recently become available. It detects unique specific rRNA sequences for *Streptococcus pyogenes* using an acridium ester-labeled single-stranded DNA probe. Compared to the gold standard culture method, sensitivities and specificities >90% have been reported [17].

For group B streptococci the gold standard method for detection is to culture onto blood agar (BA) from a swab grown overnight in selective broth [18]. Commercially available rapid detection tests for group B streptococci use the principles of those for group A streptococci. While specificity is generally high, sensitivity of group B detection tests compared to selective broth culture has been measured at <40% [19]. Since sensitivity increases in the presence of heavy group B colonization, in some obstetrical situations, when culturing is not feasible, rapid detection tests may play a vital role.

Isolation Methods

Although fastidious in their nutrient requirements, beta-hemolytic streptococci are not difficult to grow. Many commonly used nonselective solid media will support their growth. Most patient specimens may be streaked directly onto BA, which also allows observation of hemolysis. Hemolysis may vary with the animal source for the blood or the type of basal medium used. Sheep blood or horse blood is usually used at a concentration of 5%. In some parts of the world, particularly where there is difficulty with supply of sheep or horse blood, outdated human blood may be used. This is not recommended as the blood may contain antibodies or antimicrobial agents that can prevent growth of streptococci, and there is a lack of consistency in the product.

A supplementary method, ensuring recovery of *Streptococcus pyogenes* from swabs, involves seeding a Todd-Hewitt broth with the cut-off tip of the swab. After overnight incubation the swab broth is plated on to BA. This broth-enhanced culture method has been shown to be valuable for increasing the yield of streptococci but is not often used because of the added workload, material cost, and time. The most commonly used liquid medium is Todd-Hewitt broth, with or without supplementary neopeptone. The addition to Todd-Hewitt broth of gentamicin (8 g/L) and nalidixic acid (15 g/L), or colistin (10 g/L) and nalidixic acid (15 g/L) is recommended to enhance recovery of group B streptococci from vaginal or anorectal swabs [19].

Blood agar containing crystal violet (1 μg/ml) is selective and therefore helpful, particularly in situations where cultures are likely to contain staphylococci, as may be found in skin lesions. Media containing antibiotics have been advocated to selectively inhibit normal flora or gram-negative organisms. Columbia 5% BA with colistin (10 μg/ml) and nalidixic acid (15 μg/ml) inhibits gram-negative organisms [20]. The use of oxolinic acid (5 μg/ml) in place of nalidixic acid will be inhibitive to staphylococci and corynebacterium as well as gram-negative organisms [21]. The use of 5% sheep BA containing trimethoprim (1.25 μg/ml)-sulfamethoxazole (23.75 μg/ml) has been shown to increase the recovery of beta-hemolytic streptococci [22].

Swab specimens should be rolled over approximately one-half of the plate to deposit bacteria onto the surface of the culture medium. A heat-sterilized loop is then used to streak out the inoculum to obtain well-isolated colonies. Other specimens such as aspirates may be streaked directly.

Streptococci are aerobic or facultatively anaerobic. Growth is stimulated by an atmosphere of 5% to 10% CO_2 or by anaerobic conditions. However, the use of CO_2-supplemented atmosphere is also conducive to the growth of other bacteria that are facultative anaerobes and this can lower the likelihood of recovery of *Streptococcus pyogenes* from throat swabs [7]. Anaerobic incubation is favored because it enhances hemolysis but is also more costly and time-consuming. Aerobic conditions are quite satisfactory and reduction in oxygen tension to enhance hemolysis can be achieved if cuts are made in the surface of the agar at the time of streaking. The optimum temperature of incubation is 35°–37°C. There is now general acceptance that cultures negative for *Streptococcus pyogenes* following overnight incubation should be incubated for another 24 h. Increases in the recovery of streptococci of up to 46% have been reported [7].

Identification of Beta-Hemolytic Streptococci

Typically beta-hemolytic streptococci are gram-positive cocci, around 0.8 to 1.0 mm in diameter. They usually appear singularly and in pairs, or in chains, particularly when grown in liquid media. Beta hemolysis on BA is observed as complete clearing (lysis) of the red blood cells surrounding colonies, resulting in a clear zone. Alphahemolysis occurs when blood cells are only partially lysed, producing a green appearance around colonies.

Colonies of *Streptococcus pyogenes* may be quite opaque or grayish in color, and appear flat, dry, glossy, matt, or mucoid. Mucoid colonies appear large, wet, and glistening and are formed by colonies producing large amounts of hyaluronic acid. Glossy colonies are the smallest and appear domed. Beta hemolysis is the single most important feature observed. However, considerable variations do occur and many opacity factor–

producing group A streptococci appear alpha-hemolytic [23]. Nonhemolytic *Streptococcus pyogenes* have also been reported [24]. Although colonies of groups C and G can be confused with group A streptococci, group C streptococci often produce large brilliant zones of beta hemolysis on BA and colonies can be small. Group G streptococci tend to be domed and white in appearance and the zone of beta hemolysis is wider than for group A. Colonies of group B streptococci usually are gray and have very narrow zones of beta hemolysis, sometimes barely visible. The appearance of colonies of different morphological or hemolytic characteristics on the same plate may indicate a mixed culture of two different serogroups.

In culture, *Streptococcus pyogenes* can be presumptively identified using a 0.04 unit bacitracin differential disc. Inappropriate results will be achieved if the higher-dose antibiotic sensitivity discs are used in error. Bacitracin is strongly inhibitory to *Streptococcus pyogenes* but not usually to other streptococci, although it has been shown that streptococci of groups B, C, and G, can be as sensitive as *Streptococcus pyogenes* [25]. Erroneous results may be obtained if bacitracin discs are placed on primary cultures, rather than pure cultures, and it has been suggested that up to 50% of *Streptococcus pyogenes* may be missed by this practice.

Group A streptococci can be presumptively identified by the PYR test, which measures the enzymatic hydrolysis of the substrate L-pyrroli-donyl-β-napthylamide [26]. However, positivity is not a property of *Streptococcus pyogenes* alone, and enterococci, *Gemella* spp., and aerococci have been shown to be positive. The PYR test is available commercially. A distinguishing test for group B strepococci is the CAMP reaction. Group B streptococci produce a diffusible extracellular protein (CAMP factor) that acts synergistically with staphylococcal beta lysin to cause lysis of erythrocytes [27].

Serogrouping of Beta-Hemolytic Streptococci

Many streptococci, regardless of their hemolytic ability or whether they are pyogenic, possess group-specific polysaccharide that can be detected with antibody. Rebecca Lancefield was the first to demonstrate the presence of both group- and type-specific soluble antigens in acid extracts of streptococcal cells [28]. She developed the method for classifying streptococci into serogroups that remains the standard for group determination today. Groups have been labelled from A through V (excluding I and J), plus the provisional groups W–Z [29]. Grouping is of greatest value for differentiating *Streptococcus pyogenes* (group A streptococcus) from the other beta-hemolytic streptococci (groups B, C, G). Among human streptococci only *Streptococcus agalactiae* identify as a single species based on the group antigen. Taxonomic significance does not apply to other groups as they contain more than one species. For example, four distinct streptococcal species possess the group C carbohydrate antigen, although almost all human infection with group C involves only *Streptococcus equisimilis*. Some species belong to more than one group [30].

The Lancefield hot-acid extraction technique is only one of a number of methods that are used to extract group carbohydrate. Others include extraction with formamide, nitrous acid, or autoclaving the suspension of streptococci in saline. Enzyme extraction techniques have also been used [31]. The group-specific reaction of extracted polysaccharide can be demonstrated by precipitation, agglutination, immunofluorescence, or enzyme-linked immunosorbant assay (ELISA) and with group-specific antiserum.

Commercially available grouping kits, equivalent to the direct antigen tests used for throat swabs, enable streptococci in culture to be extracted and grouped very rapidly. Group-specific hyperimmune rabbit antiserum or isolated IgG that has been bound either to latex particles (latex agglutination) or to a treated cell suspension of protein A–rich *Staph. aureus* strain (co-agglutination) is used in these tests.

Diagnostic Serum Antibody Tests

Streptococcal antibodies are measured to indicate current or recent streptococcal infection and to differentiate true infection from the carrier state. They are important for establishing antecedent streptococcal infection, particularly when the diseases rheumatic fever (RF) or acute glomerulonephritis (AGN) are being considered. True group A streptococcal infections involve a specific immunologic response measured by a significant increase in the titer of antibodies to at least one of the extracellular antigens, streptolysin O (SLO), deoxyribonuclease B, hyaluronidase, streptokinase, and nicotinamide adenine dinucleotidase. The neutralization of enzyme by specific antibodies present in a patient's serum is the basis of each streptococcal antibody test used.

Antibody raised against extracellular enzyme antigens reaches a peak from 3 to 8 weeks after acute infection. The level of antibody reached is generally governed by idiosyncratic differences within individuals, the site of infection, and will be determined by the existing level of that antibody from previous infections [32]. Antibody is maintained for 2 to 3 months before declining [33]. The magnitude of the immune response can be modified by antibiotic therapy. A serum antibody is judged to be elevated if it exceeds the upper limit of normal (ULN) for the community. The ULN is taken as the titer exceeded by no more than 20% of the particular population at a given time [34]. As the level varies with age, season, and population studied it should be determined for the population being tested [35]. An antibody standard or reference serum with a known titer should be used as a control with each set of antibody determinations.

Since RF and AGN are sequelae of a group A streptococcal infection and there is a lag period between a streptococcal infection and onset of disease, serum taken at disease onset is convalescent and a rising titer will not usually be demonstrated. However, antibody titers are likely to be elevated compared with the 'norm' of the population. Over time, a measured decrease in the antibody titer may serve to indicate likely recovery from a streptococcal infection. Failure to demonstrate at least one elevated streptococcal antibody titer makes the diagnosis of ARF or AGN unlikely.

Storage of Human Serum

As human serum may contain pathogens such as hepatitis B or human immunodeficiency virus, the utmost care should be taken in handling serum from patients. Serum is best kept at 4°C in the short term and at -20°C for longer term. Frozen aliquots should be thawed rapidly to prevent shearing forces affecting antibodies. Frequent freeze thawing of serum should be avoided.

Anti-Streptolysin O

Anti-streptolysin O (ASO) is the most widely used and the most easily standardized of the serological tests available. Streptolysin O is antigenic. Neutralizing antibodies to SLO are found elevated after infection with group A streptococci and may also be elevated following infection with groups C and G streptococci. The test has been found to have limited usefulness for the measurement of antibodies when skin infections are involved [36].

Commercial kits are available and the test can be undertaken using micro- or macromethods. The test uses the property that SLO in its reduced form will hemolyse red blood cells. Known dilutions of a patient's serum are reacted with a standardized concentration of SLO. Residual SLO is detected using red blood cells as the indicator. The end point is the highest dilution showing no hemolysis. False-positive results may be recorded if the SLO becomes oxidized or if the serum being tested is either contaminated or hyperlipemic [33]. Streptolysin O titers are often reported as Todd units which represent the highest dilution of serum showing complete inhibition of hemolysis [37]. For a given population, normal levels should be established for the adult population and separately for children of different age bands [35,38].

Anti-Deoxyribonuclease B

Group A streptococci produce four deoxyribonucleases (DNases) designated A, B, C, and D. During infection response is greatest against DNase B. The presence of antibodies against DNase B provides evidence of recent infection with *Streptococcus pyogenes* [34], although some isolates of group C and G streptococci also produce DNase B. The anti–DNase B test is usually used in parallel with the ASO test. Unlike ASO, infection of the skin yields a good anti–DNase B response. In patients with AGN following a skin infection, the anti-DNase B test is the most reliable indicator of antecedent streptococcal infection [34]. Peak levels of anti–DNase B may be slower to occur but may remain elevated for longer periods than ASO.

In the test, anti–DNase B antibodies neutralize the enzymatic activity of DNase B, preventing it from depolymerizing DNA that has been coupled to an indicator dye. In the absence of antibodies depolymerization is detected through a color change. The anti–DNase B test has the advantage that the reagents are stable, purified antigen can be stored for long periods of time without losing potency, and false-positive tests are not recorded. The test is available commercially and can be performed as a micro- or macrotest. Currently, no standard international reference serum for anti–DNase B is available. In countries with high rates of skin infection upper limits of normal for school-aged children may be as high as 600 units [38].

Anti-Hyaluronidase Titer

Hyaluronidase is an enzyme expressed by group A streptococci that hydrolyses hyaluronic acid. The anti-hyaluronidase (AHT) test measures the level of antibody in a patient's serum that will neutralize hyaluronidase, preventing hydrolysis of the substrate potassium hyaluronate [39]. Hyaluronidase produced by group A streptococci is antigenically distinct from hyaluronidases of other streptococcal serogroups and its neutralization by antibody is considered specific for group A. The AHT responses occur with similar frequency to anti–DNase B responses and follow both throat and skin infections. The AHT can be performed as a micro- or macrotest.

Other Antibody Tests

Anti-nicotinamide adenine dinucleotidase (NADase) and anti-streptokinase (ASK) tests currently are uncommonly used for determination of streptococcal antibodies.

NONPYOGENIC STREPTOCOCCI

The nonpyogenic streptococci contribute significantly to the flora of the mouth, oropharynx, and gastrointestinal tract. Included is *Streptococcus pneumoniae*, the nutritionally variant species of streptococci, and a heterogeneous group of species collectively referred to as the viridans group.

Isolation and Identification of *Streptococcus pneumoniae* (Pneumococcus)

Streptococcus pneumoniae is the most important pathogen contributing to community-acquired pneumonia, often accompanied by bacteremia. Other pneumococcal infections include meningitis (particularly in infants), otitis media, and sinusitis. In clinically significant infection *Streptococcus pneumoniae* (pneumococcus) will most often be recovered from blood and cerebrospinal fluid (CSF) in pure culture. Recovery of pneumococci from sputum is suspect, as the organism is a commensal of the oropharynx.

Cultured on BA, colonies of pneumococci typically appear as round, flat, smooth, and translucent, often with a central pitting giving a poached egg appearance. Alpha hemolysis on BA is usually clearly seen. Pneumococci are facultative anaerobes and some strains are CO_2-dependent on isolation from clinical specimens [40]. Pneumococci are observed in gram stain as lanceolate diplococci with a clear capsule surrounding the cells. Noncapsulated pneumococci are occasionally observed.

Pneumococci can be differentiated from other alpha-hemolytic streptococci by their sensitivity to optochin and by bile solubility. Sensitivity to optochin (ethylhydrocupreine hydrochloride) is tested using commercially available discs. Bile solubility is demonstrated by the incubation of the organism in a 10% solution of sodium desoxycholate. Pneumococci are dissolved within 15 min [27]. Rapid molecular based testing procedures have been developed for identifying pneumococcal DNA. Molecular methods are more sensitive than culture, results are obtained faster, and pneumococcal involvement can be detected even after administration of antibiotics. A PCR assay based on the penicillin-binding protein gene *PBP2B* has been described [41].

Serogrouping/Serotyping of Pneumococci

Capsular typing involves the Neufeld test, in which serogroup-specific or serotype-specific antibody, when reacted with specific capsular antigen, renders the capsule visible [40]. Common antigenic determinants are shared by some pneumococci. Those pneumococci sharing antigens can be differentiated into serotypes using absorbed antisera. A limited number of serogroups/serotypes cause most cases of pneumococcal invasive disease. Monitoring of capsular types is being undertaken worldwide to ensure inclusion of important serogroups/serotypes in pneumococcal vaccines being developed for prevention of pediatric and adult disease. Multiple-antimicrobial resistance has been associated with specific clones of certain serogroups or serotypes [42].

Identification of Other Nonpyogenic Streptococci

Other nonpyogenic streptococci may be recovered from deep-seated abscesses, blood, vegetations on heart valves, and urine. Unless recovered in pure culture from a patient, their involvement in an infection is difficult to interpret.

The viridans group has undergone many taxonomic classifications [43]. Attempts to construct a comprehensive scheme for their serological classification have failed, as many do not have a detectable carbohydrate antigen. Until recently speciation of the group had been based on physiological reactions and much time and effort put into establishing batteries of individual physiological tests to define species [44]. Commercially available identification systems now allow rapid speciation within 4 h of incubation, instead of days. In these systems, metabolic end products are indicated by color reactions demonstrated either spontaneously or by the addition of reagents. Reactions are read automatically or visually by referring to a color table produced by the manufacturer.

While rapid tests have enabled speciation to be made, there has been general confusion about the names of some species with assignations varying in different parts of the world. Furthermore, the names of some species have been amended and new taxonomic names introduced. Increasingly, efforts are being focused on the application of nucleic acid–based diagnostic techniques for the identification and classification of nonpyogenic streptococci [43,45]. Speciation has already identified disease associations—for example, the association of *Streptococcus angi-*

nosus with liver or brain abscesses and the association of *Streptococcus bovis* bacteremia and endocarditis with colonic cancer. Improved taxonomy will enable recognition of those species most important in human infections. For further detail refer to Chapters 14 and 18.

TYPING METHODS FOR SUBSPECIES DISCRIMINATION OF STREPTOCOCCI

Discriminatory typing at the subspecies level enables recognition of outbreak strains or measurement of the frequency, spread, and temporal variation of streptococcal populations (clones). Either phenotypic or genotypic methods can be used. Phenotypic typing methods include recognition of differences in the expression of cell products (biochemical properties), antigenic differences on particular molecules (serotyping) [30,31,40,46], phage typing [47], and bacteriocin typing [48].

Methods using molecular discrimination are based on recognition and distinction of sequence variations. Sequence variation may alter recognition sites for restriction enzymes, creating differences in fragment size and numbers, following restriction by specific enzymes. This is known as restriction fragment length polymorphism (RFLP) analysis. This analysis can be used to define differences within specific genes, segments of genetic material, or the total chromosome. Amplification of genetic material using the PCR prior to RFLP analysis is a common approach, sometimes referred to as PCR-AREA (PCR–amplicon restriction endonuclease analysis). Other molecular approaches involve direct comparisons of sequence data obtained for a particular gene or segment of DNA or hybridisation with specific probes following amplification of target DNA by PCR.

The advantages of molecular typing methods are a greater typeability, better reproducibility, and increased discriminatory power. Molecular methods allow estimation of genetic relatedness or diversity and permit tracing of the evolution of streptococcal strain populations. Molecular epidemiology provides a framework for investigating the distribution of virulence factors and disease associations among clonal populations.

Phenotypic Discrimination of Streptococci

Phage Typing

Subtyping of group A streptococci by use of phage typing was used to subtype M type 49 isolates [47] but has had limited other use.

Bacteriocin Typing

Group A streptococci produce bacteriocin-like inhibitory substances. A method measuring the inhibitory action of a test strain against a set of nine defined indicator strains of various bacterial species has been developed for subtyping streptococci [48]. With a few exceptions, bacteriocin types (P types) are not M type–specific. Used in association with M typing, this method provides a useful epidemiological tool.

Serologic Typing of Beta-Hemolytic Streptococci

The classification into specific serotypes is based on the detection and identification of cell-surface protein or carbohydrate antigens. In the case of group A streptococci, the proteins M, T, and opacity factor (OF) are used. M protein is the most important marker of clonality. T antigen typing is also useful for group C and G streptococci [49]. Group C and G streptococci isolated from humans express M or M-like proteins that have biologic, immunochemical, and genetic properties similar to those expressed by group A streptococci [50,51]. Serologic characterization of group B streptococci involves identifying serotype-specific polysaccharide and protein antigens on isolates [46]. R protein antigens occur on some strains of *Streptococcus pyogenes* as well as group B, C, and G streptococci [52]. R proteins are not associated with virulence and the antibodies they elicit do not appear to have a role in immunity. These antigens provide little discrimination.

For group A streptococci M protein is an important virulence factor by nature of its antiphagocytic properties [53]. It exists as a dimeric filament protruding outward from the cell surface. The epitopes denoting M type specificity are found within the amino-terminal region distal from the cell membrane [53]. M type is usually defined by precipitation of extracted M protein using M type–specific antisera prepared against reference type strains [31]. Over 80 distinct M types have been identified internationally. Many more remain undesignated. Most studies on the epidemiology and strain characterization of group A streptococci have been conducted and interpreted in relation to the M protein type of the streptococci studied. T antigens, also found on the surface of cells, have no known relationship with virulence or protection but are useful in assisting with the characterization of group A streptococci, particularly when the streptococci are not typeable with existing M antisera. The information gained is less useful in that T antigen types are not as specific as M type. A single T antigen may be found in strains belonging to different M types, and streptococci belonging to the same M type may carry more than one T antigen, referred to as the T antigen pattern rather than T type. T antigens are recognized by agglutination of trypsinized cells [31].

Group A streptococci belonging to certain M types produce opacity in mammalian sera by the action, on high-density lipoproteins, of an apoproteinase known as opacity factor (OF) [54,55]. The OF can be detected in supernatants of broth cultures of OF-producing M types and in HCl or SDS extracts of cells. The OF type of a strain is determined by the OF-inhibition test using antisera produced in rabbits [56]. Since the antigenic specificity of OF parallels that of M protein, OF typing is considered equivalent to direct identification of the M type [56]. Specific correlations between Tantigen pattern, M type and OF result have been reviewed by Johnson and Kaplan [57].

The valuable information obtained from serologic typing of group A streptococci is tempered by the fact that few laboratories in the world have a comprehensive range of typing antisera and in some countries the percentage of streptococci not typeable with the existing range of antisera is high [31].

Molecular Typing Methods for Discriminating Streptococci

Sequencing of *emm* and Other Genes

The *emm* gene of *Streptococcus pyogenes* is the gene that encodes the M protein. The 5′ ends of the *emm* genes are heterogeneous and encode the serotype specificity detected by the M serotyping of streptococci. A method for typing streptococci using sequencing of *emm*-specific PCR products has been described [58]. The discriminatory power of this genotypic *emm* sequence-typing scheme approximates that of the phenotypic M-serotyping scheme [58,59]. Most M serotypes have a unique *emm* sequence type and isolates of that M type will show ≥95% sequence identity with the comparable *emm* sequence of the reference M serotype strain. A few discrepancies have been documented to date and further such discrepancies are to be expected as the method is more extensively used [59]. *Emm* sequence typing has the advantage that isolates not typeable using serologic methods, can be genotyped by *emm* sequence determination. To enable appropriate biologic interpretation of *emm* sequence typing results, investigative studies need to be undertaken to determine relationships between specific *emm* sequences, serotype-specific epitopes on the expressed M proteins they encode, and the type-specific antibodies elicited by these proteins.

An alternative method for genetically determining the M type, uses DNA–DNA hybridization with type-specific oligonucleotide probes to detect type-specific sequences in the PCR product of the *emm* gene [60]. This method requires a comprehensive array of sequence specific probes. A disadvantage of this method is that sequences for which probes are not available cannot be identified.

A method using multilocus sequence typing for seven housekeeping genes has recently been validated and described for *Streptococcus pneumoniae* [61]. This method has the potential to discriminate large numbers of pneumococcal genotypes and to provide useful information such as monitoring the global spread of antibiotic resistant clones. The method is applicable to other streptococci, particular *Streptococcus pyogenes.*

Sequence polymorphism analysis of the *sic* gene and a region of the chromosome with DR sequences was recently used to discriminate clonally related M type I streptococci [62].

Multilocus Enzyme Electrophoresis

Multilocus enzyme electrophoresis (MEE) detects different alleles of genes by scoring the electrophoretic mobilities of the enzymes they encode. Isolates with the same multilocus enzyme type (ET) are referred to as clones. Similarity of type is taken to reflect descent from a common ancestor. A strong correlation between ETs and M types studied has been shown, indicating the clonal nature of certain M types and emphasizing the important role that M typing has had in "pigeonholing" streptococci [63,64]. Correlation between group B streptococci causing neonatal sepsis, serotype, and ET type has been described [65].

Restriction Fragment Length Polymorphism Analysis

Restriction fragment length polymorphism (RFLP) analysis, also referred to as restriction endonuclease analysis (REA), is a valuable method for discriminating strains at the subtype or subspecies level. Restriction enzymes are used to cut DNA or RNA generating a number of different-sized fragments that are visualized as a pattern of discrete bands by gel electrophoresis. The fragment patterns or profiles produced for different isolates or strains are then compared. The use of frequently cutting restriction enzymes on total genomic DNA results in a large number of small fragments that are resolvable by standard agarose gel electrophoresis but patterns are difficult to interpret. Rarely cutting enzymes produce fewer but larger fragments which, because of their size, require resolution using pulsed field gel electrophoresis (PFGE) or field inversion gel electrophoresis (FIGE).

RFLP OF TOTAL CHROMOSOMAL DNA

Various methods have been reported for extraction of total chromosomal DNA from streptococci. The most favored method involves lysis of streptococci embedded in agarose plugs followed by macrorestriction using rarely cutting restriction enzymes [66]. Genetic profiles produced are conserved among most isolates from the same M type [67,68]. Within M types clear genetic heterogeneity among group A streptococci has also been shown [64,66,68]. Recently, RFLP analysis was used to identify the intercontinental spread of a subclone of M type1 streptococci causing episodes of invasive disease

[64]. Analysis by RFLP has been found useful for discriminating streptococci belonging to groups B, C, and G [69,70].

RIBOTYPING

This method uses RFLP analysis of ribosomal RNA genes to characterize streptococci. It provides information on specific regions within the genome. It appears less discriminatory than other methods for group A streptoccocci [63]. The method has been used to discriminate among group B streptococci although shown to be less discriminatory than RFLP analysis of the chromosome [69].

VIR TYPING

This application of RFLP typing measures changes in the region of the genome encoding major virulence factors [72,73]. Most of the 5–7 kb variable Vir regulon is amplified, prior to RFLP analysis. Because M types are represented by distinct Vir types, but not all Vir types represent distinct M types, the method does not replace M typing.

Arbitrary Primed Polymerase Chain Reaction

This method, also known as random amplified polymorphic DNA (RAPD), uses low-stringency PCR amplification with single primers of arbitrarily selected nucleotide sequences to generate strain-specific arrays of amplified DNA fragments. The method gives similar discrimination to RFLP analysis and is a useful tool in association with M typing [74]. Problems in reproducibility of banding patterns linked to difficulties in standardization of concentrations of reagents have been reported. The RAPD method has been used to discriminate among isolates of groups A, C, and G and recently among isolates of group B [75].

Subtyping Using the Intergenic Spacer

The 16S–23S RNA gene intergenic spacer has been used for identification and subtyping of a number of species of bacteria. This method was recently applied to isolates of group C streptococci. Different combinations of variant regions within the intergenic spacer were found providing a basis for species subtyping and evolutionary tracking of strains [76].

COMMENTS

Molecular techniques are proving to be extraordinarily important both as tools for unraveling poorly understood mechanisms of pathogenicity and for descriptive molecular epidemiology. However, traditional and standardized methods for the isolation, identification, and serotyping of streptococci still have a significant role in defining the cause of infections and in disease control. It is just as important to recognize the changes in the phenotypes of important streptococci which may affect their behavior, as it is to be able to understand the implications of variation at the genetic level. The importance of using appropriate laboratory methodology is stressed.

REFERENCES

1. Schleifer KH, Kilpper-Balz R. Molecular and chemotaxonomic approaches to the classification of streptococci, enterococci and lactococci: a review. Syst Appl Microbiol 1987; 10:1–19.
2. Bouvet A, Grimont F, Grimont PAD. *Streptococcus defectivus* sp. nov. and *Streptococcus adjacens* sp. nov., nutritionally variant streptococci from human clinical specimens. Int J Syst Bacteriol 1989; 39:290–294.
3. Denny FW, Wannamaker LW, Brink WR, Rammelkamp CH, Custer EA. Prevention of rheumatic fever. Treatment of preceding streptococcic infection. JAMA 1950; 143:151–153.
4. van Cauwenberge PB, van der Mijnsbrugge A. Pharyngitis: a survey of the microbiologic etiology. Pediatr Infect Dis J 1991; 10:S39–S42.
5. Breese BB, Disney FA, Talpey WB, Green JL. Beta-hemolytic streptococcal infection. Am J Dis Child 1970; 119:18–26.
6. Gerber MA, Randolph MF, Chanatry J, Wright LL, DeMeo KK, Anderson LR. Antigen detection test for streptococcal pharyngitis: evaluation of sensitivity with respect to true infections. J Pediatr 1986; 108:654–657.
7. Kellogg JA. Suitability of throat culture procedures for detection of group A streptococci and as reference standards for evaluation of streptococcal antigen detection kits. J Clin Microbiol 1990; 28:165–169.
8. Redys JJ, Hibbard EW, Borman EK. Improved dry-swab transportation for streptococcal specimens. Public Health Rep 1968; 83:143–149.

9. Hollinger NF, Lindberg LH, Russell EL, Sizer HB, Cole RM, Browne AS, Updyke EL. Transport of streptococci on filter paper strips. Public Health Rep 1960; 75:251–259.

10. Gerber MA, Spadaccini LJ, Wright LL, Deutsch L. Latex agglutination tests for rapid identification of group A streptococci directly from throat swabs. J Pediatr 1984; 105:702–705.

11. Christensen P, Kahlmeter G, Jonsson S, Kronvall G. New method for the serological grouping of streptococci with specific antibodies adsorbed to protein A–containing staphylococci. Infect Immun 1973; 7:881–885.

12. Knigge KM, Babb JL, Firca JR, Ancell K, Bloomster TG, Marchlewicz BA. Enzyme immunoassay for the detection of group A streptococcal antigen. J Clin Microbiol 1984; 20:735–741.

13. Harbeck RJ, Teague J, Crossen GR, Maul DM, Childers PL. Novel, rapid optical immunoassay technique for detection of group A streptococci from pharyngeal specimens: comparison with standard culture methods. J Clin Microbiol 1993; 31:839–844.

14. Kaltwasser G, Diego J, Welby-Sellenriek PL, Ferrett R, Caparon M, Storch GA. Polymerase chain reaction for *Streptococcus pyogenes* used to evaluate an optical immunoassay for the detection of group A streptococci in children with pharyngitis. Pediatr Infect Dis J 1997; 16:748–753.

15. Roe M, Kishiyama C, Davidson K, Schaefer L, Todd J. Comparison of BioStar Strep A OIA Opitical Immune Assay, Abbott TestPack Plus Strep A, and culture with selective media for diagnosis of group A streptococcal pharyngitis. J Clin Microbiol 1995; 33:1551–1553.

16. Lieu Ta, Fleischer GR, Schwartz JS. Cost-effectiveness of rapid latex agglutination testing and throat culture for streptococcal pharyngitis. Pediatrics 1990; 85:246–256.

17. Heelan JS, Wilbur S, Depretis G, Letourneau C. Rapid antigen testing for group A *Streptococcus* by DNA probe. Diagn Microbiol Infect Dis 1996; 24:65–69.

18. Centers for Disease Control and Prevention. Prevention of perinatal group B streptococcal disease: a public health perspective. MMWR Morb Mortal Wkly Rep 1996; 45(No RR-7):16–17.

19. Baker CJ. Inadequacy of rapid immunoassays for intrapartum detection of group B streptococcal carriers. Obstet Gynecol 1996; 88:51–55.

20. Ellner PD, Stoessel CJ, Drakeford E, Vasi F. A new culture medium for medical bacteriology. Am J Clin Pathol 1966; 45:502–504.

21. Petts DN. Colistin-oxolinic acid-blood agar: a new selective medium for streptococci. J Clin Microbiol 1984; 19:4–7.

22. Gunn BA, Ohashi DK, Gaydos CA, Holt ES. Selective and enhanced recovery of group A and B streptococci from throat cultures with sheep blood agar containing sulfamethoxazole

and trimethoprim. J Clin Microbiol 1977; 5:650–655.

23. Pinney AM, Widdowson JP, Maxted WR. Inhibition of β-haemolysis by opacity factor in group A streptococci. J Hyg 1977; 78:355–362.

24. James L, McFarland RB. An epidemic of pharyngitis due to a nonhemolytic group A streptococcus at Lowry Air Force Base. N Engl J Med 1971; 284:750–752.

25. Maxted WR. The use of bacitracin for identifying group A haemolytic streptococci. J Clin Pathol 1953; 6:224–226.

26. Facklam RR, Thacker LG, Fox B, Eriquez L. Presumptive identification of streptococci with a new test system. J Clin Microbiol 1982; 15:987–990.

27. Ruoff KL. Streptococcus. In: Manual of Clinical Microbiology, 6th ed. PR Murray, EJ Baron, MA Pfaller, FC Tenover, RH Yolken (eds.) Washington, DC: American Society for Microbiology, 1995; 299–307.

28. Lancefield RC. A serological differentiation of human and other groups of hemolytic streptococci. J Exp Med 1933; 57:571–595.

29. Facklam RR, Edwards LR. A reference laboratory's investigations of proposed M-type strains of *Streptococcus pyogenes*, capsular types of *S. agalactiae*, and new group antigens of streptococci. In: Parker MT (ed). Pathogenic Streptococci. Chertsey, Surrey: Reedbooks, 1979; 251–253.

30. Facklam RR. Serologic identification of streptococci: how useful is serologic grouping? Clin Microbiol Newslett 1985; 7:91–94.

31. Johnston DR, Kaplan EL, Sramek J, Bicova R, Havlicek J, Havlickova H, Motlova J, Kriz P. Laboratory Diagnosis of Group A Streptococcal Infections. Geneva: World Health Organisation, 1996; 23–53.

32. Kaplan EL, Anthony BF, Chapman SS, Ayoub EM, Wannamaker LW. The influence of the site of infection on the immune response to group A streptococci. J Clin Invest 1970; 49:1405–1414.

33. Ayoub EM. Streptococcal antibody tests in rheumatic fever. Clin Immunol Newslett 1982; 3:107–111.

34. Ayoub EM, Wannamaker LW. Evaluation of the streptococcal desoxyribonuclease B and diphosphopyridine nucleotidase antibody tests in acute rheumatic fever and acute glomerulonephritis. Pediatrics 1962; 29:527–538.

35. Kaplan EL, Rothermel CD, Johnson DR. Antistreptolysin O and anti-deoxribonuclease B titers: normal values for children ages 2 to 12 in the United States. Pediatrics 1998; 101:86–88.

36. Kaplan EL, Wannamaker LW. Streptolysin O: supression of its antigenicity by lipids extracted from skin. Proc Soc Exp Biol Med 1974; 146:205–208.

37. Todd E. Antigenic streptococcal hemolysis. J Exp Med 1932; 55:267–280.

38. Dawson KP, Martin DR. Streptococcal involvement in childhood acute glomerulonephritis: a re-

view of 20 cases at admission. NZ Med J 1982; 95:373–376.

39. Murphy RA. Improved antihyaluronidase test applicable to the microtitration technique. Appl Microbiol 1972; 23:1170–1171.

40. Lund E, Henrichsen J. Laboratory diagnosis, serology and epidemiology of *Streptococcus pneumoniae*. Methods Microbiol 1978; 12:242–262.

41. Isaacman DJ, Zhang Y, Rydquist-White J, Wadowsky RM, Post JC, Ehrlich GD. Identification of a patient with *Streptococcus pneumoniae* bacteremia meningitis by the polymerase chain reaction (PCR). Mol Cell Probes 1995; 9:157–160.

42. Klugman KP. Pneumococcal resistance to antibiotics. Clin Microbiol Rev 1990; 3:171–196.

43. Coykendall AL. Classification and identification of the viridans streptococci. Clin Microbiol Rev 1989; 2:315–328.

44. Facklam RR. Physiological differentiation of viridans streptococci. J Clin Microbiol 1977; 5:184–201.

45. Bentley RW, Leigh JA. Development of PCR-based hybridization protocol for identification of streptococcal species. J Clin Microbiol 1995; 33:1296–1301.

46. Henrichsen J, Ferrieri P, Jelinkova J, Köhler W, Maxted WR. Nomenclature of antigens of group B streptococci. Int J Syst Bacteriol 1984; 34:500.

47. Skjold SA, Wannamaker LW. Method for phage typing group A type 49 streptococci. J Clin Microbiol 1976; 4:232–238.

48. Tagg JR, Martin DR. Evaluation of a typing scheme for group A streptococci based upon bacteriocin-like inhibitor production. Zentralbl Bakteriol Hyg [A] 1984; 257:60–67.

49. Efstratiou A. Outbreaks of human infection caused by pyogenic streptococci of Lancefield groups C and G. J Med Microbiol 1994; 32:1312–1317.

50. Bisno AL, Collins CM, Turner JC. M proteins of group C streptococci isolated from patients with acute pharyngitis. J Clin Microbiol 1996; 34:2511–2515.

51. Schnitzler N, Podbielski A, Baumgarten G, Mignon M, Kaufhold A. M or M-like protein gene polymorphisms in human group G streptococci. J Clin Microbiol 1995; 33:356–363.

52. Wilkinson HW. Comparison of streptococcal R antigens. Appl Microbiol 1972; 24:669–670.

53. Fischetti VA. Streptococcal M protein: molecular design and biological behavior. Clin Microbiol Rev 1989; 2:285–314.

54. Ward HK, Rudd GV. Studies on haemolytic streptococci from human sources: the cultural characteristics for potentially virulent strains. Aust J Exp Biol Med Sci 1938; 16:181–192.

55. Saravani GA, Martin DR. Opacity factor from group H streptococci is an apoproteinase. FEMS Microbiol Letters 1990; 68:35–40.

56. Maxted WR, Widdowson JP, Fraser CAM, Ball LC, Bassett DCJ. The use of the serum opacity reaction in the typing of group-A streptococci. J Med Microbiol 1973; 6:83–90.

57. Johnson DR, Kaplan EL. A review of the correlation of T-agglutination patterns and M-protein typing and opacity factor production in the identification of group A streptococci. J Med Microbiol 1993; 38:311–315.

58. Beall B, Facklam R, Thompson T. Sequencing *emm*-specific polymerase chain reaction products for routine and accurate typing of group A streptococci. J Clin Microbiol 1996; 34:953–958.

59. Facklam R, Beall B, Efstratiou A, Fischetti V, Johnson D, Kaplan E, Kriz P, Lovgren M, Martin D, Schwartz B, Totolian A, Bessen D, Hollingshead S, Rubin F, Scott J, Tyrell G. Emm typing and validation of provisional M types for group A streptococci. Emerging Infect Dis 1999; 5:247–253

60. Saunders NA, Hallas G, Gaworzewska ET, Metherell L, Efstratiou A, Hookey JV, George RC. PCR-enzyme immunosorbent assay and sequencing as an alternative to serology for M-antigen typing of *Streptococcus pyogenes*. J Clin Microbiol 1997; 35:2689–2691.

61. Enright MC, Spratt BG. A multilocus sequence typing scheme for *Streptococcus pneumoniae*: identification of clones associated with serious invasive disease. Microbiol 1998; 144:3049–3060.

62. Hoe N, Nakashima K, Grigsby D, Pan X, Dou SJ, Naidich S, Garcia M, Kahn E, Bergmire-Sweat D, Musser JM. Rapid molecular genetic subtyping of serotype MI group A *Streptococcus* strains. Emerg Infect Dis 1999; 5:254–263.

63. Musser JM, Hauser AR, Kim MH, Schlievert PM, Nelson K, Selander RK. Streptococcus pyogenes causing toxic-shock-like syndrome and other invasive diseases: clonal diversity and pyrogenic exotoxin expression. Proc Natl Acad Sci USA 1991; 88:2668–2672.

64. Musser JM, Kapur V, Szeto J, Pan X, Swanson DS, Martin DR. Genetic diversity and relationships among *Streptococcus pyogenes* strains expressing serotype M1 protein: recent intercontinental spread of a subclone causing episodes of invasive disease. Infect Immun 1995; 63:994–1003.

65. Quentin R, Huet H, Wang F-S, Geslin P, Goodeau A, Selander RK. Characterisation of *Streptococcus agalactiae* strains by multilocus enzyme genotype and serotype: identification of multiple virulent clone families that cause invasive neonatal disease. J Clin Microbiol 1995; 33:2576–2581.

66. Single LA, Martin DR. Clonal differences within M-types of the group A streptococcus revealed by pulsed field gel electrophoresis. FEMS Microbiol Lett 1992; 91:85–90.

67. Cleary PP, Kaplan EL, Livdahl C, Skjold S. DNA fingerprints of *Streptococcus pyogenes* are

M type specific. J Infect Dis 1988; 158:1317–1323.

68. Martin DR, Single LA. Molecular epidemiology of group A streptococcus M type 1 infections. J Infect Dis 1993; 167:1112–1117.

69. Blumberg HM, Stephens DS, Licitra C, Pigott N, Facklam R, Swaminathan B, Wachsmuth IK. Molecular Epidemiology of group B streptococcal infection: use of restriction endonuclease analysis of chromosomal DNA and DNA restriction fragment length polymorphisms of ribosomal RNA genes (ribotyping). J Infect Dis 1992; 166:574–579.

70. Bert F, Branger C, Lambert-Zechovsky N. Pulsed-field gel electrophoresis is more discriminating than multilocus enzyme electrophoresis and random amplified polymorphic DNA analysis for typing pyogenic streptococci. Curr Microbiol 1997; 34:226–229.

71. Seppälä H, Vuopio-Varkila J, Österblad M, Jahkola M, Rummukainen M, Holm SE, Huovinen P. Evaluation of methods for epidemiological typing of group A streptococci. J Infect Dis 1994; 169:519–525.

72. Gardiner D, Hartas J, Currie B, Mathews JD, Kemp DJ, Sriprakash K. Vir typing: a long-PCR typing method for group A streptococci. PCR Methods Appl 1995; 4:288–293.

73. Hookey JV, Saunders NA, Clewley JP, Efstratiou A, George RC. Virulence regulon polymorphism in group A streptococci revealed by long PCR and implications for epidemiological and evolutionary studies. J Med Microbiol 1996; 45:285–293.

74. Seppälä H, Qiushui H, Österblad M, Huovinen P. Typing of group A streptococci by random amplified polymorphic DNA analysis. J Clin Microbiol 1994; 32:1945–1948.

75. Chatellier S, Ramanantsoa C, Harriau P, Rolland K, Rosenau A, Quentin R. Characterization of *Streptococcus agalactiae* strains by randomly amplified polymorphic DNA analysis. J Clin Microbiol 1997; 35:2573–2579.

76. Chanter N, Collin N, Holmes N, Binns M, Mumford J. Characterization of the Lancefield group C streptococcus 16S–23S RNA gene intergenic spacer and its potential for identification and sub-specific typing. Epidemiol Infect 1997; 118:125–135.

16

Enterococcal Infections

LARRY J. STRAUSBAUGH
MICHAEL S. GILMORE

Enterococci were first described at the turn of the century. Thiercelin used the term "enterocoque" in an 1899 French publication to delineate a gram-positive diplococcus of intestinal origin isolated from patients with enteritis, appendicitis, and meningitis [1]. The common genus designation derived from his term. In 1906 Andrewes and Horder coined the name *Streptococcus faecalis* for an isolate recovered from the blood of a patient with endocarditis [2]. These authors appreciated its similarity to other bacteria of intestinal origin and also reported identifying similar isolates from urinary tract infections. Subsequently, others confirmed the association of enterococci with endocarditis and also linked enterococci with puerperal sepsis and purulent abdominal infections following trauma [3]. Wound infections caused by enterococci were reported by several authors during World War I [4].

For most of this century enterococci were classified with the group D streptococci on the basis of their common morphology and reaction with group-specific antiserum. However, the identification of fundamental genetic differences in the 1980s prompted the establishment of a separate *Enterococcus* genus for these bacteria, which differ substantially from *Streptococcus bovis* and the other group D streptococci [5]. *Enterococcus faecalis* and *Enterococcus faecium* are the two species most frequently associated with human disease. Their role in community-acquired infections such as endocarditis and pyelonephritis has been recognized for decades. During the last decade, enterococci have emerged as common causes of nosocomial infections including bacteremia. The propensity of these bacteria to acquire antimicrobial resistance suggests that their role as pathogens in hospitalized patients will continue to increase as they enter their second century as a recognized cause of human disease.

IDENTIFICATION

Morphology

Like many streptococci, enterococci occur in pairs, short chains, or singly, depending on cultivation conditions and age of culture, and stain gram positive [4,6,7]. Enterococcal cells are typically lancet shaped to coccobacillary.

Culture and Biochemical Characteristics

The genus *Enterococcus* currently includes 19 species, but the status of several of these species is in question [6]. Enterococci generally produce well-circumscribed, smooth, raised colonies about 2 mm in diameter on primary isolation media such as blood agar. Zones of hemolysis may be observed around enterococcal colonies if the agar contains horse, rabbit, bovine, or human erythrocytes, but sheep erythrocytes are largely refractory to the effects of the enterococcal hemolysin [8]. Enterococci may also appear alpha-hemolytic, or nonhemolytic on these media. Selective media, including bile-esculin azide agar or Pfizer selective enterococcus agar, can be used to enrich enterococci from samples that are polymicrobic or cultured from nonsterile sites.

Enterococci are facultatively anaerobic and typically grow at temperatures from 10°C to 42°C. They are regarded generally as catalase negative; however, strains of E. faecalis and possibly other species may be weakly positive when grown on blood agar or other media with added hematin. Enterococci have been presumptively identified by their ability to grow in 6.5% NaCl at pH 9.6, and to grow and hydrolyze esculin in the presence of 40% bile salts, but these reactions are not exclusive to this genus [4,6]. Enterococci do not produce gas from glucose in Mann, Rogosa, Sharpe Lactobacillus broth, but do produce a pyrrolidonyl arylamidase and a leucine aminopeptidase [4,6,7]. Members of the Streptococcus bovis group of group D streptococci ferment esculin on bile esculin agar, but are distinguishable from Enterococcus species because they do not grow in the presence of NaCl, do not grow at 10°C, and do not hydrolyze pyrrolidonyl-beta-naphthylamide.

Species-level identification is required to confirm that an isolate is an Enterococcus. Although presumptive identification together with antibiotic susceptibility tests may provide sufficient information for making initial treatment decisions, species-level identification is extremely valuable in generating epidemiological data of increasing importance in infection control of these nosocomial pathogens. Most clinical isolates that are presumptively identified as Enterococcus are E. faecalis (80%–90%) or, less commonly, E. faecium (5%–10%). Remaining species constitute only a few percent of clinical isolates. Enterococcal species have been divided into four groups based on biochemical reactions [6], with members of groups I–III being isolated from human sources. Biochemical reactions of value in identifying enterococci from human sources are shown in Table 16.1. Interestingly, E. casseliflavus, E. flavescens, and E. gallinarum are motile, and E. casseliflavus, E. flavescens, and E. mundtii are pigmented. E. casseliflavus has been reported to form acid from ribose, which permits its differentiation from E. flavescens [6].

Relationships Among Isolates

The epidemiology of nosocomial outbreaks is of increasing concern, especially in light of the occurence of vancomycin-resistant enterococci (VRE) and the prospect of acquisition of the van-

Table 16.1 Biochemical Reactions of Enterococci from Human Sources

Species	MAN	SBL	SOR	ARG	ARA	RAF	TEL	MOT	PIG	SUC	PYU
Group I											
E. avium	+	+	+	−	+	−	−	−	−	+	+
E. raffinosus	+	+	+	−	+	+	−	−	−	+	+
Group II											
E. faecalis	+	+	−	+	−	−	+	−	−	+/−	+
E. faecium	+	−/+	−	+	+	−/+	−	−	−	+/−	−
E. casseliflavus	+	−/+	−	+	+	+	−/+	+	+	+	−/+
E. mundtii	+	−/+	−	+	+	+	−	−	+	+	−
E. flavescens	+	−/+	−	+	+	+	−	+	+	+	−
E. gallinarum	+	−	−	+	+	+	−	+	−	+	−
Group III											
E. durans	−/+	−	−	+	−	−	−	−	−	−	−
E. hirae	−	−	−	+	−	+	−	−	−	+	−
E. faecalis (var)	−	−	−	+	−	−	+	−	−	−	+

Biochemical tests: fermentation of mannitol (MAN), sorbitol (SBL), sorbose (SOR), arginine (ARG), arabinose (ARA), raffinose (RAF), sucrose (SUC), and pyruvate (PYR); growth in the presence of tellurite (TEL); production of pigment (PIG); and motile (MOT). Symbols: +, >90% positive; −, >90% negative; −/+, generally negative with a few exceptions; +/−, generally positive with a few exceptions.

From Facklam and Sahm [6], with permission.

comycin resistance phenotype by staphylococci. Although phage typing has been used to classify enterococci, no broadly applied typing schemes using readily accessible reagents have been described. Epidemiological studies have instead relied on genetic fingerprinting. Enterococci are extremely adept at exchanging extrachromosomal elements among each other and among other genera. This, together with the technical difficulty of purifying and resolving enterococcal plasmids, which are frequently 60 kb or larger, has limited the use of plasmid profiles for following the relationship among clinical isolates. Instead, genomic fingerprinting has been adapted for this purpose. Pulsed field electrophoresis techniques have been used to generate relatively simple and easily interpretable genomic fingerprints from enterococcal strains. These studies have shown the clonality of a large proportion of isolates from different patients at a single location over an extended period of time, indicating that the strain is endemic to that institution [9,10]. This approach has also been used to document the spread of new resistant phenotypes among geographically diverse institutions [11]. Pulsed field gel electrophoresis requires specialized equipment that is increasingly available. Standard electrophoresis, however, can also be used to generate meaningful, although much more complex, fingerprints for epidemiologic studies [12,13].

EPIDEMIOLOGY

Description

Enterococci are common causes of human disease in the community and in the hospital. In the community they account for 5% to 15% of infective endocarditis cases and 1% to 5% of urinary tract infections [4,7,14,15]. They are often isolated from patients presenting with polymicrobial infections arising from the normal flora of the vagina or gut, including salpingitis, tuboovarian abscess, cholecystitis, diverticulitis, and periappendiceal abscess. Rarely, in the community or the hospital, enterococci are isolated from central nervous system, upper and lower respiratory tract, ocular, dental, and cutaneous infections.

In the hospital, enterococci account for approximately 15% of nosocomial urinary tract infections [4,7,14–17]. As either sole pathogen or participant in mixed infections, they account for 10% to 15% of surgical site infections, 5% to 10% of nosocomial bacteremias, and 5% to 10% of nosocomial cutaneous infections unrelated to surgery, e.g., those involving burn wounds. The Centers for Disease Control and Prevention's National Nosocomial Infection Study has identified enterococci as the fourth leading cause of nosocomial infections; it accounts for approximately 10% of all nosocomial infections in the country [18]. Reports from three medical centers have documented increases in the frequency of hospital-acquired bacteremias and urinary tract infections caused by enterococci during the last two decades [19–21].

The emergence of highly resistant strains of enterococci and the development of better strain typing methods in recent years have facilitated recognition of enterococcal outbreaks and strain transmission in hospitals and other health-care settings [22]. A 1990 report described rapid dissemination of a beta-lactamase-producing, aminoglycoside-resistant strain of E. faecalis among patients and staff on an infant-toddler surgical ward at a Boston hospital [23]. Colonization was detected in 8 staff members and 78 patients during a 17-month period. A 1992 report described 18 cases of colonization or infection with a vancomycin-resistant strain of E. faecium occurring in the medical-surgical intensive care unit of a university hospital in Philadelphia [24]. Restriction endonuclease analysis of plasmid DNA suggested that all clinical isolates were identical. Another 1992 report described an epidemic of 19 nosocomial infections caused by an ampicillin-resistant strain of E. faecium at a university-affiliated hospital in Providence, RI during an 18-month period [25]. Analysis of plasmid and chromosomal DNA helped identify the epidemic at a time when other nosocomial enterococcal infections were also on the rise. Lastly, a 1993 report described nine cases of infection caused by a multiply resistant strain of E. faecium occurring in an intensive care unit over a 6-month period in an acute care hospital in New York City [26]. An additional eight patients and four staff members were found to harbor the outbreak strain. Analysis of restriction endonuclease digests of chromosomal DNA from outbreak isolates suggested dissemination of a single strain throughout the intensive care unit.

Sources and Reservoirs

Enterococci can be recovered from water, soil, food, and a variety of animals; and they constitute part of the normal microbial flora of healthy humans. Enterococci are most numerous in the large intestine where concentrations of 10^5 to 10^7 bacteria per gram of feces are typical. In 5% to 35% of healthy individuals they may also be isolated from vagina, anterior urethra, skin, and other portions of the gastrointestinal tract including oropharynx and bile ducts [4,7,14,27]. Concentrations of enterococci in vaginal secretions approach those in stool, but concentrations are much lower at other sites. In the hospital, patients with cutaneous ulcers, soft tissue wounds, endotracheal tubes, or rectal carriage constitute an additional source of enterococci [28–32]. Several studies have also indicated that enterococci can be recovered from environmental surfaces within the hospital, but the role of the inanimate environment in strain transmission remains to be clarified [29,33].

Age, diet, underlying disease, and prior antimicrobial therapy appear to influence the kinds and numbers of enterococci recovered from various parts of the body [4,14]. In general, *E. faecalis* is the species isolated most frequently and in highest numbers. *E. faecium* is isolated less frequently and in smaller numbers, and other enterococcal species are infrequently detected in the normal flora of humans. In most studies of the normal human flora *E. faecalis* has been recovered from most individuals whereas *E. faecium* has been isolated from only 20% to 40% of the study population. Vancomycin-resistant strains of *E. faecium* are recovered from stools of hospitalized patients with increasing frequency [31,32].

Transmission

Traditionally, enterococcal infections were thought to arise from a patient's endogenous microbial flora [34]. Notwithstanding this viewpoint, documentation of nosocomial outbreaks and spread of colonization with resistant strains in hospitalized patients has prompted a new look at transmission. As noted earlier, patients in the hospital readily acquire new strains of resistant enterococci during outbreaks. Endemic spread of resistant strains has also been noted in several studies. For example, in a prospective study of enterococci with high-level gentamicin-resistance at one Veterans Affairs (VA) medical center, 10% of the patients at risk became colonized with these strains during a 2-month period [35]. Similarly, in another prospective study examining acquisition of ampicillin-resistant strains in 100 consecutive admissions to one ward, 18% of patients became colonized with resistant enterococci during their hospitalization [36]. In these and other studies nosocomial acquisition of resistant strains was clearly demonstrated, as was spread within hospitals. Spread between hospitals has also been documented [25].

In one outbreak, strain transmission was linked to the use of electronic thermometers whose rectal probe handles were repeatedly found to be contaminated with *E. faecium* [24]. In other outbreak and endemic transmission studies, however, person-to-person spread has been the rule [23,27,35,37]. The isolation of identical strains from patients and the hands of their caregivers suggest that this is the primary means of spread. In many respects the epidemiology of enterococci in the hospital appears similar to that of methicillin-resistant *Staphylococcus aureus* and multiply resistant gram-negative bacilli. As with these bacteria, the role of contaminated environmental surfaces, which are frequently detected, in strain transmission remains to be clarified.

The duration of colonization following acquisition of a new enterococcal strain may be brief, but in hospitalized patients it often persists for weeks to months, especially when stool carriage is present [24,32,38,39]. Prolonged colonization and stool carriage have been documented in at least one health-care worker who was thought to be instrumental in the spread of a multiply resistant strain on an infant-toddler surgical ward [23]. Data from both outbreak and endemic transmission studies indicate that colonization precedes overt infection in most cases.

Little is known about strain transmission or exchange outside the hospital, but the recent observation in one study that 7% of enterococcal infections caused by multiply high-level aminoglycoside-resistant strains were acquired in the community suggests that transmission occurs in that setting [40]. One case report describes human-to-human enterococcal transmission in the community, possibly through shared injection paraphernalia in intravenous drug addicts with endocarditis [41].

Risk Factors

Virtually all studies regarding risk factors for colonization or infection with enterococci have involved hospitalized patients and strains that are highly resistant to antimicrobial agents. The extent to which these risk factors are applicable to colonization or infection developing in the community, or involving more susceptible strains of enterococci, has not been explored. Hence, the results of hospital studies with resistant strains cannot be readily extrapolated to other situations. In general, risk factors for colonization and infection with unusually resistant enterococci in the hospital include measures indicative of poor patient functional status, presence of invasive devices, antimicrobial therapy, and prolonged lengths of stay [9,21,23–27,33,36,37,42–48]. Location and proximity to other cases have also been important in outbreaks.

Risk factors for mortality associated with enterococcal bacteremia have been examined in several studies. In a study reported by Stroud and co-workers that included mostly non-VRE bacteremias, independent predictors of mortality included indices of severity of illness, age, use of third-generation cephalosporin antibiotics or metronidazole during the week prior to infection, and female gender [49]. Other studies have highlighted the risk posed by serious underlying disease in patients with enterococcal bacteremia [44,48]. In the study reported by Stroud and colleagues as well as the one reported by Shay and associates, vancomycin resistance was not an independent predictor of death [48,49]. However, in two other series of bacteremic cases, VRE infection was a strong predictor of death [44,50]. Moreover, in the analysis by Edmond and colleagues, the attributable mortality for VRE bacteremia was 37% (90% confidence interval [CIs], 10% to 64%); patients who had VRE bacteremia were twice as likely to die as closely matched controls [51].

CLINICAL INFECTIONS

Most of the medical literature on enterococcal infections describes those caused by E. faecalis and, to a lesser extent, those caused by E. faecium. Neither gives rise to a unique clinical syndrome, but each is capable of causing a variety of infections in different organ systems. Other enterococcal species such as E. avium and E. durans appear to have a similar range but reports are scanty [25,52]. Regardless, no specific clinical feature or constellation of features distinguishes enterococcal infections from those due to other infectious agents. Consequently, determination of an enterococcal etiology always rests on culture results. Isolation of enterococci in pure culture from a normally sterile body site generally provides a definitive diagnosis. The diagnostic significance of enterococci isolated from a mucosal surface exudate or their presence in a mixed culture from a normally sterile body site is more difficult to interpret and has occasioned many an argument regarding the relative virulence of these bacteria [4,7,53–58]. These arguments notwithstanding, the following categories of enterococcal infections are widely recognized.

Endocarditis

Even in intravenous drug addicts, enterococcal endocarditis usually involves either aortic or mitral valves [53,59,60]. Approximately 50% of patients have antecedent valvular abnormalites. Prosthetic valves are occasionally infected [61]. As a rule, the valves become infected during the course of bacteremias arising from abdominal or genitourinary sources. Such bacteremias are often transient and clinically silent. Men are affected twice as frequently as women. Male patients are older, 50 to 70 years of age as a rule, and they frequently report prior urinary tract infections or procedures. In contrast, female patients are often in their childbearing years, and they describe antecedent obstetrical or gynecological conditions that may have triggered their bacteremias.

Enterococcal endocarditis most commonly presents in a subacute manner; i.e., patients have been ill for several weeks before they seek medical attention [59–61]. Clinical features are highly variable and usually encompass manifestations from three principal categories. Constitutional findings, which reflect the systemic inflammatory response to the local infection, may include fatigue, fever, weight loss, night sweats, pallor, anemia, leukocytosis, and elevated sedimentation rate. Fever and elevated erythrocyte sedimentation rates are present in 90% of patients, and anemia is present in 70% to 90% of patients [59].

Findings referable to cardiac valve dysfunction, which results from destruction of the valve by the infectious process, may include heart murmur or features of progressive congestive heart failure—dyspnea, orthopnea, edema, elevated jugular venous pulse, gallop rhythm, rales, and even pulmonary edema. Murmurs are present in 85% of patients, and signs of congestive heart failure are present in up to one-third of patients [59]. Lastly, so-called peripheral manifestations may include skin findings such as petechiae, purpura, splinter hemorrhages, Janeway's lesions or Osler's nodes; splenomegaly; symptoms or signs of cerebrovascular disease such as aphasia, hemiparesis, or Babinski reflex; subarachnoid hemorrhage; myocardial infarction; renal or splenic pain; hematuria; proteinuria; azotemia; and ischemic injury involving the upper or lower extremities. Some of these peripheral manifestations are due to embolization of cardiac vegetations and some are due to deposition of immune complexes. The percentage of patients with any given peripheral manifestation is highly variable and ranges from 2% to 40% in most case series [59–61].

Untreated enterococcal endocarditis invariably leads to death. Progressive congestive heart failure and renal failure were the usual causes of death in the pre-antibiotic era. Less common causes of death in that era included stroke, subarachnoid hemorrhage, and myocardial infarction. Today, appropriate antimicrobial therapy is curative for most patients with this disease, and the overall prognosis has improved considerably: case fatality rates average <20% and relapse rates are generally <10% [59–61]. Nevertheless, valve replacement surgery is required by a fair number of patients whose valves are significantly injured by either the infection or scarring during the healing process. Complications such as stroke, congestive heart failure, and subarachnoid hemorrhage also continue to cause morbidity in the antibiotic era.

Bacteremia without Endocarditis

Depending upon the series, 20% to 40% of enterococcal bacteremias that are not associated with endocarditis occur as secondary events in patients with community-acquired infections [4,7,14,15,20,53,62]. These include cholecystitis and other biliary tract infections, urinary tract infections, and other infections arising from colonic or genitourinary tract flora, e.g., diverticulitis, appendicitis, and salpingitis.

Up to 80% of enterococcal bacteremias that are not associated with endocarditis are hospital acquired. A growing number of case series indicate that both men and women, especially those over 50 years of age, with severe underlying diseases and life-threatening conditions are afflicted most frequently [9,15,20,48,62–71]. Such diseases and conditions include cancer, renal failure, congestive heart failure, diabetes mellitus, major trauma, complicated surgical procedures, vascular and urinary catheterizations, and the like. These bacteremias often occur after 2 or 3 weeks of hospitalization and after prolonged administration of antimicrobial agents, especially broad-spectrum cephalosporin antibiotics. Although the source of the bacteremia may be obscure in up to 30% of patients, in the majority it is secondary to primary infection at another site. Common locations for the primary infection include the urinary tract, burn wounds and other cutaneous lesions such as pressure ulcers or intravascular catheter insertion sites, the biliary tree, and various intra-abdominal and pelvic sites, especially those perturbed by recent surgery.

Twenty-five to forty-five percent of enterococcal bacteremias are polymicrobial. Staphylococci and gram-negative enteric bacilli are isolated with enterococci from blood cultures most commonly, but occasionally, anaerobic bacteria or fungi crop up [15,20,62–71]. Patients with polymicrobial bacteremias tend to be sicker and often manifest more systemic toxicity than those with only enterococci in the bloodstream. Otherwise, clinical features and outcomes of enterococcal bacteremia correspond to those of the primary infection. Shock, respiratory or renal failure, and disseminated intravascular coagulation seldom complicate isolated enterococcemia. Metastatic foci of infection, i.e., abscess or suppuration at a distant site seeded via the bloodstream, rarely appear as a consequence of the bacteremia. Nevertheless, mortality associated with enterococcal bacteremia ranges between 25% and 50% in most case series [9,15,20,48,49–51,62–71].

Urinary Tract Infections

Urinary tract infections are the most commonly encountered enterococcal infections [4,7,14,53, 72]. Healthy young women and older men with prostatic hypertrophy occasionally present with urinary tract infections caused by enterococci, but this infection occurs more commonly in hospitalized patients with obstructive uropathies or urinary catheters, or in patients who have undergone urological procedures [19]. Clinical manifestations range from asymptomatic bacteriuria to pyelonephritis accompanied by bacteremia. In adults symptoms commonly include dysuria, urgency, and frequency. Fever and flank pain are indicative of upper tract disease. Urinalysis discloses pyuria and bacteriuria, and urine cultures yield enterococci in quantities ranging from 10^3 to $>10^5$ colony-forming units (cfu) per milliliter of urine. Urinary tract infections caused by strains of E. faecalis that actually require vancomycin for growth in vitro have been reported [73].

As a rule, enterococcal urinary tract infections are easily treated and complications are rare. Even untreated infections may resolve spontaneously. Rarely, enterococcal urinary tract infections lead to prostatitis or perinephric abscess [4].

Intra-abdominal and Pelvic Infections

Cultures of clinical specimens obtained from patients with peritonitis, intra-abdominal or pelvic abscesses, biliary tract disease, surgical site infections, endomyometritis, pelvic inflammatory disease, and other infections arising from bowel or vaginal flora often yield enterococci, usually in association with other members of the resident flora [4,7,14,15,53–58]. In patients treated with broad-spectrum antibiotics, enterococci may be the sole isolates. Although hotly debated, the relative contribution of enterococci to polymicrobial infections remains unsettled. However, its pathogenecity is well established in immunosuppressed patients with intra-abdominal or pelvic infections associated with enterococcal breakthrough bacteremia [65].

Clinical manifestations of these diverse, albeit typically acute, infections include fever, prostration, anorexia, nausea, vomiting, abdominal pain and tenderness, some degree of ileus, and leukocytosis [15,20,64,66]. Imaging studies, especially computerized axial tomography, are helpful in localizing the pathologic process. Percutaneous drainage and surgery play a crucial role in the therapy of these conditions. Antimicrobial therapy specifically directed against enterococci has been recommended for patients with persistent or recurrent intra-abdominal infection, for patients hospitalized for a prolong period with such infections, and, possibly, for immunocompromised patients, e.g., liver transplant recipients, at risk for enterococcal infection [4,54–56].

Skin and Soft Tissue Infections

Cultures of burn wounds, pressure ulcers, diabetic foot infections, and wounds at the sites of abdominal or pelvic surgery often yield enterococci in mixed culture with staphylococci, other streptococci, enteric gram-negative bacilli, or anaerobes [4,7,14,15,28,53]. In this setting enterococci are clearly opportunists, filling a niche created by tissue injury. It is difficult to ascertain the relative contribution of enterococci to these processes except when enterococcal bacteremia ensues [20,62–71]. Clinical features of these diverse entities from which enterococci are isolated are highly variable and generally correlate with the amount of tissue destruction and the relative virulence of associated microbes. Findings in surgical site infections tend to be acute and dramatic—fever, wound pain, wound dehiscence—whereas other cutaneous infections involving enterococci tend to be more chronic and indolent. Management of symptomatic infections frequently requires drainage, debridement, amputation, or other surgical procedures as well as antimicrobial therapy.

Neonatal Infections

Both endemic and epidemic cases of neonatal sepsis caused by enterococci have been reported in the medical literature [4,7,14,53,74]. Infections within the first week of life generally occur in full-term infants without obvious predisposing factors or evidence of nosocomial acquisition. In this group, illness tends to be mild, with respiratory difficulties, lethargy, poor feeding, diarrhea, and fever being the chief manifestations. Local infection is uncommon.

In contrast, infants developing enterococcal sepsis after the first week of life are usually premature, exhibit lower birth weights, and have more invasive devices [74]. They usually acquire their infection from a nosocomial source, and several outbreaks have been described. These infants are sicker, demonstrating severe apnea, bradycardia, circulatory collapse, and increased ventilatory requirements. Focal infections including meningitis, pneumonia, and scalp abscesses are also common in this group. Case fatality rates range from 8% to 17% in these infants, being highest in those with necrotizing enterocolitis-associated infections.

Miscellaneous Infections

Case reports and small case series describing enterococcal involvement in a variety of other infections continue to appear. From this literature enterococci can be recognized as rare causes of meningitis, pneumonia, empyema, otitis, sinusitis, and septic arthritis [4,7,14,15,53,75–77]. In the patients reported, debilitating illness, trauma, recent surgery, invasive devices, and antecedent antimicrobial therapy are recurrent themes. Enterococci appear to be an increasingly prevalent cause of endophthalmitis [8,78]. Not surprisingly, enterococci, alone or in combination with other pathogens, also account for a small percentage of infections involving orthopedic prostheses, central nervous system shunts, peritoneal dialysis catheters, and other medical devices [4,7,79].

PATHOGENESIS

As commensals, enterococci have evolved to a point where their presence is well tolerated by the host and other co-inhabitants of the gastrointestinal tract. This equilibrium requires that enterococci possess few traits that would precipitate their rejection by the host. Therefore, virulence, in principle, is largely incompatible with the stable relationship that exists between enterococci and humans. These observations notwithstanding, enterococci have emerged as important causes of serious nosocomial infection that often pose a significant therapeutic challenge. Developing an understanding of the normal relationship between enterococci and humans, and elucidating the factors capable of destabilizing this balance, represent challenges that have assumed an element of urgency during the past decade.

Adherence to Host Tissues

The stable existence of enterococci as minor species of the gut flora suggests that enterococci possess a mechanism for adherence within the intestine. Otherwise, enterococci would be expected to be eliminated from the intestine by the bulk flow of the luminal contents. However, specific mechanisms of enterococcal adherence and colonization of the gut remain poorly understood. One enterococcal adhesin, aggregation substance, has been studied in some detail. Aggregation substance is a surface protein that is encoded within the transfer region of pheromone-responsive enterococcal plasmids and is expressed upon pheromone induction [80]. In conjugative plasmid transfer, aggregation substance produced on the surface of the donor cell binds to a ubiquitous substance on the surface of a potential recipient (now believed to be lipoteichoic acid [LTA]), resulting in formation of a stable mating aggregate. Aggregation substance has been observed to contain potential integrin-binding RGD (arginine-glycine-aspartic acid) motifs that appear to be functional in contributing to attachment of renal epithelial cells [81]. Aggregation substance has also been shown to contribute to vegetation size in an endocarditis model [82]. Additionally, aggregation substance was found to contribute to the ability of enterococci to invade HT-29 enterocytes [83]. However, since aggregation substance is produced only by a subpopulation of enterococcal strains possessing pheromone-responsive plasmids, and the presence of these plasmids is not a prerequisite for the ability of enterococcus to colonize the intestine or to infect, aggregation substance may contribute to adherence, but other cell-surface properties undoubtedly play an important role as well. Other enterococcal binding factors have been implicated, but they have yet to be physically defined [84–86].

Invasion

A large percentage of enterococcal infections are obscure in origin and presumably originate from the intestinal tract. One strain of *E. faecalis*, which expresses aggregation substance as discussed above, was observed to be as invasive for HT-29 enterocytes as *Listeria monocytogenes* and *Salmonella typhimurium* [87]. However, greater variation in invasion ability was observed among different *E. faecalis* strains not expressing aggregation substance than was observed between isogenic strains differing in aggregation substance expression, indicating that enterococcal traits, in addition to aggregation substance, are critical for invasion [87]. In a separate study, enterococci were observed to translocate across a histologically normal intestinal epithelium in mice treated with broad-spectrum antibiotics [88]. Enterococci were subsequently recovered in mesenteric lymph nodes, liver, and spleen. Whether this dissemination involved invasion of epithelial cells or migration in phagocytes remains open to speculation, although these investigators demonstrated that the preferred site of translocation in monoassociated mice was the cecum or colon [89].

Modulation of Host Immunity

Enterococcal LTA stimulates the production of proinflammatory cytokines by cultured human monocytes at levels comparable to that observed for lipopolysaccharide [90]. Whether enterococci shed LTA into the environment, as is known for *Streptococcus pyogenes*, remains to be determined. Enterococcal LTA was observed to inhibit pheromone-induced aggregation of enterococcal mating pairs [91], and the mutagenesis, cloning, and analysis of genes related to enterococcal LTA expression have been reported [92,93].

Interactions between complement, human neutrophils, and enterococci have been examined [94–96]. Enterococci appear to be efficiently opsonized by the alternate complement pathway, although the studies differed with respect to conclusions on the involvement of hyperimmune rabbit serum in augmenting neutrophil mediated clearance. Strains capable of expressing protease, cytolysin, or aggregation substance proved no more resistant to phagocytosis than strains lacking these traits [85]. However, it is unclear whether these traits are expressed under the assay conditions employed. The fate of phagocytized enterococci has not been studied extensively. The intrinsic ruggedness of the organism may favor survival in the otherwise hostile environment of the phagolysosome. Enterococci express a flavin containing NADH peroxidase and an oxygen-inducible superoxide dismutase [97, 98], which may be of value in neutralizing peroxide and superoxide formed in the phagolysosome.

Enterococcal pheromones, small hydrophobic oligopeptides that induce a mating response from a potential donor, have been found to be capable of acting as neutrophil chemoattractants and elicit granule enzyme secretion and an oxidative burst [99,100]. The biological relevance of these observations in focal or systemic infections remains to be determined.

Extracellular Products

Cytolysin

Evidence exists for the contribution of two secreted products of enterococci to lethality, toxicity, or loss of organ function in infection: *(1)* the cytolysin, a novel cytolytic toxin that appears to be related structurally to "lantibiotics" expressed by many gram-positive bacteria of industrial importance [101]; and *(2)* coccolysin (formerly gelatinase), a metalloendopeptidase [102]. The *E. faecalis* cytolysin is typically encoded by large transmissible plasmids [8]. This highly post-translationally modified and extracellularly activated cytolysin possesses unusually broad-membrane lytic activity, in that it lyses eukaryotic cells (hemolysin) as well as prokaryotic cells (bacteriocin).

An enrichment for the cytolytic phenotype among infection-derived enterococcal isolates [103], particularly those from the bloodstream [9], has been observed. Moreover, a tight linkage between antibiotic resistance and the hemolytic phenotype was noted [9,103]. The molecular basis and selection forces for the association between a transposon-mediated [104] antibiotic resistance and the hemolytic phenotype were investigated. Since the *E. faecalis* hemolysin is also a bacteriocin, two mechanisms were considered through which it may contribute to the pathogenesis of enterococcal disease: (1) it may serve in its bacteriocin capacity as a colonization factor, conferring upon invading strains a selective advantage; and/or (2) it may contribute directly to the disease, or to a propensity to cause disease, through a toxic activity that results from its ability to act as a eukaryotic cell lysin.

To determine the contribution of the hemolysin/bacteriocin (or more generally, cytolysin) to the ecology of the organism, the competitive growth of isogenic pairs of strains varying only in various aspects of cytolysin expression were compared in mice [105]. In broth culture it was observed that hypercytolytic enterococci were capable of outpopulating wild-type or hypersusceptible enterococci, but normally cytolytic strains were capable only of outpopulating hypersusceptible enterococci, but not wild-type, susceptible strains. In vivo in the gastrointestinal tract of mice, hypercytolytic derivatives were observed to be at a surprising growth disadvantage, and no significant or lasting growth advantage was observed for any of the cytolytic derivatives tested (even though mouse-derived enterococci were used as the hosts for the various plasmid derivatives). These studies showed that, within the parameters tested, no selective advantage was conferred by cytolysin expression in antibiotic-treated but otherwise healthy animals.

No established models exist for assessing the role of the enterococcal cytolysin in the common form of enterococcal infection—bacteremia of obscure origin—as is frequently observed among intensive care unit patients. To assess the role of the cytolysin for its ability to be produced and act as a virulence factor in vivo, an endophthalmitis model was developed. Endophthalmi-

tis provides an exquisitely sensitive infection system where organ function can be directly assessed and where organ function can be compromised without triggering a confounding cascade of end-stage events. Again, in comparing infections caused by a wild-type cytolytic strain to those produced by isogenic noncytolytic derivatives, two easily distinguishable types of infection were observed: (1) one caused by the cytolytic *E. faecalis* strain, which exhibited a precipitous, irretrievable loss of retinal function and was totally unresponsive to antibiotic and anti-inflammatory therapy; and (2) infection caused by specifically attenuated *E. faecalis* strains, which was characterized by a more moderate loss of vision, and an infection that responded well to antibacterial and anti-inflammatory therapy [106].

Coccolysin

Coccolysin, formerly gelatinase, is an extracellular metalloendopeptidase that is the principal distinguishing feature of *E. faecalis* strains formerly identified as *Streptococcus faecalis* subsp. *liquefaciens*. In a large study employing a rabbit model of catheter-induced endocarditis, coccolysin-producing strains were found to be associated with a more rapidly fatal course of disease. Vegetations involving coccolysin-producing strains of *E. faecalis* were typically smaller and more friable, and these infections were associated with a higher level of bacteremia and a higher frequency of kidney infarcts when compared in aggregate to infections caused by non-coccolysin-producing strains [102]. Moreover, it was observed that coccolysin-producing strains constituted 63.7% of 618 enterococci isolated from two intensive care units in Germany [107]. These results were confirmed for enterococcal isolates from the U.S., where 54% of 192 clinical isolates were observed to produce coccolysin [108].

Coccolysin was recently observed to be capable of hydrolyzing and inactivating human endothelin [109]. As endothelin is a highly vasoactive peptide, one mechanism through which coccolysin may contribute to the pathogenicity of enterococcal disease is through direct effects on vasoconstriction as a result of endothelin inactivation [109]. Alternatively, it has been proposed that the coccolysin protease may directly or indirectly effect the partial dissolution of enterococcal heart valve vegetations, resulting in a higher level of dissemination of the organism throughout the body, causing an increase in the frequency of systemic sequalae including kidney infarcts [102]. This evidence indicates a probable role for coccolysin in enterococcal disease, however, its precise contribution remains to be tested directly.

Genetic Exchange

Enterococci possess an efficient capacity to exchange genetic material among themselves and with other genera [100,101]. This facile genetic exchange confers enterococci with a unique ability to collect antibiotic resistance determinants, culminating in the existence of pan-resistant enterococcal strains, as discussed in the following section. Furthermore, the accretion of resistance determinants coupled with active exchange mechanisms threatens the broader dissemination of these determinants to the staphylococci and other medically important gram-positive bacteria. Two conjugative systems exist by which enterococci naturally transfer genetic elements: (1) narrow host-range, sex pheromone–responsive systems for plasmid transfer [80]; and (2) broad host-range, pheromone-independent systems for transfer of plasmids and transposons [110–113]. Although relatively efficient protocols have been described for the electrotransformation of E. faecalis [114–117], natural transformation of enterococci has not been reported or suggested to play an important role in the accretion of antibiotic resistances.

ANTIMICROBIAL RESISTANCE

Enterococci number among the most antimicrobial-resistant human pathogens [4,7,118–120]. Enterococcal resistance is classified as intrinsic or acquired. Intrinsic resistance, an inherent property grounded in the basic physiology of enterococci, is universal. In contrast, the occurrence of acquired resistance is more variable as it depends upon acquisition of new genetic traits through mutation or conjugation by individual strains [110]. The following descriptions are based on studies of E. faecalis and E. faecium, the major human pathogens.

Intrinsic Resistance

Enterococci are innately resistant to antistaphylococcal penicillin antibiotics, cephalosporins and the related beta-lactam antibiotics, polymyxin, and aztreonam [4,7,72,118,119]. They also possess low-level resistance to aminoglycoside and lincosamide antibiotics. The low-level resistance to aminoglycoside antibiotics reflects the inability of these agents to penetrate through the cell envelope. Several other resistance features are noteworthy. Enterococci are tolerant to the bactericidal effect of virtually all antimicrobial agents; i.e., they are not killed by concentrations many-fold higher than the minimum inhibitory concentration (MIC). Although susceptible to benzylpenicillin, ampicillin, mezlocillin, piperacillin, and imipenem, enterococci are less susceptible than streptococci, requiring concentrations of these agents for inhibition that are up to 100-fold higher than those needed for bactericidal effects against most streptococci. This requirement for higher concentrations derives from diminished affinity of penicillin-binding proteins (PBP), especially of PBP 5, for these antibiotics. In general, E. faecium exhibits a greater degree of intrinsic resistance to beta-lactam antibiotics than E. faecalis.

E. faecium natively produces low levels of aminoglycoside 6'-actetyltransferase, a chromosomally encoded enzyme that accounts for the higher MICs of kanamycin, netilimicin, tobramycin, and sisomicin for this species [4,7,72,118,119]. Combinations of these aminoglycosides with penicillin also fail to exert a synergistic bactericidal effect against E. faecium isolates. Lastly, the ability of enterococci to use thymidine and mammalian folate intermediates in their metabolism appears to render them resistant in vivo to trimethoprim-sulfamethoxazole, an antimicrobial combination that usually inhibits clinical isolates in laboratory susceptibility tests [121–123].

The presence of intrinsic resistances in enterococci has a number of important therapeutic consequences [4,7,72,118,119]. First, it limits the number of therapeutic alternatives. Secondly, it necessitates that high dosages of beta-lactam antibiotics be used. Third, it requires the use of synergistic combinations that possess bactericidal activity for the therapy of endocarditis, meningitis, and other severe infections. Lastly, it necessitates the use of gentamicin combinations for the treatment of severe infections caused by *E. faecium* because other aminoglycoside antibiotics fail to synergize with either beta-lactam antibiotics or vancomycin.

Acquired Resistance

Both *E. faecalis* and *E. faecium* have a remarkable capacity to acquire resistance to antimicrobial agents [4,7,72,118,119]. Most forms of acquired resistance in enterococci derive from production of enzymes that inactivate antimicrobial agents or from changes in the molecular targets (Table 16.2). The prevalence of resistant enterococci varies considerably from time to time

and place to place. Resistance to teracycline, erythromycin, and chloramphenicol has been common throughout the world for several decades [4,7,118,119], as has high-level resistance to streptomycin and kanamycin. In contrast, ciprofloxacin resistance has only been noted recently [124], and beta-lactamase producing strains of enterococci, which first appeared in the early 1980s, remain rare [125–127]. Beta-lactam resistance in *E. faecium*, which is not mediated by beta-lactamases, has disseminated widely in the last several years and is present in 25% to 50% of isolates in some U.S. medical centers [128–130]. High-level resistance to gentamicin and other aminoglycoside antibiotics appeared in the early 1980s, and it has become widespread since then [9,131–133]. It is present in up to 60% of clinical isolates in some centers. Although vancomycin resistance was first noted in 1969, it did not emerge as a

Table 16.2 Acquired Antimicrobial Resistances of *E. faecalis* and *E. faecium*

Antimicrobial Agent	Mechanism of Resistance	Mode of Acquisition
Beta-lactams		
Benzylpenicillin, ampicillin, mezlocillin, and piperacillin	Beta-lactamase production	Plasmid transfer
Benzylpenicillin, ampicillin, mezlocillin, piperacillin, and imipenem	Altered PBP 5 or overproduction of PBP 5 in *E. faecium*	Unknown
Aminoglycosides (high-level)		
Gentamicin, kanamycin, tobramycin, amikacin, and netilmicin	bifunctional 6'-acetyltransferase/2"-phosphotransferase	Plasmid or transposon transfer; possibly transduction
Streptomycin	(1) altered ribosomal protein	Spontaneous mutation
	(2) adenyltransferase production	Plasmid transfer
Kanamycin	3'-phosphotransferase production	Plasmid transfer
Glycopeptides		
Vancomycin (VanB phenotype)	Possibly same mechanism as for VanA but different regulation	Transposon transfer
Vancomycin, teicoplanin, and others (VanA phenotype)	Production of ligase with altered specificity that results in synthesis of cell-wall precursors that fail to bind glycopeptides	Plasmid or transposon transfer
Miscellaneous		
Ciprofloxacin	Unknown	Unknown
Tetracyclines	(1) protection of ribosome from tetracyline inhibition	Plasmid or transposon transfer
	(2) induction of active transport system to remove tetracycline from cell	Plasmid or transposon transfer
Chloramphenicol	Chloramphenicol Acetyltransferase production	Plasmid or transposon transfer
Erythromycin and clindamycin (high-level)	Methylation of ribosomal RNA	Plasmid or transposon transfer

problem until the late 1980s in Western Europe [12,120,134–143]. It has since spread widely throughout the U.S. during the 1990s.

There are three known phenotypes of vancomycin resistance, which are designated VanA, VanB, and VanC, respectively [120,139,140]. The VanC phenotype, which yields only moderate levels of resistance to vancomycin, is found in *E. gallinarum* and *E. casseliflavus*. The genes responsible for this phenotype appear to be natural constituents of these two species. In contrast, VanA and VanB phenotypes arose from new gene clusters not previously found in enterococci. Avoparcin, a glycopeptide antimicrobial drug used in Europe as a growth promoter in food-producing animals, may have led to their emergence [139,141]. These genes are found in both *E. faecalis* and *E. faecium*. The VanA phenotype is characterized by high-level resistance to both vancomycin and teicoplanin [120,139,140]. It is inducible and transferable and has been found in several other enterococcal species. The VanB phenotype is characterized by variable levels of resistance to vancomycin, but susceptibility to teicoplanin is preserved. Enterococcal strains with the VanA or VanB phenotype do not produce the terminal D-alanine-D-alanine cell-wall precursor that binds vancomycin in susceptible cells. Resistant cells make precursors with a different terminus, and they either do not make or modify the D-alanine-D-alanine terminus so that vancomycin cannot bind to the precursor and prevent cell wall synthesis [120,139].

The addition of acquired resistance to a high level of intrinsic resistance further complicates the treatment of enterococcal infections. Beta-lactam resistance precludes the use of these agents in some infections. Synergistic combinations are no longer available for enterococci that possess high-level resistance to all available aminoglycoside antibiotics. Vancomycin and ciprofloxacin resistance take away other therapeutic options. Moreover, the capacity for certain strains of *E. faecium* to acquire multiple forms of resistance has given rise to a new generation of "superbugs". These multiply resistant strains of *E. faecium*, which are resistant to all commercially available antimicrobial agents including all glycopeptide antibiotics, all beta-lactam antibiotics, and all fluoroquinolone antibiotics, have rightly been dubbed the "nosocomial

pathogen of the 1990s" [144]. Such strains have been encountered with increasing frequency throughout the U.S. during the last few years [145,146].

Detection of these various forms of acquired resistance is an important part of the diagnostic evaluation. It is not always straightforward [4,7,118,119,120,147]. For example, penicillinase production is most reliably detected by a chromogenic cephalosporin test, and not conventional susceptibility assays. Similarly, high-level aminoglycoside resistance requires use of either high-content disks in diffusion assays or dilution tests with both streptomycin and gentamicin in concentrations ranging from 500 to 2000 μg/ml [4,147]. Agar dilution and broth microdilution methods most reliably establish the presence of vancomycin resistance, especially for strains with the VanB phenotype, which may yield equivocal results in disk diffusion assays.

MANAGEMENT

Enterococcal endocarditis and probably both meningitis and severe infections in patients with compromised host defenses require bactericidal synergistic combinations of antimicrobial agents [4,7,72,118,119,147]. Therapeutic recommendations for infections caused by strains of *E. faecalis* or *E. faecium* that are not resistant to beta-lactam or glycopeptide antibiotics and do not exhibit high-level resistance to aminoglycoside antibiotics are listed in Table 16.3. Less severe infections caused by these strains may be treated with a single agent such as ampicillin or vancomycin. When therapy must be selected before the identity and susceptibility patterns of the infecting organism are known, several considerations influence the empiric choice: *(1)* the likelihood of encountering an ampicillin- or vancomycin-resistant strain; *(2)* the patient's history regarding drug allergies; *(3)* the need for synergistic bactericidal therapy and the probability that either *E. faecium* or a strain with high-level aminoglycoside resistance is present; and *(4)* the concurrent necessity to treat other bacteria likely to be present in a polymicrobial infection, e.g., the need to cover gram-negative bacilli and anaerobes in a patient with a peritonitis. Percutaneous drainage and other surgi-

Table 16.3 Antimicrobial Therapy of Enterococcal Infections[a]

Type of Infection	First Choices	Alternatives
Endocarditis, meningitis, and serious infections in patients with compromised host defenses	Ampicillin (2 g IV q4h) *or* vancomycin (1 g IV q12h) *plus* gentamicin (1 mg/kg IV q8h) *or* streptomycin (500 mg IM q12h)	Benzylpenicillin (20 to 24 × 10^6 units IV q24h), mezlocillin 5 g IV q6h, *or* piperacillin 3 g IV q4h for ampicillin or vancomycin, *and* tobramycin (1 mg/kg IV q8h), amikacin (5 mg/kg IV q12h), or netilmicin (1 mg/kg IV q8h) for gentamicin or streptomycin
Bacteremia, cholecystitis, and other serious pelvic, abdominal, or wound infections in patients with normal host defenses	Ampicillin (2 g IV IV 4qh) *or* vancomycin (1 g IV q12h)	Mezlocillin (5 g IV q6h), piperacillin (3 g IV q4h), imipenem (500 mg IV q6h), *or* ciprofloxacin (400 mg IV q12h)
Uncomplicated urinary tract infection or wound infection with minimal systemic toxicity	Amoxicillin (500 mg PO tid) *or* ampicillin (500 mg PO qid) *or* ciprofloxacin (250–500 mg PO bid)	Norfloxacin (400 mg PO bid), ofloxacin (400 mg PO bid), *or* nitrofurantoin[b] (100 mg PO q6h)

[a]See text for therapy of highly resistant strains of *E. faecalis* and *E. faecium*.

[b]Urinary tract infection only.

cal procedures also play an important role in the management of the intra-abdominal and pelvic conditions associated with enterococcal infection [54–56].

The therapy of infections caused by the more resistant strains of enterococci is problematic. Ampicillin/sulbactam, piperacillin/tazobactam, or imipenem provide alternatives to vancomycin for beta-lactamase-producing strains of *E. faecalis*, but offer no help for treating beta-lactam-resistant strains of *E. faecium*. Instead, vancomycin or a fluoroquinolone may be useful against such strains. Experience with ciprofloxacin and other fluoroquinolones is limited, yet they may be the only choice for patients with either life-threatening penicillin allergies and infection by a vancomycin-resistant strain, or infection by strains of *E. faecium* resistant to both vancomycin and beta-lactam antibiotics.

Two types of enterococcal infections are especially worrisome because there is no proven antimicrobial agent or antimicrobial regimen available. The first is endocarditis caused by enterococci that possess high-level resistance to all aminoglycoside antibiotics [4,7,72,118,119,147]. In the absence of synergistic bactericidal combinations this form of endocarditis may be incurable. Therapeutic considerations include, if

the organism is susceptible, prolonged (8 to 12 weeks) therapy with ampicillin or vancomycin [4,7,72]. On the basis of experimental studies, administration of ampicillin by continuous infusion is recommended by some authorities [148]. Surgical excision of the infected valve may ultimately be required. Regardless, consultation with infectious diseases specialists who have experience with these difficult enterococcal infections is highly recommended. The same recommendation applies to the management of any severe infection caused by multiply resistant strains of *E. faecium* that are resistant to beta-lactam, glycopeptide, and fluoroquinolone antibiotics. Some of these strains are susceptible in vitro to tetracycline antibiotics or chloramphenicol, but limited clinical experience suggests that resistance to these agents can emerge rapidly during therapy [149]. Combinations of ampicillin plus vancomycin plus gentamicin are bacteriostatic for some strains and may warrant consideration [4,7,150]. Nitrofurantoin is a consideration for urinary tract infections caused by VRE but cannot be used for infections at other sites [151].

Several investigational agents hold promise for the treatment of infections caused by multiply resistant strains of *E. faecium*. Quinupristin-dalfopristin (Synercid®), a semi-synthetic, injectable streptogramin derivative, will probably be released in late 1999 [151–154]. This combination has bacteriostatic activity against most strains of vancomycin-resistant *E. faecium* with minimum inhibitory concentrations ranging from 1 to 8 μg/ml. Published data indicate efficacy in many VRE infections, and adverse effects have been minor. Emergence of enterococcal resistance to quinupristin-dalfopristin during therapy has already been documented [155]. In vitro studies with novel glycopeptide derivatives [156,157], and a new ketolide antibiotic [158] suggest that other agents may become available for multiply resistant strains of *E. faecium* during the next several years.

PREVENTION

Antimicrobial agents are used to prevent enterococcal infections in two settings. First, anti-enterococcal therapy such as ampicillin and gentamicin is administered to patients with cardiac lesions who are at risk for developing endocarditis when they undergo procedures such as colonoscopy, which predispose them to enterococcal bacteremia, and, hence, endocarditis. Detailed recommendations for this practice have been provided by the American Heart Association [159]. Secondly, anti-enterococcal therapy is often administered to patients undergoing abdominal or pelvic surgery in an effort to prevent postoperative surgical site infections. This practice is controversial because perioperative prophylaxis directed at only gram-negative enteric bacilli and anaerobes without specific enterococcal coverage often appears to be sufficient [4,7]. Nevertheless, in one study of patients undergoing surgery after abdominal trauma, antimicrobial prophylaxis including specific enterococcal coverage proved superior to that without it in the prevention of postoperative wound infections [160]. The frequency of enterococcal bacteremias after procedures on the biliary tract has also argued for anti-enterococcal prophylaxis in that setting too [161].

The appearance and spread of multiply resistant strains of VRE has prompted the adoption of new strategies to prevent infection with these enterococci in hospitalized patients. Formal recommendations have been made by the Centers for Disease Control and Prevention's Hospital Infection Control Practices Advisory Committee (HICPAC) [162]. The Surgical Infection Society and others have endorsed them [163,164]. The recommendations include (1) guidelines for prudent use of vancomycin; (2) education of hospital staff; (3) early detection and prompt reporting of new VRE cases; and (4) implementation of barrier precautions to interrupt nosocomial transmission, especially that mediated by the hands of health-care workers.

Vancomycin use in the hospital may foster the spread of resistance, and it is frequently used inappropriately [165,166]; hence, the HICPAC recommendations promote better usage. In one center, implementation of these guidelines and restriction of vancomycin use appeared to reduce not only the frequency of its use but also the incidence of new VRE cases [167]. In another hospital manipulations of the hospital antimicrobial formulary were thought to be key factors in reducing the prevalence of VRE colonization [168]. In these and other studies [169], however, it has been difficult to sort out the relative value of the various components of the control effort. Nevertheless, it appears that one or more of these actions in combination offer some hope of limiting spread.

Education of hospital staff is essential for any VRE control effort. The importance of person-to-person spread requires emphasis as does the potential role of contaminated surfaces. Fortunately, VRE strains are susceptible to most environmental disinfectants, but they must be used in accordance with the manufacturers' recommended time of exposure [170,171]. Housekeeping protocols may need to be reviewed with this consideration in mind.

Over the last few years, methods for detecting vancomycin-resistant strains have been refined and widely promulgated [120,140]. Most hospital laboratories can identify them easily. Notwithstanding, facilities that haven't tested enterococcal isolates routinely still may need encouragement to implement the newer methodologies for all isolates.

Some controversy surrounds the recommendations for barrier precautions. In one well-controlled study in a medical intensive care unit, universal use of gloves and gowns was no better than universal use of gloves alone in preventing rectal colonization by VRE [172]. In another hospital, use of gowns with gloves was thought to be essential in terminating a nosocomial outbreak [25]. While awaiting additional information on this topic, most authorities continue to recommend maximum use of barrier precautions for VRE cases in hospitals.

REFERENCES

1. Thiercelin ME. Sur un diplocoque saprophyte de l'intestin susceptible de devenir pathogene. C R Soc Biol 1899; 5:269–271.
2. Andrewes FW, Horder TJ. A study of streptococci pathogenic for man. Lancet 1906; 2:708–713.
3. Sherman JM. The streptococci. Bacteriol Rev 1937; 1:3–97.
4. Murray BE. The life and times of the enterococcus. Clin Microbiol Rev 1990; 3:46–65.
5. Schleifer KH, Kilpper-Balz R. Transfer of *Streptococcus faecalis* and *Streptococcus faecium* to the genus *Enterococcus* nom. rev. as *Enterococcus faecalis* comb. nov. and *Enterococcus faecium* comb. nov. Int J Syst Bacteriol 1984; 34:31–34.
6. Facklam RR, Sahm DF. Enterococcus. In: Murray PR, Baron EJ, Pfaller MA, Tenover FC, Yolken RH (eds). Manual of Clinical Microbiology, 6th ed. Washington, DC: American Society for Microbiology, 1995; 308–314.
7. Moellering RC. *Enterococcus* species, *Streptococcus bovis*, and *Leuconostoc* species. In: Mandell GL, Bennett JE, Dolin R (eds). Principles and Practice of Infectious Diseases, 4th ed. New York: Churchill Livingstone, 1995; 1826–1835.
8. Jett BD, Huycke MM, Gilmore MS. Virulence of enterococci. Clin Microbiol Rev 1994; 7:462–478.
9. Huycke M, Spiegel CA, Gilmore MS. Bacteremia caused by hemolytic, high-level gentamicin-resistant *Enterococcus faecalis*. Antimicrob Agents Chemother 1991; 35:1626–1634.
10. Patterson JE, Singh KV, Murray BE. Epidemiology of an endemic strain of β-lactamase-producing *Enterococcus faecalis*. J Clin Microbiol 1991; 29:2513–2516.
11. Murray BE, Singh KV, Markowitz SM, Lopardo HA, Patterson JE, Zervos MJ, Rubeglio E, Eliopoulos GM, Rice LB, Goldstein FW, Jenkins SG, Caputo GM, Nasnas R, Moore LS, Wong ES, Weinstock G. Evidence for clonal spread of a single strain of β-lactamase-producing *Enterococcus (Streptococcus) faecalis* to six hospitals in five states. J Infect Dis 1991; 163:780–785.
12. Frieden TR, Munsiff SS, Low DE, Willey BM, Williams G, Faur Y, Eisner W, Warren S, Kreiswirth B. Emergence of vancomycin-resistant enterococci in New York City. Lancet 1993; 342:76–79.
13. Willey BM, McGeer AJ, Ostrowski MA, Kreiswirth BN, Low DE. The use of molecular typing techniques in the epidemiologic investigation of resistant enterococci. Infect Control Hosp Epidemiol 1994; 15:548–556.
14. Chenoweth C, Schaberg D. The epidemiology of enterococci. Eur J Clin Microbiol Infect Dis 1990; 9:80–89.
15. Patterson JE, Sweeney AH, Simms M, Carley N, Mangi R, Sabetta J, Lyons RW. An analysis of 110 serious enterococcal infections: epidemiology, antibiotic susceptibility, and outcome. Medicine 1995; 74:191–200.
16. George RC, Uttley AH. Susceptibility of enterococci and epidemiology of enterococcal infection in the 1980's. Epidemiol Infect 1989; 103:403–413.
17. Terpenning MS, Zervos MJ, Schaberg DR, Kauffman CA. Enterococcal infections: an increasing problem in hospitalized patients. Infect Control Hosp Epidemiol 1989; 9:457–461.
18. CDC NNIS System. National Nosocomial Infections Surveillance (NNIS) report, data summary from October 1986–April 1996, issued May 1996. Am J Infect Control 1996; 24:380–388.
19. Morrison AJ, Wenzel RP. Nosocomial urinary tract infections due to enterococcus—ten year's experience at a university hospital. Arch Intern Med 1986; 146:1549–1551.
20. Maki DG, Agger WA. Enterococcal bacteremia: clinical features, the risk of endocarditis, and management. Medicine 1988; 67:248–269.
21. Montecalvo MA, Shay DK, Patel P, Tacsa L, Maloney SA, Jarvis WR, Wormser GP. Bloodstream infections with vancomycin-resistant enterococci. Arch Intern Med 1996; 156:1458–1462.
22. Quale J, Landman D, Atwood E, Kreiswirth B, Willey BM, Ditore V, Zaman M, Patel K, Saurina G, Huang W, Oydna E, Burney S. Experience with a hospital-wide outbreak of vancomycin-resistant enterococci. Am J Infect Control 1996; 24:372–379.
23. Rhinehart E, Smith NE, Wennersten C, Gorss E, Freeman J, Eliopoulos GM, Moellering RC Jr, Goldmann DA. Rapid dissemination of β-lactamase-producing, aminoglycoside-resistant *Enterococcus faecalis* among patients and staff on an infant-toddler surgical ward. N Engl J Med 1990; 323:1814–1818.
24. Livornese LL Jr, Dias S, Samel C, Romanowski B, Taylor S, May P, Pitsakis P, Woods G, Kaye D, Levison ME, Johnson CC. Hospital-acquired infection with vancomycin-resistant *Enterococcus faecium* transmitted by electronic thermometers. Ann Intern Med 1992; 117:112–116.
25. Boyce JM, Opal SM, Potter-Bynoe G, LaForge

RG, Zervos MJ, Furtado G, Victor G, Medeiros AA. Emergence and nosocomial transmission of ampicillin-resistant enterococci. Antimicrob Agents Chemother 1992; 36:1032–1039.

26. Handwerger S, Raucher B, Altarac D, Monka J, Marchione S, Singh KV, Murray BE, Wolff J, Walters B. Nosocomial outbreak due to *Enterococcus faecium* highly resistant to vancomycin, penicillin, and gentamicin. Clin Infect Dis 1993; 16:750–755.

27. Patterson JE, Zervos MJ. High-level gentamicin resistance in *Enterococcus*: microbiology, genetic basis, and epidemiology. Rev Infect Dis 1990; 12:644–652.

28. Horvitz RA, von Graevenitz A. A clinical study of the role of enterococci as sole agents of wound and tissue infection. Yale J Biol Med 1977; 50:391–395.

29. Bonten MJM, Hayden MK, Nathan C, van Voorhis J, Matushek M, Slaughter S, Rice T, Weinstein RA. Epidemiology of colonisation of patients and environment with vancomycin-resistant enterococci. Lancet 1996; 348:1615–1619.

30. Beezhold DW, Slaughter S, Hayden MK, Matushek M, Nathan C, Trenholme GM, Weinstein RA. Skin colonization with vancomycin-resistant enterococci among hospitalized patients with bacteremia. Clin Infect Dis 1997; 24: 704–706.

31. Rafferty ME, McCormick MI, Bopp LH, Baltch AL, George M, Smith RP, Rheal C, Ritz W, Schoonmaker D. Vancomycin-resistant enterococci in stool specimens submitted for *Clostridium difficile* cytotoxin assay. Infect Control Hosp Epidemiol 1997; 18:342–344.

32. Lai KK, Fontecchio SA, Kelley AL, Melvin ZS, Baker S. The epidemiology of fecal carriage of vancomycin-resistant enterococci. Infect Control Hosp Epidemiol 1997; 18:762–765.

33. Weber DJ, Rutala WA. Role of environmental contamination in the transmission of vancomycin-resistant enterococci. Infect Control Hosp Epidemiol 1997; 18:306–309.

34. Gross PA, Harkavy LM, Barden GE, Flower MF. The epidemiology of nosocomial enterococcal urinary tract infection. Am J Med Sci 1976; 272:75–81.

35. Zervos MJ, Kauffman CA, Therasse PM, Bergman AG, Mikesell TS, Schaberg DR. Nosocomial infection by gentamicin-resistant *Streptococcus faecalis*—an epidemiologic study. Ann Intern Med 1987; 106:687–691.

36. Chirurgi VA, Oster SE, Goldberg AA, McCabe RE. Nosocomial acquisition of β-lactamase-negative, ampicillin-resistant enterococcus. Arch Intern Med 1992; 152:1457–1461.

37. Zervos MJ, Dembinski S, Mikesell T, Schaberg DR. High-level resistance to gentamicin in *Streptococcus faecalis*: risk factors and evidence

for exogenous acquisition of infection. J Infect Dis 1986; 1075–1082.

38. Montecalvo MA, de Lencastre H, Carraher M, Gedris C, Chung M, VanHorn K, Wormser GP. Natural history of colonization with vancomycin-resistant *Enterococcus faecium*. Infect Control Hosp Epidemiol 1995; 16:680–685.

39. Bonten MJM, Hayden MK, Nathan C, Rice TW, Weinstein RA. Stability of vancomycin-resistant enterococcal genotypes isolated from long-term-colonized patients. J Infect Dis 1998; 177:378–382.

40. Nachamkin I, Axelrod P, Talbot GH, Fischer SH, Wennersten CB, Moellering RC Jr, MacGregor RR. Multiply high level aminoglycoside-resistant enterococci isolated from patients in a university hospital. J Clin Microbiol 1988; 26:1287–1291.

41. Hall RW, Bayer AS, Mayer WP, Pitchon HE, Yoshikawa TT, Guze LB. Infective endocarditis following human-to-human enterococcal transmission—a complication of intravenous narcotic abuse. Arch Intern Med 1976; 136:1173–1174.

42. Wells VD, Wong ES, Murray BE, Coudron PE, Williams DS, Markowitz SM. Infections due to beta-lactamase-producing, high-level gentamicin-resistant *Enterococcus faecalis*. Ann Intern Med 1992; 116:285–292.

43. Zervos MJ, Terpenning MS, Schaberg DR, Therasse PM, Medendorp SV, Kauffman CA. High-level aminoglycoside-resistant enterococci—colonization of nursing home and acute care hospital patients. Arch Intern Med 1987; 147:1591–1594.

44. Papanicolaou GA, Meyers BR, Meyers J, Mendelson MH, Lou W, Emre S, Sheiner P, Miller C. Nosocomial infections with vancomycin-resistant *Enterococcus faecium* in liver transplant recipients: risk factors for acquisition and mortality. Clin Infect Dis 1996; 23:760–766.

45. Weinstein JW, Roe M, Towns M, Sanders L, Thorpe JJ, Corey GR, Sexton DJ. Resistant enterococci: a prospective study of prevalence, incidence, and factors associated with colonization in a university hospital. Infect Control Hosp Epidemiol 1996; 17:36–41.

46. Tornieporth NG, Roberts RB, John J, Riley LW. Risk factors associated with vancomycin-resistant *Enterococcus faecium* infection or colonization in 145 matched case patients and control patients. Clin Infect Dis 1996; 23:767–772.

47. Bonten MJM, Gaillard CA, van Tiel FH, van der Geest S, Stobberingh EE. Colonization and infection with *Enterococcus faecalis* in intensive care units: the role of antimicrobial agents. Antimicrob Agents Chemother 1995; 39:2783–2786.

48. Shay DK, Maloney SA, Montecalvo M, Banerjee S, Wormser GP, Arduino MJ, Bland LA, Jarvis WR. Epidemiology and mortality risk of

vancomycin-resistant enterococcal bloodstream infections. J Infect Dis 1995; 172:993–1000.

49. Stroud L, Edwards J, Danzig L, Culver D, Gaynes R. Risk factors for mortality associated with enterococcal bloodstream infections. Infect Control Hosp Epidemiol 1996; 17:576–589.

50. Linden PK, Pasculle AW, Manez R, Kramer DJ, Fung JJ, Pinna AD, Kusne S. Differences in outcomes for patients with bacteremia due to vancomycin-resistant *Enterococcus faecium* or vancomycin-susceptible *E. faecium*. Clin Infect Dis 1996; 22:663–670.

51. Edmond MB, Ober JF, Dawson JD, Weinbaum DL, Wenzel RP. Vancomycin-resistant enterococcal bacteremia: natural history and attributable mortality. Clin Infect Dis 1996; 23:1234–1239.

52. Patel R, Keating MR, Cockerill FR III, Steckelberg JM. Bacteremia due to *Enterococcus avium*. Clin Infect Dis 1993; 17:1006–1011.

53. Lewis CM, Zervos MJ. Clinical manifestations of enterococcal infections. Eur J Clin Microbiol Infect Dis 1990; 9:111–117.

54. Dougherty SH. Role of enterococcus in intraabdominal sepsis. Am J Surg 1984; 148:308–312.

55. Barie PS, Christou NV, Dellinger EP, Rout WR, Stone HH, Waymack JP. Pathogenicity of the enterococcus in surgical infections. Ann Surg 1990; 212:155–159.

56. Nichols RL, Muzik AC. Enterococcal infections in surgical patients: the mystery continues. Clin Infect Dis 1992; 15:72–76.

57. Burnett RJ, Haverstock DC, Dellinger EP, Reinhart HH, Bohnen JM, Rotstein OD, Vogel SB, Solomkin JS. Definition of the role of enterococcus in intraabdominal infection: analysis of a prospective randomized trial. Surgery 1995; 118:716–723.

58. de Vera ME, Simmons RL. Antibiotic-resistant enterococci and the changing face of surgical infections. Arch Surg 1996; 131:338–342.

59. Megran DW. Enterococcal endocarditis. Clin Infect Dis 1992; 15:63–71.

60. Wilkowske CJ. Enterococcal endocarditis. Mayo Clin Proc 1982; 57:101–105.

61. Rice LB, Calderwood SB, Eliopoulos GM, Farber BF, Karchmer AW. Enterococcal endocarditis: a comparison of prosthetic and native valve disease. Rev Infect Dis 1991; 13:1–7.

62. Shlaes DM, Levy J, Wolinsky E. Enterococcal bacteremia without endocarditis. Arch Intern Med 1981; 141:578–581.

63. Malone DA, Wagner RA, Myers JP, Watanakunakorn C. Enterococcal bacteremia in two large community teaching hospitals. Am J Med 1986; 81:601–606.

64. Garrison RN, Fry DE, Berberich S, Polk HC Jr. Enterococcal bacteremia—clinical implications and determinants of death. Ann Surg 1982; 196:43–47.

65. Dougherty SH, Flohr AB, Simmons RL. Breakthrough enterococcal septicemia in surgical patients. Arch Surg 1983; 118:232–238.

66. Barrall DT, Kenney PR, Slotman GJ, Burchard KW. Enterococcal bacteremia in surgical patients. Arch Surg 1985; 120:57–63.

67. Rimailho A, Lampi E, Riou B, Richard C, Rottman E, Auzepy P. Enterococcal bacteremia in a medical intensive care unit. Crit Care Med 1988; 16:126–129.

68. Gulberg RM, Homann SR, Phair JP. Enterococcal bacteremia: analysis of 75 episodes. Rev Infect Dis 1989; 11:74–84.

69. Hoge CW, Adams J, Buchanan B, Sears SD. Enterococcal bacteremia: to treat or not to treat, a reappraisal. Rev Infect Dis 1991; 13:600–605.

70. Noskin GA, Till M, Patterson BK, Clarke JT, Warren JR. High-level gentamicin resistance in *Enterococcus faecalis* bacteremia. J Infect Dis 1991; 164:1212–1215.

71. Graninger W, Ragette R. Nosocomial bacteremia due to *Enterococcus faecalis* without endocarditis. Clin Infect Dis 1992; 15:49–57.

72. Moellering RC Jr. Emergence of enterococcus as a significant pathogen. Clin Infect Dis 1992; 14:1173–1178.

73. Fraimow HS, Jungkind DL, Lander DW, Delso DR, Dean JL. Urinary tract infection with an *Enterococcus faecalis* isolate that requires vancomycin for growth. Ann Intern Med 1994; 121:22–26.

74. Dobson SRM, Baker CJ. Enterococcal sepsis in neonates: features by age at onset and occurrence of focal infection. Pediatrics 1990; 85:165–171.

75. Stevenson KB, Murray EW, Sarubbi FA. Enterococcal meningitis: report of four cases and review. Clin Infect Dis 1994; 18:233–239.

76. Berk SL, Verghese A, Holtsclaw SA, Smith JK. Enterococcal pneumonia—occurrence in patients receiving broad-spectrum antibiotic regimens and enteral feeding. Am J Med 1983; 74:153–154.

77. Zwillich SH, Hamory BH, Walker SE. Enterococcus: an unusual cause of septic arthritis. Arthritis Rheum 1984; 27:591–595.

78. Mao LK, Flynn HW Jr, Miller D, Pflugfelder SC. Endophthalmitis caused by streptococcal species. Arch Ophthalmol 1992; 110:798–801.

79. Dickinson GM, Bisno AL. Infections associated with indwelling devices: infections related to extravascular devices. Antimicrob Agents Chemother 1989; 33:602–607.

80. Clewell D. Bacterial sex pheromone-induced plasmid transfer. Cell 1993; 73:9–12.

81. Kreft B, Marre R, Schramm U, Wirth R. Aggregation substance of *Enterococcus faecalis* mediates adhesion to cultured renal tubular cells. Infect Immun 1992; 60:25–30.

82. Chow JW, Thal LA, Perri MB, Vazquez JA, Don-

abedian SM, Clewell DB, Zervos MJ. Plasmid-associated hemolysin and aggregation substance production contributes to virulence in experimental enterococcal endocarditis. Antimicrob Agents Chemother 1993; 37:2474–2477.

83. Olmsted, SB, Dunny GM, Erlandsen SL, Wells CL. A plasmid-encoded surface protein on *Enterococcus faecalis* augments its internalization by cultured intestinal epithelial cells. J Infect Dis 1994; 170:1549–1556.

84. Guzman CA, Pruzzo C, Lipira G, Calegari L. Role of adherence in pathogenesis of *Enterococcus faecalis* urinary tract infection and endocarditis. Infect Immun 1989; 57:1834–1838.

85. Guzman CA, Pruzzo M, Plate M, Guardati M, Calegari L. Serum-dependent expression of *Enterococcus faecalis* adhesins involved in the colonization of heart cells. Microb Pathog 1991; 11:399–409.

86. Shorrock PJ, Lambert PA. Binding of fibronectin and albumin to *Enterococcus* (*Streptococcus*) *faecalis*. Microb Pathog 1993; 6:61–67.

87. Olmsted SB, Dunny GM, Erlandsen SL, Wells CL. A plasmid-encoded surface protein on *Enterococcus faecalis* augments its internalization by cultured epithelial cells. J Infect Dis 1994; 170:1549–1556.

88. Wells CL, Jechorek RP, Erlandsen SL. Evidence for the translocation of *Enterococcus faecalis* across the mouse intestinal tract. J Infect Dis 1990; 162:82–90.

89. Wells CL, Erlandsen SL. Localization of translocating *Escherichia coli*, *Proteus mirabilis*, and *Enterococcus faecalis* within cecal and colonic tissues of monoassociated mice. Infect Immun 1991; 59:4693–4697.

90. Bhakdi S, Klonisch T, Nuber P, Fischer W. Stimulation of monokine production by lipoteichoic acids. Infect Immun 1991; 59:4614–4620.

91. Ehrenfeld EE, Kessler RE, Clewell DB. Identification of pheromone-induced surface proteins in *Streptococcus faecalis* and evidence of a role for lipoteichoic acid in the formation of mating aggregates. J Bacteriol 1986; 169:3473–3481.

92. Trotter KM, Dunny GM. Mutants of *Enterococcus faecalis* deficient as recipients in mating with donors carrying pheromone-inducible plasmids. Plasmid 1990; 24:57–67.

93. Bensing BA, Dunny GM. Cloning and molecular analysis of genes affecting expression of binding substance, the recipient-encoded receptor(s) mediating mating aggregate formation in *Enterococcus faecalis*. J Bacteriol 1993; 175:7421–7429.

94. Arduino RC, Murray BE, Rakita RM. Roles of antibodies and complement in phagocytic killing of enterococci. Infect Immun 1994; 62:987–993.

95. Harvey BS, Baker CJ, Edwards MS. Contributions of complement and immunoglobulin to neutrophil-mediated killing of enterococci. Infect Immun 1992; 60:3635–3640.

96. Novak RM, Holzer TJ, Libertin CR. Human neutrophil oxidative response and phagocytic killing of clinical and laboratory strains of *Enterococcus faecalis*. Diagn Microbiol Infect Dis 1993; 164:1212–1215.

97. Poole LB, A Claiborne. Interactions of pyridine nucleotides with redox forms of the flavin-containing NADH peroxidase from *Streptococcus faecalis*. J Biol Chem 1986; 261:14525–14533.

98. Britton L, Malinowski DP, Fridovich I. Superoxide dismutase and oxygen metabolism in *Streptococcus faecalis* and comparisons with other organisms. J Bacteriol 1978; 134:229–236.

99. Ember JA, Hugli TE. Characterization of the human neutrophil response to sex pheromones from *Streptococcus faecalis*. Am J Pathol 1989; 134:797–805.

100. Sannomiya PA, Craig RA, Clewell DB, Suzuki A, Fujino M, Till GO, Marasco WA. Characterization of a class of nonformylated *Enterococcus faecalis*–derived neutrophil chemotactic peptides: the sex pheromones. Proc Natl Acad Sci USA 1990; 87:66–70.

101. Gilmore MS, RA Segarra, LR Hall, MC Booth, CP Bogie, DB Clewell. Structure and mutagenesis of the *Enterococcus faecalis* cytolysin operon and its relationship to those encoding lantibiotics. J Bacteriol 1994; 176:7335–7344.

102. Gutchik E, Moller S, Christensen N. Experimental endocarditis in rabbits. 3. Significance of the proteolytic capacity of the infecting strains of *Streptococcus faecalis*. Acta Pathol Microbiol Scand B Microbiol 1979; 87:353–362.

103. Ike Y, Hashimoto H, Clewell DB. High incidence of hemolysin production by *Enterococcus* (*Streptococcus*) *faecalis* strains associated with human parenteral infections. J Clin Microbiol 1987; 25:1524–1528.

104. Hodel-Christian SL, Murray BE. Characterization of the gentamicin resistance transposon Tn5281 from *Enterococcus faecalis* and comparison to staphylococcal transposons Tn4001 and Tn4031. Antimicrob Agents Chemother 1991; 35:1147–1152.

105. Huycke MM, Joyce WD, Gilmore MS. The *Enterococcus faecalis* cytolysin does not confer an in vivo growth advantage. J Infect Dis 1995; 172:273–276.

106. Jett BD, Jensen HG, Atkuri R, Gilmore MS. Evaluation of therapeutic measures for treating endophthalmitis caused by isogenic toxin producing and toxin non-producing *Enterococcus faecalis* strains. Invest Ophthalmol Vis Sci 1995; 36:9–15.

107. Kuhnen E, Richter F, Richter K, Andries L. Establishment of a typing system for group D streptococci. Zentralbl Bakteriol Mikrobiol Hyg Ser A 1988; 267:322–330.

108. Coque TM, Patterson JE, Steckelberg JM, BE Murray. Incidence of hemolysin, gelatinase, and aggregation substance among enterococci iso-

lated from patients with endocarditis and other infections and from feces of hospitalized and community-based persons. J Infect Dis 1995; 171:1223–1229.

109. Makinen P-L, Makinen KK. The *Enterococcus faecalis* extracellular metalloendopeptidase (EC 3.4.24.30; Coccolysin) inactivates human endothelin at bonds involving hydrophobic amino acid residues. Biochem Biophys Res Commun 1994; 200:981–985.

110. Clewell D. Moveable genetic elements and antibiotic resistance in enterococci. Eur J Clin Microbiol Infect Dis 1990; 9:90–102.

111. Schaberg DR, Zervos MJ. Intergeneric and interspecies gene exchange in gram-positive cocci. Antimicrob Agents Chemother 1986; 30:817–822.

112. Franke AE, Clewell DB. Evidence for a chromosome-borne resistance transposon (Tn*916*) in *Streptococcus faecalis* that is capable of "conjugal" transfer in the absence of a conjugative plasmid. J Bacteriol 1981; 145:494–502.

113. Scott JR. Sex and the single circle: conjugative transposition. J Bacteriol 1992; 174:6005–6010.

114. Fiedler S, Wirth R. Transformation of bacteria with plasmid DNA by electroporation. Anal Biochem 1988; 170:38–44.

115. Cruz-Rodz AL, Gilmore MS. High efficiency introduction of plasmid DNA into glycine treated *Enterococcus faecalis* by electroporation. Mol Gen Genet 1990; 224:152–154.

116. Friesenegger A, Fiedler S, Devriese LA, Wirth R. Genetic transformation of various species of *Enterococcus* by electroporation. FEMS Microbiol Lett 1991; 63:323–327.

117. Dunny GM, Lee LN, LeBlanc DJ. Improved electroporation and cloning vector system for gram-positive bacteria. Appl Environ Microbiol 1991; 57:1194–1201.

118. Eliopoulos GM, Eliopoulos CT. Therapy of enterococcal infections. Eur J Microbiol Infect Dis 1990; 9:118–126.

119. Herman DJ, Gerding DN. Antimicrobial resistance among enterococci. Antimicrob Agents Chemother 1991; 35:1–4.

120. Murray BE. Vancomycin-resistant enterococci. Am J Med 1997; 101:284–293.

121. Goodhart GL. In vivo and in vitro susceptibility of enterococcus to trimethoprim-sulfamethoxazole—a pitfall. JAMA 1984; 252:2748–2749.

122. Chenoweth CE, Robinson KA, Schaberg DR. Efficacy of ampicillin versus trimethoprim-sulfamethoxazole in a mouse model of lethal enterococcal peritonitis. Antimicrob Agents Chemother 1990; 34:1800–1802.

123. Grayson ML, Thauvin-Eliopoulos C, Eliopoulos GM, Yao JD, DeAngelis DV, Walton L, Woolley JL, Moellering RC Jr. Failure of trimethoprim-sulfamethoxazole therapy in experimental enterococcal endocarditis. Antimicrob Agents Chemother 1990; 34:1792–1794.

124. Schaberg DR, Dillon WI, Terpenning MS, Robinson KA, Bradley SF, Kauffman CA. Increasing resistance of enterococci to ciprofloxacin. Antimicrob Agents Chemother 1992; 36:2533–2535.

125. Patterson JE, Zervos MJ. Susceptibility and bactericidal activity studies of four β-lactamase-producing enterococci. Antimicrob Agents Chemother 1989; 33:251–253.

126. Coudron PE, Markowitz SM, Wong ES. Isolation of a β-lactamase-producing, aminoglycoside-resistant strain of *Enterococcus faecium*. Antimicrob Agents Chemother 1992; 36:1125–1126.

127. Murray BE. β-lactamase-producing enterococci. Antimicrob Agents Chemother 1992; 36:2355–2359.

128. Bush LM, Calmon J, Cherney CL, Wendeler M, Pitsakis P, Poupard J, Levison ME, Johnson CC. High-level penicillin resistance among isolates of enterococci—implications for treatment of enterococcal infections. Ann Intern Med 1989; 110:515–520.

129. Oster SE, Chirurgi VA, Goldberg AA, Aiken S, McCabe RE. Ampicillin-resistant enterococcal species in an acute-care hospital. Antimicrob Agents Chemother 1990; 34:1821–1823.

130. Grayson ML, Eliopoulos GM, Wennersten CB, Ruoff KL, DeGirolami PC, Ferraro M-J, Moellering RC Jr. Increasing resistance to β-lactam antibiotics among clinical isolates of *Enterococcus faecium*: a 22-year review at one institution. Antimicrob Agents Chemother 1991; 35:2180–2184.

131. Mederski-Samoraj BD, Murray BE. High-level resistance to gentamicin in clinical isolates of enterococci. J Infect Dis 1983; 751–757.

132. Patterson JE, Masecar BL, Kauffman CA, Schaberg DR, Hierholzer WJ Jr, Zervos MJ. Gentamicin resistance plasmids of enterococci from diverse geographic areas are heterogeneous. J Infect Dis 1988; 158:212–216.

133. Eliopoulos GM, Wennersten C, Sighelboim-Daum S, Reiszner E, Goldmann D, Moellering RC Jr. High-level resistance to gentamicin in clinical isolates of *Streptococcus (Enterococcus) faecium*. Antimicrob Agents Chemother 1988; 32:1528–1532.

134. Leclercq R, Derlot E, Duval J, Courvalin P. Plasmid-mediated resistance to vancomycin and teicoplanin in *Enterococcus faecium*. N Engl J Med 1988; 319:157–161.

135. Nicas TI, Wu CYE, Hobbs JN Jr, Preston DA, Allen NE. Characterization of vancomycin resistance in *Enterococcus faecium* and *Enterococcus faecalis*. Antimicrob Agents Chemother 1989; 33:1121–1124.

136. Sahm DF, Olsen L. In vitro detection of enterococcal vancomycin resistance. Antimicrob Agents Chemother 1990; 34:1846–1848.

137. Handwerger S, Perlman DC, Altarac D, McAuliffe V. Concomitant high-level vancomycin and penicillin resistance in clinical isolates of enterococci. Clin Infect Dis 1992; 14:655–661.

138. Arthur M, Courvalin P. Genetics and mechanisms of glycopeptide resistance in enterococci. Antimicrob Agents Chemother 1993; 37:1563–1571.

139. Leclercq R, Courvalin P. Resistance to glycopeptides in enterococci. Clin Infect Dis 1997; 24:545–556.

140. Noskin GA. Vancomycin-resistant enterococci: clinical, microbiologic, and epidemiologic features. J Lab Clin Med 1997; 130:14–20.

141. McDonald LC, Kuehnert MJ, Tenover FC, Jarvis WR. Vancomycin-resistant enterococci outside the health-care setting: prevalence, sources, and public health implications. Emerg Infect Dis 1997; 3:311–317.

142. Coque TM, Tomayko JF, Ricke SC, Okhyusen PC, Murrary BE. Vancomycin-resistant enterococci from nosocomial, community, and animal sources in the United States. Antimicrob Agents Chemother 1996; 40:2605–2609.

143. Van der Auwera P, Pensart N, Korten V, Murray BE, Leclercq R. Influence of oral glycopeptide on the fecal flora of human volunteers: selection of highly glycopeptide-resistant enterococci. J Infect Dis 1996; 173:1129–1136.

144. Spera RV Jr, Farber BF. Multiply-resistant *Enterococcus faecium*—the nosocomial pathogen of the 1990s. JAMA 1992; 268:2563–2564.

145. Centers for Disease Control and Prevention. Nosocomial enterococci resistant to vancomycin—United States, 1989–1993. JAMA 1993; 270:1796.

146. Morris JG, Shay DK, Hebden JN, McCarter RJ, Perdue BE, Jarvis W, Johnson JA, Dowling TC, Polish LB, Schwalbe RS. Enterococci resistant to multiple antimicrobial agents, including vancomycin—establishment of endemicity in a university medical center. Ann Intern Med 1995; 123:250–259.

147. Herman DJ, Gerding DN. Screening and treatment of infections caused by resistant enterococci. Antimicrob Agents Chemother 1991; 35:215–219.

148. Eliopoulos GM, Thauvin-Eliopoulos C, Moellering RC Jr. Contribution of animal models in the search for effective therapy for endocarditis due to enterococci with high-level resistance to gentamicin. Clin Infect Dis 1992; 15:58–62.

149. Norris AH, Reilly JP, Edelstein PH, Brennan PJ, Schuster MG. Chloramphenicol for the treatment of vancomycin-resistant enterococcal infections. Clin Infect Dis 1995; 20:1137–1144.

150. Shlaes DM, Etter L, Guttmann L. Synergistic killing of vancomycin-resistant enterococci of classes A, B, and C by combinations of vancomycin, penicillin, and gentamicin. Antimicrob Agents Chemother 1991; 35:776–779.

151. Lai KK. Treatment of vancomycin-resistant *Enterococcus faecium* infections. Arch Intern Med 1996; 156:2579–2584.

152. Fuller RE, Drew RH, Perfect JR. Treatment of vancomycin-resistant enterococci, with a focus on quinupristin-dalfopristin. Pharmacotherapy 1996; 16:584–592.

153. Bryson HM, Spencer CM. Quinupristin-dalfopristin. Drugs 1996; 52:406–415.

154. Bouanchaud DH. In-vitro and in-vivo antibacterial activity of quinupristin/dalfopristin. J Antimicrob Chemother 1997; 39(Suppl A):15–21.

155. Chow JW, Donahedian SM, Zervos MJ. Emergence of increased resistance to quinupristin/dalfopristin during therapy for *Enterococcus faecium* bacteremia. Clin Infect Dis 1997; 24:90–91.

156. Jones RN, Barrett MS, Erwin ME. In vitro activity and spectrum of LY333328, a novel glycopeptide derivative. Antimicrob Agents Chemother 1996; 41:488–493.

157. Nicas TI, Mullen DL, Flokowitsch JE, Preston DA, Snyder NJ, Stratford RE, Cooper RD. Activities of the semisynthetic glycopeptide LY191145 against vancomycin-resistant enterococci and other gram-positive bacteria. Antimicrob Agents Chemother 1995; 39:2585–2587.

158. Schulin T, Wennersten CB, Moellering RC Jr, Eliopoulos GM. In vitro activity of RU 64004, a new ketolide antibiotic, against gram-positive bacteria. Antimicrob Agents Chemother 1997; 41:1196–1202.

159. Dajani AS, Taubert KA, Wilson W, Bolger AF, Bayer A, Ferrieri P, Gewitz MH, Shulman ST, Nouri S, Newburger JW, Hutto C, Pallasch TJ, Gage TW, Levison ME, Peter G, Zuccaro G Jr. Prevention of bacterial endocarditis. Recommendations by the American Heart Association. JAMA 1997; 277:1794–1801.

160. Weigelt JA, Easley SM, Thal ER, et al. Abdominal surgical wound infection is lowered with improved perioperative enterococcus and bacteroides therapy. J Trauma 1993; 34:579–585.

161. Clark CD, Picus D, Dunagan WC. Bloodstream infection after interventional procedures in the biliary tract. Radiology 1994; 191:495–499.

162. Hospital Infection Control Practices Advisory Committee. Recommendations for preventing the spread of vancomycin resistance. Infect Control Hosp Epidemiol 1995; 16:105–113.

163. Davis JM, Huycke MM, Wells CL, Bohnen JMA, Gadaleta D, Fichtl RE, Barie PS. Surgical infection society position on vancomycin-resistant *Enterococcus*. Arch Surg 1996; 131:1061–1068.

164. Boyce JM. Vancomycin-resistant enterococci: pervasive and persistent pathogens. Infect Control Hosp Epidemiol 1995; 16:676–679.

165. Evans ME, Kortas KJ. Vancomycin use in a university medical center: comparison with Hospital Infection Control Practices Advisory Committees guidelines. Infect Control Hosp Epidemiol 1996; 17:356–359.

166. Logsdon BA, Lee KR, Luedtke G, Barrett FF. Evaluation of vancomycin in a pediatric teaching hospital based on the CDC criteria. Infect Control Hosp Epidemiol 1997; 18:780–782.

167. Anglim AM, Klym B, Byers KE, Scheld WM, Garr BM. Effect of a vancomycin restriction policy on ordering practices during an outbreak of vancomycin-resistant *Enterococcus faecium*. Arch Intern Med 1997; 157:1132–1136.
168. Quale J, Landman D, Saurina G, Atwood E, Di-Tore V, Patel K. Manipulation of a hospital antimicrobial formulary to control an outbreak of vancomycin-resistant enterococci. Clin Infect Dis 1996; 23:1020–1025.
169. Dembry LM, Uzokwe K, Zervos MJ. Control of endemic glycopeptide-resistant enterococci. Infect Control Hosp Epidemiol 1996; 17:286–292.
170. Saurina G, Landman D, Quale JM. Activity of disinfectants against vancomycin-resistant *Enterococcus faecium*. Infect Control Hosp Epidemiol 1997; 18:345–348.
171. Anderson RL, Carr JH, Bond WW, Favero MS. Susceptibility of vancomycin-resistant enterococci to environmental disinfectants. Infect Control Hosp Epidemiol 1997; 18:195–199.
172. Slaughter S, Hayden MK, Nathan C, Hu T-C, Rice T, Van Voorhis J, Matushek M, Franklin C, Weinstein RA. A comparison of the effect of universal use of gloves and gowns with that of glove use alone on acquisition of vancomycin-resistant enterococci in a medical intensive care unit. Ann Intern Med 1996; 125:448–456.

17

Streptococcus pneumoniae Infections

BARRY M. GRAY

For over a hundred years *Streptococcus pneumoniae* has been recognized as one of the most important bacterial pathogens causing disease in humans. Many of the efforts to subvert the pneumococcus have been associated with major developments in antibiotics, genetics, and immunology. Readers interested in the history of the pneumococcus are encouraged to consult White's *The Biology of the Pneumococcus* [1], published originally in 1938, and Heffron's *Pneumonia with Special Reference to Pneumococcus Lobar Pneumonia* [2], published a year later, both of which have been reprinted. More recent readings should include Austrian's accounts of the first 100 years of the pneumococcus [3], and a description of the organism's panoply of scientific discovery by Watson and colleagues [4].

The pneumococcus is the prototypic encapsulated extracellular pathogen. It is able to resist phagocytosis, in the absence of type-specific antibodies, and replicate in mammalian tissue, causing pneumonia, otitis media, meningitis, and a multitude of other clinical manifestations. Historically, the pneumococcus is most closely associated with lobar pneumonia, having been first visualized in bronchial secretions and tissue sections by Klebs in 1875 and later identified as the major cause of that disease. Its pathogenic potential was not yet appreciated when first iso-

lated in 1880 by Sternberg, who recovered it in a rabbit injected with his own saliva, and nearly simultaneously by Pasteur, who isolated it from a rabbit injected with saliva of a rabies victim. Identification of the organism was facilitated by Gram, who developed the Gram stain in 1884. Within a few years many infections were shown to be due to the pneumococcus, and a number important developments were begun in immunology and pathology. Immunization with killed pneumococci was found to be protective in animals, and this heralded the later therapeutic use of specific antiserums. The role of type-specific antibodies and nonspecific factors later known as complement was demonstrated as necessary to the process of opsonization that allows phagocytes to engulf and kill the organisms.

The pneumococcus was the first organism against which a specific antimicrobial agent—the quinine derivative, optochin—was used in animal models as a therapeutic antibiotic [4]. It did not prove to be useful in treating pneumonia in humans because it had significant optic toxicity and because pneumococci rapidly became resistant to therapeutic doses. The sulfonamides were used successfully to treat pneumococcal infections for several years until resistance became increasingly frequent in the mid-1940s. The advent of penicillin was a great turning point in the history of medicine. Penicillin and other β-lactam antibiotics remain the cornerstones of antibiotic therapy, but the development and spread of resistant strains over the past two decades has complicated the clinician's approach to pneumococcal infections.

The pneumococcus enjoys distinction as a seminal player in the discovery of the "transforming principle," brought to light in experiments by Griffith in 1928, and later shown to be DNA by Avery, MacLeod, and McCarty in 1944 [4]. Since that time, the understanding of pneumococcal genetics has lagged behind that of other more cooperative species. Recent molecular and genetic studies have focused on antibiotic resistance and on biosynthesis of capsular materials. The pneumococci have much in common with other streptococci and have several distinct features of their own. Streptococcal genetics is further discussed in Chapter 3.

The first pneumococcal vaccines used in humans were made from whole, killed organisms by Wright and colleagues in 1911, prior to the delineation of capsular serotypes and long before the "specific soluble substance" was shown to be the capsular polysaccharide [3,4]. A vaccine consisting of purified capsular polysaccharides of four common serotypes was developed in the 1940s by MacLeod, Hodges, and Heidelberger and shown to be effective in one of the first carefully controlled efficacy trials. After World War II, a hexavalent vaccine was licensed in the United States, but it was not extensively used, because many physicians had already turned to antibiotics as a facile cure for pneumococcal disease. Vaccines containing 14 capsular polysaccharides were eventually introduced in 1977, followed by a 23-valent formulation in 1983. These vaccines have remained underutilized, despite reasonable assessments of efficacy in adult populations. Young infants do not respond well to pneumococcal polysaccharides; however, vaccines consisting of the polysaccharides coupled to protein carriers are proving to be sufficiently immunogenic in this age-group in ongoing clinical trials. These and other approaches to pneumococcal immunization are further discussed in Chapter 22.

The pneumococcus remains a major human pathogen. Current U.S. estimates suggest a yearly disease burden of 3000 cases of meningitis, 50,000 cases of bacteremia, 500,000 pneumonias, and 7,000,000 cases of otitis media [5]. In many areas of the United States a quarter of pneumococcal isolates are penicillin-intermediate or -resistant, and resistance rates are higher in parts of Europe and Africa. Case fatality rates have not improved significantly over the past decade or more. Resistant strains and compromised hosts add further complications to clinical approaches to this "captain of the men of death."

LABORATORY METHODS

Culture and Presumptive Identification

The pneumococci are gram-positive cocci described as lancet-shaped diplococci but often appear as streptococcal chains in blood cultures or liquid media. They are fastidious organisms that require rich culture media or a live animal for growth and do not survive drying at room temperature or sitting in physiologic saline. Like other streptococci, they do not produce catalase but use oxygen via a flavoenzyme system to make H_2O_2. Because they cannot degrade H_2O_2, they do not grow well in the absence of catalase, which may be supplied by erythrocytes in culture media or by host tissue during infection.

Pneumococci may be isolated in the clinical laboratory on commercial tryptic soy-based agar containing 5% sheep blood. Sometimes pneumococci in blood cultures autolyze before they can be recovered, but automated blood culture monitoring systems facilitate early sampling and help avoid this problem. Recovery of pneumococci from sputum, nasopharynx, and other sites likely to be mixed with "normal flora" is often difficult because of competing growth of other species, especially other green streptococci. Care must be taken to pick a sufficient number of representative colonies for subculture and presumptive identification. For colonization studies a selective blood agar containing 5 mg/liter gentamicin sulfate has proved especially useful [6]. Growth is good at temperatures of 35°–37°C and is further improved by 3%–5% CO_2 or a candle jar.

Colonies are smooth, shiny, and dome shaped when young. As they age and begin to autolyze, their centers form wide craters, often with the appearance of a checker piece. The pneumoccci vary considerably in colony morphology, but subtle differences may be apparent only with magnification. Type 3 colonies are characteristically very large (>3 mm) and mucoid; some type 19 strains are quite mucoid but not as large, whereas type 1 and type 14 are usually much smaller (<1 mm). Although pneumcocci are referred to as alpha hemolytic, this is not actually due to true hemolysis but to breakdown of hemoglobin to form the green pigment that colors and surrounds the colonies on blood or chocolate agar. Presumptive identification is accomplished on agar by demonstrating a zone of inhibition around a "P" disk containing optochin (ethylhydrocupreine). A few other streptococci may occasionally show optochin sensitivity, and a few pneumococci may be optochin-resistant. In such cases pneumococci may be identified using the bile solubility test. A heavy suspension of fresh pneumococcal growth is made in a small amount of water; equal volumes (a few drops) of this are added to give visible turbidity in a 10% aqueous solution of deoxycholate (or ox bile) and in a similar tube with plain water as a control; the deoxycholate will lyse pneumococci within a few minutes, causing a visually apparent reduction of turbidity, relative to the control tube. A "quick-and-dirty" method is simply to put a drop of the deoxycholate directly onto freshly grown colonies on a blood agar plate and look for dissolution of the colonies after a few minutes of incubation. Bile-insensitive pneumococci have been reported but are extremely rare.

Serologic Typing and Other Methods of Identification

There are 90 distinct pneumococcal serotypes, which are based upon the reactions of rabbit antisera with the type-specific capsular polysaccharides on the bacterial cell surface. The Danish typing system developed by Lund in the 1940s is now nearly universally accepted and has recently been updated with a complete listing of types and their cross-reactions [7]. All of the distinct types in the American system are included, but cross-reactive types are combined into groups of two or more types. For example, types 1–5, 8, and 14 exist as single types; group 6 in-

cludes types 6A and 6B (American types 6 and 26); group 9 includes types 9V and 9N, along with the rarer types 9A and 9L (American types 68, 9, 33, and 49). This system simplifies the numbering but has led to the invention of the unfortunate term "groups/types" to denote them collectively.

Serotyping is done by the Neufeld reaction, or quellung, in which capsular swelling is observed under the microscope. This is actually due to changes in water content of the capsule as antibodies bind to the surface polysaccharides and alter the refraction of light passing through the capsule. Typing may also be done by slide agglutination, but equivocal results must be confirmed by quellung. Types within groups (sometimes called subtypes), may be identified using factor sera raised against one type, such as 6A, and cross-absorbed with the cross-reacting type, 6B in this instance. The factor sera are then used in the quellung. Because this process requires carefully prepared reagents and considerable technical expertise, it is only done at the Centers for Disease Control and Prevention in Atlanta, the Statens Seruminstitut in Copenhagen, and a few other research and reference laboratories. During the late 1930s and early 1940s, serotyping was done routinely at centers that used horse or rabbit antisera for treatment of pneumococcal disease. Today, it remains an indispensable epidemiologic tool for tracking serotypes according to disease states, multidrug resistance, and patient populations. It was used to select the types included in the original 14-valent vaccines in 1977, in the present formulation of the 23-valent vaccines [8], and in selection of the seven or so types in the conjugate vaccines currently undergoing clinical trials in children [9].

Multilocus enzyme electrophoresis (MLEE) analysis is a very discriminating method that detects subtle mutations in a panel of up to 20 metabolic enzymes encoded throughout the chromosome. Determination of electrophoretic type (ET) has been especially useful when coupled with serotyping and other methods in studies of population genetics and epidemiology [10–13].

Several techniques of DNA fingerprinting and ribosomal RNA typing have been used for molecular identification of strains for epidemiological purposes. One ribotyping technique involves hybridization of endonuclease restricted DNA fragments with a cDNA probe complementary to 16 and 23S rRNAs [14]. Other methods include pulse-field gel electrophoresis (PFGE) of large DNA restriction fragments, BOX fingerprinting using the *Streptococcus pneumoniae* BOX repetitive DNA element as a DNA probe, PCR fingerprinting with an enterobacterial repetitive intergenic consensus sequence primer, and restriction fragment length polymorphism (RFLP) by end-labeling of small DNA fragments [12,15]. The method selected may depend upon the kind of information desired. For example, ribotyping may be best for investigating long-term epidemiologic events and genetic relatedness. For distinguishing among closely related strains, BOX fingerprinting or RFLP may be more suitable [15].

Gram's Stain, Antigen Detection, and Molecular Methods

The Gram stain of sputum samples for diagnosis of pneumonia has been marked by controversy since its introduction over a century ago. Detractors cite the interference by normal flora and the poor correlation of the Gram stains with culture results. According to some authorities, sputa are useful only if positive for tuberculosis bacilli or *Legionella*, and seldom, if ever, for pneumococci. Proponents attribute poor specificity to poorly collected sputum samples and to prior administration of antibiotics [16–18]. Sputum culture can be useful in areas where penicillin- or multiresistant pneumococci are common. The sputum should show an abundance of neutrophils (>25 per low-power field) and very few (<10) squamous epithelial cells. In positive samples diplococci are usually present in numbers >25 per field; when >10 diplococci are seen per field, cultures are positive about 60% of the time [17]. In children, good sputum samples are difficult to obtain, and the high frequency of asymptomatic colonization further diminishes their utility in etiologic diagnosis. In patients with moderate to severe pneumonia, bronchoscopy may be indicated; here the use of the protected specimen brush or bronchoalveolar lavage in conjunction with semiquantitative bacterial cultures has a

much higher yield but still remains controversial [17–19].

Gram stains of cerebrospinal fluid (CSF) samples are subject to fewer vagaries of interpretation and remain an essential part of every evaluation for meningitis. Bacteria may be concentrated by centrifugation of the CSF sample, but conventional speeds of 2000 rpm or cytocentrifuges using slower speeds do not bring organisms down nearly as well as a microfuge at >5000 rpm. Care must be taken not to over- or under-decolorize the slide, lest pneumococci be mistaken for meningococci or vice versa. Gram stains of CSF may become negative soon after antibiotic administration [20].

Latex and co-agglutination methods of detection of pneumococcal antigens in cerebrospinal fluid usually offer no advantage over the Gram stain for diagnosing meningitis. These reagents vary considerably in their sensitivity to different pneumococcal serotypes, and CSF may have to be heated to 100°C for a few minutes to eliminate false-positive reactions. Nevertheless, antigen detection can be helpful in patients who have already received antibiotics and whose cultures and Gram stains are negative [20]. The test is also useful in confirming an etiology when applied to pleural fluid in the diagnosis of pneumonia [21]. Latex agglutination requires concentrations 10^6–10^7 pneumococci/ml, about the same as the numbers needed for visualization microscopically or for growth of colonies on agar plates [22]. Commercially available methods for detection of antigens in urine are not reliable, although some research applications are promising.

Polymerase chain reaction (PCR) methods may offer additional ways of detecting pneumococci in clinical materials. Pneumococci have been identified in sputum samples by PCR amplification of the autolysin gene [23] and in middle ear fluids with amplification of the pneumolysin gene [24]. A PCR assay based on amplification of the gene (*pbp2B*) coding for penicillin-binding protein 2B (PBF 2B) was found to lack the sensitivity and specificity needed for clinical use [25], but a semi-nested PCR for the *pbp2B* gene was highly successful for detection of pneumococci in CSF and was able to predict penicillin resistance from the size of the amplified gene fragments [26]. Some of these techniques are quite promising but none have yet been adapted for routine clinical use. Recovery of organisms by culture is necessary for serotyping and testing against various antibiotics of clinical relevance.

Antibiotic Susceptibility Testing

Before the advent of penicillin resistance there was little need for clinical laboratories to perform routine susceptibility testing on pneumococci [27]. Up until the mid-1970s quantitative dilution tests found minimal inhibitory concentrations (MICs) uniformly in the range of <0.03 μg/ml for penicillin G. As penicillin-intermediate (MIC 0.1–1.0 μg/ml) and -resistant strains (MIC >1.0 μg/ml) began to appear, it was found that screening with the conventional 10 μg penicillin disk often failed to detect resistance by the Kirby-Bauer method. This problem was largely solved by use of the 1.0 μg oxacillin disk introduced by Dixon et al. in 1977 and further validated by Swenson et al. [28]. Properly performed, the oxacillin screening test rarely fails to detect resistant strains, although up to 40% of strains with inhibition zones <20 mm may prove to be susceptible at borderline MICs of 0.06 μg/ml [28–30]. Current methods for oxacillin screening and disk susceptibility testing of pneumococci have been recommended by the National Committee for Clinical Laboratory Standards (NCCLS) [31]. Disk tests are done using Mueller-Hinton agar supplemented with 5% sheep blood and incubated at 35°C in a 5% CO_2 atmosphere. The problems encountered with disk testing mostly involve careless errors, such as using out-of-date disks or failing to check them with control strains, preparing the inoculum with old cultures, failing to adjust the inoculum to the 0.5 McFarland density standard, inoculating unevenly with a loop instead of a swab, and not allowing the inoculum to dry sufficiently before applying the disks.

The E test (AB Biodisk, Solna, Sweden, and Piscataway, NJ) is an ingenious variation on the disk diffusion method and is performed in much the same way [32–34]. Instead of a disk, a plastic strip is used to deliver a gradient of antibiotic from low to high concentration along the strip, which is calibrated to give the approximate MIC at the point where growth reaches the edge of the strip. Although the E test does not always delineate minor differences between intermediate and resistant strains, it performs much better than the oxacillin test in separating penicillin-sensitive strains from penicillin-intermediate or -resistant strains. E tests have been developed and evaluated for cefotaxime, cefuroxime, ceftriaxone, chloramphenicol, erythromycin, and tetracycline.

Quantitative measurment of MIC is done either by broth microdilution or agar dilution methods [29,31,33,35]. Pneumococci are especially finicky when it comes to susceptibility testing, and as yet there is no universal agreement on growth conditions and supplementation of media. Most authorities now recommend using a 5% CO_2 atmosphere because growth is better and fewer discrepancies are noted. Broth media are supplemented with 3%–5% lysed horse blood. Several commercially available broth microdilution systems are now in use, but these vary considerably in their reliablility, and some are not recommended [33,34].

Testing for resistance to chloramphenicol can be problematic. Some strains appear sensitive by disk diffusion or MIC testing but are actually quite tolerant, because the chloramphenicol acetyl transferase may not be induced by disk test methods. In cases where chloramphenicol susceptibility is critical, an alternative is to assay for the acetyltransferase directly using a simple 90-min colorometric method [36].

Antibody Measurement

For many years, studies of pneumococcal antibody levels relied upon a Farr-type radioimmunoassay (RIA), in which total antibody (IgG, IgM, and IgA) was allowed to bind to endogenously labeled pneumococcal antigens, then precipitated and counted [37]. Solid-phase enzyme-linked immunosorbant assays (ELISA, or EIA-enzyme immunoassay) were later developed that are capable of measuring isotype-specific responses, including IgG, IgM, IgA, and IgG subclasses. However, it was noted that measurement of the anticapsular antibodies was complicated by the presence of C-polysaccharide contaminating the capsular antigens, resulting in falsely elevated antibody measurements [38]. Many variations of the

ELISA are now in use, most of which incorporate a step to neutralize anti-C-polysaccharide antibodies. Ongoing efforts to standardize ELISA methodology are being coordinated by George Carlone at the Centers for Disease Control (CDC) in Atlanta. Farr assays are now being reevaluated and improved, and appear to have some advantages as well as disadvantages compared to ELISA techniques [39]. Some commercial laboratories now offer pneumococcal antibody measurements, but the reliability and comparability of results vary enormously. For clinical purposes, when antibody levels are needed for immunological evaluations, it is prudent to send paired acute and convalescent (or postvaccine) sera for testing in the same assay run.

Assays for opsonization and phagocytosis have chiefly been employed in research aspects of pneumococcal virulence, mechanisms of complement action, and evaluation of functional activity of antibodies [40,41]. Antibodies to capsular polysaccharides have repeatedly been shown to be required for opsonization of most encapsulated strains. Although antibodies to C-polysaccharide and phosphorylcholine may be protective in animal models, evidence from opsonization studies suggest that human antibodies to C-polysaccharide are poorly opsonic and probably do not play a significant role in protection of humans [42].

MICROBIOLOGY AND VIRULENCE FACTORS

Pneumococcal Capsules

The defining structural and antigenic feature of pneumococci is a polysaccharide capsule [43,44]. Despite the depiction of the cell body being surrounded by a wall of capsular material like a candy-coated peanut, the capsule is actually a tangle of capsular polysaccharide polymers, covering and intermingled with surface proteins, strands of peptidoglycan, teichoic acids, C-polysaccharide, and other constituents of the cell wall. The capsule is the major pneumococcal virulence factor; without it, the pneumococcus is naked and defenseless against nonspecific killing mechanisms.

The capsular polysaccharides confer resistance to opsonization and phagocytosis [41,45]. Unencapsulated strains have "activator" surface structures, especially teichoic acids, that bind C3 directly via the alternative complement pathway. Some serotypes (e.g., 6, 18, and 23) can be readily opsonized via the alternative pathway [40], and yet these types are common in serious human disease. Opsonization of most types requires the addition of anticapsular antibody. Encapsulated pneumococci have much larger surface areas that must be coated with opsonins, and the capsule makes covalent binding of C3 and conversion to active C3b more difficult. The alternative pathway is activated less efficiently because there is less binding of factor B to C3b, much of which is converted to the inactive form iC3b. There is also evidence that a pneumococcal proteinase associated with the cell wall degrades unbound C3 [46]. When type-specific antibodies are present, 2 to 4 times as much C3 is deposited on the capsular surface [41]. This greatly aids phagocytic recognition, attachment, ingestion, and killing. Virulence, however, is not entirely dependent upon capsular type or on site of infection and may be strongly affected by properties of the host species. In a reevaluation of mouse virulence only about 30% of fresh human disease isolates were lethal in mice. Type 4 isolates and some type 3 and group 6 strains were virulent; type 1, which is common in severe human disease, was marginally virulent; and strains of groups/types 14, 19, and 23 were consistently avirulent [47]. Genetic switching of capsular types suggests that although capsular type exerts a major influence, other factors in the genetic background of a given strain are also important [48].

Capsular polysaccharides are composed of long polymers of repeating units of 2 to 7 monosaccharides [8,43]. As illustrated in Table 17.1, some of the repeating units are linear polysaccharides, and some have branched chains. Others have phosphodiester linkages and resemble teichoic acids. Types 6A and 6B are identical except for their ribose-ribitol linkages; immunization with either type gives about 80% cross-protection with the other, allowing for a satisfactory vaccine containing 6B alone. Types 9V and 9N are similar except for the *O*-acetyl groups added to 9V; however, because there is much less cross-

Table 17.1 Polysaccharide Repeating Units of Common Pneumococcal Types

Type 3	→ 3)-β-D-Glc-(1 → 4)-β-D-Glc$p$A-(1 →
Type 6A	→ 2)-α-D-Gal$p$-(1 → 3)-α-D-Glc$p$-(1 → 3)-α-L-Rha$p$-(1 → 3)-D-ribitol-5-PO$_4$ →
Type 6B	→ 2)-α-D-Gal$p$-(1 → 3)-α-D-Glc$p$-1 → 3)-α-L-Rha$p$-(1 → 4)-D-ribitol-5-PO$_4$ →
Type 9N	→ 4)-α-D-Glc$p$-(1 → 3)-α-D-Glc$p$-(1 → 3)-β-D-Man$p$NAc-(1 → 4)-α-D-Glc$p$-(1 → 4)-β-D-Glc$p$NAc-(1 →

Type 9V → 4)-α-D-Glc$p$A-(1 → 3)-α-D-Glc$p$-(1 → 3)-β-D-Man$p$NAc-(1 → 4)-α-D-Glc$p$-(1 → 4)-β-D-Glc$p$NAc-(1 →
    | |
    OAc   OAc

Type 14 → 6)-β-D-GlcNAc-(1 → 3)-β-D-Gal-(1 → 4)-β-D-Glc-(1 →
    β|4
    Gal

Type 19F → 4)-β-N-Man$p$NAc-(1 → 4)-β-D-Glc$p$-1 → 3)-α-L-Rha$p$-(1 → PO$_4$ →

Type 19A → 4)-β-N-Man$p$NAc-(1 → 4)-β-D-Glc$p$-1 → 3)-α-L-Rha$p$-(1 → PO$_4$ →
                                  |2 |2
                                  PO$_4$ PO$_4$
                                  |1 |1
                                  β-D-Gal α-L-Fuc
                                  |3
                                  β-D-GlcNAc

Type 23F → 3)-β-D-Glc$p$-(1 → 4)-β-D-Gal$p$-(1 → 4)-α-L-Rha$p$-(1 →
    | |2
    PO$_4$ α-L-Rha$p$

p = pyranose form (5-carbon ring); Glc, glucose; Glc$p$A, glucuronic acid; GlcNAc, N-acetylglucosamine; Gal, galactose; Fuc, fucose; Rha, rhamnose; ManNAc, N-acetylmannosamine.

reactivity, both types were included in the 23-valent vaccine (see Table 17.2; [8]). Type 9V was selected for a heptavalent conjugate vaccine because it is more common in children. There is a tendency for some types to predominate in certain kinds of infections, as further described in the epidemiology section (below). In children, for example (Table 17.3), group 6 (6A and 6B) strains are most common in meningitis, type 14, in bacteremia, and group 19 (19F and 19A), in otitis media. The biochemical reasons for this are not known, nor is it clear that this is even a func-

Table 17.2 Common Pneumococcal Groups/Types, as represented in 23-Valent Purified Polysaccharide Vaccine and Heptavalent Protein-Conjugate Vaccines

Types in 23-Valent Vaccine	Types in Heptavalent Conjugate Vaccine	Cross-reacting Types in Group (% occurrence of disease caused by type[s] in group)
1		None
2		None
3		None
4	4	None
5		None
6B	6B	6B (61%), 6A (39%)
7F		7F (96%), 7A, 7B, 7C
8		None
9V, 9N	9V	9V (57%), 9N (34%), 9A, 9L
10A		10A (89%), 10F
11A		11A (78%), 11B, 11C
12F		12F (84%),12A
14	14	None
15B		15B (22%), 15C (39%),15F, 15A
17F		17F (88%),17A
18C	18C	18C (83%),18F, 18A, 18B
19F, 19A	19F	19F (65%), 19A (34%)
20		None
22F	23F	22F (99%), 22A
23F		23F (90%), 23A, 23B
33F		33F (79%), 33A, 33B, 33C

Data mostly from Robbins et al. [8] (Tables 1–3), compiled from CDC and WHO surveys including mainly blood and CSF isolates.

tion of serotype, rather than some other associated factor.

The more complex polysaccharides are probably assembled from repeating oligosaccharide subunits synthesized in the cytoplasm from monosaccharide precursors. The polymers elongate by addition of subunits to the proximal end of the chain and are finally anchored to peptidoglycan and C-polysaccharide on the cell wall. An exception to this is type 3, which produces copious amounts of capsular material, of which little if any is covalently attached to cell wall structures [44].

The Pneumococcal Cell Wall

Pneumococcal cell walls, like those of other streptococci, are composed mainly of cross-linked layers of peptidoglycan [44,49]. Interspersed with peptidoglycan is the C-polysaccharide, an unusual, teichoic-like polymer containing phosphorylcholine determinants. This corresponds to the "group" antigens of group A, group B, and other Lancefield streptococci. The Forssman, or F-antigen is essentially C-polysaccharide attached to lipid components of the cell membrane. Peptidoglycan is synthesized intracellularly from disaccharide precursors of N-acetylglucosamine (GlcNAc) and N-acetylmuramic acid (MurNAc). A stem peptide and an undecaprenolpyrophosphate (a 55-carbon lipid carrier) are then added to the muramic acid. The undecaprenol anchors the disaccharide temporarily to the cell membrane, and 20 or so disaccharides are linked together and extruded to the outside. There, about every tenth muramic acid is cross-linked to other chains via a bridge of glycine units connecting the stem peptides.

The enzymes responsible for cross-linking peptidoglycan chains include six transpeptidases and transcarboxylases better known as the penicillin-binding proteins (PBPs) 1a, 1b, 2a, 2b, 2x, and 3 [27,50]. The PBPs 1a and 1b are bifunctional, catalyzing the linkage of disaccharide subunits at one enzymatic site and cross-linking stem peptides at another site. The PBPs 2b and 2x are essential to growth and are important to penicillin-resistant strains. PBP 3 is a low-molecular-weight enzyme that functions mainly in cell division.

The prototypic stem peptide consists of the pentapeptide L-alanine-D-isoglutamine-L-lysine-D-alanine-D-alanine. Pneumococci, however, utilize a wide array of stem peptides, including branched peptides, which are important in resistance to β-lactam antibiotics [51]. Cell walls are constantly being remodeled during periods of growth and cell division. The breakdown of peptidoglycan is controlled by autolytic enzymes, described below. The muramyl dipeptide (MurNAc-D-alanyl-D-isoglutamine) is the minimal active unit of a tribe of peptidoglycan breakdown products. Many of these are highly inflammatory and are responsible for most of the toxic effects that characterize pneumococcal infections [52–55].

Enzymes

Autolysin, an autolytic amidase (N-acetyl-muramoyl-L-alanine amidase), normally functions to separate daughter cells into diplococci at the end of cell division, to break down the organisms at the end of exponential growth, and perhaps to render cells competent for transformation [56,57]. Mutants with defective amidases fail to divide into normal diplococci or lyse when exposed to penicillins. A second autolytic enzyme is a glycosidase that breaks down the saccharide units of the peptidoglycan [58]. Both enzymes are inhibited by teichoic acids and choline, which are breakdown products of the C-polysaccharide. This negative feedback mechanism presumably serves to modulate autolysis and favor the survival of some cells within a population that is normally beginning to self-destruct at the end of the exponential growth phase. Autolysin-negative strains are less virulent in mice, and antibodies to the enzyme confer a modicum of protection [59]. In natural infections the regulation of autolytic activity appears to be important in the timing and magnitude of pneumococcal cell breakdown, and in turn, determining the inflammatory response in the host. The human host may induce autolytic activity of the amidase by the action lysozyme [60], and the host's physician may provoke widespread lysis of organisms by the administration of penicillin. Some clinical isolates, especially those resistant to penicillins, exhibit various defects in lytic activity that may contribute to different clinical manifestations relating to the magnitude of the inflammatory response [61]. Lysis-defective organisms continue to grow while releasing less cell wall material and provoking initially delayed and diminished inflammation, but ultimately causing worse disease.

Pneumolysin is a thiol-activated cytotoxin similar to the group A streptolysin O and to listeriolysin [62]. This polypeptide occurs in the cytoplasm and does not exert any pathological effect until it is released by cell lysis. Studies with defined point mutations suggest that its major effects are due to its cytolytic properties, although it may also induce human monocytes to produce tumor necrosis factor (TNF) and interlukin-1 (IL-1). Pneumolysin appears to have a limited role in the pathogenesis of meningitis, as determined in rabbits by intracisternal inoculation of isogenic pneumolysin-positive or -negative pneumococci or by instillation of recombinant pneumolysin [63]. This model, however, was designed to test effects within the brain and does not assess the activity of pneumolysin in earlier stages of the disease process. In a rat model of pneumonia induced by intranasal inoculation of isogenic mutants, pneumolysin-negative strains showed slower growth, delayed onset of bacteremia, and fewer of the severe histological changes seen in the lungs of animals infected with the pneumolysin-positive strain. Immunofluorescent staining showed that pneumolysin was produced in vivo and was present in areas of pulmonary inflammation [57].

IgA proteases cleave serum and secretory IgA1 (but not IgA2) at the hinge region, releasing Fc, Fab, and secretory component fragments [64]. The Fab fragments retain their ability to bind antigens, but they can no longer induce microbial agglutination, inhibit adherence, or perform other effector functions that depend upon an intact IgA molecule. The pathogenic role of IgA proteases is not clear, but essentially all important respiratory bacteria secrete them, and humans make antibodies that neutralize their activity, presumably in an effort to limit colonization and invasion.

At least two distinct neuraminidases are produced by pneumococci [65]. These enzymes remove terminal sialic acids from glycoconjugates on host cell surfaces, exposing underlying Glc-NAc-Gal determinants thought to be important in the adherence of pneumococci and other respiratory bacteria [66–68]. Cells of the choroid plexus and the central nervous system are heavily covered with sialic acid–rich surface structures. Alteration of these protective barriers may help explain the propensity of certain pneumococci for causing meningitis. Another much rarer disease associated with neuraminidase-producing pneumococci is a peculiar but devastating form of hemolytic uremic syndrome [69]. Neuraminidase secreted into the circulation exposes the T (Thomsen-Freidenreich) antigen on red blood cells, platelets, and glomeruli, inducing hemolysis, thrombocytopenia, and deposition of immune complexes. The extent to which this process may contribute to other severe pneumococcal infections is not known.

Hyaluronidase is produced by a majority of clinical pneumococcal isolates [62,70]. This enzyme appears to be more closely related to the hyaluronidase of group B streptococci than to the phage-mediated spreading factor of *Streptococcus pyogenes* [71]. The presumed pathogenic role is to facilitate colonization and promote translocation of organisms from tissues, such as the lung, to the vascular system.

Pneumococcal Surface Proteins

Pneumococcal surface protein A (PspA) is found on essentially all clinically important isolates [72,73]. PspA is a coiled protein that is quite variable among serotypes with respect to molecular size and antigenic epitopes but is genetically stable for any given strain. The surface location and its accessibility to antibodies has been demonstrated by immunogold electron microscopy [27]. PspA plays a role in virulence of pneumococci, and antibodies elicited to several of the more common epitopes protect mice from experimental infection [74]. Candidate PspA vaccines are under development and are further described in Chapter 22 and in a recent review [73]. A second protein, PspB, exhibits properties similar to those of the R antigen of group A streptococcus type 28. Antibodies to this protein were not protective in mice, and its physiologic role is uncertain [75].

Antibiotic Resistance

Penicillin kills pneumococci both by inhibiting cell wall synthesis and by triggering the autolytic activity of amidase. The mechanisms of resistance to penicillin and other β-lactam antibiotics have been reviewed elsewhere [27,76]. Development of resistance has been a slow process involving multiple transformation and recombination events [77]. Resistance requires both multiple subtle alterations in the enzymatic sites of the PBPs and complementary changes in the structures of stem peptides used to cross-link peptidoglycan. The changes in stem peptide utilization are metabolically costly to the organism [51], which may help explain the observation that resistance rates tend to reach some balance with the amount of exposure to penicillins in different localities [78]. At the genetic level some PBP genes have been shown to have regions in their nucleotide sequences that are strongly divergent, suggesting that they have been borrowed from other streptococcal species [77].

Vancomycin, teichoplanin, and related glycopeptides have two completely different mechanisms of action, the combination of which makes development of resistance extremely difficult [27,79]. Vancomycin binds reversibly but with high affinity to the stem peptides. This inhibits the transglycosylase that normally couples GlcNAc-MurNAc disaccharide subunits, preventing elongation of the peptidoglycan. It also hinders recognition of the stem peptides by the PBPs, thus interfering with the enzymatic reactions that cross-link peptidoglycan chains. Because peptidoglycans are cross-linked via a small number of available stem peptides, the concentration of vancomycin must be high enough to saturate most of the potential binding sites to be effective. This may provide an explanation for the importance of dosage and bioavailability in clinical use of this drug.

Pneumococcal resistance to chloramphenicol is attributed to an inducible acetyltransferase present alone or in association with multiple resistance factors. Alterations in dehydrofolate metabolism confer resistance to sulfonamides and trimethoprim-sulfamethoxazole (TMP-SMX) by yet undetermined mechanisms [76]. Resistance to some antibiotics can occur readily by simple deletions or mutations involving as few as a single nucleotide or one to several amino acid substitutions. Examples of this include rifampin, which inhibits RNA polymerase; streptomycin, which acts on ribosomes; and ciprofloxacin, which interferes with DNA gyrase [77]. Resistance to kanamycin, erythromycin, and tetracycline is encoded in a transposon [80]. Some newer quinolones are quite active against pneumococci, especially clinafloxacin, sparfloxacin, and trovofloxacin [81]. Clindamycin (related to lincomycin) and the newer macrolides are still effective against most strains in the United States, but up to 40% of highly penicillin-resistant pneumococci may be resistant to clarithromycin and azithromycin. Meropenem, one of several new carbapenem antibiotics, has recently been approved for treatment of meningitis and may be particularly useful against penicillin-resistant pneumococci [82].

Genetics

The pneumococcus has been a stellar contributor to the understanding of bacterial genetics, including the seminal discoveries of transformation and of DNA as the transforming principle—key concepts that opened the way for molecular biology [4]. Early genetic work revealed considerable evidence that the genes responsible for capsule production are closely linked on the chromosome and can be transferred as a functioning unit by genetic transformation [83]. Some aspects of the organization, function, and regulation of capsule genes were proposed decades ago. But only very recently have DNA sequencing and analysis of a few of these genes been published, including types 1, 3, 14, and 19F [83–87]. The interested reader should seek additional information in the proceedings of a recent symposium on streptococcal genetics [88].

The genes required for capsule biosynthesis are organized in a cassette-like cluster unique to a particular type and situated between flanking regions that are highly conserved among strains of all capsular types studied thus far. The type 3 capsule locus contains four genes: UDP-glucose dehydrogenase, polysaccharide synthetase, UTP-glucose-1-phosphate-uridyltransferase, and a phosphoglucomutase. The genes immediately upstream have not been identified. The gene just downstream may have a regulatory role affecting virulence. Both of these flanking elements could also be involved in recombination and transformation events affecting capsular type [83]. The type 19F capsule locus contains at least seven genes with functions deduced from sequence similarities with known enzymes of other bacterial species [87]. Also of note is that the capsule locus is located very close to the genes encoding PBP 2x and PBP 1a.

The genes encoding enzymes for the type 3 capsule appear to have little similarity in hybridization experiments to those from other types that also use glucuronic acid, e.g., 2, 5, 8, 9, and 22, suggesting that those types evolved independently of type 3. However, the type 3 locus has considerable sequence homology with the group A streptococcus hyaluronic acid (has) locus, which also includes genes for glucuronic acid in the capsule [83]. Several of the type 19F capsule genes are probably shared by a number of serologically unrelated pneumococcal types that may have some mechanisms of biosynthesis in common [87]. Four of the 19F genes had significant homology (46%–63% identity) with genes involved in the group B streptococcus type III capsule, along with similarities to genes from Bacillis subtilis and Rhizobium meliloti. Interspecies recombinational events have been postulated in the evolution of pbp2x and possibly pbp2b genes in penicillin-resistant pneumococci [77].

The extent to which horizontal transfer of capsular genes has contributed to the diversity of serotypes is unknown. Horizontal transfer of genes encoding PBP 2b has occurred several times as independent transformation events, giving rise to distinct classes of penicillin-resistant pneumococci [11,89]. Resistance is independent of serotype but is most common in groups/types 6, 14, 19, and 23, probably because these types are commonly carried by children and others who are exposed to frequent or unnecessary antibiotic treatments. One group of pbp2b genes originated in Papua, New Guinea, perhaps as early as the 1950s. These genes are now distributed worldwide and occur in strains of various serotypes, although most are in groups/types 6, 14, 19, and 23. They have developed considerable sequence diversity, whereas the pbp2b genes from sensitive strains are quite uniform [89]. In a more detailed study, the pbp2b genes were found to differ by up to 170 nucleotide substitutions, resulting in 38 amino acid substitutions but conserving several sequences essential for enzymatic activity [90]. A more recent pbp2b gene probably arose in Spain in the late 1970s, bearing mainly capsular types 6B and 23F. Although several distinct clones have been stable long enough for them to spread geographically [11,12], the population structure pneumococci is characterized by frequent horizontal genetic exchange, as recently shown in a study of the antigenic diversity of IgA1 protease [13]. Several factors favor genetic exchange among pneumococcal strains: carriage of more than one type occurs frequently in humans (up to 6% of colonization among infants less than 2 years of age [6]); pneumococci naturally autolyse, releasing DNA; and pneumococci are naturally competent for DNA uptake. Immune responses of the host and environmental pressures, such as use of antibiotics, no doubt foster antigenic and metabolic diversity in this genetically adept species.

PATHOGENESIS AND HOST DEFENSES

The pathogenesis of pneumococcal disease is a complex process of multiple interacting bacterial and host factors. Several excellent reviews provide further details, references, and speculation [45,52,55,62,91,92].

Most human encounters with pneumococci are essentially benign, and pathologic processes appear to begin innocently with adherence to epithelial cells of the host. Neuraminidases may aid the organisms in breaching the protective mucus layer and in uncovering specific receptors, which in turn aid in attachment directly to β-GalNAc-$(1 \rightarrow 3)$-β-Gal- or β-GalNAc-$(1 \rightarrow 4)$-β-Gal- on respiratory glycolipids [68, 93] or indirectly via a "sandwich" adhesin molecule [67]. In vitro studies of adherence have suggested that pneumococci isolated from the middle ear adhered more proficiently to human epithelial cells than strains isolated in cases of bacteremia or meningitis [94]. This notwithstanding, we also found in a study of pneumococci from infants with and without otitis media that the strains associated with otitis media did not have any special propensity for adherence compared to other nasopharyngeal isolates [66]. Adherence may be required for establishing and maintaining colonization, but this was not a property that distinguished between infecting strains and those associated with asymptomatic carriage.

Additional factors must be involved in determining whether a colonizing strain is able to breach mucosal defenses and cause disease. These might include concomitant viral infections causing local inflammation, impairment of macrophage function, dysfunction of ciliated epithelia, and impaired mucociliary transport. A role for viral–bacterial interaction involving these and other mechanisms has been well established in acute otitis media [95,96]. Inflammation and congestion of eustachian tube epithelia results in obstruction and failure to clear secretions from the middle ear. Bacteria from colonization sites in the nasopharynx become entrapped, multiply in the middle ear fluid, and may invade the submucosa producing further inflammation. Pneumococcal peptidoglycan and teichoic acid (C-polysaccharide) are the principle initiators of middle ear inflammation [53]. These cell wall breakdown products activate the alternative complement pathway, induce cytokines, and lead to recruitment of neutrophils. One presumes a similar course of events in the development of acute sinusitis.

The pathogenesis of pneumonia includes some of the mechanisms just described. In addition, an impaired cough reflex, anesthesia and narcotics, ethanol, smoking, chronic pulmonary diseases, and immune suppression, have all been noted in experimental and clinical pneumococcal pneumonia [16,62,91,97]. Classic pathologic descriptions of lobar pneumonia [91] begin with engorgement of alveoli by bacteria, which multiply and spread in the edema fluid. This is followed by "red hepatization," named for its resemblance to raw liver. Alveolar capillaries become congested, promoting the infiltration of erythrocytes and neutrophils, and deposition of fibrin within the alveoli. As exudate increases, capillaries are compressed, fewer red blood cells get into the alveoli, but neutrophils continue to accumulate, giving rise to "gray hepatization."

These overlapping stages are also present simultaneously in advancing disease: there is an outer edema zone containing numerous pneumococci in the edema fluid, a middle zone of early leukocytic infiltration, and an inner zone of consolidation with many phagocytes and no organisms [98]. If host defenses have succeeded in killing the pneumococci, resolution ensues with dissolution and removal of cells and fibrin from the alveoli, and the lung clears. This process is greatly enhanced by exogenous antibody or by the development of a timely antibody response.

It remains unclear how pneumococci gain entrance into the bloodstream to cause bacteremia [62]. In studies done in the 1930s, animals became bacteremic within minutes after intranasal challenge, suggesting that organisms can invade directly through the olfactory mucosa. Other experiments suggested that pneumococci from the nasopharynx first entered the submucosa and were picked up in the cervical lymphatics, where they multiplied and eventually entered the bloodstream. In experimental pneumonia pneumococci are rapidly cleared by the normal lung, but organisms that escape phagocytosis may go from the alveoli to the regional lymphatics and appear in the blood after 6 to 24 h [98]. Once in the circulation pneumococci are filtered out by the spleen and liver. Mice challenged intravenously clear their bacteremia quickly, but organisms that are able to multiply in the reticuloendothelial system eventually break out to cause a more sustained bacteremia some hours later.

Invasion of the blood-brain barrier is the least understood aspect of pneumococcal invasion. It has been shown in vitro that pneumococci attach to human umbilical vein endothelial cells, cause progressive widening of intracellular junctions, and preferentially adhere to the borders of separating cells on the monolayers [54]. The attachment may be blocked by pretreatment of monolayers with purified pneumococcal cell wall material, suggesting that cell wall components on the bacteria normally mediate adherence. Although endothelial cells are not professional phagocytes, some bacteria are taken up and are visible within cytoplasmic vacuoles. Cytopathic changes induced by the pneumococci could be attenuated by antibodies to IL-1 and TNF-α, implicating the response of host tissues in their own destruction. Other studies show that IL-1 and TNF-γ induce human endothelial cells to promote transendothelial passage of neutrophils. Platelet activating factor and IL-8 are released in response to IL-1 and may also affect neutrophil adhesion and diapedesis. IL-1 and TNF-α also induce expression of selectins and other adhesion molecules on the neutrophils. Presumably, events of this kind are operating in the choroid plexus and other areas where bacteria are thought to sneek through the blood-brain barrier [52].

Once pneumococci have entered the meninges, they multiply to about 10^5 bacteria per ml, in a rabbit model, before clinical symptoms are apparent [55,99]. The inflammatory response begins as pneumococci die and release cell-wall, pneumolysin, and other components. The degree of inflammation and course of disease varies depending on the infecting strain or serotype, probably because of differences in virulence, cell wall metabolism, and the capacity for inciting inflammation. When pneumococci are killed rapidly by treatment with penicillin, their breakdown products provoke release of IL-1 and TNF, resulting in an intense inflammatory response. As described by Tuomanen, "bacterial corpses do not kill directly; instead they stir the body into a self-destructive frenzy that leads to the symptoms and consequences of disease" [55]. The inflammatory responses provoke the generation of oxygen intermediates in the microvasculature, causing an initial increase cerebral blood flow. Later in the course of disease, cerebral blood flow is diminished by cerebral edema and by the increasing intercranial pressure. The cerebral vasculature eventually loses its normal autoregulatory functions, at which point cerebral blood flow fluctuates directly with the arterial blood pressure and becomes especially sensitive to underperfusion by hypovolemia or lowered blood pressure [52].

Adjunctive therapies, such as administration of steroids and supportive care to maintain euvolemia and adequate cerebral blood flow, are directed toward blocking or compensating for the pathophysiologic responses of the host [52]. Dexamethasone given prior to or at the time of antibiotic administration in experimental animals reduces release of CSF IL-1 but not TNF, and this has also been observed in human dis-

ease. Unfortunately, for reasons that are not entirely clear, this does not translate directly into clinical practice, and adjunctive steroid therapy remains controversial, as discussed below. Nonsteroidal anti-inflammatory drugs, such as indomethacin, reduce cerebral edema but not inflammation. Targeting the adhesion-promoting receptors of the neutrophil with monoclonal antibodies to the CD18 integrin molecule reduced inflammation and brain edema and improved survival in rabbits [55]. In the same vein, mortality in a pig model of septicemia was associated with high levels of IL-6, whereas mortality was zero in pigs pretreated with a monocyte activator that prevented the rise in IL-6 [100]. These are useful research tools, but it is still uncertain if similar strategies can be applied to humans.

It has been known for years that nonspecific host-defense mechanisms play a critical protective role, including the mucus blanket covering respiratory epithelia, the mucociliary clearance of bacteria and debris, and the cough reflex. Pulmonary macrophages, and probably tissue macrophages, are capable of trapping and killing virulent pneumococci in the absence of antibody and with little or no participation of complement. Nonspecific opsonins may include fibronectin, human pulmonary surfactant protein, and C-reactive protein (CRP). CRP is an acute-phase protein that binds to phosphoryl choline determinants of pneumococci and other bacteria and to damaged host cell surfaces. It activates the classical complement pathway and promotes phagocytosis [101]. Exogenous human CRP can protect mice from pneumococcal challenge, but its role in defense against human pneumococcal infection is probably limited. It should be noted that experimental models reveal striking differences among animal species [102]. Rabbits clear aerosolized pneumococci from the lungs almost as fast as they are deposited, phagocytizing and killing them intracellularly. Rats also clear pneumococci quickly, but killing is slower and occurs at the outside surface of the macrophage. Humans appear to be more like rabbits in this respect. Animal models of bacteremia also show that the spleen and liver clear pneumococci from the blood much more efficiently in the presence of type-specific opsonization, and that higher antibody levels are necessary in the absence of a functioning spleen. In humans the risk for over-whelming pneumococcal sepsis is greatly increased by splenectomy or by the functional asplenia of sickle cell disease [103,104].

The major defense against pneumococcal infection is acknowledged to be the combined activity of type-specific anticapsular antibody and complement (opsonization), followed by efficient phagocytosis and killing by neutrophils [45]. Humoral immunity was extensively studied in humans and laboratory animals in the years before penicillin [2]. Investigators focused mainly on the curative and protective aspects of antibody function. The role of the capsular polysaccharide in evoking type-specific immunity was established by the early 1930s, and protection against bacterial challenge was demonstrated in animals with either active immunization or passive administration of antibody. Exogenous antibody was efficacious in curing experimental pneumonias, and the application of this approach to human disease, using horse or rabbit antisera, was quite well developed just prior to World War II [2,105].

Antibodies begin to appear in the serum of adults about 7 days after immunization or natural infection. Older studies found that two-thirds of adults and about a quarter of infants and children made responses after recovering from pneumococcal pneumonia [2,106]. A recent study of two pneumonia outbreaks in military camps found that most infected individuals made antibody to the infecting serotype and that type-specific responses also occurred in one-third to two-thirds of recruits with asymptomatic colonization, depending upon the serotype involved [107]. Children under 2 years of age are known to respond poorly to pneumococcal infection or immunization, especially against such types as 6, 19, and 23. Type 3 strains and a few other types evoke much better responses [38, 108–111]. Serotypic differences in response may be related to the patterns of complement deposition and degradation [41]. The slow development of immune responsiveness may be related to delayed maturation of certain B cell populations [45]. Responses to pneumococcal and other polysaccharides are commonly described as thymus-independent, because T helper function is not required, as in responses to protein antigens. One characteristic of T-independent

antigens exemplified by pneumococcal polysaccharides is failure to induce a booster effect after revaccination. Still, antibody levels may persist for 6 to 10 years after primary immunization [112]. In contrast, pneumococcal vaccines composed of polysaccharide coupled to a protein carrier behave more like T-dependent antigens and evoke good responses in infants [113,114].

Young children have little antibody against common pneumococcal types, compared to adolescents [110]. Young adults may have antibody to a limited number of types but make responses to about 75% of types after immunization with the 23-valent vaccine. IgM and IgG antibodies appear at about the same time, but IgM levels typically remain rather low, whereas IgG continues to rise, peaking 4 to 12 weeks later [112]. The level of vaccine-induced antibody required for protection against invasive disease in humans has not been determined, but most instances of vaccine failure occur at levels below 2 μg/ml (300 ng antibody nitrogen/ml) [115].

Data on IgG subclass responses have been varied and often conflicting, perhaps because of differences among IgG subclass reagents and the small numbers of subjects tested against a very few pneumococcal serotypes. The predominant response seems to be in the IgG2 subclass, but IgG1 and IgG3 figure prominently in several investigations [45,116,117]. Opsonization also appears to favor IgG2 antibodies. Studies of twins suggest that the level of antibody response is under genetic control, with high correlations of IgG2 levels for homozygous twins of certain G2m allotypes [118].

Little is known about the role of mucosal immunity in human colonization or disease. Type-specific anticapsular antibodies have been detected in saliva and at low levels in human milk, but there is no apparent relationship between these antibody levels and colonization or development of otitis media in infants [119,120]. Mucosal responses may be induced independently of a systemic response, and type-specific secretory IgA antibodies may appear as early as 6 months of age in nasal secretions of infants with pneumococcal otitis media [121]. The primacy of the mucosal response is further supported by the detection of specific IgA-secreting B cells in the peripheral blood of infants soon after onset of pneumococcal otitis media [122]. Secretory antibodies probably play a role in modulating adherence and preventing colonizing pneumococci from invasion at the mucosal surface.

EPIDEMIOLOGY

The pneumococci are considered part of the normal flora of the human upper respiratory tract and may be cultured from the nasopharynx of 5%–10% of healthy adults and 40%–50% of healthy infants under 2 year of age. Asymptomatic colonization with a given serotype may persist for a year or more, but the duration of carriage decreases with age and thus tends to be longer in children than adults [2,6,123]. Colonization rates fluctuate somewhat during the year with a modest decrease during the summer months. Pneumococci spread relatively slowly among family members and among children in day-care settings, usually without the development of more than occasional isolated infections [124,125]. Nevertheless, invasive disease is more frequent among infants attending day care and among children with other siblings [126]. Outbreaks of pneumococcal disease are unusual but do occur in day-care centers, military training centers, overcrowded jails, and similar settings [127–129]. A uniquely human pathogen, pneumococci rarely colonize or cause disease in laboratory rodents, primates, and horses [130,131]. Animals are not a reservoir or vector but rather appear to acquire pneumococci accidentally from their human caretakers.

In temperate climates the exchange and acquisition of new types increase dramatically during the winter and early spring. This also corresponds with the seasonal occurrence of viral respiratory disease, which may play a role in facilitating spread of respiratory bacteria [132]. Otitis media in children is strongly seasonal, with most cases occurring from November through May; the seasonal component is less pronounced in the occurrence of bacteremia and meningitis [133]. The most striking seasonal feature is perhaps not so much a seasonal peak as a summer nadir, also observed in a recent study from Houston [134]. In that investigation modest but statistically significant correlations were found for association of invasive pneumococcal disease with the occurrence of respiratory viruses and SO_2 levels as an index of air pollution. The association with viral respiratory illnesses was less marked for children and subject to a 4-week lag period. In children, but not adults, invasive disease was also associated with ragweed pollen counts.

Colonization rates do not correlate well with attack rates; however, seasonal attack rates do follow rates of acquisition, defined as the onset of colonization by a new serotype [6]. Hodges and MacLeod, studying epidemic pneumonia at an Air Force training school, found and that new recruits became colonized by the "epidemic" types prevalent on the base within 4 to 6 weeks of arrival. This coincided with the time of onset of pneumonia from the newly acquired strains [127]. Children in our prospective study frequently carried pneumococci for long periods of time. Regardless of serotype, infections (mainly otitis media) were seldom caused by strains associated with prolonged carriage but were usually due to new types that were acquired within the preceding month [6]. In these studies, pneumococci did not appear to be opportunistic in the sense that disease would develop from any pneumococcus that happens to reside in one's nasopharynx; rather, infections were mostly due to new strains with which the host had had little previous immunologic experience.

Such a close relationship between acquisition and infection was not observed by Smith et al. among Papua New Guinea children, who frequently developed bacteremia due to pneumococci. These children were exposed to less common, more virulent serotypes (e.g., 1, 2, 5, 7, and 16) and also had constant, very heavy colonization by the less virulent childhood types (e.g., 6, 19, and 23) [135]. There is some evidence that pneumococci act more opportunistically in elderly adults, 80% of whom have some factor predisposing them to pneumonia [16,17]. Opportunism is also suggested by the high frequency of adults with pneumococcal pneumonia who had recently undergone endotracheal intubation [136]. Environmental conditions and perturbations of the hosts may thus push the balance in favor of disease.

Most pneumococcal infections occur in otherwise healthy infants younger than 2 years of age or in adults older than 65 years of age. Recent population-based studies of pneumococcal bacteremia in the United States reveal the following approximate age-specific attack rates per 100,000 population: infants <1 year, 160–180; children 1–5 years, 40–60; young adults 20–55 years, 5–10; and elderly adults >65 years, 50–80 [137–139]. Within these populations, however, attack rates among African Americans were 4 to 5 times higher than among white Americans. The effect of race could not be removed by controlling for socioeconomic status by census tract income data [137], although differences in access to health care, crowding, associated underlying conditions, and other environmental and biological factors remain possible explanations [138]. Even larger discrepancies have been reported among Alaskan populations, where Native children <2 years of age have bacteremia rates of 624 per 100,000, and among Apache children in Arizona, where rates are 1800 per 100,000 [140]. The highest contemporary attack rates have been reported among Australian Aborigines, with 1025 per 100,000 <5 years of age and >2000 per 100,000 for infants younger than 24 months [141].

Persons with underlying host defense problems are at increased risk for pneumococcal disease, especially those with asplenia, hypogammaglobulinemia, and deficiency of early complement factors (C2, C3, factor I) [91,142]. The risks from splenectomy and the functional asplenia of sickle cell disease are now well appreciated [103,104]. Case fatality rates of 43% have been reported for adult sickle cell disease patients with pneumococcal bacteremia [143]. Pneumococci are the most common cause of serious bacterial infection among HIV-infected children [144]. Rates of bacteremia in adults with HIV infection are about 100 times that of the age-matched population [145]. Pneumococcal pneumonia may be the first manifestation in up to half of HIV-infected adults, and HIV infection was found subsequently in 70% of those under 40 years of age presenting with pneumococcal pneumonia [146].

The distribution of serotypes causing infections are similar throughout the United States, including Alaska and Arizona, and do not differ much from that in most industrialized countries. Infants are infected by a limited number of serotypes that are commonly carried in childhood (e.g., groups/types 6, 14, 19, and 23), whereas older children and adults are less frequently colonized but over time are exposed to and infected by a broader range of strains, some of which have been described as "adult" or "epidemic" serotypes (e.g., groups/types 1, 3, 4, 7, 8, and 12). The distribution of types varies to some extent with disease syndrome and site of infection [142]. This is illustrated in Table 17.3, showing types observed in children with meningitis, bacteremia, and otitis media over a 15-year period in Birmingham, Alabama [133,142,147]. Group 6 (types 6A + 6B) was by far the leading cause of meningitis with 28% of cases, and the five groups/types—6, 14, 18, 19, and 23—accounted for about 70% of all cases of bacteremia or meningitis. The same types were common in otitis media, but group 19 was by far the leading offender with 29%. Types 1 and 4 were especially common in cases of bacteremic pneumonia. The serotypes causing disease in this one community were remarkably similar to those seen in the U.S. as a whole [9]. The distribution of types in adult disease, compiled from various other studies (see Table 17.3), show a wider variety of types with none accounting for more than about 10% of the total.

The 23 types listed in Table 17.2 are those included in the current pneumococcal polysaccharide vaccine and could potentially protect against 86% of adult infections. The protein-conjugated polysaccharide vaccines under investigation in children currently contain seven types (4, 6B, 9V, 14, 18C, 19F, and 23F), potentially covering up to 80% of childhood infection (assuming cross-protection against all types within groups).

There is a strong though still poorly understood association of respiratory viral infections and pneumococcal disease [127,130]. An important part of this may have to do with facilitating the spread and acquisition of strains, but viral infection may also favor the pneumococcus by altering cell surfaces, phagocyte function, and other features of normal host-defense mechanisms.

Table 17.3 Serotype Distribution of Pneumococci Causing Meningitis, Bacteremia, and Otitis Media in Children in Birmingham, Alabama, 1975–1989,[a] and Serotypes in Adult Infections[b]

Groups/ Types[c]	Infections in Children[a]			Infections[b] in Adults (N = 281)
	Meningitis (N = 12)	Bacteremia (N = 521)	Otitis Media (N = 1411)	
1	—	3	2	2
2	—	—	1	<1
3	3	<1	9	11
4	6	5	3	11
5	—	<1	<1	2
6	28	18	13	5
7	2	<1	2	4
8	2	<1	1	7
9	4	7	5	8
10	4	<1	1	1
11	1	<1	2	3
12	2	1	<1	2
14	12	25	12	4
15	—	<1	3	6
17	—	<1	1	3
18	11	10	3	3
19	7	12	29	4
20	—	—	<1	3
22	—	<1	1	3
23	13	7	12	4
33	1	<1	<1	3
Included in 23-valent vaccine (%)[c]	94	95	96	86
Included in 7-valent vaccine (%)[c]	80	85	77	40

[a]Compiled from three reports from Birmingham, Alabama, 1975–1989 [133,142,147]

[b]Compiled from five reports [15,16,18,21,24] in Hager et al. [196].

[c]Groups/types not subtyped; percentages of types included in vaccines assumes the possibility of cross-reactive protection.

CLINICAL MANIFESTATIONS OF PNEUMOCOCCAL DISEASE

There is no particular disease process that can be described as uniquely characteristic of the pneumococcus. True, pneumococcal pneumonia has earned the adjective "classical," but other organisms are well known to cause pneumonia with the same presenting signs, symptoms, and radiological features. Similarly, pneumococcal otitis media, sinusitis, and meningitis share clinical manifestations with infections due to other predominantly respiratory bacteria. From the clinician's point of view, the pneumococcus may be the best bet in many situations, but an etiologic diagnosis and antibiotic susceptibility testing is requisit to optimal management of the patient. A diagnosis is relatively straightforward when cultures are positive from blood, CSF, or other normally sterile sites. It is considerably more difficult in nonbactreremic pneumonia, otitis media, and sinusitis, or when cultures have been compromised by prior administration of antibiotics.

Pneumonia, Pleural Effusion, and Empyema

Pneumonia is the classical disease caused by the pneumococcus, and in the era before the advent of antibiotics, this organism accounted for about 80% of cases. Although a pneumococcal etiology can be confirmed in only 10%–15% of adults and about 25% of children with pneumonia, a recent analysis of 122 reports published between 1966 and 1995 found that pneumococci accounted for two-thirds of more than 7000 cases for which an etiological diagnosis could be determined and for two-thirds of pneumonia-related deaths [148].

Historically, morbidity and mortality were always highest in older adults and lowest in children. This could probably be accounted for in part by the lower virulence of the common "childhood" serotypes (6, 14, 19, and 23), compared to the "epidemic types" seen in adults (1, 2, 4, 5, 7, 8, and 12) [142]. Up to a third of children with pneumococcal bacteremia have pneumonia, but the best estimates suggest that only about 1 in 10 children with pneumococcal pneumonia is bacteremic. Bacteremia also occurs in 15%–25% of adults with pneumonia; these patients tend to have lobar consolidations and generally have a worse outcome than those who present with bronchopneumonia [17,136].

Mortality from uncomplicated pneumonia is low among outpatients, but adults admitted to the hospital have a mortality rate of 10%–25%. The best indicators of a poor outcome, as validated in a pneumonia prognostic index, are age >65 years, pleuritic chest pain, vital sign abnormalities, altered mental status, associated neoplastic disease, and high-risk bacterial etiology, especially pneumococcus, *Legionella*, and *Staphylococcus aureus* [18,149]. As noted below, cases complicated by bacteremia and other risk factors have a poorer prognosis.

The likelihood of a pneumococcal etiology varies, depending on the circumstances of infection. Clinically, pneumonias are divided into three major categories: community-acquired pneumonia, hospital-acquired pneumonia, and ventilator-associated pneumonia, known respectively as CAP, HAP, and VAP [18,19]. A pneumococcal etiology can be confirmed in about 15% of CAP cases, but this is considered an underestimate because of the difficulty of assigning a cause in a large proportion of pneumonias. Pneumococci are less frequent but included among the "core" organisms in HAP, especially in cases diagnosed within 5 days of hospital admission. Pneumococci are not as common in VAP, but a fair number of adults with pneumococcal pneumonia are noted to have been recently intubated for either anesthesia or respiratory arrest [136]. There are scant data on VAP in children. It does not appear that endotracheal

intubation itself substantially increases the risk of pneumococcal disease in healthy children undergoing elective procedures, but pneumonia or bacteremia occasionally occur after intubation of debilitated or critically ill children, possibly because children have a high rate of asymptomatic colonization, which is disturbed during intubation.

Patients with pneumococcal pneumonia are usually ill-appearing with symptoms of fever and cough productive of sputum. Most patients will have an increased respiratory rate out of proportion to fever or lung involvement, and most will have crackles (râles) on auscultation. A hyperacute (sometimes called "classic") presentation begins with an episode of shaking chills, followed later by sustained fevers, cough, and production of purulent rust- or blood-tinged sputum. This is typical of older children and young adults with lobar consolidations. In older adults the disease is more often insidious, developing over several days, even without much fever, sputum production, or more than minimal cough. The most common associated or predisposing factors in adult pneumonias are preexisting pulmonary disease, smoking, alcoholism, heart disease, malignancy, and diabetes mellitus [17,136]. Chest pain may suggest empyema or extension to visceral pleura, but pleural effusions do not produce respiratory embarrassment unless they become quite large. Pneumonias adjacent to the diaphragm may present with vomiting and abdominal pain before pulmonary symptoms become apparent. Upper lobe pneumonias can be associated with neck pain or meningismus, sometimes accompanied by cerebrospinal pleocytosis in the absence of positive bacterial or viral cultures [150]. Although it is a common practice to obtain a chest X-ray on febrile infants evaluated for possible sepsis, the yield of positive radiographs is extremely low in the absence of pulmonary findings on history or physical examination [151].

Radiographic findings in hospitalized patients with pneumococcal pneumonia reveal classic segmental or lobar infiltrates in only about 40% of patients, while most will have a bronchopneumonic pattern characterized by multifocal patchy air space shadows [136]. Lobar or segmental consolidations are more frequent in previously healthy young adults and are more often associated with bacteremia. Most infiltrates involve less than a full segment, beginning peripherally, sometimes with a typical round lesion expanding to adjacent areas. Although few clinicians claim to be able to reliably distinguish bacterial from viral pneumonias by X-rays alone, some generalities are often made. Pneumococcal infiltrates are characteristically unilateral and occupy contiguous alveolar areas (air space disease) with little change in overall lung volume. Infiltrates associated with viral infection usually involve bronchioles and surrounding interstitial tissue (airway disease), giving rise to a more diffuse pattern on X-ray, often with some hyperexpansion. In a study of pneumonias in children, a pattern of alveolar infiltration was a good predictor of bacterial, mainly pneumococcal pneumonia. However, a diffuse interstitial pattern was not very good at predicting viral pneumonias. About half of these cases appeared to have a bacterial or mixed viral–bacterial etiology, reinforcing the importance of other clinical and laboratory findings when making decisions concerning antibiotic therapy [152].

Pneumococcal pneumonias often present with an associated pleural effusion, but only about 1 in 10 are large enough to require drainage, and fewer still develop empyema. Because the pleural fluid may yield a definitive diagnosis, most clinicians recommend diagnostic thoracentesis, especially if there is >10 mm of effusion on a lateral dicubitus radiograph or if the patient appears toxic. The presence of pleural fluid on X-ray may be confirmed, if necessary, with ultrasound [17].

Pneumococcal empyema is an uncommon but serious complication in adults and children [153,154]. Differentiation from pleural thickening and lung abscess has been greatly facilitated by ultrasound and computed tomography (CT). Empyemas rarely resolve without both antibiotic and surgical intervention. Chest tube drainage is the mainstay of therapy; intrapleural infusion of thrombolytics, such as urokinase, is often used adjunctively in adults. When this fails, thoracotomy and decortication may be needed, although video-assisted thorascopic methods are now being used as alternative approaches to this problem. Necrotizing pneumococcal pneumonias with lobar liquification or lung abscess may also

be difficult to detect radiographically but are easily diagnosed on CT. A possible role for anaerobic bacteria has been suggested in such cases, but anaerobes have been isolated concomitantly in only a few reported cases. In contrast to the high morbitity and mortality in adults, complete recovery is usually anticipated in children with necrotizing pneumococcal pneumonia [155].

Otitis Media and Sinusitis

Acute otitis media, defined by fluid in the middle ear space accompanied by signs of acute illness, is the most frequent bacterial infection in childhood [96]. Diagnosis is made most reliably using pneumatic otoscopy, which allows the clinician to assess not only the color and degree of translucency of the ear drum but also its position and mobility. Too often the finding of a red ear in a screaming child is used merely as an excuse to prescribe antibiotics. A bulging or immobile opaque drum usually yields a definitive diagnosis upon myringotomy or typmanocentesis. Pneumococci account for 40% to 50% of cases for which an etiology can be assigned on the basis of middle ear cultures. Other important organisms are *Hemophilus influenzae* and *Moraxella* (*Branhamella*) *catarrhalis* and occasionally group A streptococci. Over the past several years, penicillin-resistant pneumococci have become an increasing cause of therapeutic failures [156]. Even when the acute infection is controlled by antibiotic treatment, residual middle ear fluid may persist for weeks or months, causing few symptoms other than mild to moderate conductive hearing loss. This condition, known as otitis media with effusion (OME), may be associated with delay in speech development and lower scores on test of cognitive ability. Acute otitis media in adults is caused by the same organisms as those seen in childhood [157].

Sinusitis may be classified as acute (symptoms for <1 month), subacute (1 to 3 months), or chronic (>3 months) [158]. Pneumococcus and *H. influenzae* account for about 70% of isolates from maxillary sinus punctures in acute and subacute cases. Clinical diagnosis is often difficult, especially in young children and when ethmoid and sphenoid sinuses may be involved. Conventional X-ray views are most helpful when the sinuses are normal. Mucosal thickening (>5 mm) is a sensitive but not particulary specific finding in maxillary or frontal sinusitis confirmed by culture, but only about 60% of patients will have opacification or air-fluid levels. Computed tomography (CT) is not generally recommended for diagnosis in primary care settings because mucosal abnormalities are frequently revealed even in the absence of symptoms or suspicion of sinus disease.

Bacteremia and Sepsis

Bacteremia, the finding of organisms in the bloodstream, may be associated incidentally with mild disease or may reflect serious uncontrolled infection. Sepsis connotes severe disease adversely affecting multiple organ systems. Bacteremia and sepsis are proportionately more common and more lethal in patients with underlying conditions. In otherwise normal children no focus of infection is found in up to half of bacteremic children [126,142,147,159]. About a quarter of bacteremias are associated with otitis media. Another third occur in conjunction with pneumonia or other discrete focal infections, such as arthritis, cellulitis, or peritonitis. With the exception of occasional reports of fulminant pneumococcal sepsis with hemorrhagic shock [160], pneumococcal bacteremia is surprisingly well tolerated in children. When recalled to the clinic because of a positive blood culture, as many as 10% to 20% may have a negative repeat blood culture, prior to antibiotic administration.

In contrast, adults with pneumococcal bacteremia have average fatality rates of 20% to 35%. The mortality rates increase with age and do not appear to have improved over the past half century [139,143]. The vast majority of adult bacteremias are associated with pneumonia, and less than 10% of cases have no apparent focus of infection. Important risk factors include alcoholism, malignancy, HIV infection, sickle cell disease, and asplenia. Outcome is worst for patients with low body temperature, leukopenia, thrombocytopenia, and low blood pressure.

Meningitis

The pneumococcus accounts for about a third of all community-acquired meningitis in adults [161], and probably for at least as much in children in localities where infection due to *H. influenzae* type b has been reduced by immunization. Most cases of meningitis are thought to develop from blood-borne infection with bacteria probably entering via the choroid plexus. A few cases are associated with direct communications with middle ear, mastoids, sinuses, orbits, and areas affected by trauma or fractures. This is especially true in patients with recurrent meningitic infections. One of the record holders is a child who had 19 episodes of meningitis before a CSF leak was found: pneumococci were recovered in 6 of 11 episodes in which bacteria were isolated from the CSF [162]. Although some patients may have concurrent otitis media, most are also bacteremic, and autopsy studies have rarely revealed evidence of direct extension from the middle ear.

The typical clinical presentation with fever, stiff neck, and changes in mental status occurs in about two-thirds of adult cases [161,163]. Elderly patients may present insidiously with lethargy, obtundation, little or no fever, and varying degrees of meningismus. Infants often have little or no meningismus, and only about a third develop a bulging fontanelle, usually late in the course of illness. They generally have vague nonspecific symptoms, such as irritability, lethargy, crying, vomiting, and seizures. Focal neurologic deficits involving cranial nerves are relatively uncommon, and papilledema is quite rare. In such cases a CT scan may be warranted to rule out a mass lesion, prior to performing a lumbar puncture, but antibiotic therapy should nevertheless be started without delay [163].

The diagnosis of meningitis depends on examination and culture of the CSF [163,164]. Pleocytosis is present in nearly all cases in school age children and adults; the few patients with low or normal CSF white cell counts in the face of bacteria on the Gram stain generally have a poor prognosis. Some infants, up to several months of age, may have little or delayed pleocytosis.

Although some patients may show an initial preponderance of lymphocytes on the differential count, most (86%) will shift to predominantly neutrophils within 48 h. The total white cell count generally increases somewhat during the first 24 to 48 h of antibiotic therapy, then declines. However, inflammatory markers may be altered by early treatment with dexamethasone. The CSF protein is usually elevated initially (>100 mg/dl) even in the absence of significant pleocytosis. Hypoglycorrhachia is also a common but less reliable finding. Partial treatment with oral antibiotics given prior to the lumbar puncture rarely interferes with the interpretation CSF parameters. Although culture results may sometimes be compromised, the Gram stain and antigen detection tests may still be positive.

Other Pneumococcal Infections

The capacity of pneumococci for infecting almost any tissue or organ system has been observed from the pre-antibiotic era [2]. Most large medical centers will occasionally see a case of pneumococcal endocarditis, pericarditis, endophthalmitis, epiglottitis, or soft tissue infection [165–167]. Although such infections occur in normal hosts, unusual infections with this organism are often associated with immunocompromising conditions, such as systemic lupus erythematosis, malignancy, or HIV infection. Osteomyelitis and septic arthritis have remained fairly common infections in children [168] and are sometimes seen in adults with prosthetic joints or rheumatoid arthritis. The pneumococcus causes about 8% of spontaneous peritonitis in adults, mainly in association with liver disease [169], but in children peritonitis is more often associated with nephrotic syndrome [170]. Peritonitis can also be associated with tubo-ovarian abscess [171] and other infections of the female genital tract [172]. Pneumococcal sepsis in neonates, noted sporadically, is essentially indistinguishable from the more common infections caused by group B streptococci [172,173]. A rare but serious complication of pneumococcal infection is a form of hemolytic uremic syndrome (described above in the section on enzymes) that results from alterations of human cell-surface antigens by the action of pneumococcal neuraminidases [174].

TREATMENT

The most common pneumococcal infections, pneumonia and otitis media, are usually treated empirically, except for the occasional patient with a positive blood, ear, or sputum culture. The selection of antibiotics is influenced by the possibility of other bacterial causes, the severity of illness, age, and underlying disorders [149,175,176]. Several recent reviews address these problems in detail [177–179], and the Infectious Diseases Society of America (IDSA) has issued a comprehensive management guideline for community-acquired pneumonia (CAP) [18]. Whereas the IDSA emphasizes efforts to obtain an etiologic diagnosis, the American Thoracic Society (ATS) is more empirical, but both arrive at similar recommendations for initial treatment of adult outpatients with pneumonia: erythromycin or one of the newer macrolides, with tetracycline being the alternative drug. The assumption is that the macrolide will cover hemophilus, legionella, and mycoplasma, in addition to the pneumococcus. The British Thoracic Society bases their recommendations on essentially the same data but prefers amoxicillin or ampicillin, with erythromycin as an alternative if legionella or mycoplasma are specifically suspected. When penicillin-resistant pneumococci are suspected, a floroquinolone may be more appropriate. In more severe cases, and in hospitalized or older patients, both societies recommend a second- or third-generation cephalosporin, with various alternative options, depending on suspected etiologies. A definitive diagnosis of pneumococcal pneumonia makes the selection of a penicillin or cephalosporin much easier. Although β-lactam resistance is now common, resistant pneumococci do not appear to be associated with any increase in mortality among patients treated with penicillin G or ampicillin [175]. The same has been shown for bacteremic children with nonmeningitic illnesses [176,180]. In most of these cases pneumococci had penicillin or cephalosporin MICs of ≤ 2 μg/ml, which is easily surpassed in lung tissue and blood. However, prospective efficacy trials have yet to be done, and it is not known how effective the same antibiotics are for pneumonias due to strains with MICs of ≥ 4 μg/ml. For this reason many authorities now advocate use or addition of alternative drugs, such as vancomycin or imepenem, when resistant pneumococci are encountered.

Acute otitis media is also treated empirically, usually with oral antibiotics selected on the basis of known common pathogens and their susceptibilities [96]. In addition to the pneumococcus, therapy is directed to nontypable *H. influenzae* and *M. catarrhalis*. The latter two species are frequently β-lactamase producers, but they pose less of a clinical problem in that they are rarely associated with systemic disease. Despite the occurrence of various resistant organisms, amoxicillin remains the drug of choice because of its general efficacy, acceptability and safety, and low cost [96,178]. Patients who do not respond to initial therapy may require another antibiotic or a diagnostic tympanocentesis for culture and sensitivity. Cefuroxime axetil and cefprozil have activity against many penicillin-intermediate pneumococci and are considered better by in vitro testing than loracarbef, cefpodoxime, cefterbutin, and cefixime. However, most efficacy studies show little difference among treatment regimens, in part because otitis media may resolve spontaneously in about half of cases caused by hemophili and a fifth of those caused by pneumococci [96]. Penicillin-intermediate and -resistant pneumococci are frequently recovered from middle ear aspirations in cases after an initial treatment failure [156]. In a small number of patients, efficacies of about 70% were observed for a second round of therapy using amoxicillin at higher dosage (80 mg/kg/day), amoxicillin/clavulanate, clindamycin, or parenteral ceftriaxone (50 mg/kg daily for 3 to 5 days) [156,181]. Trimethoprim-sulfamethoxazole has become less useful because of increased resistance, and success with erythromycin-sulfonamide combinations seems to depend more on the macrolide component. Azithromycin is now coming into wider use, but many penicillin-resistant pneumococci are also resistant to this drug as well.

Therapy for meningitis is more difficult because initial treatment must take into account the possibility of penicillin-resistant pneumococci, as well as other pathogens. Definitive therapy is complicated by the poor penetration of most agents into the CSF [182] and by even poorer penetration of some antibiotics when

dexamethasone is used adjunctively to reduce inflammation [163,178]. When pneumococci are known to be sensitive, penicillin G and ampicillin remain the drugs of choice. For historical reasons, recommended dosages have not always been equivalent, and relatively low penicillin doses are still listed in many textbooks. Penicillin G is commonly measured in international units (1595 units = 1 mg); thus 100,000 units is about 63 mg, and 300,000–600,000 units/kg/day is roughly equivalent to ampicillin doses of 200–400 mg/kg/day. Potassium penicillin G has 1.7 mEq K+ per million units, which may have to be figured into fluid and electrolyte orders. Sodium penicillin or ampicillin may be used instead. The usual maximum or adult doses are 24 million units (15 g) for penicillin G and 12 g for ampicillin, but higher doses have been used.

At present there is no completely satisfactory recommendation for empirical or definitive treatment of meningitis due to multiresistant pneumococci. Ceftriaxone or cefotaxime are currently preferred, despite occasional reports of treatment failures [163,178]. Cefotaxime doses in the range of 250–350 mg/kg/day have been used successfully. In localities where cephalosporin resistance (MIC >1 μg/ml) has become common, the addition of vancomycin or rifampin has also been advocated. Patients infected with a strain showing reduced sensitivity to penicillins or cephalosporins should have a repeat lumbar puncture done 24 to 48 h into therapy to confirm sterilization of the CSF. Repeating the lumbar puncture should also be done for any patient not responding as expected, regardless of the antibiotic susceptibility results.

Pneumococci remain susceptible to vancomycin, but vancomycin penetrates poorly and unpredictably into the CSF, even when meninges are inflamed [182]. The practice of monitoring serum concentrations has been challenged, because vancomycin levels have never been shown to correlate with either clinical efficacy or reduction in possible toxic side effects [183]. Current vancomycin preparations do not have significant oto- or nephrotoxicity, but the "red man syndrome," characterized by erythema and pruritis, occasionally occurs when the drug is administered too rapidly. Controlled experience with vancomycin for pneumococcal is quite limited, and it is not certain if concomitant use of dexamethasone may have contributed to treatment failures by reducing inflammation and entry of vancomycin into the CSF [163].

Combination therapies and other antibiotics have been used on the basis of case reports or animal experiments. Cefotaxime or ceftriaxone plus vancomycin has been recommended for use in children, with or without adjunctive treatment with dexamethasone [178]. Ceftriaxone plus rifampin has been preferred in adults [52], but there are no controlled studies to confirm this recommendation. Although imipenem/cilastatin also penetrates poorly into CSF, several patients have been successfully treated with doses up to 400 mg/kg/day. The major problem with imipenem is the increased frequency of seizures, but it may sometimes be difficult to distinguish drug-induced seizures from those associated with the underlying meningitis. Meropenem, a new carbapenem with fewer side effects, has recently been approved for treatment of meningitis, but published experience remains sparse [82]. Cefapime is a broad-spectrum cephalosporin with properties similar to those of cefotaxime and ceftriaxone, but there is little experience treating meningitis due to penicillin-resistant pneumococci [178].

Resistance to chloramphenicol is uncommon, but treatment failures have occurred, especially in parts of the world where use of the drug is widespread. Anecdotal evidence has found the clinical efficacy of chloramphenicol to be fair to poor, and it is not generally recommended for pneumococcal meningitis [76,163,178].

Adjunctive therapies, principally the use of steroids to decreased the detrimental effects of the host's inflammatory response, have been extensively reviewed [52,163,178,184–186]. Although animal data clearly demonstrate improvement in outcome, clinical studies have been more difficult to control or have been entirely retrospective with only incidental information on pneumococcal disease. To be optimally effective, dexamethasone must be given just before or with the first dose of antibiotic.

PREVENTION

Pneumococcal vaccines have been studied for nearly 80 years. Their history and newer developments are further discussed in Chapter 22. Clinical use of purified polysaccharides vaccines began in 1977 with a vaccine containing capsular antigens of the 14 most common pneumococcal serotypes; the current vaccine formulation licensed in 1983 contains polysaccharides of 23 types accounting for about 90% of disease isolates [8]. Estimates of vaccine efficacy have ranged from 50% to 80% against bacteremic infections in adults [187]. Current recommendations for immunization include those patients 65 years of age and older, those older than 2 years with chronic or immunocompromising disorders, and those living in high-risk areas or social settings [188]. Until the past few years, utilization surveys found that fewer than 20% of elderly Americans received the vaccine when indicated. However, concern about the spread of antibiotic-resistant strains and changes in recommendations and funding have been prompting an increase in use in the United States and some other developed countries [189]. Although there is still some skepticism regarding the efficacy of vaccines in preventing adult pneumococcal disease [190], a preponderance of evidence, mostly from retrospective and case–control studies, falls in favor of the vaccines and for expansion of their use [187,189].

Infants and children less than 2 years of age respond poorly to most bacterial polysaccharides, and the pneumococcal polysaccharide vaccine is not recommended for this age-group. Following the lead of the spectacularly successful vaccines against Hemophilus influenzae type b (Hib), a new generation of protein-conjugated pneumococcal vaccines has been developed for children and is currently in clinical trials [113,191]. These vaccines contain polysaccharides of the seven or so most common types in childhood infections (types 1 or 4, 6B, 9V, 14, 18C, 19F, and 23F) [9] coupled to either meningococcal outer membrane protein complex (Merck) or to diphtheria toxin mutant protein (Lederle-Praxis), similar to the licensed Hib vaccines.

Vaccines based on prevalent epitopes of the surface protein PspA are under development and would be expected to elicit good immunologic responses in children. This approach is further described in a recent review and in Chapter 22 of this volume [73].

Passive immunotherapy was used briefly but

with considerable success in the treatment of pneumococcal pneumonia just prior to the advent of penicillin [105]. More recently, a specialized hyperimmune globulin has been developed from plasma donors immunized with pneumococcal and *H. influenzae* type b, and meningococcal vaccines. Called "bacterial polysaccharide immune globulin," BPIG has been effective in reducing the number of pneumococcal and *H. influenzae* type b infections in high-risk Native American infant populations [192], and it has been evaluated with some success in preventing pneumococcal otitis media in suburban middle-class infants [193].

Antibiotic prophylaxis against pneumococcal infections has been practiced for years in patients with sickle cell disease, nephrotic syndrome, and other immunocompromising conditions. Though generally effective, the emergence of penicillin- and multiply resistant pneumococci has raised serious concerns about this approach [104]. Sickle cell patients may safely discontinue penicillin prophylaxis at 5 years of age, so long as parents are counseled appropriately and they have ready access to medical evaluation for acute febrile illnesses [194]. Children may remain colonized by pneumococci even after conventional antibiotic treatment [6], and attempts to eradicate carriage or spread in day-care environments by administration of rifampin have not proved to be effective [128,160]. Some success has been reported after intranasal administration of the topical antibiotic mupirocin in sickle cell patients carrying penicillin-resistant pneumococci [195].

With no simple solutions in the immediate future, efforts have been directed toward minimizing the impact of pneumococcal infections through strategies being developed by The Drug-Resistant *Streptococcus pneumoniae* Working Group [5]. Their focus is on implementing an effective national surveillance system, improving the identification of risk factors, increasing pneumococcal immunization, and promoting judicious use of antibiotics through better treatment guidelines to avoiding their inappropriate or unnecessary use. The pneumococci are likely to be with us for many years to come. Improvements in prevention and treatment will require a concerted effort and a better understanding of this resourceful organism.

REFERENCES

1. White B (with the collaboration of Robinson ES and Barnes LA). The Biology of the Pneumococcus: The Bacteriological, Biochemical and Immunological Characters and Activities of *Diplococcus pneumoniae*. New York: Commonwealth Fund, 1938; reprinted by Harvard University Press, 1979.
2. Heffron R. *Pneumonia with Special Reference to Pneumococcus Lobar Pneumonia*. New York: Commonwealth Fund, 1939; reprinted by Harvard University Press, 1979.
3. Austrian R. Pneumococcus: the first one hundred years. Rev Infect Dis 1981; 3:183–189.
4. Watson DA, Musher DM, Jacobson JW, Verhoef J. A brief history of the pneumococcus in biomedical research: a panoply of scientific discovery. Clin Infect Dis 1993; 17:913–924.
5. Jernigan DB, Cetro MS, Breiman RF. Minimizing the impact of drug-resistant *Streptococcus pneumoniae* (DRSP). JAMA 1996; 275: 206–209.
6. Gray BM, Converse GM III, Dillon HC Jr. Epidemiologic studies of *Streptococcus pneumoniae* in infants: acquisition, carriage, and infection during the first 24 months of life. J Infect Dis 1980; 142:923–933.
7. Henrichsen J. Six newly recognized types of *Streptococcus pneumoniae*. J Clin Microbiol 1995; 33:2759–2762.
8. Robbins JB, Austrian R, Lee C-J, Rastogi SC, Schiffman G, Henrichsen J, Makala PH, Broome CV, Facklam RR, Tiesjema RH, Park JC, Jr. Considerations for formulating the second-generation pneumococcal capsular polysaccharide vaccine with emphasis on the cross-reactive type within groups. J Infect Dis 1983; 148:1136–1159.
9. Butler JC, Breiman RF, Lipman HB, Hofmann J, Facklam RR. Serotype distribution of *Streptococcus pneumoniae* infections among preschool children in the United States, 1978–1994: implications for development of a conjugate vaccine. J Infect Dis 1995; 171:885–889.
10. McDougal LK, Facklam R, Reeves M, Hunter S, Swenson JM, Hill BC, Tenover FC. Analysis of multiply antimicrobial-resistant isolates of *Streptococcus pneumoniae* from the United States. Antimicrob Agents Chemother 1992; 36:2176–2184.
11. Muñoz R, Musser JM, Crain M, Briles DE, Marton A, Parkinson AJ, Sorensen U, Tomaz A. Geographic distribution of penicillin-resistant clones of *Streptococcus pneumoniae*: characterization by penicillin-binding protein profile, surface protein A typing, and multilocus enzyme analysis. Clin Infect Dis 1992; 15:112–118.
12. Soares S, Kristinsson KG, Musser JM, Tomasz A. Evidence for the introduction of a multiresistant clone of serotype 6B *Streptococcus pneu-*

moniae from Spain to Iceland in the late 1980's. J Infect Dis 1993; 168:158–163.

13. Lomholt H. Evidence of recombination and an antigenically diverse immunoglobulin A1 protease among strains of *Streptococcus pneumoniae*. Infect Immun 1995; 63:4238–4243.

14. Harakeh H, Bosley GS, Keihlbaugh JA, Fields BS. Heterogeneity of rRNA gene restriction patterns of multiresistant serotype 6B *Streptococcus pneumoniae* strains. J Clin Microbiol 1994; 32:3046–3048.

15. Hermans PWM, Sluijter M, Hoogenboezem T, Heersma H, van Belkum A, de Groot R. Comparative study of five different DNA fingerprint techniques for molecular typing of *Streptococcus pneumoniae* strains. J Clin Microbiol 1995; 33:1606–1612.

16. Musher DM. Pneumococcal pneumonia including diagnosis and therapy of infections caused by penicillin-resistant strains. Infect Dis Clin North Am 1991; 5:509–521.

17. Marrie TJ. Community acquired pneumonia. Clin Infect Dis 1994; 18:501–515.

18. Bartlett JG, Breiman RF, Mandell LA, File TM Jr. Community-acquired pneumonia in adults: guidelines for management. Clin Infect Dis 1998; 26:811–838.

19. American Thoracic Society. Hospital-acquired pneumonia in adults: diagnosis, assessment of severity, inital antimicrobial therapy, and preventive strategies. Am J Respir Crit Care Med 1995; 153:1711–1725.

20. Maxson S, Lewno MJ, Schutze GE. Clinical usefulness of cerebrospinal fluid bacterial antigen studies. J Pediatr 1994; 125:235–238.

21. Boersma WG, Löwenberg A, Holloway Y, Kuttschrütter H, Snijder JAM, Koëter GH. Rapid detection of pneumococcal antigen in pleural fluid of patients with community acquired pneumonia. Thorax 1993; 48:160–162.

22. Holloway Y, Boersma WG, Kuttschrütter H, Snijder JAM. Minimum number of pneumococci required for capsular antigen to be detectable by latex agglutination. J Clin Microbiol 1992; 30:517–519.

23. Gillespie SH, Ullman C, Smith MD, Emery V. Detection of *Streptococcus pneumoniae* in sputum samples by PCR. J Clin Microbiol 1994; 32:1308–1311.

24. Virolainen A, Salo O, Jero J, Karma P, Eskola J, Leinoen M. Comparison of PCR assay with bacterial culture for detecting *Streptococcus pneumoniae* in middle ear fluid of children with otitis media. J Clin Microbiol 1994; 32:2667–2670.

25. Isaacman DJ, Zhang Y, Reynolds EA, Ehrlich GD. Accuracy of a polemerase chain reaction-based assay for detection of pneumococcal bacteremia in children. Pediatrics 1998; 101:813–816.

26. Du Plessis M, Smith AM, Klugman KP. Rapid detection of penicillin-resistant *Streptococcus*

pneumoniae in cereabrospinal fluid by a semi-nested-PCR strategy. J Clin Microbiol 1998; 36:453–457.

27. Gray BM. Pneumococcal infections in an era of multiple antibiotic resistance. Adv Pediatr Infect Dis 1996; 11:55–99.

28. Swenson JM, Hill BC, Thornsberry C. Screening pneumococci for penicillin resistance. J Clin Microbiol 1986; 24:749–752.

29. Willett LD, Dillon HC Jr, Gray BM. Penicillin-intermediate pneumococci in a children's hospital. Am J Dis Child 1985; 139:1054–1057.

30. Mason EO, Kaplan SL, Lamberth LB, Tillman J. Increased rate of isolation of penicillin-resistant *Streptococcus pneumoniae* in a children's hospital and in vitro susceptibilities to antibiotics of potential therapeutic use. Antimicrob Agents Chemother 1992; 36:1703–1707.

31. National Committee for Clinical Laboratory Standards (NCCLS). Performance standards for antimicrobial susceptibility testing. Fifth informational supplement M100-S5. Villanova, PA: National Committee for Clinical Laboratory Standards, 1994.

32. Jacobs MR, Bajaksouzian S, Appelbaum PC, Bolmstrom A. Evaluation of the E-test for susceptibility testing of pneumococci. Diagn Microbiol Infect Dis 1992; 15:473–478.

33. Clark RB, Giger O, Mortensen JE. Comparison of susceptibility test methods to detect penicillin-resistant *Streptococcus pneumoniae*. Diagn Microbiol Infect Dis 1993; 17:213–217.

34. Krisher KK, Linscott A. Comparison of three commercial MIC systems, E test, fastidious antimicrobial susceptibility panel, and FOX fastidious panel, for confirmation of penicillin and cephalosporin resistance in *Streptococcus pneumoniae*. J Clin Microbiol 1994; 32:2242–2245.

35. Jorgensen JH, Swenson JM, Tenover FC, Ferraro MJ, Hindler JA, Murray PR. Development of interpretive criteria and quality control limits for broth microdilution and disk diffusion antimicrobial susceptibility testing of *Streptococcus pneumoniae*. J Clin Microbiol 1994; 32:2448–2459.

36. Walker CW, Brown DFJ. A rapid technique for detection of resistance to chloramphenicol in *Streptococcus pneumoniae* and comparison with minimum inhibitory concentration and disk diffusion methods. J Med Microbiol 1990; 31:133–136.

37. Schiffman G, Douglas RM, Bonner MJ, Robbins M, Austrian R. A radioimmunoassay for immunologic phenomena in pneumococcal disease and for the antidody response to pneumococcal vaccine. I. Method for the radioimmunoassay of anticapsular antibodies and comparison with other techniques. J Immunol Methods 1981; 33:133–144.

38. Koskela M, Leinonen M, Häivä VM, Timonen

M, Mäkelä H. First and second dose antibody responses to pneumococcal polysaccharide vaccine in infants. Pediatr Infect Dis J 1986; 5:45–50.

39. Nahm MH, Siber GR, Olander JV. A modified Farr assay is more specific than ELISA for measuring antibodies to *Streptococcus pneumonae* capsular polysaccharides. J Infect Dis 1996; 173:113–118.

40. Giebink GS, Verhoe J, Peterson PK, Quie PG. Opsonic requirements for phagocytosis of *Streptococcus pneumoniae* types VI, XVIII, XXIII, and XXV. Infect Immun 1977; 18:291–297.

41. Hostetter MK. Serotypic variation among virulent pneumococci in deposition and degradation of covalently bound C3b: implications for phagocytosis and antibody production. J Infect Dis 1986; 153:682–693.

42. Vixarsson G, Jonsdottir I, Jonsson S, Valdimarsson H. Opsonization and antibodies to capsular and cell wall polysaccharides of *Streptococcus pneumoniae*. J Infect Dis 1994; 170:592–599.

43. van Dam JEG, Fleer A, Snippe H. Immunogenicity and immunochemistry of *Streptococcus pneumoniae* capsular polysaccharides. Antonie Van Leeuwenhoek 1990; 58:1–47.

44. Sørensen UBS. Pneumococcal polysaccharide antigens: capsules and C-polysaccharide. Dan Med Bull 1995; 42:47–52.

45. Bruyn GAW, Zegers BJM, van Furth R. Mechanisms of host defense against infection with *Streptococcus pneumoniae*. Clin Infect Dis 1992; 14:251–262.

46. Angel CSW, Ruzek M, Hostetter MK. Degradation of C3 by *Streptococcus pneumoniae*. J Infect Dis 1994; 170:600–608.

47. Briles DE, Crain MJ, Gray BM, Yother J. Strong association between capsular type and virulence for mice among human isolates of *Streptococcus pneumoniae*. Infect Immun 1992; 60:111–116.

48. Kelly T, Dillard JP, Yother J. Effect of genetic switching of capsular type on virulence of *Streptococcus pneumoniae*. Infect Immun 1994; 62:1813–1819.

49. Shockman GD, Barrett JF. Structure, function and assembly of gram-positive bacteria. Annu Rev Microbiol 1983; 37:501–527.

50. Ghuysen JM. Serine β-lactamases and penicillin-binding proteins. Annu Rev Microbiol 1991; 45:37–67.

51. Garcia-Bustos J, Tomasz A. A biological price of antibiotic resistance: major changes in the peptidoglycan structure of penicillin-resistant pneumococci. Proc Natl Acad Sci USA 1990; 87:5415–5419.

52. Quagliarello V, Scheld WM. Bacterial meningitis: pathogenesis, pathophysiology, and progress. N Engl J Med 1992; 327:864–872.

53. Carlsen BD, Kawana M, Kawana C, Tomasz A, Giebink GS. Role of the bacterial cell wall in middle ear inflammation caused by *Streptococcus pneumoniae*. Infect Immun 1992; 60:2850–2854.

54. Geelen S, Bhattacharyya C, Tuomanen E. The cell wall mediates pneumococcal attachment to and cytopathology in human endothelial cells. Infect Immun 1993; 61:1538–1543.

55. Tuomanen E. Breaching the blood-brain barrier. Sci Am 1993; 268:80–84.

56. Ronda C, Garcia JL, Garcia E, Sanchez-Puelles JM, Lopez R. Biological role of the pneumococcal amidase. Eur J Biochem 1987; 164: 621–624.

57. Canvin JR, Marvin AP, Sivakumaran M, Paton JC, Boulnois GJ, Andrew PW, Mitchell TJ. The role of pneumolysin and autolysin in the pathology of pneumonia and septicemia in mice infected with type 2 pneumococcus. J Infect Dis 1995; 172:119–123.

58. Garcia P, Garcia JL, Garcia E, Lopez L. Purification of the autolytic glycosidase of *Streptococcus pneumoniae*. Biochem Biophys Res Commun 1989; 158:251–256.

59. Lock RA, Hansman D, Paton, JC. Comparative efficacy of autolysin and pneumolysin as immunogens protecting mice against infections by *Streptococcus pneumoniae*. Microb Pathog 1992; 12:137–143.

60. Cottagnoud P, Tomasz A. Triggering of pneumococcal autolysis by lysozyme. J Infect Dis 1992; 167:684–690.

61. Tuomanen E, Pollack H, Parkinson A, Davidson M, Facklam R, Rich R, Zak O. Microbiological and clinical significance of a new property of defective lysis in clinical strains of pneumococci. J Infect Dis 1988; 158:36–43.

62. Boulnois GJ. Pneumococcal proteins and the pathogenesis of disease caused by *Streptococcus pneumoniae*. J Gen Microbiol 1992; 138:249–259.

63. Friedland IR, Paris MM, Kickey S, Shelton S, Olsen K, Paton JC, McCracken GH. The limited role of pneumolysin in the pathogenesis of pneumococcal meningitis. J Infect Dis 1995; 172:805–809.

64. Killian M, Mestecky J, Russell MW. Defense mechanisms involving Fc-dependent functions of immunoglobulin A and their subversion by bacterial immunoglobulin A proteases. Microbiol Rev 1988; 52:296–303.

65. Camara M, Mitchell TJ, Andrew PW, Boulnois GJ. *Streptococcus pneumoniae* produces at least two distinct enzymes with neuraminidase activity: cloning and expression of a second neuraminidase gene in *Escherichia coli*. Infect Immun 1991; 59:2856–2858.

66. Andersson B, Gray BM, Dillon HC Jr, Bahrmand A, Svanborg EC. Role of adherence of *Streptococcus pneumoniae* in acute otitis media. Pediatr Infect Dis J 1988; 7:476–480.

67. Andersson B, Beachy EH, Tomaz A, Tuomanen

E, Svanborg-Eden C. A sandwich adhesin on Streptococcus pneumoniae attaching to human oropharyngeal epithelial cells in vitro. Microb Pathog 1988; 4:267–278.

68. Krivan HC, Roberts DD, Ginsberg V. Many pulmonary pathogenic bacteria bind specifically to the carbohydrate sequence GalNAcβ1-4Gal found in some glycolipids. Proc Natl Acad Sci USA 1988; 85:6157–6161.

69. Novak RW, Martin CR. Hemolytic-uremic syndrome and T-cryptantigen exposure by neuraminidase-producing pneumococci: an emerging problem? Pediatr Pathol 1983; 1:409–413.

70. Berry AM, Lock RA, Thomas SM, et al. Cloning and nucleotide sequence of the *Streptococcus pneumoniae* hyaluronidase gene and purification of the enzyme from recombinant *Escherichia coli*. Infect Immun 1994; 62:1101–1108.

71. Pritchard DG, Lin B, Willingham TR, Baker JR. Characterization of the group B streptococcal hyaluronate lyase. Arch Biochem Biophys 1994; 315:431–437.

72. Crain MJ, Waltman WD II, Turner JS, Yother J, Talkington DF, McDaniel LS, Gray BM, Briles DE. Pneumococcal surface protein A (PspA) is serologically highly variable and is expressed by all clinically important capsular serotypes of *Streptococcus pneumoniae*. Infect Immun 1990; 58:3293–3299.

73. Briles DE, Tart RC, Swiatlo E, Dillard JP, Smith P, Benton KA, Ralph BA, Brooks-Walter A, Crain MJ, Hollingshead SK, McDaniel LS. Pneumococcal diversity: considerations for new vaccine strategies with emphasis on pneumococcal surface protein A (PspA). Clin Microbiol Rev 1998; 11:645–57.

74. McDaniel LS, Sheffield JS, Delucchi P, Briles DE. PspA, a surface protein of *Streptococcus pneumoniae*, is capable of eliciting protection against pneumococci of more than one capsular type. Infect Immun 1991; 59:222–228.

75. McDaniel LS, Briles DE. A pneumococcal surface protein (PspB) that exhibits the same protein sensitivity as streptococcal R antigen. Infect Immun 1988; 56:3001–3003.

76. Klugman KP. Pneumococcal resistance to antibiotics. Clin Microbiol Rev 1990; 34:171–196.

77. Spratt BG. Resistance to antibiotics mediated by target alterations. Science 1994; 264:388–393.

78. Baquero F, Martinez-Beltran J, Loza E. A review of antibiotic resistance patterns of *Streptococcus pneumoniae* in Europe. J Antimicrob Chemother 1991; 28:31–38.

79. Reynolds PE. Structure, biochemistry and mechanism of action of glycopeptide antibiotics. Eur J Clin Microbiol Infect Dis 1989; 8:943–950.

80. Caillaud F, Trieu-Cuot P, Carlier C, Courvalin P. Nucleotide sequence of the kanamycin resistance determinant of the pneumococcal trans-

poson TN*1545:* evolutionary relationships and transcriptional analysis of *aphA-3* genes. Mol Gen Genet 1987; 207:509–513.

81. Waites K, Brookings E, Nix S, Robinson A, Gray B, Swiatlo E. Comparative in vitro activities of four new floroquinolones against *Streptococcus pneumoniae* determined by E test. Int J Antimicrob Agents 1998; 9:215–218.

82. Klugman KP, Dagan R, and the Meropenem Meningitis Study Group. Randomized comparison of meropenem with cefotaxime for treatment of bacterial meningitis. Antimicrob Agents Chemother 1995; 39:1140–1146.

83. Dillard JP, Vandersea MW, Yother J. Characterization of the cassette containing genes for type 3 capsular polysaccharide biosynthesis in *Streptococcus pneumoniae*. J Exp Med 1995; 181:973–983.

84. Muñoz R, Mollerach M, López R, Garcia E. Molecular organization of the genes required for the synthesis of type 1 capsular polysaccharide of *Streptococcus pneumoniae:* formation of binary encapsulated pneumococci and identification of cryptic dTDP-rhamnose biosynthesis genes. Mol Microbiol 1997; 25:79–92.

85. Watson DA, Kapur V, Musher DM, Jacobson JW, Musser JM. Identification, cloning, and sequencing of DNA essential for encapsulation of *Streptococcus pneumoniae*. Curr Microbiol 1995; 31:251–259.

86. Kolkman MA, Morrison DA, van der Zeijst AAM, Nuitjen PJM. The capsule polysaccharide synthesis locus of *Streptococccus pneumoniae* serotype 14: identification of the glycosyl transferase gene *cps14E*. J Bacteriol 1996; 178:3736–3741.

87. Morona JK, Morona R, Paton JC. Characterization of the locus encoding the *Streptococcus pneumoniae* type 19F capsular polysaccharide biosynthetic pathway. Mol Microbiol 1997; 23:751–763.

88. Ferretti JJ, Gilmore MS, Klaenhammer TR, Brown F (eds). Genetics of Streptococci, Enterococci and Lactococci. Dev Biol Stand 1995; 85.

89. Dowson CG, Hutchinson A, Brannifan JA, George RC, Hansman D, Linares J, Tomasz A, Maynard-Smith J, Spratt BG. Horizontal transfer of penicillin-binding protein genes in penicillin-resistant clinical isolates of *Streptococcus pneumoniae*. Proc Natl Acad Sci USA 1989; 86:8842–8846.

90. Smith AM Klugman KP. Alterations in penicillin-binding protein 2B from penicillin resistant wild-type strains of *Streptococcus pneumoniae*. Antimicrob Agents Chemother 1995; 39:859–867.

91. Johnston RB Jr. Pathogenesis of pneumococcal pneumonia. Rev Infect Dis 1991; 13:S509–S517.

92. Watson DA, Musher DM, Verhoef J. Pneumococcal virulence factors and host immune re-

sponses to them. Eur J Clin Microbiol Infect Dis 1995; 14:479–490.

93. Andersson B, Dahmén J, Frejd T, Leffler H, Magnusson G, Noori G, Svanborg Edén C. Identification of an active disaccharide unit of a glycoconjugate receptor for pneumococci attaching to human pharyngeal epithelial cells. J Exp Med 1983; 158:559–570.

94. Andersson B, Eriksson B, Falsen E, Fogh A, Hanson LA, Nylen O, Peterson H, Svanborg Eden C. Adhesion of *Streptococcus pneumoniae* to human pharyngeal epithelial cells in vitro: differences in adhesive capacity among strains isolated from subjects with otitis media, septicemia, or meningitis or from healthy carriers. Infect Immun 1981; 32:311–317.

95. Ruuskanen O, Heikkinen T. Viral-bacterial interaction in acute otitis media. Pediatr Infect Dis J 1994; 13:1047–1049.

96. Klein JO. Otitis media. Clin Infect Dis 1994; 19:823–833.

97. Davis CC, Mellencamp MA, Preheim LC. A model of pneumococcal pneumonia in chronically intoxicated rats. J Infect Dis 1991; 163:799–805.

98. Wood WB. Studies on the mechanism of recovery in pneumococcal pneumonia. J Exp Med 1941; 73:201–222.

99. Täuber MG, Burroughs M, Neimöller UM, Kuster H, Borschberg U, Tuomanen E. Differences of pathology in experimental meningitis caused by three strains of *Streptococcus pneumoniae*. J Infect Dis 1991; 163:806–811.

100. Zeiglerr-Heightbrock HWL, Passlick B, Käfferlein E, Coulie PG, Izbicki JR. Protection against lethal pneumococcal septicemia in pigs is associated with decreased levels of interlukin-6 in blood. Infect Immun 1992; 60:1692–1694.

101. Agrawal A, Kilpatrick JM, Volanakis JE. Structure and function of human C-reactive protein. In: Mackiewicz A, Kushner I, Baummann H (eds). Acute Phase Proteins: Molecular Biology, Biochemistry, and Clinical Applications. Ann Arbor, MI: CRC Press, 1993; 79–92.

102. Coonrod JD, Varble R, Jarrels MC. Species variation in the mechanism of killing of inhaled pneumococci. J Lab Clin Med 1990; 116:354–362.

103. Styrt B. Infection associated with asplenia: risks, mechanisms, and prevention. Am J Med 1990; 88(5N):33N–42N.

104. Wong WY, Overturf GD, Powars DR. Infection caused by *Streptococcus pneumoniae* in children with sickle cell disease: epidemiology, immunologic mechanisms, prophylaxis, and vaccination. Clin Infect Dis 1992; 14:1124–1136.

105. Casadevall A, Scharff MD. Serum therapy revisited: animal models of infection and development of passive antibody therapy. Antimicrob Agent Chemother 1994; 38:1695–1702.

106. Finland M, Shuman HI. The type-specific ag-

glutinin response of infants and children with pneumococcal pneumonias. J Immunol 1942; 45:215–222.

107. Musher DM, Groover JE, Reichler MR, Reido FX, Schwartz B, Watson DA, Baughn RE, Breiman R. Emergence of antibody to capsular polysaaccharides of *Streptococcus pneumoniae* during outbreaks of pneumonia: association with nasopharyngeal colonization. Clin Infect Dis 1997; 24:441–446.

108. Prober CG, Frayha H, Klein M, Schiffman G. Immunologic responses of children to serious infections with *Streptococcus pneumoniae*. J Infect Dis 1983; 148:427–435.

109. Barrett DJ, Lee CG, Ammann AJ, Ayoub EM. IgG and IgM pneumococcal polysaccharide antibody responses in infants. Pediatr Res 1984; 18:1067–1071.

110. Gray BM, Converse GM III, Huhta N, Johnston RB Jr, Pichichero ME, Schiffman G, Dillon HC Jr. Epidemiologic studies of *Streptococcus pneumoniae* in infants: antibody response to nasopharyngeal carriage of types 3, 19, and 23. J Infect Dis 1981; 144:312–318.

111. Gray BM, Dillon HC Jr. Epidemiological studies of *Streptococcus pneumoniae* in infants: antibody to types 3, 6, 14, and 23 in the first two years of life. J Infect Dis 1988; 158:948–955.

112. Musher DM, Groover JE, Rowland JM, Watson DA, Struewing JB, Baughn RE, Mufson MA. Antibody to capsular polysaccharides of *Streptococcus pneumoniae*: prevalence, persistence, and response to revaccination. Rev Infect Dis 1993; 17:66–73.

113. Giebink GS. Immunology: promise of new vaccine. Pediatr Infect Dis J 1994; 13:1064–1068.

114. Siber GR. Pneumococcal disease: prospects for a new generation of vaccines. Science 1994; 265:1385–1387.

115. Landesman SH Schiffman G. Assessment of the antibody response to pneumococcal vaccine in high-risk populations. Rev Infect Dis 1981; 3(Suppl):S184–S196.

116. Bardardottir E, Jonsson S, Jonsdottir I, Sigfusson A, Valdimarsson H. IgG subclass response and opsonization of *Streptococcus pneumoniae* after vaccination of healthy adults. J Infect Dis 1990; 162:482–488.

117. Lortan JE, Kaniuk AS, Monteil MA. Relationship of in vitro phagocytosis of serotype 14 *Streptococcus pneumoniae* to specific class and IgG subclass antibody levels in healthy adults. Clin Exp Immunol 1993; 91:54–57.

118. Konradsen HB, Oxelius V-A, Hanson LÅ. The importance of G1m and 2 allotypes for the IgG2 antibody levels and avidity against pneumococcal polysaccharide type 1 within mono- and dizygotic twin-pairs. Scand J Immunol 1994; 40:251–256.

119. Gray BM, Polhill RB, Reynolds DW. Antibodies to *Steptococcus pneumoniae* in sera and se-

cretions of mothers and their infants. Adv Exp Med Biol 1991; 310:331–341.

120. Andersson I, Rosen V, Håkansson A, Aniansson G, Hansson C, Anderson B, Nylén O, Sabharwal H, Svanborg C. Antibodies to pneumococcal polysaccharides in human milk: lack of relationship to colonization and acute otitis media. Pediatr Infect Dis J 1996; 15:498–507.

121. Virolainen A, Jero J, Käyhty H, Karma P, Leinoen M, Eskola J. Nasopharyngeal antibodies to pneumococcal capsular polysaccharides in children with acute otitis media. J Infect Dis 1995; 172:1115–1118.

122. Nieminen T, Virolainen A, Käyhty H, Jero J, Karma P, Leinonen M, Eskola J. Antibody-secreting cell and their relation to humoral antibodies in serum and in nasopharyngeal aspirates in children with pneumococcal acute otitis media. J Infect Dis 1995; 173:136–141.

123. Gray BM, Turner ME, Dillon HC Jr. Epidemiologic studies of Streptococcus pneumoniae in infants: the effects of season and age on pneumococcal acquisition and carriage in the first 24 months of life. Am J Epidemiol 1982; 116:692–703.

124. Hendley JO, Sande MA, Stewart PM, Gwaltney JM. Spread of Streptococcus pneumoniae in families. I. Carriage rates and distribution of types. J Infect Dis 1975; 132:55–61.

125. Loda FA, Collier AM, Glezen WP, Strangert K, Clyde WA, Denny FW. Occurrence of Diplococcus pneumoniae in the upper respiratory tract of children. J Pediatr 1975; 87:1087–1093.

126. Takala AK, Jero J, Kela E, Rönnberg P-R, Koskeniemmi E, Eskola J. Risk factors for invasive penumococcal disease among children in Finland. JAMA 1995; 273:859–864.

127. Hodges RG, MacLeod CM. Epidemic pneumococcal pneumonia. Am J Hyg 1946; 44:183–243.

128. Cherian T, Steinhoff MC, Harrison LH, Rohn D, McDougal LK, Dick J. A cluster of invasive pneumococcal disease in young children in child care. JAMA 1994; 271:695–697.

129. Hoge CW, Reichler MR, Dominguez EA, Bremer JC, Mastro TD, Hendricks KA, Musher DM, Elliott JA, Facklam RR, Breiman RF. An epidemic of pneumococcal disease in an overcrowded, inadequately ventilated jail. N Engl J Med 1994; 331:643–648.

130. Jones EE, Alford PL, Reingold AL, Russell H, Keeling ME, Broome CV. Predisposition to invasive pneumococcal illness following parainfluenza type 3 virus infection in chimpanzees. JAVM 1984; 185:1351–1353.

131. Fallon MT, Reinhard MK, Gray BM, Davis TW, Lindsey JR. Inapparent Streptococcus pneumoniae type 35 infections in commercial rats and mice. Lab Animal Sci 1988; 38:129–132.

132. Brimblecombe FSW, Cruicshank R, Masters PL, Reid DD, Stewart GT. Family studies of respiratory infections. BMJ 1958:119–128.

133. Gray BM, Converse GM III, Dillon HC Jr. Serotypes of Streptococcus pneumoniae causing disease. J Infect Dis 1979; 140:979–983.

134. Kim PE, Musher MD, Glezen WP, Rodriguez-Barradas MC, Nahm WK, Wright CE. Association of invasive pneumococcal disease with season, atmospheric conditions, air pollution and isolation of respiratory viruses. Clin Infect Dis 1996; 22:100–106.

135. Smith T, Lehmann D, Montgomery J, Gratten M, Riley JD, Alpers MP. Acquisition and invasiveness of different serotypes of Streptococcus pneumoniae in young children. Epidemiol Infect 1993; 111:27–39.

136. Ort S, Ryan RL, Barden G, D'Esopo N. Pneumococcal pneumonia in hospitalized patients. JAMA 1983; 249:214–218.

137. Breiman RF, Spika JS, Navarro VJ, Daden PM, Darby CP. Pneumococcal bacteremia in Charleston county, South Carolina. Arch Intern Med 1990; 150:1401–1405.

138. Bennett NM, Buffington J, LaForce FM. Pneumococcal bacteremia in Monroe County, New York. Am J Public Health 1992; 82:1513–1516.

139. Plouffe JF, Breiman RF, Facklam RR. Bacteremia with Streptococcus pneumoniae: implications for therapy and prevention. JAMA 1996; 275:194–198.

140. Davidson M, Parkinson AJ, Bulkow LR, Fitzgerald MA, Peters HV, Parks DJ. The epidemiology of invasive pneumococcal diesase in Alaska, 1986–1990—ethnic differences and opportunities for prevention. J Infect Dis 1994; 170:368–376.

141. Trotman J, Highes B, Mollison L. Invasive pneumococcal disease in central Australia. Clin Infect Dis 1994; 20:1553–1556.

142. Gray BM, Dillon HC Jr. Clinical and epidemiologic studies of pneumococcal infection in children. Pediatr Infect Dis J 1986; 5:201–207.

143. Afessa B, Greaves WL, Frederick WR. Pneumococcal bacteremia in adults: a 14-year experience in an inner-city university hospital. Clin Infect Dis 1995; 21:345–351.

144. Mao C, Harper M, McIntosh K, Reddington C, Cohen JR, Caldwell B, Hsu HW. Invasive pneumococcal infections in human immunodeficiency virus–infected children. J Infect Dis 1995; 173:870–876.

145. Janoff AN, Breiman RF, Daley CL, Hopewell P. Pneumococcal disease during HIV infection. Ann Intern Med 1992; 117:314–324.

146. Garcia-Leoni ME, Moreno S, Rodeno P, Cercenado E, Vocente T, Bouza E. Pneumococcal pneumonia in adult hospitalized patients infected with human immunodeficiency virus. Arch Intern Med 1992; 152:1808–1812.

147. Orange M, Gray BM. Pneumococcal serotypes causing disease in children in Alabama. Pediatr Infect Dis J 1993; 12:244–246.

148. Fine MJ, Smith MA, Carson CA, Mutha SS, Sankey SS, Weissfeld LA, Kapoor WN. Progno-

sis and outcomes of patients with community-acquired pneumonia. JAMA 1996; 275.

149. Fine MJ, Singer DE, Hanusa BH, Lave JR, Kapoor WN. Validation of a pneumococcal prognostic index using the MedisGroups comparative hospital database. Am J Med 1993; 94:153–159.

150. Nussinovitch M, Cohen HA, Frydman M, Varsano I. Cerebrospinal fluid pleocytosis in children with pneumonia but lacking evidence of meningitis. Clin Pediatr 1993; 32:372–373.

151. Bransom RT, Meyer TL, Silbiger ML, Blickman JG, Halpern E. The futility of chest radiograph in the febrile infant without respiratory symptoms. Pediatrics 1993; 92:524–526.

152. Korppi M, Kiekara O, Heiskanen-Kosma T, Soimakallio S. Comparison of radiological findings and microbial aetiology of childhood pneumonia. Acta Paediatr 1993; 82:360–363.

153. Bryant ER, Salmon CJ. Pleural empyema. Clin Infect Dis 1996; 22:747–764.

154. Stovroff M, Teague G, Heiss KF, Parker P, Ricketts RR. Thoracostomy in the management of pediatric empyema. J Pediatr Surg 1995; 30:1211–1215.

155. Karem E, Bar Ziv Y, Rudenski B, Katz S, Kleid D, Branski D. Bacteremic necrotizing pneumococcal pneumonia in children. Am J Respir Crit Care Med 1993; 149:242–244.

156. Block S, Harrison CJ, Hedrick J, Tyler RD, Smith RA, Keegan E, Chartrand SA. Penicillin-resistant *Streptococcus pneumoniae* in acute otitis media: risk factors, susceptibility patterns and antimicrobial management. Pediatr Infect Dis J 1995; 14:751–759.

157. Celin SE, Bluestone CD, Stephenson J, Yilmaz HM, Collins JJ. Bacteriology of acute otitis media in adults. JAMA 1991; 266:2249–2252.

158. Willett LR, Carson JL, Williams JW. Current diagnosis and management of sinusitis. J Gen Intern Med 1994; 9:38–45.

159. Dagan R, Englehard D, Piccard E. Epidemiology of invasive childhood pneumococcal infections in Israel. JAMA 1992; 268:3328–3332.

160. Nims L, Hatch K, Gallaher M, Voorhees R, Tanuz M, Vold I. Hemorrhage and shock associated with invasive pneumococcal infection in healthy infants and children—New Mexico, 1993–1994. MMWR Morb Mortal Wkly Rep 1995; 43:949–952.

161. Durand ML, Calderwood SB, Weber DJ, Miller SI, Southwick FS, Caviness VS, Swartz MN. Acute bacterial meningitis in adults. N Engl J Med 1993; 328:21–28.

162. Spitz EB, Wagner S, Satalof J, Hoffman NP, Hope JW. Cerebrospinal fluid otorrhea and recurrent meningitis. J Pediatr 1961; 59:397–401.

163. Tunkel AR, Scheld MW. Acute bacterial meningitis. Lancet 1995; 346:1675–1680.

164. Bonadio W. The cerebrospinal fluid: physiologic aspects and alterations associated with bacterial meningitis. Pediatr Infect Dis J 1992; 11:423–432.

165. Aronin SI, Mukherjee SK, West JC, Cooney EL. Review of pneumococcal endocarditis in adults in the penicillin era. Clin Infect Dis 1998; 26:165–171.

166. Kessler HA, Schade R, Trenholme GM, Jupa JE, Levin S. Acute pneumococcal epiglottitis in immunocompromised adults. Scand J Infect Dis 1980; 12:207–210.

167. Patel M, Ahrens JC, Moyer DV, DiNubile MJ. Pneumococcal soft-tissue infections: a problem deserving more recognition. Clin Infect Dis 1994; 19:149–151.

168. Jacobs NM. Pneumococcal osteomyelitis and arthritis in children. Am J Dis Child 1991; 145:70–74.

169. Wilcox CM, Dismukes WE. Spontaneous bacterial peritonitis. Medicine 1987; 66:447–456.

170. Gorensek MJ, Lebel MH, Nelson JD. Peritonitis in children with nephrotic syndrome. Pediatrics 1988; 81:849–846.

171. Sirotnak AP, Eppes SC, Klein JD. Tuboovarian abscess and peritonitis caused by *Streptococcus pneumoniae* serotype 1 in young girls. Cin Infect Dis 1996; 22:993–996.

172. Westh H, Skibsted L, Korner B. *Streptococcus pneumoniae* infections of the female genital tract and in the neonate. Rev Infect Dis 1990; 12:416–422.

173. Jacobs J, Garmyn K, Verhaegen J, Devlieger H, Eggermont E. Neonatal sepsis due to *Streptococcus pneumoniae*. Scand J Infect Dis 1990; 22:493–497.

174. Feld LG, Springate JE Jr, Darraugh R, Fildes RD. Pneumococcal pneumonia and hemolytic uremic syndrome. Pediatr Infect Dis J 1987; 6:693–695.

175. Pallares R, Linares J, Vadillo M, Cabellos C. Resistance to penicillin and cephalosporins and mortality from severe pneumococcal pneumonia in Barcelona, Spain. N Engl J Med 1995; 333:474–480.

176. Tan TQ, Mason EO, Barson WJ, Wald ER, Schutze GE, Bradley JS, Arditi M, Givner LB, Yogev R, Kim KS, Kaplan SL. Clinical characteristics and outcome of children with pneumonia attributable to penicillin-susceptible and penicillin-nonsusceptible *Streptococcus pneumoniae*. Pediatrics 1998; 102:1369–1375.

177. American Academy of Pediatrics. Therapy for children with invasive pneumococcal infections. Pediatrics 1997; 99:289–299.

178. Kaplan SL, Mason EO. Management of infections due to antibiotic-resistant *Streptococcus pneumoniae*. Clin Microbiol Rev 1998; 11:628–44.

179. Campbell GD, Silberman R. Drug-resistant *Streptococcus pneumoniae*. Clin Infect Dis 1998; 26:1188–1195.

180. Deeks SL, Palacio R, Ruvinsky R, Kertesz DA, Hortal M, Rossi A, Spika JS, Di Fabio JL. Risk

factors and course of illness among children with invasive penicillin-resistant *Streptococcus pneumoniae*. Pediatrics 1999; 103:409–413.

181. Leibovitz E, Piglansky L, Raiz S, Greenberg D, Yagupsky P, Press J, Fliss DM, Leiberman A, Dagan R. Bacteriologic efficacy of a three-day intramuscular ceftriaxone regimen in nonresponsive acute otitis media. Pediatr Infect Dis J 1998; 17:1126–1131.

182. Ristuccia AM, LeFrock JL. Cerebrospinal fluid penetration of antimicrobials. Antibiot Chemother 1992; 45:118–152.

183. Cantú TG, Yamanak-Yuen NA, Lietman PS. Serum vancomycin concentrations: reappraisal of their clinical value. Clin Infect Dis 1994; 19:533–543, [correspondence] 1180–1182.

184. Prober CG. The role of steroids in the management of children with bacterial meningitis. Pediatrics 1995; 95:29–31.

185. Schaad UB, Kaplan SL, McCracken GH. Steroid therapy for bacterial meningitis. Clin Infect Dis 1995; 20:685–690.

186. McIntyre PB, Berkey CS, King SM, Schaad UB, Kilpi T, Kanta GY, Perez CM. Dexamethasone as adjunctive therapy in bacterial meningitis. A meta-analysis of randomized clinical trials since 1988. JAMA 1997; 278:925–931.

187. Fedsen DS, Shapiro ED, LaForce FM, Muffson MA, Musher DM, Spika JS, Breiman RF, Broome CV. Pneumococcal vaccine after 15 years of use: another view. Arch Intern Med 1994; 154:2531–2535.

188. Centers for Disease Control. Pneumococcal polysaccharide vaccine. MMWR Morb Mortal Wkly Rep 1997; 46(RR-8):1–24.

189. Fedson DS. Pneumococcal vaccination in the United States and 20 other developed countries, 1981–1996. Clin Infect Dis 1998; 26:1117–1123.

190. Hirschmann JV, Lipsky BA. The pneumococcal vaccine after 15 years of use. Arch Intern Med 1994; 154:373–377.

191. Rennels KB, Edwards KM, Keyserling HL, Reisinger KS, Hogerman DA, Madore DV, Chang I, Pardiso PR, Malinowski FJ, Kimura A. Safety and immunogenicity of heptavalent pneumococcal vaccine conjugated to CRM_{197} in United States infants. Pediatrics 1998; 101:604–611.

192. Siber GR, Thompson C, Reid GR, Almeido-Hill J, Zacher B, Wolff M, Santosham M. Evaluation of bacterial polysaccharide immune globulin for the treatment of prevention of *Haemophilus influenzae* type b and pneumococcal disease. J Infect Dis 1992; 165(Suppl 1):S129–133.

193. Shurin PA, Rehmus JM, Johnson CA, Marchant CD, Carlin SA, Super DM, Van Hare GF, Jones PK, Ambrosino DM, Siber GR. Bacterial polysaccharide immune globulin for prophylaxis of acute otitis media in high risk children. J Pediatr 1993; 123:801–810.

194. Falletta JM, Woods GM, Verter JI, Buchanan GR, Pegelow CH, Iyer RV, Miller ST, Holbrook CT, Kinney TR, Vichinsky E. Discontinuing penicillin prophylaxis in children with sickle cell anemia. J Pediatr 1995; 127:685–690.

195. Workman MR, Layton M, Hussein M, Philpott-Howard J, George RC. Nasal carriage of penicillin-resistant pneumococcus in sickle-cell patients. Lancet 1993; 342:746–747.

196. Hager HL, Wooley TW, Berk SL. Review of recent pneumococcal infections with attention to vaccine and nonvaccine serotypes. Rev Infect Dis 1990; 12:267–272.

18

Oral Streptococci in Health and Disease

MARK C. HERZBERG

Many species of streptococci are members of the indigenous flora of the oral cavity. Most are benign commensals that cause no apparent disease in their native niches. When colonizing other niches, however, commensals may behave as pathogens, expressing a strikingly diverse set of virulence traits. In foreign niches, environmental signals regulate the expression of virulence factors, enabling these commensal bacteria to behave as pathogens. In the oral cavity, certain oral streptococci cause or are associated with a variety of endemic oral infections, including dental caries, periodontal diseases, and apthous stomatitis.

Generally considered to be Lancefield nontypeable, the taxonomy of the oral streptococci has been refined in recent years through use of DNA riboprobes and cluster analysis (Fig. 18.1; [1,1a]) The genus *Streptococcus* is divided into the pyogenic beta-hemolytic group and the alpha-hemolytic viridans group. Virtually all species in the viridans groups are found in the oral cavity and are considered to be oral streptococci. The viridans streptococci can be subdivided into the mutans, bovis, salivarius, mitis, and anginosus groups. Some species in the mitis and anginosus groups are recognized as pathogenic in tissues and organs other than the oral cavity, whereas the mutans group are generally associated with dental caries only. The taxonomy remains in flux. Research and clinical laboratories classify new isolates by using the best available information, often relying on less-refined commercial typing kits. Strains maintained in culture collections are sometimes reclassified when investigators need to reestablish gold standards for reference comparisons. Consequently, there is often little consistency in the species identification of strains reported in the literature. With the exception of *Streptococcus mutans* and dental caries, specific species cannot yet be reliably associated with certain infections. It is helpful to recognize that a reported species assignation using a more primitive taxonomic scheme reasonably allows retrospective and tentative classification into one of the five groups of viridans streptococci. Species identified in this review will rely on the original assignation published by the authors, acknowledging reclassification if the information is available.

The oral or viridans streptococci colonize selectively the hard and soft tissues of the oral cavity, oropharynx, and gastrointestinal (GI) tract (Fig. 18.2). While their functions outside of the oral cavity are less well understood, much is known about the oral streptococci of the tooth surface and proximal surfaces. On the tooth surface, certain species of streptococci reside in complex colonial biofilms called dental plaque. In some dental environments, including the pits and fissures of the enamel and protected interproximal surfaces, mutans streptococci can pro-

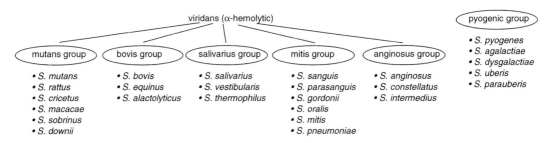

Figure 18.1 A taxonomy of the genus *Streptococcus*.

liferate and are considered the primary etiological agent in coronal dental caries and are strongly suspected in root surface caries. Root surface caries is generally a sequellae of periodontitis, in which chronic, ulcerative inflammation of the gingiva is associated with necrosis of the alveolar bony socket and ligamentous attachment that support the teeth. With loss of periodontal ligament and alveolar bone, root surfaces become exposed to cariogenic pathogens. While coronal caries of the enamel and dentin are primarily a disease of childhood and adolescence, root surface caries primarily affect the aged.

In periodontitis, the subgingival dental plaque harbors a plethora of gram-negative pathogens, but the viridans streptococci and other gram-positive bacteria also colonize in high numbers. Consequently, the subgingival plaque contains likely pathogens in coronal caries. In this protected crevice between the tooth and the gingiva, the commensal viridans streptococci are ex-

posed to ulcerated gingival epithelium, breaches in the capillary circulation, and entry to the blood (Fig. 18.3). Similarly, ulcerative lesions of the mucous membranes, which are frequently associated with immunosuppression, result in viridans streptococcal bacteremias of clinical significance. The association of oral streptococci with sepsis, disseminated intravascular coagulation, and infections such as infective endocarditis, indicates that this generally benign group of bacteria must be viewed as endogenous pathogens.

The prevalence and morbidity associated with oral streptococcal infections are a major international public health concern. In developed countries, the incidence of oral diseases associated with streptococci is declining, largely because of education, performance of personal dental hygiene, improved access to professional care, and fluoridation. For some populations within developed countries and elsewhere, these strategies have been less effective. One strategy

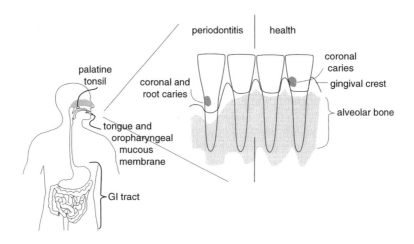

Figure 18.2 Tissues and anatomic sites typically colonized by viridans streptococci.

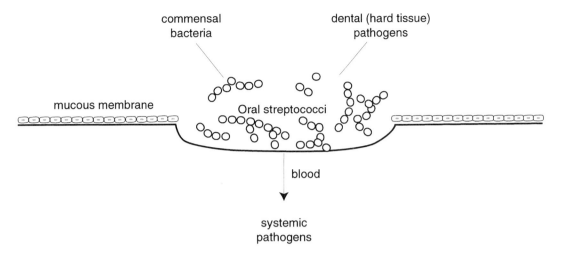

Figure 18.3 Viridans streptococci enter the blood through breaches in mucous membranes (or abscess contiguous with the dental pulp). Viridans streptococci that colonize mucous membranes or dental plaque can enter the circulation as single cells, chains of cocci or fragments of biofilm. In the blood, the viridans streptococci may behave as systemic pathogens. Generally the resulting bacteremias are polymicrobial, given the genus and species complexity of the oral and mucosal microfloras. While virulence traits are inferred from *in vitro* studies and other experimental models using pure cultures of bacteria, gene expression *in vivo* may alter substantially the potential of viridans streptococci to infect and cause disease at sites other than the oral cavity.

to control diseases associated with oral streptococci in these select populations is the design of effective streptococcal vaccines. Investigators have taken on the challenges of vaccine development. By analysis of potential antigens and design of immunogens, investigators have contributed substantial fundamental knowledge about streptococcal biology. Uncovering mechanisms to modulate the mucosal immune response has promoted new, clinically useful concepts in the development of transmucosal adjuvants. With further study these and other approaches may permit control of the oral streptococci in mucosal and systemic settings to promote health and treat disease.

HISTORY

The threads of discovery linking oral streptococci to human diseases span thousands of years. That dental caries might be caused by submacroscopic viable organisms was suspected by the ancient Babylonians ("tooth worm") [2]. In 1677, to the disbelief of the members of the Royal Society, van Leeuwenhoek revealed for the first time through magnifying lenses the

complex mixture of microbial forms in dental plaque and demonstrated that motility of some was lost upon contact with hot coffee [3]. About 50 years later, Pierre Fauchard advocated that the cause of dental caries was eliminated by cleansing of the teeth [4]. By the first half of the twentieth century, streptococci were recognized to be a major constituent of the microbiota of dental plaque sampled from the enamel surface and within the gingival crevice, and replenished rapidly on the shedding mucosal surfaces of the cheeks and tongue [5]. In health, the oral streptococci reside with other indigenous flora in these environments and exhibit low virulence. Hence, in the oral cavity, the streptococci exist as benign commensals, with the exception of cariogenic species such as *Streptococcus mutans*. Colonization and increasing numbers of *Streptococcus mutans* at or near their commensal intra-oral niche is associated with dental caries.

The connection between streptococci and dental caries was made first and most convincingly by the landmark studies of Keyes and Fitzgerald (reviewed in Tanzer [6]). Keyes had shown in animals that sucrose-rich diets promoted caries, while fluoride was inhibitory. Meanwhile, McClure and Hewitt [7] showed that penicillin prevented experimental caries. Paul Keyes teamed up with Robert Fitzgerald in the 1950s, as they both hypothesized that caries must be infectious and transmissible. To dissect the contributions of environment and genetics to dental caries, the two investigators monoinfected gnotobiotic rats, varied their diet, and introduced suspected inhibitors. While sucrose exacerbated the effects of the streptococci, penicillin or erythromycin prevented the occurrence of lesions. Together, Keyes and Fitzgerald demonstrated that the evidence of a streptococcal etiology of experimental caries fulfilled Koch's postulates. Certain oral streptococci were shown to create a transmissible cariogenic flora in rodents of differing genetic backgrounds, initiating demineralizing lesions of the hardest tissue in the human body, dental enamel.

Theodor Roseberry conceptualized the oral streptococci to be "endogenous pathogens" [5]. As endogenous pathogens, the oral streptococci multiply and cause diseases in tissues and organs removed from the dental and mucosal tissues. For example, multiplication of certain streptococci on heart valves causes infective endocarditis. In the case of *Streptococcus mutans*, the transformation of a commensal to a pathogen may result from merely a loss of restraint on growth. If oral streptococci breach the mucous membrane barrier to enter the systemic compartment, the new environment may trigger the expression of otherwise unexpressed genes and new virulence factors.

While not currently considered to be a primary pathogen in human periodontal diseases, the streptococci are a major constituent of dental plaques exposed in the oral cavity and subgingivally [8,9]. The streptococci constitute 30% to 60% of the bacteria colonizing supragingival and subgingival dental plaques and predominate also on the tongue, buccal mucosa, and in saliva [10,11]. Employing various adhesive mechanisms, the species of oral streptococci show selective tropisms for colonization of the various mucosal tissues and sites in the mouth as shown by Ronald Gibbons and co-workers [12,13]. These pioneering studies established conceptual paradigms for others studying the microbial inhabitants of other complex mammalian ecosystems. From an ecological point of view, the oral

streptococci have favored curiosity because they are among the first colonizers of clean teeth [14–16]. Colonizing streptococci resist displacement from these sites and hold together many species in the plaque community by producing soluble and insoluble dextrans, which are gelatinous and sticky in texture [17,18].

STREPTOCOCCI IN DENTAL PLAQUE

The oral cavity is a challenging and often hostile environment for microorganisms. While streptococci typically predominate as colonizers of dental plaque, their clearance and retention in the oral cavity are mediated by interactions with salivary constituents. To colonize, the streptococci resist the ebb and flow of saliva, hydration and desiccation, shedding mucosal surfaces, wide swings in ambient temperature, osmolarity, pH and oxygen tension, abrasive foodstuffs and maceration, systemic antibiotics and microbial antagonisms, periodic personal and professional oral hygiene, mucosal immune and non-immune antibacterial mechanisms, and swallowing. Virtually all surfaces in the mouth are coated with saliva. The salivary film will vary in composition depending on complex factors including the interfacial chemistry of specific oral surfaces, proximity of the surface to the ductal orifices of the different major and minor salivary glands, gustatory changes in concentrations and structures of salivary proteins and glycoproteins, lipids, and electrolytes, and modification by earlier resident flora. Not unlike algae in a fast-moving stream, streptococci, bathed in saliva, colonize the oral cavity because they bind or adhere to saliva-coated teeth and mucosal surfaces and cope and adjust with great facility to the complex and challenging environment.

To survive in the presence of many environmental stressors, the oral flora express sophisticated regulatory and response mechanisms [19]. For example, strains can be transmitted from host to host, with clonotypes expressing specific characteristics to enhance colonization and survival. Survival is enhanced by the cooperative fabrication of dental plaque, which provides a biofilm structure to offer an additional level of protection against rapid or wide fluctuations in growth conditions. Dental plaque also facilitates colonization of the species near "friends" and away from adversarial competitors.

Adherence Leads to Colonization

The oral streptococci employ several strategies to promote their adherence to the various hard and soft tissues of the oral cavity and, indeed, recapitulate with fidelity the known tissue tropisms. Since the species tend to segregate into intraoral niches, microbial strategies have evolved to overcome charge-charge repulsion with oral surfaces, bind the appropriate surface with selectivity, and stabilize adhesion to create anchorage. To bring the microbial surface to within molecular distances to the saliva-coated tooth, for example, hydrophobic interactions probably prevail. When the interfacial proximity is less than the van der Waals radius, specific streptococcal adhesins appear to mediate binding to stereochemically complimentary sites on the salivary film. If complimentary binding does not occur, the streptococcus may detach and remain resuspended in saliva until swallowed or there is sufficient contact with the specific niche. To colonize the niche, streptococci may require additional adhesive stabilization. To increase adhesion, many oral streptococci synthesize, process, and colonize within gummy extracellular polysaccharides, a process that is greatly enhanced by the presence of dietary sucrose.

While the specific mechanisms may differ, proteinaceous adhesins, physicochemical forces, and dextran biosynthesis each appear to contribute to the process of adhesion. The adhesins facilitate specific binding to sites on the soft tissues or saliva-coated tooth. The complimentary sites on the tooth are not well characterized, but likely consist of determinants formed by salivary proteins and other macromolecules and modified from their solution conformations by adsorption to the hydroxylapatite mineral of enamel. The genes for several adhesins of the oral streptococci have been identified. Some are conserved across species in this group of streptococci and others are known to be distributed more widely within the genus. Adhesins are generally considered to be proteins, although glycoproteins, lipoproteins, and polysaccharides have been described. Indeed, a single strain may express more than one adhesin or adhesins with more than one adhesive epitope (oligospecific).

Promotion of adhesion increases the ability to colonize. Among the prominent constituents of the salivary film that coats the teeth, candidate binding sites for streptococci include specific secretory immunoglobulin A (IgA) antibodies, mucin glycoproteins, and proline-rich proteins. While cell surface dextrans do not appear to serve as adhesins nor explain the specificity for binding of the oral streptococci in their niches, their production facilitates colonization. Indeed, agglutination by certain polymeric salivary macromolecules with binding specificity for streptococci and affinity for hydroxylapatite may also promote adhesion and colonization [20]. Small aggregates of streptococci appear to bind to saliva-coated hydroxylapatite more readily than single cells or large clumps. Agglutination of streptococci into larger aggregates may limit the potential for adhesion and colonization. The mass of the aggregate may exceed the strength of adhesive forces. Clearance from the oral cavity is promoted by swallowing.

Between birth and 2 months of age, infant saliva manifests specific secretory IgA1 titers primarily against strains of *Streptococcus mitis*, followed by antibodies against *Streptococcus salivarius* (reviewed in Smith and Taubman [21]). By 1 year, secretory IgA2 titers are also evident and with the eruption of the primary teeth, anti-*Streptococcus sanguis* antibodies are also identified. Certain species of "pioneer" early colonizing oral streptococci, predominately *Streptococcus mitis* and *Streptococcus oralis* [22] express secretory IgA1 proteases [23,24]. Strains expressing secretory IgA proteases may adhere preferentially to the saliva-coated tooth surface, particularly during infancy. While secretory IgA in the salivary film may promote adhesion of certain streptococci, specific antibodies in the saliva serve to agglutinate and clear them from the oral cavity by swallowing. Given the dipeptidyl peptidase specificity of cloned enzyme [25], secretory IgA1 proteases have been suggested to digest specific agglutinating antibodies in vivo, favoring pioneer colonization of strains that are less likely to be swallowed. Yet it is unclear to what extent this mechanism may actually work in the mouth. Recent evidence [26] indicates that anti-*Streptococcus mitis* secretory IgA antibodies are virtually intact in infant saliva. Indeed, some antibody may neutralize the secretory IgA protease, thus the oral tissues become colonized by *Streptococcus mitis* and other species nonetheless. The consensus of data indicates that specific secretory IgA antibodies control the levels of colonization by agglutination and swallowing of streptococci but may promote adhesion to the saliva-coated surfaces of the mouth and subsequent colonization.

Expression of Adhesins and Colonization

Adhesins (Table 18.1) may be defined in terms of their purported function as streptococcal surface macromolecules that promote binding of microbes to receptors in a biochemically specific manner. Selective adhesion characterizes the oral streptococci and reflects known tissue tropisms for colonization with *Streptococcus mutans* adhering best to dextran-coated hydroxyapatite, *Streptococcus sanguis* and *Streptococcus mitis* competing in part to bind saliva-coated hydroxyapatite (sHA), and *Streptococcus salivarius* showing the lowest affinity for these substrates [27]. Such interactions do not explain how charge-charge and van der Waals repulsion between the microbial surface and the tooth are surmounted, nor how the sheer of the tongue or salivary flow would be resisted. Indeed, the negative charge-charge repulsion of the apatitic and streptococcal cell surfaces needs to be surmounted and suggests that electrostatic interactions do not explain the specificity and stability of adhesion [28]. Arguably, adhesin–receptor interactions best explain the specific tissue tropisms so characteristic of the streptococci in the oral cavity.

Analysis of adhesins is complex and several lines of experimental evidence is required for verification. As described by Jenkinson [29], adhesins should be *(1)* expressed on the cell surface of adhering strains, blocked by *(2)* specific antibodies and *(3)* isolated purified homologues, and *(4)* unexpressed when the specific gene is inactivated. Often, inactivation of a putative adhesin gene is considered sufficient evidence for the identification of adhesins. Since the loss or alteration of more than one surface protein (pleiotropic phenotype) may occur when a putative adhesin gene is unexpressed [30], gene inactivation is not sufficient to identify an adhe-

sion [29]. Clearly, when an adhesin is blocked or unexpressed, adhesion should be inhibited or abrogated.

The best-characterized putative adhesins of the oral streptococci are the antigen I/II family of proteins [31,32]. Members of this family (having a deduced protein mass of 158 to 166 kDa) are expressed on most species of oral streptococci and include the proteins I/II, B, P1, SR, PAc, IF, SpaA, PAg, SSP-5, and p130 (Table 18.1; [33]). While there are strain and species differences, adhesins in the antigen I/II family generally contribute to hydrophobicity of the cell surface and facilitate co-aggregation with *actinomyces* ssp. and binding to sHA, an in vitro model of the enamel surface.

The molecular identity of the I/II family adhesin binding site on sHA is unclear. In the presence of calcium, these I/II family adhesins bind selectively to sialic acid residues available on a high-molecular-weight ($\sim$400 kDa) glycoprotein from parotid saliva, facilitating streptococcal agglutination in the fluid phase [34]. When sHA is treated with neuraminidase, the binding of certain strains is reduced while others are unaffected [35]. It is unclear whether the I/II adhesins actually bind the parotid agglutinin in salivary pellicle. Adhesins from the I/II family appear to employ two different internal epitopes or domains (N-terminal alanine-rich and central proline-rich regions) when reacting with fluid or immobilized (e.g., HA, nitrocellulose) salivary proteins [36–38]. Binding to the salivary agglutinin is confined to residues 186 to 469 of the alanine-rich region [39]. Furthermore, monoclonal antibodies specific for either protein or carbohydrate epitopes on high-molecular-weight glycoproteins present in saliva from the parotid and submaxillary glands both interfere with adherence of *Streptococcus mutans* serotype c to sHA [40]. Salivary proteins (or domains) other than parotid agglutinin are probably bound by many oral streptococci, and potentially, by group A (pyogenic) streptococci [41]. Clearly, several salivary proteins may serve as binding sites on sHA for oral streptococci.

Several well-characterized salivary macromolecules are likely binding sites on oral tissues and surfaces for streptococcal adhesins. Macromolecules such as mucin glycoproteins [42], for example, mediate sialic acid–dependent agglutination [43], and adhesion [44] of *Streptococcus sanguis*. *Streptococcus sanguis* appears to express a lectin with more restricted specificity than SSP-5, binding NeuNAc(α)2,3gal(β)1,3galNAc O-linked carbohydrate chains on salivary mucins [45] and buccal epithelial cells [46]. *Streptococcus gordonii*, which generally expresses family I/II adhesins, appears to bind to segments of adsorbed salivary proline-rich proteins on hydroxylapatite [47]. Indeed, several other immobilized salivary proteins [44], including low-molecular-weight mucin, glycosylated proline-rich proteins, and α-amylase [48], may selectively bind different oral streptococci. Furthermore, secretory IgA in salivary pellicle promotes adhesion of certain streptococci [49], perhaps in a complex with a high-molecular-mass salivary glycoprotein [50] or salivary α-amylase [51].

Taking advantage of the many different molecular determinants that might be attractive for binding to oral surfaces, the oral streptococci express adhesins other than antigen I/II. As putative adhesins with strong homology to both the ATP binding AmiA family of oligopeptide transporters [52,53] and an inducible high-affinity ABC transporter for Mn^{2+} uptake [54], the SsaB family of membrane-linked lipoproteins are widely expressed among the oral streptococci and include SarA, ScaA, SsaB, and FimA [55,56]. Although pleiotropic effects may confound interpretation, SarA deletion mutants show loss of adhesion to Actinomyces [30], whereas specific antibodies against the ScaA adhesin block binding [57]. Similarly, SsaB deletion results in reduced adhesion to sHA [58] and Actinomycetes [59]. While expected to be membrane linked, FimA immunolocalizes to the tips of the fimbriae [53]. The fimbriae are apparently unaltered in mutated strains. FimA behavior as an adhesin may therefore require that it be released from the membrane to be associated with fimbriae or polymerize into a fimbrial-associated structure. Together, FimA and antigen I/II only partially explain the repertoire of adhesins expressed by a strain of oral streptococci.

Oral streptococci show multiple adhesin specificities, with individual strains being able to bind to carbohydrate and protein targets. Some differences in specificity across strains and species may be explained by post-translational modifications in adhesin structure. Alternative expression of polymorphic forms of the same adhesin may alter specificity, perhaps in response to environmental pressure [60]. Individual strains appear oligospecific, however, expressing more than one adhesin [61]. For example, *Streptococcus sanguis* 133-79 expresses at least three independent adhesive determinants [62]. Each determinant and its contribution to adhesion to sHA can be inhibited independently with increasing doses of specific antibodies, defining surface antigens of 150, 130, (P1) and 87 kDa as adhesins. The 150 kDa adhesin contains two distinct adhesive domains. These data fulfill the prediction [63–65] that adhesion of some strains to sHA requires at least two cooperative sites of interaction complemented by nonspecific interfacial forces [66].

Adhesion of streptococci and other oral flora to intra-oral sites would appear to precede colonization or infection. Colonization and infection require access and retention in a preferred niche, availability of nutrients, companionable microbial neighbors, and freedom from antagonism. Retention and colonization on oral surfaces appear to be promoted when small aggregates or agglutinates of streptococci rather than single cells are bound [67]. Chained together, these small aggregates may adhere to oral surfaces with sufficient force to resist desorption by saliva and its constituents or the sheer created by the thrashing of the tongue or abrasive foodstuffs. For *Streptococcus gordonii*, colonization appears to depend upon the expression of the 290 kDa surface protein, CshA, which does not appear to be a major adhesin as identified and characterized in vitro [60,68]. How this protein promotes colonization is unclear.

CshA, however, appears to be environmentally regulated [69]. *Streptococcus gordonii cshA* promoter activity was enhanced when cells were incubated in conditioned medium. Since promoter activity was unaffected by growth in fresh medium, the adhesin appeared to be regulated by a product of growing *Streptococcus gordonii*. When the oligopeptide permease hppA was insertionally inactivated, expression of CshA and adhesion of *Streptococcus gordonii* to a co-aggregation partner (see below) were both reduced. The viridans streptococci express competence-stimulating peptides during growth, which are released into the medium and regu-

Table 18.1 Putative Adhesins of Oral Streptococci

Adhesin Protein	Gene (if known)	Location	Mass, kDa	Strain	Mutant Phenotype	Adherence-Specific Antibody	Purified Protein	Reference
I/II		Wall-associated	190	mutans				Russell et al. [338]
	PAc		163	MT8148	Reduced adhesion to sHA			Koga et al. [339]
B						Inhibited by specific monoclonal antibodies	Inhibited by residues 816–1161 [1213]	Russell [390], Lehner et al. [341], Munro et al. [37], Forester et al. [342], Lee et al. [343]
P1	spaP		166	NG5	Reduced binding to salivary agglutinin			
SR	sr		171	OMZ175				Ackermanns et al. [344]; Ogier et al. [345]
PAc IF	pac			MT8148				Okahashi et al. [346]; Hughes et al. [347]
SpaA	sspA	Wall-associated	210	sobrinus 6715	Reduced adhesion			Holt et al. [348]; Takahashi et al. [399]
			200	gordonii DL1	Reduced binding to salivary agglutinin; Actinomyces ssp			Jenkinson et al. [83]
PAg			210	sobrinus	Reduced binding to salivary agglutinin		Inhibited by residues 39–864	Okahashi et al. [350]; Nakai et al. [38]
SSP-5		Wall-associated	205	sanguis	Reduced binding to salivary agglutinin			Demuth et al. [34,351]
p130		Wall-associated	130	sanguis 133–79		Cross-reacts with P1; partially inhibits adhesion to sHA		Brady et al. [352]; Gong and Herzberg [62]
CshA/CshB	cshA/cshB	Wall-associated	259/245	gordonii DL1	Reduced colonization in vivo; co-aggregation with Actinomyces spp; hydrophobicity			McNab et al. [60]

Protein	Gene	Location	MW (kDa)	Species	Function/Property	Comments	Reference
Protein A	uvapA	Wall-associated	45	mutans GS-5	Reduced sucrose-dependent adhesion to smooth surfaces		Qian and Dao [151]
	AgA [uvapA]	Wall-associated	45	mutans LT11	Unchanged adhesion to sHA		Harrington and Russell [151a]
	AgB	Wall-associated	185	mutans LT11	Reduced adhesion to sHA; increased adhesion to glucan pellicle		Harrington and Russell [151a]
SsaB	ssaB	Wall-associated	36	sanguis	Reduced adhesion to sHA		Ganeshkumar et al. [58,59]
SarA	sarA	Wall-associated	76 Lipoprotein	gordonii DL1	Reduced coaggregation with Actinomyces ssp. hydrophobicity		Jenkinson [353]
ScaA	scaA	Wall-associated	38 Lipoprotein	gordonii PK488	Reduced coaggregation with Actinomyces spp. hydrophobicity		Andesen et al. [57]
FimA	fimA	Wall-associated	34	para sanguis FW213			Fives-Taylor et al. [354]; Fenno et al. [355]
PsaA	psaA	Wall-associated	37	Streptococcus pneumoniae			Sampson et al. [356]
LFP		Wall-associated	300	sanguis	Adhesion???		Morris et al. [357]
Adhesin		Wall-associated	70–90	sanguis			Liljemark and Bloomquist [358]
Fap1	fap1	Wall-associated	200	para sanguis FW213	Reduced adhesion to sHA; loss of long peritrichous fimbriae		Wu et al. [359]
C9B adhesin		Wall-associated	84	sanguis	Reduced adhesion to sHA; expresses fibrils	Inhibit adhesion to sHA	Lamont et al. [360,361]; Rosan et al. [362]
Amylase-binding protein	abpA	Wall-associated	20	gordonii	Reduced binding to amylase		Rogers et al. [363]
IgA-binding protein			39	sobrinus		Adsorbed by putative adhesin	Frithz et al. [364]; Tokuda et al. [365]
IgG-binding protein			65	sanguis			Kronvall [366]; Bjorck et al. [367]
Sialic acid–binding		Wall-associated	96, 70 (red); 65	sanguis; mitis	Sialic acid–binding lectin	Adhesion inhibited by NeuAc(α)2,3Gal(β)1,3GalNAc	Levine et al. [43]; Murray et al. [45,368]
Glucan-binding		Extracellular	74		Glucan-binding lectin		Russell [195]; Banas et al. [150]; Cox et al. [99]

late the ability of cells to take up naked DNA via a related two-component receptor system [70]. These oral streptococci may therefore regulate expression of some adhesins in response to environmental conditions.

Co-aggregation Partners

The oral streptococci may choose their neighbors from among noncompeting gram-positive and -negative bacteria and other microorganisms. In the oral cavity, a low frequency of intergenera co-aggregation may occur [71], facilitating microbial access to a preferred niche by carriage on a commensal neighbor. Intergenera microbial co-aggregations ascertained in vitro appear attenuated by saliva [72], although multivalent salivary agglutinin-like molecules may bind any microorganism that expresses the requisite adhesin [73]. In plaque, streptococci appear to bind selectively and become coated with proteins such as α-amylase and secretory IgA from saliva [74]. If amylase, for example, denatures, the specificity of binding favors *Streptococcus sanguis* [75]. Yet, compelling morphological evidence for co-aggregation in dental plaque is the frequent visualization of "corncobs" formed by streptococci (the kernels) bound to rod-shaped *Fusobacterium nucleatum* or *Bacterionema matruchotii* (the cobs) [76–78]. Furthermore, germ-free mice monoinfected with *Streptococcus mutans* supported subsequent colonization by Veillonellae, which would not sustain as a primary infection [79]. Veillonella co-aggregate in vitro with many species of oral streptococci [80].

Indeed, many common genera of oral bacteria show lactose-reversible co-aggregation [81]. To interact with Actinomyces [82], *Streptococcus sanguis* and *Streptococcus gordonii* employ SsaB/SspA/ScaA as an adhesin [57,59,83]. Other cohabiting pairs suggested by in vitro data include oral streptococci and lactobacilli [84], *Candida albicans* [85], or *Porphyromonas gingivalis* [86]. Intragenera galactosyl-specific co-aggregation between species of oral streptococci is also documented [87]. Pairing with selected early colonizing streptococci, the co-aggregation partners generally lack an adhesin system for an oral surface. *C. albicans* adhesins for sHA and *Streptococcus gordonii* are environmentally co-

regulated, which increases the probability of adhesion to the tooth if and when needed [88] to supplement or compliment integrin receptor-like binding to iC3b on epithelial cells [89,90]. The co-aggregation partners instead express adhesins for streptococci, which are able to immobilize in the preferred niche.

Specific Salivary Components May Promote Oral Clearance

Perhaps the greatest threat to microbial colonization is clearance promoted by swallowing of saliva. About 1 ml/min of saliva is swallowed. During normal turnover and renewal, epithelial cells and attached streptococci awash as flotsam into the saliva. Some bacteria may suspend freely in the fluid and others may desorb competitively from binding sites on the oral surfaces by interactions with salivary constituents. Salivary constituents that bind streptococci in the fluid phase may be the same molecules that serve as binding sites on the tooth. Some of these salivary proteins are multivalent, binding more than one streptococcal cell. Agglutination of streptococci by salivary components may promote colonization at the tooth surface [67], but clearance in the salivary fluid. For example, salivary mucins will bind and agglutinate *Streptococcus sanguis* [43]. Among the specificities in the mucosal repertoire, secretory IgA will also agglutinate species of oral streptococci [49] and contribute to antigen disposal by swallowing. Other salivary components have been suggested to serve as endogenous agglutinins, including the high-molecular-weight parotid agglutinin, which contains a sialic acid–containing binding domain for *Streptococcus sanguis* [34], secretory IgA [91], and mucin glycoprotein 2 (MG2) [92]. Alpha amylase may serve as a binding site for *Streptococcus sanguis* on the tooth [48]. While not an agglutinin, amylase in saliva may competitively desorb selected streptococci from the tooth. The proline-rich proteins (PRPs), a major family of secretory proteins, may bind *Streptococcus gordonii* to the tooth [47]. In the saliva, however, the streptococcal binding domains of the PRPs are in an inaccessible conformation termed cryptitopes [47,72]. For the glycosylated PRPs, expression of alternatively spliced alleles may either promote or selectively delete specific microbial colonization in the plaque flora [93]. Gene expression for these major salivary proteins is regulated by a highly conserved system in response to neurogenic stimuli [94,95]. Consequently, gustatory stimuli and chronic dietary patterns may influence the expression and availability of these streptococcal binding proteins and thus the tendency to adhere and colonize.

Salivary clearance of streptococci may also be promoted by foodstuffs and dietary substances that mix with saliva during eating. For example, milk and casein-containing proteins appear to competitively and selectively desorb streptococci from teeth in vivo [96] and saliva-coated hydroxylapatite in vitro [97,98]. In addition to the more familiar effects on acid metabolism in streptococci and the solubility of apatitic mineral of enamel, fluoride in drinking water may promote desorption of certain streptococci from teeth by interfering with the glucan-binding lectin [99]. Expression of the glucan-binding lectin may be up- or down-regulated by the presence of low concentrations of certain antibiotics [100]. The hydrophobicity of the streptococcal cell appears inversely related to expression of this lectin. Consequently, physical and biochemically specific adhesion may be modified passively at the substrate interface and at the level of adhesin expression by the action of dietary substances.

Saliva and Nonimmune Antibacterials May Inhibit or Control Colonization

Saliva is produced and swallowed at the rate of about 1 ml of fluid per minute. Without a large residual volume in the oral cavity, the frank growth of streptococci in saliva is precluded. Some salivary constituents may be directly antimicrobial. These salivary antimicrobials may originate in the salivary fluid or be released from other tissues in the oral cavity including the epithelium. Consequently, proteins such as lactoferrin, lactoperoxidase, and lysozyme, the defensins, and S100 calcium-binding proteins, including calprotectin [S100A8/9], are all effectively expressed in the saliva. Although these nonimmune antimicrobials may not be needed to limit the growth of microorganisms in the salivary fluid, they may limit the growth of the resident flora and control the extent of colonization

on the teeth and mucosal surfaces. People express differing amounts or isoforms of these antimicrobials and the oral flora vary in sensitivity. Hence, these proteins may limit colonization and protect against intraoral infections in otherwise healthy individuals, and altered expression or intrusion of resistant microorganisms may permit oral infections as seen, for example, in patients with AIDS.

Intermicrobial Antagonisms

The streptococci compete with each other and other oral species to colonize. Colonization may be restricted by competition for nutrients or by thwarting competitors by the elaboration of bacteriocins, which are similar to peptide antibiotics. Streptococci elaborate species-specific antibacterial lantibiotics generally targeting other gram-positive bacteria. These compounds appear to limit the growth of other streptococci attempting to colonize the same niche. Within dental plaque, such antagonisms by dominant species may limit the colonial growth of unwanted competing neighbors. For example, isolates of *Streptococcus salivarius* produce a lantibiotic that inhibits the growth of Mycobacteria, Corynebacteria, *Streptococcus pneumonia*, and groups A, C, and F streptococci [101,102]. This antagonistic mechanism may allow *Streptococcus salivarius* to become among the earliest and eventually the most prominent colonizer of oral mucosal surfaces, protecting its niche effectively against putative respiratory pathogens. The commensal streptococci are resistant to *Streptococcus salivarius* lantibiotic. Expressed by *Streptococcus salivarius*, salivaricin A has a mass of 2315 Da and contains the lantibiotic-specific amino acid, lanthionine [103]. Analogues are produced by other oral streptococci and include the mutacins of *Streptococcus mutans* [104–106] and compounds elaborated by other streptococci that inhibit *Streptococcus mutans* [107]. In the human oral cavity, *Streptococcus mutans* bacteriocin can modulate its ability to colonize in the complex competitive flora [104]. Indeed, the engineering of lantibiotic-like inhibitors of putative pathogens in commensal streptococci is an intriguing strategy for the prevention of infectious diseases such as caries and periodontal diseases [108].

Colonization of Mucosal and Dental Surfaces

In the first year of life, the oral streptococci colonize in a species-specific manner [109]. *Streptococcus mitis* biovar I colonizes the mucosal surfaces of most infants in the highest numbers. *Streptococcus salivarius* also colonizes at high prevalence, but as a very low percentage of the total flora. One-third of infants are colonized by *Streptococcus oralis* or *Streptococcus anginosus*. After eruption, the teeth of many infants are colonized by *Streptococcus sanguis*. *Streptococcus mutans*, if present, generally colonizes below detectable levels. Exclusive of *Streptococcus mutans*, the pioneer species colonize prominently into adulthood, with *Streptococcus mitis* establishing on the mucosal surfaces [110–111], *Streptococcus salivarius* dominating over time on the tongue [112–114], and *Streptococcus sanguis* on the tooth [110,115]. Like *Streptococcus sanguis*, *Streptococcus mutans* appears only on teeth after eruption, but appears to be transmitted from mothers [116] within a discrete window of infectivity at about 26 months of age [117].

The ability to transport and metabolize dietary sucrose is a major factor contributing to the retention of many groups of streptococci in the oral cavity. Sucrose is the specific substrate for the synthesis of dextrans and related polymers. Dextrans serve to make the streptococcal surface sticky. Alternatively, when dextrans are released and coat an approximating surface, adhesion of streptococci is facilitated through glucan-binding lectins. Considered a primary virulence factor in the etiology of dental caries, sucrose and sugar metabolism will be discussed more completely in a later section.

Given these many competing factors that may promote or antagonize colonization, the rates and patterns of growth are complex in this diverse ecosystem [118]. Growth varies between linear and exponential patterns, yet the weight (including water) of the dental plaque biomass is proportional to the protein concentration. Growth depends most strongly on the founder species, dominance over the various competitive factors, and the specific environment, including the formation and spatial organization of microcolonies of newly acquired microorganisms in a maturing or mature plaque [71,81,119,120]. Viability appears to depend most strongly on nutritional shifts, which may produce substantial, rapid increases in cell numbers [15,121]. The mass of plaque is limited in the oral cavity by the abrasive sheer of opposing surfaces and foodstuffs, and oral hygiene measures.

STREPTOCOCCUS MUTANS, THE INTRAORAL PATHOGEN

Streptococci as Etiological Agents in Dental Caries

Streptococcus mutans is generally accepted to cause caries of the coronal aspect of the tooth [122]. This lesion is among the most prevalent of human infections and reflects the complex virulence of this group of streptococci. The lesion initiates with the demineralization of enamel, the hardest mineral in the body. Progression into dentin is accompanied by further demineralization and dissolution of the organic matrix. Older adults incur root caries, with a microbial etiology that is still being defined [123–125], but, as in coronal caries, microorganisms including *Streptococcus mutans*, which bind [126,127] and enzymatically modify [128] dentinal collagen, may have a selective advantage. Expression of proteases appear to facilitate further demineralization and provide a protected environment for colonization by pathogens.

The carious lesion results from complex interplay between exogenous fermentable sugars from the diet, products of acidogenic and aciduric bacteria, and susceptible hard tissue surfaces. To demineralize enamel or dentin, the mutans streptococci export protons and lactic acid, which lower the pH in the oral microenvironment to 4. The drop in plaque pH is driven by the metabolism of fermentable sugars, particularly dietary sucrose and fructose [129], and by acidogenic, aciduric mutans streptococci and other bacteria (see reviews by Hamada and Slade [11], Macrina et al. [130], Kuramitsu [131], van Houte [132], LeBlanc [133], and Russell [134]). Fermentation appears to be regulated in part by the enzyme pyruvate-formate lyase, which controls the metabolism of sugar alcohols, such as sorbitol and mannitol [135].

Salivary constituents serve as the major buffer of plaque acids [132,136]. In the presence of buffering, nitrogen-rich amino acids and small peptides found in saliva, *Streptococcus mutans* grows well. The ever-adaptable *Streptococcus mutans* imports amino acids and small peptides via specialized oligopeptide permeases and related transport systems, including perhaps an ATP-dependent glutamine transport system that allows intracellular catabolism of peptides and amino acids to glutamate and ammonia [137]. Ammonia is also produced through catabolism of urea, which reduces acid production during fermentation and the occurrence of carious lesions [138]. Streptococci that colonize the mucous membranes, such as *Streptococcus salivarius*, express substantial urease activity [139], possibly contributing to the neutralization of plaque acids. Neutralization of plaque acids appears to antagonize the emergence of acidogenic and aciduric streptococci in nearby dental plaque [140,141] and reduce or reverse the demineralization of the hard dental tissues [142–144]. Restriction of fermentable sugars in the diet appears to reduce the levels of cariogenic streptococci in the saliva and in dental plaque [145]. By mitigating the presence of cariogenic microorganisms and specific substrate for acid production, the risk of caries declines.

In human caries, *Streptococcus mutans* may not act alone. Like *Streptococcus mutans*, *Lactobacillus casei* shows cariogenic potential, but may be even more acidogenic and aciduric [132]. The cariogenicity of lactobacilli has been confirmed in animal models [7] and epidemiological studies [146–148]. Since the work of Fitzgerald and Keyes in the 1950s and 1960s (reviewed by Tanzer [6]), a consensus has emerged to suggest that *Streptococcus mutans* is the major initiating pathogen [122], yet lactobacilli can be isolated from carious lesions about two-thirds as frequently as *Streptococcus mutans* [149] and may coexist in dental plaque. *Lactobacillus* species may colonize dental plaque through the selective co-aggregation noted in vitro with several commensal pioneer species of oral streptococci including *Streptococcus sanguis* and *Streptococcus gordonii* [84]. Upon colonization, *Lactobacillus* species can contribute to the progression of the demineralizing lesions [147].

To promote dental caries, major virulence factors expressed by *Streptococcus mutans* and related microorganisms include adhesins, specialized transports systems for fermentable sugars, synthesis of soluble and insoluble dextrans and fructans, and acidogenesis and aciduricity (reviewed in Kuramitsu [131]).

Adhesins

Streptococcus mutans generally expresses adhesins in the antigen I/II family, which probably promotes adhesion to the salivary film or pellicle that coats the teeth. Since expression of this adhesin is common to the pioneer species that predominate in dental plaque at most dental anatomic sites, cariogenic streptococci may use additional strategies to attach and facilitate colonization at preferred sites. On interproximal smooth surfaces and in the pits and fissures of teeth, salivary flow is minimal and weakly immobilized mutans streptococci may resist dislodgment. In these protected dental areas, the soluble dextrans synthesized by immobilized streptococci may locally incorporate and modify the salivary pellicle. *Streptococcus mutans* expresses glucan-binding proteins [150], including the wall-associated protein A [151,151a]. To stabilize its adhesion, *Streptococcus mutans* appears to produce both the needed adhesins and the complimentary binding sites.

Specialized Transport Systems and Metabolism of Fermentable Sugars

The ability of mutans group streptococci in dental plaque to import and ferment dietary sucrose, produce and tolerate acid, and synthesize soluble and insoluble polymers of glucose and fructose appears pivotal to their virulence as cariogenic microorganisms (reviewed by LeBlanc [133]). Survival of these microorganisms may depend on metabolism of dietary sucrose and other fermentable sugars in conditions of substrate limitation. Caries and the virulence of certain streptococci, on the other hand, often reflect metabolism during sucrose surfeit. Cariogenic streptococci import sucrose and other fermentable sugars by specialized transport systems. Three sucrose transport systems in these streptococci have been identified [152]: high-

and low-affinity sucrose-specific phosphoenol-pyruvate-dependent phosphotransferase system (PTS) [153–155], and a very low–affinity non-PTS transport or multiple sugar metabolism (MSM) system [156,157]. A glucose-specific non-PTS transport system has also been identified [158].

The sugars transported and metabolized through the PTS include glucose and sucrose, fructose, mannose, lactose, maltose, N-acetyl-glucosamine, trehalose, mannitol, and sorbitol. The *msm* operon transports and metabolizes structurally diverse sugars including sucrose, raffinose, stachyose, melibiose, isomaltosaccharides, and palatinose [159,160]. Unlike the PTS, the *msm* operon controls only the transport, but not metabolism, of glucose, galactose, maltose, and maltotriose. Yet recent evidence suggests that transport of sugars unique to the MSM system, such as raffinose, may be under control of the PTS [161] with an unusual mechanism of catabolite repression [162].

The transport and metabolism of sucrose, for example, follows generally the pathways highlighted in Figure 18.4 to yield products of ecological and clinical importance. Sucrose is captured with high affinity (Km = 70 μM) and transported into the cell by the membrane-associated, sucrose-specific enzyme II (EII^{suc}; *scrA*) of the PTS [162a,163,164]. Most intracellular sucrose is rapidly phosphorylated by heat-stable phosphocarrier protein (HPr ~ P) [165,166] and hydrolyzed to fructose and glucose-6-phosphate, a reaction catalyzed by sucrose-6-phosphate hydrolase (*scrB*) [167–170]. The glucose-6-phosphate enters fermentation to be hydrolyzed to phosphoenolpyruvate (PEP), to provide high-energy phosphate to HPr, and through pyruvate, to lactate (lactic acid). Lactic acid appears then to be exported across the cell membrane in an electroneutral process without a requirement for metabolic energy [171]. In the extracellular plaque fluid, lactic acid appears to efficiently demineralize the hydroxyapatite-rich mineral of the tooth [122].

Sucrose is also hydrolyzed extracellularly by fructosyl- and glucosyltransferases. The PTS also transports the products, glucose and fructose, by specific enzymes (EII^{glc}, EII^{fru}) contained within the membrane. Upon phosphorylation of these products by HPr ~ P, additional glucose-6-phosphate and fructose-6-phosphate enter fermentation and contribute to the production of acid.

The PTS also provides a low-affinity transport system for sucrose [152,162a], which appears to be identical to the high-affinity, trehalose-specific EII^{tre} (not shown in Fig. 18.1; [155]), but different from a third transport system for sucrose with very low affinity and independent of the PTS (TTS, not shown in Fig. 18.1; [152,172]. These low-affinity systems appear to function during periods of high sucrose availability, supplementing the transport function of EII^{suc} and contributing additional production of acid through fermentation.

The very low–affinity, PTS-independent mechanism for sucrose transport is now considered to be the MSM system [133]. Whether the MSM system is intended primarily to transport and metabolize high levels of dietary sucrose or more complex sugars is yet unclear (Fig. 18.1), but it is transcribed as a single operon [173]. In the presence of more complex sugars or when the PTS is repressed, sucrose is transported, hydrolyzed, and phosphorylated in mutans streptococci by the products of the regulated *msm* operon [157,159,160]. For example, raffinose is bound and transported by a four-subunit protein binding-dependent system [157], including MsmF, MsmG, MsmE, which is linked to the cell membrane by a lipid anchor [174], and MsmK, and ATPase. Within the cell, raffinose is hydrolyzed to galactose and sucrose by an intracellular α-galactosidase (*aga*) encoded within this operon [175]. The sucrose product is then phosphorylated and hydrolyzed by sucrose-1-phosphorylase (GtfA) [176] to fructose, which is fermented, and glucose-1-phosphate, which is polymerized to glycogen for storage. Similarly, isomaltotriose, another complex sugar, can be bound and transported and then hydrolyzed by intracellular dextran glucosidase (dexB) [177]. The resulting glucose-1-phosphate can also be converted to glycogen or fructose-6-phosphate, contributing to the pool of acid-producing metabolites.

The PTS and MSM systems export lactic acid to prevent acidification of the intracellular environment [171,178] (sugar transport and metabolism reviewed by Hamilton [179]). In the presence of an exogenous carbon source (e.g.,

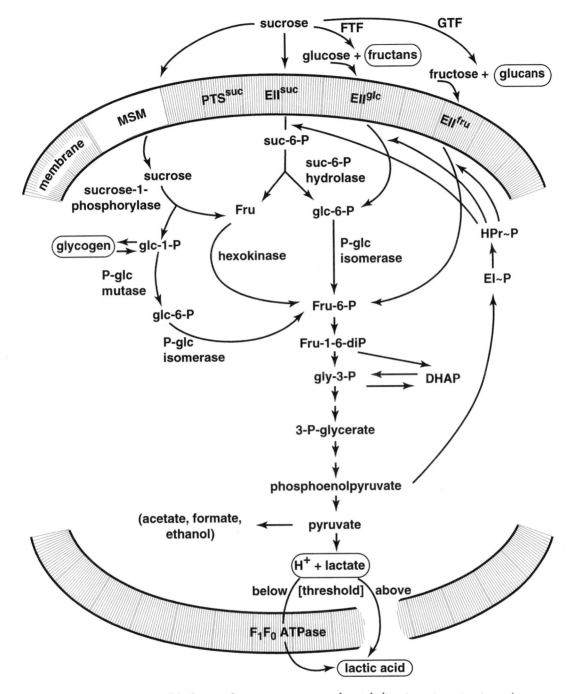

Figure 18.4 A simplified view of sucrose transport and metabolism in mutans streptococci.

glucose), the cell will maintain a pH gradient of 0.9 units from the inside to the outside. There are two mechanisms to maintain this gradient. At low concentrations of intracellular hydrogen ion and extracellular pH near neutrality, the F_1F_0 ATPase pumps out protons at a cost of ATP. At suprathreshold intracellular concentrations, lactic acid is also exported by efflux down a concentration gradient. At low extracellular pH, energy is provided by the generation of proton motive force (PMF) driven in part by chemical potential gradient created by the efflux of lactate. The sum of the resulting membrane electrical potential gradient and the pH gradient is the PMF. When external pH is low, the PMF appears to drive the cellular uptake of glucose, a high glycolytic rate, and growth. When cells lack an exogenous carbon source, the glycogen-depleted starved cell will generate little ATP and without energy the pH gradient and PMF are lost. The pH_i and pH_o approach equilibrium. Disruption of pH regulation by the membrane is a target for antimicrobial actions of salivary lysozyme [180] and fluoride [181].

Synthesis of Dextrans (and Fructans)

Mediated by availability of sucrose (and fructose) [182,183], mutans streptococci synthesize extracellular polysaccharides [184–186]. The dextran-synthetic glucosyltransferase enzymes are expressed on cell [122] and, upon release from the streptococcus, on tooth surfaces [187] and in saliva [188]. Among the sucrose-dependent polysaccharide biosynthetic enzymes, *gtfc* encodes glucosyltransferase C (GtfC), enabling synthesis of both soluble and insoluble dextrans [189]; *gtfd* provides for primer-dependent synthesis of soluble glycans [190], whereas *gtfb* encodes an enzyme that synthesizes soluble glucans exclusively [191]. Interestingly, the biosynthetic linkage specificity and substrate utilization of the enzymes appear to be modified by activity in different environments [192]. For example, GtfC activity in solution yields primarily α-1,6-linked glucose, while on hydroxyapatite surfaces, α-1,3-linked glucose predominates. Furthermore, the Gtf appear to inhibit salivary amylase activity on hydroxyapatite surfaces, limiting the availability of starch hydrolysis products such as maltose [193]. Starch hydrolysis products enhance the activity of hydroxyapatite-immobilized GtfB, for example, and the glucan product becomes increasingly resistant to digestion by glucanohydrolases.

Glucans synthesized in experimental salivary pellicles appear to compliment the salivary macromolecules and act as specific binding sites for *Streptococcus mutans* [194], probably mediated by cell-surface glucan-binding proteins [195]. The water-insoluble products of GtfB and GtfC appear to be major contributors to the adhesion of *Streptococcus mutans* to teeth and promotion of dental caries on smooth surfaces [182,196]. Synthesis of dextran (and fructan) polymers may increase the cell colonial density [197] and also act as a diffusion barrier to localize elaborated acids against the tooth surface and restrict access by neutralizing salivary constituents [141].

Acidogenicity/Aciduricity

Mutans streptococci produce acid as a byproduct of sugar metabolism, with export of protons mediated primarily by F_1F_0 ATPases (reviewed by Carlsson [198] and Bowden and Li [197]). The glucose transport enzymes are sensitive to fluoride [199], constituting an additional cariostatic mechanism to compliment the direct action of fluoride on the mineral structure of enamel. The mutans streptococci are also aciduric, capable of surviving at the low pH they create [141,200–203]. In dental plaque, the aciduricity of these streptococci provides a survival advantage over less acid-tolerant microbial competitors.

Cariogenicity of *Streptococcus mutans* depends therefore on expression of mechanisms to demineralize enamel or cementum and dentin. In the presence of sucrose and other fermentable sugars, cells produce acid, while synthesizing soluble and insoluble dextrans and related polysaccharides. Glucans bound to the tooth surface may serve as an additional adhesion system for streptococci that express cell-surface glucan binding protein. Insoluble dextrans form structural mats that protect dividing cells and facilitate colonial growth and an increase in cell density on the tooth surface. With the acidogenic and aciduric mutans streptococci residing within, the mat of extracellular polysaccharides reduces diffusion away from the tooth surface, concentrating protons at the dental surface. Acid pH increases the solubility of enamel and other mineralized tissues, while proteases digest the organic matrix. With proportionally greater protein contents, cementum and dentin generally suffer more substantial damage from caries than enamel. Proteolysis appears to facilitate additional demineralization and protected colonization in the cavitated tooth mineral.

ORAL STREPTOCOCCI AS SOFT TISSUE AND SYSTEMIC PATHOGENS

Effects of Viridans Streptococci on Cytokine Production

Bacteria in the oral cavity express a repertoire of proinflammatory substances that have been suggested to be opposed at mucosal surfaces by elicited cytokine networks [204]. While the viridans streptococci are generally considered to be harmless commensals, it is clear that when given the opportunity, these microorganisms elicit pro-inflammatory (204a) and procoagulatory effects on a variety of target cells. *Streptococcus sanguis* has been shown to enhance tissue factor expression by monocytes in vitro and ex vivo in a rabbit model [205]. Peripheral blood mononuclear cells have been shown to produce tumor necrosis factor beta (TNF-β) and interleukin-8 (IL-8) in response to viridans streptococci [206]. Similarly, murine macrophages produce TNF-α in response to viridans streptococci [207] while lipoteichoic acid stimulates production of TNF and interferon-γ (IFN-γ), leading to the production of nitric oxide by murine macrophage [208]. *Streptococcus mutans* stimulated KB cells to produce IL-8, and endothelial cells to produce IL-6 and IL-8 [209]. In response to antigen I/II or rhamnose-glucose polymers, these cells produce the same cytokines [209]. When 59 strains of viridans streptococci were incubated independently with human peripheral blood mononuclear cells, all were found to stimulate the production of TNF-α, TNF-β, and IL-8 in vitro [210]. Not unexpectedly, then, cell walls or heat-killed *Streptococcus mitis* caused elevated levels of TNF when inoculated into the blood of mice [211]. Such inocula proved lethal and were attributed to the activity of lipoteichoic acid (LTA).

Hence, it is not surprising that viridans streptococci are the most frequent cause of septic shock associated with a neutropenia secondary to immunosuppressive protocols in patients receiving autologous bone marrow transplants [212]. During alpha-hemolytic streptococcal shock syndrome, TNF and IL-6 are both elevated, while IL-1 is undetected [213]. TNF-α and IFN-γ are the principal cytokines expressed in vitro by unsuppressed human tonsillar lymphocytes stimulated with alpha-hemolytic streptococci [214].

The viridans streptococci also elicit cytokine networks among cells in host tissues. For example, *Streptococcus mitis* and *Streptococcus oralis* culture supernatants elicit production of TNF-α, IL-6, and IFN-γ when inoculated intravenously into primed mice [215]. After chromatographic separation, one fraction (F-1) was shown to elicit production of TNF-α, IL-6, and IL-1 from monocytes and macrophage, while this fraction elicited IL-1 and IL-6 from endothelial cells and fibroblasts. Hence, cytokines expressed in vivo in response to viridans streptococci must be viewed as the products of many different contributing cells, each expressing a different set of cytokine genes. Another fraction (F-2) from the culture supernatant was found to stimulate T cell Vβ2/Vβ5.1 receptors in a manner consistent with the presence of superantigen [216,217]. The superantigen-containing fraction stimulated CD8$^+$ T cells to be directly cytotoxic to human oral epithelial carcinoma cells and human gingival keratinocytes. Human gingival fibroblasts were also stimulated by F-1 to produce cytokines that caused T cells to proliferate. In the presence of superantigen-containing F-2, cytotoxic T cells elaborated IL-2 and IFN-γ. The viridans streptococci, therefore, express several types of pro-inflammatory and pro-coagulatory substances. As noninvasive commensals, these mechanisms only manifest upon entry of the bacteria into the blood and connective tissues.

It is tempting to speculate that the viridans streptococci may contribute to the pathogenesis of local oral infections such as periodontitis. These proinflammatory bacteria represent a high proportion of the subgingival dental plaque flora associated with periodontitis. Abundant species such as *Streptococcus sanguis* express formyl-methionyl-peptides, which are chemoattractants for polymorphonuclear leukocytes (PMNs) [218]. Acute episodes of periodontitis are characterized by PMN infiltrates, which transmigrate into the gingival crevice and the oral cavity. While low-molecular-weight peptides may diffuse into the gingival epithelium, access for intact cells and larger pro-inflammatory substances probably occurs via an ulcerated crevicular lining adjacent to the tooth.

Viridans Streptococcal Bacteremia and Sepsis

The viridans streptococci gain access to the circulation frequently throughout life, taking advantage of a variety of portals of entry [219]. Virtually half of the blood culture isolates obtained after dental procedures in children [220 and adults [221] are viridans streptococci. General dental and mucosal therapeutic procedures that are associated with breach of the soft tissues result in a high frequency of detectable bacteremia within 10 min [222]. For example, detectable bacteremia is noted in virtually all cases of dental extractions and half of bilateral tonsillectomies, the latter reflecting the rather widespread anatomic sites of colonization by these microorganisms. Hence, tonsillectomy [223], tonsillitis [224], and adenoidectomy [225] commonly result in viridans streptococcal bacteremia. Viridans streptococci are identified in throat and blood cultures subsequent to upper respiratory infections and the isolated organisms are frequently found to be resistant to penicillin [226]. In children, treatment for otitis media appears to result in the emergence of antibiotic-resistant *Streptococcus sanguis* in dental plaque, including strains that show multiple resistance [227]. Months to years may be required for the antibiotic-resistant organisms to disappear from dental plaque. Penicillin-resistant oral streptococci were isolated from 40% of healthy children without antibiotic consumption for the previous 3 months, but from only 5% of adult leukemia patients [227,228]. While the emergence of antibiotic-resistant viridans streptococci is well known to be associated with refractory infective endocarditis, these microorganisms are occasionally associated with community-acquired pneumonia [229] and childhood meningitis [230].

The ability of the commensal viridans streptococci to contribute to systemic disease is observed most dramatically in patients with neutropenia. In these patients, viridans streptococcal bacteremia is frequently associated with the development of septic shock and death [212,231–233]. In patients who are neutropenic and treated in a hematology unit, 75% of the viridans streptococci isolated from blood cultures are *Streptococcus oralis* and 18% are *Streptococcus mitis*, as classified by the scheme by Beighton [234]. In the general hospital population, *Streptococcus milleri* is more commonly isolated from blood cultures than *Streptococcus anginosus*, followed by *Streptococcus constellatus* and *Streptococcus intermedius* [234]. Virtually all patients presenting with a nonpneumococcal viridans streptococcal bacteremia in association with immunocompromise or other debilitating disease show an oral or gastrointestinal origin of infection. Generally, oral and gastrointestinal mucositis [234,235] is a consequence of repeated chemotherapy resulting in profound neutropenia [236,237]. The resulting viridans streptococcal bacteremias appear to result in shock in up to 18% of patients and up to one-third show acute respiratory stress syndrome; reported mortality rates approach 30% [236]. Complicating postautologous peripheral blood stem-cell transplantation, *Streptococcus sanguis* and *Streptococcus mitis* bacteremia are reported in an average of 17.5% of cases 6 days later [238]. A recent review of 195 cases of hospital-based nosocomial blood culture isolates indicates that viridans streptococci predominate in about 3% of all cases. Nine percent of isolates are penicillin resistant and of the penicillin-resistant isolates, two-thirds are multiply resistant [239]. Therefore, the viridans streptococci must be considered to be clinically significant systemic pathogens capable of producing shock and death after gaining access to the blood.

Association of Viridans Streptococci with Infective Endocarditis

Perhaps the most widely recognized systemic consequence of viridans streptococcal bacteremia is infective endocarditis [240]. Infective endocarditis is characterized by septic platelet-rich vegetations that form on injured heart valves. Pro-inflammatory cytokines (240a) and tissue factor (205) are expressed in model systems. The associated febrile illness and sepsis is frequently refractory to antibiotic therapy. Unsuccessful intervention may result in obstruction of infected valves, dissemination of septic thrombi to other organs, and death. In different patient populations and clinical settings, up to 79% of confirmed cases of infective endocarditis are associated with repeated positive identification of viridans streptococci in blood cultures [241–245]. Among the viridans streptococci, *Streptococcus sanguis* and *Streptococcus oralis* are the predominant species recovered in infective endocarditis [243]. In culture-negative endocarditis, *Streptococcus adjacens* and *defectivus* are isolated as nutritionally variant streptococci [246].

Historically, the ability of viridans streptococci to synthesize "sticky" insoluble dextrans has been viewed as a primary virulence factor [240]. Insoluble dextran production is sucrose-dependent. Since there is no sucrose in blood, the importance of dextran production during infection of the heart valves is to be questioned.

From experiments in a rat model of endocarditis, it is likely that viridans streptococci can enter the circulation to infect the heart valve, secondary to tooth extraction [247] or periodontitis [248]. During dental manipulations, fragments of the dental biofilm and individual cells or chains of streptococci probably enter the bloodstream. In the blood, it is unclear whether viridans streptococci are equally virulent if they grew as individual cells or in close proximity to neighbors in the dental plaque biofilm. Environmentally regulated genes may impart different virulence characteristics to the viridans streptococci inoculated from disparate niches. During growth, planktonic streptococci alter expression of potentially important virulence factors. For example, in the presence of collagen, the platelet aggregation–associated protein from *Streptococcus sanguis* becomes increasingly platelet interactive, taking on characteristics of a multivalent ligand [249]. Similarly, *Streptococcus gordonii* virulence may be affected by growth in the presence of laminin, which may affect its virulence in human endocarditis [250]. The streptococci transit in the blood to selectively attach to and colonize injured heart valves. On the valves, the virulence may again change, reflecting genes that are uniquely expressed in vivo. Using a recently developed promoter-less dual reporter gene construct in a library of *Streptococcus gordonii* clones, it is also now apparent that numerous streptococcal genes are expressed on the heart valve in experimental endocarditis in rabbits, which are unexpressed in vitro [251,251a]. Approaches in molecular biol-

ogy may suggest a variety of previously unknown virulence characteristics.

Putative virulence factors of current interest merit particular mention, because they reflect the great versatility of this commensal microorganism. After recovery from viridans streptococcal infective endocarditis, patients show serologic response to an 85 kDa antigen, which is cross-reactive with hsp 90, and an 180 kDa homologue of *Streptococcus mutans* antigen I/II [252]. Indeed, recombinant human antibodies prepared against the proline repeat region of antigen I/II, or the conserved epitope LKBRK of hsp 90, protected mice against lethal *Streptococcus oralis* infection. In contrast, when a P1-(antigen I/II homologue)–negative mutant of *Streptococcus mutans* was tested in the rat model of infective endocarditis, adhesion to the heart valve and virulence was indistinguishable from the wild type [253]. It is unclear how the 85 and 180 kDa antigens of *Streptococcus mutans* confer virulence in infective endocarditis.

Virulence includes the ability to colonize and cause pathology. For example, Macrina and coworkers [254] have shown that FimA may mediate colonization of *Streptococcus parasanguis* in experimental endocarditis in rats. FimA, a membrane transporter in the Lra I family of lipoproteins [255], is a purported adhesin for platelet fibrin clots. A FimA-negative mutant shows reduced infectivity, whereas immunization with FimA appears to protect against infection of heart valves [256]. On the basis of these studies, FimA may promote adhesion to injured heart valves, but its role as a peptide transporter may also contribute to cell growth and colonization.

A key pathological feature of the heart valve lesion in infective endocarditis is the accumulation of platelets into a mural thrombus [240]. The ability of certain viridans streptococci to induce platelet aggregation in vitro appears to adversely affect the clinical outcome in patients [257,258]. Many strains of *Streptococcus sanguis* induce human platelets to aggregate in vitro [259–262]; this process is mediated by a cell wall–expressed, collagen-like antigen known as the platelet-aggregation associated protein (PAAP) [263–265]. In the rabbit model, it has been demonstrated in vivo that a PAAP$^+$ strain triggers the formation of larger platelet vegetations and a more severe course of endocarditis than a PAAP⁻ strain [266].

The platelet vegetations that form in response to PAAP⁺ *Streptococcus sanguis* are, indeed, thrombi [267]. In a rabbit model, recombinant human tissue plasminogen activator (rtPA) was used to treat endocarditis. Catalyzing the hydrolysis of fibrin, rtPA reduced the mass of the vegetation and made it more susceptible to penicillin treatment [267]. Platelet recognition of the collagen-like epitope on PAAP offers an attractive explanation for why certain strains of *Streptococcus sanguis* induce platelet aggregation and in vivo thrombosis. Yet other viridans streptococci appear to induce aggregation by still different mechanisms [260,261,268,269] and may use several strategies to promote heart valve pathology.

Some strains of viridans streptococci infect heart valves and cause experimental endocarditis only when vegetative lesions fail to develop. For example, infection of heart valves by viridans streptococci without formation of a significant thrombus occurs with pharmacological thrombocytopenia [270]. Some strains fail to infect injured heart valves when platelet function is normal. In the thrombus, platelets release a microbicidal protein (PMP) and only PMP-resistant strains of viridans streptococci are likely to colonize the interior of a platelet vegetation [271,272].

Virulence of viridans streptococci in infective endocarditis appears to require expression of adhesins [2] for injured valve tissue and platelets, [3] mediators of growth, [4] promotion of thrombus, a niche protected from immune clearance, and PMP resistance [5].

Evidence for Thrombogenic Potential of PAAP⁺ *Streptococcus sanguis*

Several lines of evidence suggest that strains of *Streptococcus sanguis* may be thrombogenic in the blood. In the rabbit model of endocarditis ([240]; see above) PAAP⁺ *Streptococcus sanguis* triggered formation of thrombotic vegetations on injured heart valves [266]. The ability of *Streptococcus sanguis* to trigger these vegetations rests on the surface expression of PAAP which carries a collagen-like domain [263,265]. The collagen-like structural motif contains the primary amino

acid sequence PGE(P/Q)GPK, which conforms to a predicted consensus motif found in virtually all platelet-interactive domains of collagens [265]. Using anti-idiotype monoclonal antibodies raised against murine anti–*Streptococcus sanguis* adhesin hybridomas, previously uncharacterized platelet membrane antigens were immunoprecipitated and predicted to be part of a complex receptor for PAAP [273]. Epitopes marking platelet receptors and binding sites on saliva-coated hydroxyapatite are immunologically related; strains able to adhere to both targets use the same adhesin and binding site epitopes [274]. The platelet receptor complex identified by the anti-idiotypic antibodies interacts with cells of *Streptococcus sanguis*, promoting adhesion to the platelet and triggering platelet aggregation. The platelet response to *Streptococcus sanguis* and collagen is clearly similar, suggesting that introduction of these microbes to the blood may trigger responses central to hemostasis and thrombosis. Hence, it is not altogether surprising that *Streptococcus sanguis* bacteremias are frequently associated with often fatal disseminated intravascular coagulation shock-like syndrome in neutropenic or otherwise immunocompromised patients [275,276].

To model thrombogenic potential, platelet-aggregating and nonaggregating (in vitro) strains of *Streptococcus sanguis* were inoculated intravenously to cause bacteremia in otherwise healthy rabbits. Platelet aggregation was induced in the blood by the in vitro aggregation promoting strain. Platelet clots occurred causing hemodynamic changes, acute pulmonary hypertension, and cardiac abnormalities including myocardial ischemia [277–279]. Evidence for platelet clotting occurred within a minute of the beginning of infusion and was not seen with identical concentrations of the nonaggregation-promoting strain of viridans streptococci. Hence, there are clinical and experimental in vitro and in vivo lines of evidence suggesting that certain strains of *Streptococcus sanguis* and other platelet-aggregating viridans streptococci may be thrombogenic agents in the circulation.

The thrombogenic potential of these organisms is also of interest, given the epidemiological association between dental infections and myocardial infarction [280–282] and stroke [280,282,283,284,284a]. *Streptococcus sanguis* represents as much as 30% of the organisms in dental plaque and is frequently recovered from blood during asymptomatic bacteremia and clinically significant sepsis. But more must be learned to establish the biologic basis for the epidemiological association between dental health and myocardial infarction and stroke in humans.

Eukaryotic Adherence Targets of Viridans Streptococci

When viridans streptococci enter the circulation and encounter normal target cells, platelets, or damaged tissue, they may behave as systemic pathogens rather than harmless oral commensals. In vitro, the viridans streptococci do not typically adhere to human endothelial cells [285]. Strains of *Streptococcus sanguis*, *Streptococcus mitis*, and *Streptococcus mutans* adhere to extracellular matrix preparations from umbilical vein epithelial cells, while the nutritionally virulent species *Streptococcus defectivus* and *Streptococcus adjacens* do not adhere well in vitro [286]. When human endothelial cell interactions with viridans streptococci occur, they appear to inhibit pro-coagulant activity [287]. Adherence of viridans streptococci to endothelial cells in vitro, however, appears to be promoted by the presence of soluble fibronectin [288], suggesting that this protein in serum may promote adhesion in vivo. Hence, it remains unclear if viridans streptococci will adhere to normal unperturbed endothelial cells in vivo.

The various species of viridans streptococci show selective tissue tropisms in the oral cavity, which highlights nicely the subtle differences in ecologic niche selection by similar but nonidentical microorganisms [12]. Niche selection by the species of viridans streptococci occurs in infancy before the eruption of teeth [289]. For example, *Streptococcus mitis* greatly exceeds *Streptococcus salivarius*, followed by *Streptococcus oralis* and *Streptococcus anginosus* in the proportion and frequency of recovery from predentate buccal mucosa and alveolar ridges. In postdentate infants up to 1 year old, *Streptococcus sanguis* can be recovered in increasing proportions in at least half of the subjects. Through maturity, *Streptococcus sanguis* becomes the predominant microorganism in dental plaque and is isolated from virtually all adults.

The viridans streptococci also colonize niches on contiguous mucosa of the oropharynx. The viridans streptococci are the most frequently cultured microorganisms from healthy palatine tonsils [290]. Indeed, it has been speculated that the viridans streptococci protect the tonsils from superinfection by respiratory pathogens. For example, acid production by viridans streptococci appears to inhibit colonization by *Hemophilus influenza* [291].

Kawasaki Disease and the Link to Viridans Streptococci

Kawasaki disease is an acute febrile systemic vasculitis most commonly seen in children under the age of 5 years [292]. Patients show a spectrum of fever, rash, cervical lymphadenopathy, bilateral nonexudative conjunctivitis, lesions of the oropharyngeal mucosa, and desquamative erythema of the hands and feet. Secondary to vasculitis, coronary aneurisms develop in 10% to 25% of cases. Thrombocytopenia and coronary thrombosis occur, promoting myocardial infarction [293]. While the etiology and pathogenesis of Kawasaki disease are unclear, intravenous gamma-globulin therapy is helpful in promoting remission and an infectious etiology is strongly associated.

The vasculitis and thrombogenesis associated with Kawasaki disease have been modeled in experimental rabbits by challenge with viridans streptococci that were isolated from patients [294]. Culture supernatants injected into rabbits increased capillary permeability and dermal redness and swelling. One-third of the *Streptococcus mitis* isolates and one-fifth of unidentified viridans streptococci induced platelet aggregation ex vivo. No strain of *Streptococcus oralis* induced aggregation. The experimental vasculitis was consistent with the production of toxic shock syndrome–like exotoxins [293,295,296], which have been isolated from many strains of viridans streptococci [216,297]. The expression of viridans streptococcal exotoxins in the infectious etiology of Kawasaki disease is consistent with the expansion of T cell clones during acute vasculitis, including the T cell receptor $V\beta$ gene selection characteristic of superantigens [298,299]. Whereas $V\beta2^+$ T cells are activated during the acute phase of Kawasaki disease and inversion of the CD4:CD8 ratio is common, these signs disappear during convalescence from vasculitis. More expansive clonal selection of CD8$^+$ T cells has also been noted in Kawasaki disease, suggesting involvement of additional antigens [299]. The thrombotic sequellae in Kawasaki disease, if promoted by certain viridans streptococci, suggest an additional virulence factor (see above). While a number of infectious agents could contribute to the pathogenesis of Kawasaki disease, a mucosal portal of entry is suggested by the histopathology of the vasculitis lesions [300]. The vascular infiltrate contains an unusual predominance of IgA-producing plasma cells, suggesting an antigen-driven immune response to mucosal microorganisms, such as viridans streptococci.

Behçet's Disease and Viridans Streptococci

Behçet's disease is multisystem vasculitis that typically affects adults between 20 and 30 years of age and may be related to Kawasaki disease. In Behçet's disease, lesions may occur in the eyes, skin, joints, blood vessels, central nervous system, and oral cavity. The major organs and gastrointestinal tract are less frequently affected, in contrast to Kawasaki disease, which shows clinically significant lesions primarily in the coronary arteries. Similar geographic and ethnic populations are at risk for Kawasaki disease [293,301] and Behçet's disease [302], with a high prevalence in Japan and in Mediterranean countries. Fully half of patients with Behçet's disease show mucocutaneous lesions, one-quarter have ocular involvement, and about 15% show musculoskeletal or vascular disease [303]. Approximately 30% of patients with Behçet's disease develop thrombosis of arteries and veins [304].

Streptococcus sanguis has been implicated as an etiological agent in Behçet's disease [305]. Patients with confirmed Behçet's disease yielded "uncommon" serotypes from dental plaque. Half of the isolates induced human platelets to aggregate in comparison to 30% of the isolates from healthy control subjects. Plasma isolated from patients whose platelets did not aggregate also failed to support aggregation of platelets from healthy controls. Products of the uncommon serotypes of *Streptococcus sanguis* were suggested to directly or indirectly inhibit platelet function and contribute to vasculitis. Some of the uncommon isolates of *Streptococcus sanguis* have been shown to be related to ATCC 10556, while others may be related to strains isolated from patients with Kawasaki disease and ATCC 10557 [306,306a]. Strains of *Streptococcus sanguis* isolated from patients with Behçet's disease show a high prevalence of IgA protease activity, suggesting that persistence may be associated with cleavage and dysfunction of specific secretory IgA antibodies in the oral cavity [307]. Interestingly, serum IgA titers against both *Streptococcus sanguis* and IgA protease in patients with Behçet's disease were significantly higher than IgG titers or titers from healthy controls. In general, patients show higher antibody titers to antigens from Behçet syndrome strains of *Streptococcus sanguis* than strains from healthy control individuals [308].

A T cell abnormality has been postulated for Behçet's disease. In response to *Streptococcus sanguis* antigens, T cells from Behçet syndrome patients show significantly greater stimulation than patients with other rheumatic disease or healthy individuals [309]. Stimulated Behçet's T cells produce IL-6 in a monocyte-dependent and HLA-B51-independent manner. The principal immunogenic antigen in this preparation has been cloned and identified as the *bes-1* gene, which predicts a polypeptide of 95 kDa with a domain of high homology to human intraocular peptide, Brn-3b [310]. These data suggest that T cell hypersensitivity to a *Streptococcus sanguis* antigen may have autoimmune characteristics.

That patients with Behçet's disease may manifest an autoimmune response to streptococcal infection is supported by the identification of a *Streptococcus sanguis* 65 kDa heat shock protein (HSP), which is immunologically cross-reactive with human mitochondrial HSP expressed in mucosal epithelium [311]. The *Streptococcus sanguis* HSP65 also cross-reacts with HSP65 from *Mycobacterium tuberculosis* [312]. Using synthetic peptides modeled from segments of *M. tuberculosis* HSP65, putative T cell epitopes were identified that are capable of inducing uveitis in Lewis rats after foot pad injection. Several *M. tuberculosis* peptides and their human mitochondrial HSP60 analogues were shown to preferentially stimulate IgA-producing B cells, which suggests that class-specific antibody titers may rise during ocular manifestations [313]. Selected *M. tuberculosis* HSP peptides stimulate γδ T cells isolated from 25 of 33 Behçet's patients in contrast to 2 of 55 controls. Human HSP peptide analogs also stimulated T cells, but less effectively [314]. The extent of stimulation appeared to be related to the severity of disease, ranging from no apparent lesions to recurrent oral ulcers and systemic disease. *Streptococcus sanguis* HSP 65 has been cloned and is highly homologous to HSP65 of *M. tuberculosis* [315]. Four HSP65 peptides from *M. tuberculosis* show the greatest ability to stimulate γδ T cells from patients with Behçet's syndrome and these peptides show the highest homologies with regions of human HSP60 [311]. Th2-type T cell lines have been established from epidermal lesions of patients with Behçet's disease [316]. The existence of these lines suggests that self-reactive T cells may be expressed in Behçet's disease. Since patients express significant antibody titers against *Streptococcus sanguis* antigens, including HSP65 (as modeled by *M. tuberculosis* HSP65), streptococcal antigens may elicit autoimmune mechanisms that promote cross-reactivity with host proteins in Behçet's disease [317].

DEVELOPMENT OF A VACCINE FOR DENTAL CARIES

Dental caries is a disease with a high prevalence in selected populations, but low morbidity and virtually no mortality. Proponents of development of a caries vaccine recognize that the prevalence of dental caries is greatest in populations with the least access to dental care and personal hygiene education. Historically, the strategy to target mutans streptococci as etiologic agents in dental caries confronts the same challenge encountered in the development of other streptococcal vaccines: the potential of eliciting host cross-reactive antibodies [318,319]. A myosin cross-reactive epitope of group A streptococcal M protein may be conserved within the genus [320]. Now that this epitope is known, characterized streptococcal immunogens can be selected to prepare vaccines that circumvent the risk. Nonetheless, much has been

learned about systemic and mucosal routes of immunization to confer immunity against mucosal microorganisms. Indeed, purified proteins and genetically engineered immunogens from *Streptococcus mutans* have been used as vaccines in laboratory animals, which appear to confer protection against dental caries without producing untoward side effects.

Caries-protective vaccines have been developed in laboratory animals using strategies targeting different prominent antigens of mutans streptococci, including a salivary interactive domain of antigen I/II [321], both the catalytic and glucan-binding sites of glucosyltransferase [322], and the glucan-binding protein [323]. Active and passive immunization strategies show promise.

In primates, passive oral administration of monoclonal antibodies against the salivary interactive domain of antigen I/II (amino acids 816–1213) reduces colonization of *Streptococcus mutans* [321]. Specific monoclonal secretory IgA (sIgA) antibodies have been engineered in tobacco plants for large-scale production [324,325]. The sIgA product from plants shows the protective features of passively administered antibodies prepared in animals.

Active immunization to elicit protective antibodies in the animal host also appears to be effective. When used to immunize mice, the domain defined by amino acids 816–1213 has been shown to be a preferred T cell antigen, when compared to the adhesin domain, amino acids 975–1044 [326,327]. A transmucosal vaccine has been developed by conjugating the B subunit of cholera toxin with antigen I/II. When conjugated, the cholera toxin B subunit serves as an adjuvant to produce a generalized elevated secretory IgA response when administered intranasally [328] or orally [329]. Similar immune responses have been obtained by mucosal immunization with *Salmonella typhimurium* engineered to express *Streptococcus mutans* antigen I/II in tandem with cholera toxin A2/B [330]. Indeed, an oral vaccine produced from epitope amino acids 816–1213 conjugated to cholera toxin B subunit elicited specific T and B cell responses in SJL mice [331]. When administered intranasally, the mucosal vaccine elicited specific IgA that reacted with antigen I/II [332].

Glucosyltransferases synthesize soluble and insoluble dextrans, which may assist mutans streptococci to bind stably to the tooth and fabricate a dense, protected niche in dental plaque. People who expressed serum antibody against glucosyltransferase in their gingival crevicular fluid showed lower oral colonization of mutans streptococci [333]. Glucosyltransferase functional domains may also be an effective target for a vaccine [109]. When the immune response against a 22 amino acid glucan-binding domain of glucosyltransferase was examined, the elevated serum antibodies inhibited isozymes of glucosyltransferase and production of insoluble glucan. These antibodies also reacted with an 87 kDa glucan-binding protein from *Streptococcus sobrinus*. The 22-mer glucan-binding domain appeared to contain both B and T cell epitopes. Similarly, a 21-mer marking the catalytic domain served as a B cell epitope eliciting antibodies that inhibited glucosyltransferase function [334]. Hence, experimental vaccines consisting of glucan-binding protein or catalytic or glucan-binding domains of glucosyltransferase have each proved effective in eliciting serum and sIgA responses that protected rats against experimental caries [335,336].

While fluoride in dentifrices and drinking water, improved nutrition and oral hygiene, and access to dental care have made a major impact on the incidence and prevalence of dental caries in many populations in developed nations, the persistence of this costly infection in many communities appears to justify continuing exploration of strategies to develop immunity against cariogenic microorganisms. Technical barriers [337] to development of an efficacious vaccine are being surmounted. Efficacy in humans must eventually be demonstrated and the risk-benefit issues for a disease of high morbidity but virtually no mortality must be addressed.

I wish to thank Ms. Urve Daigle for preparation of the illustrations and assistance with word processing. For their helpful input into the content of this manuscript, I also thank Rob Quivey, Bob Burne, Bob Marquis, and Bill Bowen, Department of Dental Research and the Center for Dental Caries Research, University of Rochester; Sue Michalek and Page Caufield, Departments of Oral Biology and Microbiology, University of Alabama at Birmingham; Lin Tao, Department of Oral Biology, University of Illinois, Chicago; Joel Rudney, Greg Germaine, and Bill Liljemark, School of Dentistry, University of Minnesota; Martin Taubman, Forsyth Dental Center, Boston; Howard Jenkinson, formerly of the Experimental Oral Biology Unit, University of Otago, New Zealand and currently at the University of Bristol, UK. The support of NIH/NIDR grants DE05501, DE08590 and DE00270 is gratefully acknowledged.

REFERENCES

1. Kawamura Y, Hou X-G, Sultana F, Miura H, Ezaki T. Determination of 16s RNA sequences of *Streptococcus mitis* and *Streptococcus gordonii* and phylogenetic relationship among members of the genus *Streptococcus*. Int J Syst Bacteriol 1995; 45:406–408.

1a. Whiley RA, Beighton D. Current classification of the oral streptococci. Oral Microbiol Immunol 1998; 13:195–216.

2. Weinberger BW. An Introduction to the History of Dentistry, Vol. 1. St. Louis: CV Mosby, 1948; 21–28.

3. De Kruif P. Microbe Hunters. New York: Harcourt Brace, 1953; 3–24.

4. Weinberger BW. Pierre Fauchard Surgeon-Dentist. Minneapolis: Pierre Fauchard Academy, 1941; 61–67.

5. Rosebury T, Sonnenwirth AC. Bacteria indigenous to man. In: Dubos RJ (ed). Bacterial and Mycotic Infections of Man, 3rd ed. Philadelphia: Lippencott, 1958; 626–653.

6. Tanzer JM. Dental caries is a transmissible infectious disease: the Keyes and Fitzgerald revolution. J Dent Res 1995; 74:1536–1542.

7. McClure FJ, Hewitt WL. The relation of penicillin to induced rat caries and oral *L. acidophilus*. J Dent Res 1946; 25:441–443.

8. Darwish S, Hyppa T, Socransky SS. Studies of the predominant cultivable microbiota of early periodontitis. J Periodontal Res 1978; 13:1–16.

9. Wolff LF, Liljemark WF, Bloomquist, Pihlstrom BL, Schaffer EM, Bandt CL. The distribution of *Actinobacillus actinomycetemcomitans* in human plaque. J Periodontol Res 1985; 20:237–250.

10. Michalek SM, McGhee JR. Oral streptococci with emphasis on *Streptococcus mutans*. In: McGhee JR, Michalek SM, Cassell GH (eds). Dental Microbiology. Philadelphia: Harper & Row, 1982; 679–690.

11. Hamada S, Slade HD. Biology, immunology, and cariogenicity of *Streptococcus mutans*. Microbiol Rev 1980; 44:331–384.

12. Gibbons RJ, van Houte J. Bacterial adherence in oral microbial ecology. Annu Rev Microbiol 1975; 29:19–44.

13. Gibbons RJ, Spinell DM, Skobe Z. Selective adherence as a determinant of the host tropisms of certain indigenous and pathogenic bacteria. Infect Immun 1976; 13:238–246.

14. Tinanoff N, Gross A, Brady JM. Development of plaque on enamel. Parallel investigations. J Periodontol Res 1976; 11:197–209.

15. Socransky SS, Manganiello AD, Propas D, Oram V, van Houte J. Bacteriological studies of developing supragingival dental plaque. J Periodontal Res 1977; 12:90–106.

16. Bowden GH, Hardie JM, Slack GL. Microbial variations in approximal dental plaque. Caries Res 1975; 9:253–277.

17. Gibbons RJ, Nygaard M. Synthesis of insoluble dextran and its significance in the formation of gelatinous deposits by plaque-forming streptococci. Arch Oral Biol 1968; 13:124–126.

18. Gibbons RJ, van Houte J. On the formation of dental plaques. J Periodontol 1973; 44:347–359.

19. Bowden GHW, Hamilton IR. Survival of oral bacteria. Crit Rev Oral Biol Med 1998; 9:54–85.

20. Liljemark WF, Bloomquist CG, Germaine GR. Effect of bacterial aggregation on the adherence of oral streptococci to hydroxyapatite. Infect Immun 1981; 31:935–941.

21. Smith DJ, Taubman MA. Emergence of immune competence in saliva. Crit Rev Oral Biol Med 1993; 4:335–341.

22. Pearce C, Bowden GH, Evans M, Fitzsimmons SP, Johnson J, Sheridan MJ, Wientzen R, Cole MF. Identification of pioneer viridans streptococci in the oral cavity of human neonates. J Med Microbiol 1995; 42:67–72.

23. Cole MF, Evans M, Fitzsimmons S, Johnson J, Pearce C, Sheridan MJ, Wientzen R, Bowden G. Pioneer oral streptococci produce immunoglobulin A1 protease. Infect Immun 1994; 62:2165–2168.

24. Tyler BM, Cole MF. Effect of IgA1 protease on the ability of secretory IgA1 antibodies to inhibit the adherence of Streptococcus mutans. Microbiol Immunol 1998; 42:503–508.

25. Gilbert JV, Plaut AG, Wright A. Analysis of the immunoglobulin A protease gene of Streptococcus sanguis. Infect Immun 1991; 59:7–17.

26. Smith DJ, King WF, Gilbert JV, Taubman MA. Structural integrity of infant salivary immunoglobulin A (IgA) in IgA1 protease-rich environments. Oral Microbiol Immunol 1998; 13:89–96.

27. Liljemark WF, Schauer SV. Competitive binding among oral streptococci to hydroxyapatite. J Dent Res 1977; 56:157–165.

28. Rao MKY, Somasundaran P, Schilling KM, Carson B, Ananthapadmanabhan KP. Bacterial adhesion onto apatite minerals-electrokinetic aspects. Colloids Surf 1993; 79:293–300.

29. Jenkinson HF. Genetic analysis of adherence by oral streptococci. J Industr Microbiol 1995; 15:186–192.

30. Jenkinson HF, Easingwood RA. Insertional inactivation of the gene encoding a 76-kilodalton cell surface polypeptide in Streptococcus gordonii challis has a pleiotropic effect on cell surface composition. Infect Immun 1990; 58:3689–3697.

31. Ma JK-C, Kelly CG, Munro G, Whiley RA, Lehner T. Conservation of the gene encoding streptococcal antigen I/II in oral streptococci. Infect Immun 1991; 59:2686–2694.

32. Bleiweis AS, Oyston PCF, Brady LJ. Molecular, immunological and functional characterization of the major surface adhesin of Streptococcus mutans. In: Ciardi JE, McGhee JR, Keith JM (eds). Genetically Engineered Vaccines. New York: Plenum Press, 1992; 229–241.

33. Moisset A, Schatz N, Lepoivre Y, Amadio S, Wachsmann D, Schöller M, Klein J-P. Conservation of salivary glycoprotein-interacting and human immunoglobulin G–cross-reactive domains of antigen I/II in oral streptococci. Infect Immun 1994; 62:184–193.

34. Demuth DR, Golub EE, Malamud D. Streptococcal-host interactions. Structural and functional analysis of a Streptococcus sanguis receptor for a human salivary glycoprotein. J Biol Chem 1990; 265:7120–7126.

35. Liljemark WF, Bloomquist CG, Fenner LJ, Antonelli PJ, Coulter MC. Effect of neuraminidase on the adherence to salivary pellicle of Streptococcus sanguis and Streptococcus mitis. Caries Res 1989; 23:141–145.

36. Brady LJ, Crowley PJ, Piacentini DA, Bleiweis AS. The interactions of cell surface P1 adhesin molecule of Streptococcus mutans with human and salivary agglutinin. J Microbiol Methods 1993; 18:181–196.

37. Munro GH, Evans P, Todryk S, Buckett P, Kelly CG, Lehner T. A protein fragment of streptococcal cell surface antigen I/II which prevents adhesion to Streptococcus mutans. Infect Immun 1993; 61:4590–4598.

38. Nakai M, Okahashi N, Ohta H, Koga T. Saliva-binding region of Streptococcus mutans surface protein antigen. Infect Immun 1993; 61:4344–4349.

39. Crowley PJ, Brady LJ, Piacentini DA, Bleiweis AS. Identification of a salivary agglutinin-binding domain within cell surface adhesin P1 of Streptococcus mutans. Infect Immun 1993; 61:1547–1552.

40. Carlen A, Olsson J. Monoclonal antibodies against a high molecular weight agglutinin block adherence to experimental pellicles on hydroxyapatite and aggregation of Streptococcus mutans. J Dent Res 1995; 74:1040–1047.

41. Courtney HS, Hasty DL. Aggregation of group A streptococci by human saliva and effect of saliva on streptococcal adherence to host cells. Infect Immun 1991; 59:1661–1666.

42. Herzberg MC, Levine MJ, Ellison SA, Tabak LA. Purification and characterization of monkey salivary mucin. J Biol Chem 1979; 254:1487–1494.

43. Levine MJ, Herzberg MC, Levine MS, Ellison SA, Stinson MW, Li HC, van Dyke T. Specificity of salivary-bacterial interactions: role of terminal sialic acid residues in the interaction of

salivary glycoproteins with *Streptococcus sanguis* and *Streptococcus mutans*. Infect Immun 1978; 19:107–115.

44. Murray PA, Prakophol A, Lee T, Hoover CI, Fisher SJ. Adherence of oral streptococci to salivary glycoproteins. Infect Immun 1992; 60:31–38.

45. Murray PA, Levine MJ, Reddy MS, Tabak LA, Bergey EJ. Preparation of sialic acid–binding protein from *Streptococcus mitis*. Infect Immun 1986; 53:359–365.

46. Nesser J-R, Grafstrom RC, Woltz A, Brassart D, Fryder V, Guggenheim B. A 23-kDa membrane glycoprotein bearing NeuNAcα2,3galβ1, 3galNAc O-linked carbohydrate chains acts like a receptor for *Streptococcus sanguis* OMZ-9 on human buccal epithelial cells. Glycobiology 1995; 5:97–104.

47. Gibbons RJ, Hay DI, Schlesinger DH. Delineation of a segment of adsorbed salivary acidic proline-rich proteins which promotes adhesion of *Streptococcus gordonii* to apatitic surfaces. Infect Immun 1991; 59:2948–2954.

48. Scannapieco FA, Torres GI, Levine MJ. Salivary amylase promotes adhesion of oral streptococci to hydroxyapatite. J Dent Res 1995; 74:1360–1366.

49. Liljemark WF, Bloomquist CG, Ofstehage JC. Aggregation and adherence of *Streptococcus sanguis*: role of human salivary immunoglobulin A. Infect Immun 1979; 26:1104–1110.

50. Oho T, Yu H, Yamashima Y, Koga T. Binding of salivary glycoprotein-secretory immunoglobulin A complex to the surface protein antigen of *Streptococcus mutans*. Infect Immun 1998; 66:115–121.

51. Gong K, Mailloux L, Herzberg MC. Salivary film expresses a complex, macromolecular binding site for *Streptococcus sanguis*. 1999 submitted.

52. Ganeshkumar N, Arora N, Kolenbrander PE. Saliva-binding protein [SsaB] from *Streptococcus sanguis* 12 is a lipoprotein. J Bacteriol 1993; 175:572–574.

53. Fenno JC, Shaikh A, Spatafora G, Fives-Taylor P. The *fimA* locus of *Streptococcus parasanguis* encodes an ATP-binding membrane transport system. Mol Microbiol 1995; 15:849–863.

54. Kolenbrander PE, Andersen RN, Baker R, Jenkinson HF. The adhesion-associated *sca* operon in *Streptococcus gordonii* encodes an inducible high-affinity ABC transporter for Mn^{2+} uptake. J Bacteriol 1998;180–290–295.

55. Jenkinson HF. Adherence and accumulation of oral streptococci. Trends Microbiol 1994; 2:209–212.

56. Sutcliffe IC, Russell RRB. Lipoproteins of gram-positive bacteria. J Bacteriol 1995; 177:1123–1128.

57. Andersen RK, Ganeshkumar N, Kolenbrander PE. Cloning of the *Streptococcus gordonii* PK488 gene, encoding an adhesin which medi-

ates coaggregation with *Actinomyces naeslundii* PK606. Infect Immun 1993; 61:981–987.

58. Ganeshkumar N, Song M, McBride BC. Cloning of a *Streptococcus sanguis* adhesin which mediates binding to saliva-coated hydroxyapatite. Infect Immun 1988; 56:1150–1157.

59. Ganeshkumar N, Hannum PM, Kolenbrander PE, McBride BC. Nucleotide sequence of a gene coding for a saliva-binding protein [SsaB] from *Streptococcus sanguis* 12 and possible role of the protein in the coaggregation with actinomyces. Infect Immun 1991; 59:1093–1099.

60. McNab R, Jenkinson HF, Loach DM, Tannock GW. Cell-surface-associated polypeptides CshA and CshB of high molecular mass are colonization determinants in the oral bacterium *Streptococcus gordonii*. Mol Microbiol 1994; 14:743–754.

61. Hasty DL, Ofek I, Courtney HS, Doyle RJ. Multiple adhesins of streptococci. Infect Immun 1992; 60:2147–2152.

62. Gong K, Herzberg MC. *Streptococcus sanguis* expresses a 150-kilodalton two-domain adhesin: characterization of several independent adhesin epitopes. Infect Immun 1997; 65:3815–3821.

63. Gibbons RJ, Etherden I, Peros W. Aspects of the attachment of oral streptococci to experimental pellicles. In: Mergenhagen SE, Rosan B (eds). Molecular Basis of Oral Microbial Adhesion. Washington DC: American Society of Microbiology 1985; 77–84.

64. Rosan B, Eifert R, Golub E. Bacterial surfaces, salivary pellicles, and plaque formation. In: Mergenhagen SE, Rosan B (eds). Molecular Basis of Oral Microbial Adhesion. Washington DC: American Society of Microbiology 1985; 69–76.

65. Doyle RJ, Oakley JD, Murphy KR, McAllister D, Taylor KG. Graphical analysis of adherence data. In: Mergenhagen SE, Rosan B (eds). Molecular Basis of Oral Microbial Adhesion, Washington DC: American Society of Microbiology 1985; 109–113.

66. Busscher HJ, Cowan MM, van der Mei MC. On the relative importance of specific and non-specific approaches to oral microbial adhesion. FEMS Microbiol Rev 1992; 8:199–209.

67. Skopek RJ, Liljemark WF. The influence of saliva on interbacterial adherence. Oral Microbiol Immunol 1994; 9:19–24.

68. Loach DM, Jenkinson HF, Tannock GW. Colonization of the oral cavity by *Streptococcus gordonii*. Infect Immun 1994; 62:2129–2131.

69. McNab R, Jenkinson HF. Altered adherence properties of a *Streptococcus gordonii* hppA (oligopeptide permease) mutant result from transcriptional effects on *cshA* gene expression. Microbiology 1998; 144:127–136.

70. Håvarstein LS, Hakenbeck R, Gaustad P. Natural competence in the genus *Streptococcus*: evidence that streptococci can change pherotype

by interspecies recombinatorial exchanges. J Bacteriol 1997; 179:6589–6594.

71. Skopek RJ, Liljemark WF, Bloomquist CG, Rudney JD. Dental plaque development on defined streptococcal surfaces. Oral Microbiol Immunol 1993; 8:16–23.

72. Stinson MW, Levine MJ. Modulation of intergeneric adhesion of oral bacteria by saliva. Crit Rev Oral Biol Med 1993; 4:309–314.

73. Lamont RJ, Demuth DR, Davis CA, Malamud D, Rosan B. Salivary agglutinin-mediated adherence of Streptococcus mutans to early plaque bacteria. Infect Immun 1991; 59:3446–3450.

74. Rudney JD, Ji Z, Larson CJ, Liljemark WF, Hickey KL. Saliva protein-binding to layers of oral streptococci in vitro and in vivo. J Dent Res 1995; 74:1280–1288.

75. Bergmann JE, Gulzow HJ. Detection of binding of denatured salivary alpha-amylase to Streptococcus sanguis. Arch Oral Biol 1995; 40:973–974.

76. Listgarten MA, Mayo HE, Tremblay R. Ultrastructure of the attachment device between coccal and filamentous microorganisms in "corn cob" formations in dental plaque. Archs Oral Biol 1973; 18:651–656.

77. Mouton C, Reynolds HS, Genco RJ. Characterization of the tufted streptococci isolated from the "corn cob" configuration of human dental plaque. Infect Immun 1980; 27:235–249.

78. Lancy P, DiRienzo JM, Applebaum B, Rosan B, Holt SC. Corncob formation between Fusobacterium nucleatum and Streptococcus sanguis. Infect Immun 1983; 40:303–309.

79. McBride BC, van der Hoeven JS. Role of interbacterial adherence in colonization of the oral cavities of gnotobiotic rats infected with Streptococcus mutans and Veillonella alcalescens. Infect Immun 1981; 33:467–472.

80. Hughes CV, Andersen RN, Kolenbrander PE. Characterization of Veillonella atypica PK1910 adhesin-mediated coaggregation with oral streptococcus spp. Infect Immun 1992; 60:1178–1186.

81. Kolenbrander PE, Ganeshkumar N, Cassels FJ, Hughes CV. Coaggregation: specific adherence among human oral plaque bacteria. FASEB J 1993; 7:406–413.

82. Ellen RP, Veisman H, Buivids IA, Rosenberg M. Kinetics of lactose-reversible coadhesion of Actinomyces naeslundii WVU 398A and Streptococcus oralis 34 on the surface of hexadecane droplets. Oral Microbiol Immunol 1994; 9:364–371.

83. Jenkinson HF, Terry SD, McNab R, Tannock GW. Inactivation of the gene encoding surface protein SspA in Streptococcus gordonii DL1 affects cell interactions with human salivary agglutinin and oral actinomyces. Infect Immun 1993; 61:3199–3208.

84. Willcox MD, Patrikakis M, Harty DW, Loo CY,

Knox KW. Coaggregation of oral lactobacilli with streptococci from the oral cavity. Oral Microbiol Immunol 1993; 8:319–321.

85. Holmes AR, Gopal PK, Jenkinson HF. Adherence of Candida albicans to a cell surface polysaccharide receptor on Streptococcus gordonii. Infect Immun 1995; 63:1827–1834.

86. Kamaguchi A, Baba H, Hoshi M, Inomata K. Coaggregation between Porphyromonas gingivalis and mutans streptococci. Microbiol Immunol 1994; 38:457–460.

87. Clemans DL and Kolenbrander PE. Isolation and characterization of coaggregation-defective [Cog-] mutants of Streptococcus gordonii DL-1 [Challis]. J Industr Microbiol 1995; 15:193–197.

88. Holmes AR, Cannon RD, Jenkinson HF. Interactions of Candida albicans with bacteria and salivary molecules in oral biofilms. J Industr Microbiol 1995; 15:208–213.

89. Bendel CM, Hostetter MK. Distinct mechanisms of epithelial adhesion for Candida albicans and Candida tropicalis. J Clin Invest 1993; 92:1840–1849.

90. Hostetter MK. Adhesins and ligands involved in the interaction of Candida spp with epithelial and endothelial surfaces. Clin Microbiol Rev 1994; 7:29–42.

91. Kilian M, Roland K, Mestecky J. Interference of secretory IgA with sorption of oral bacteria to hydroxyapatite. Infect Immun 1981; 31:942–951.

92. Levine MJ, Tabak LA, Reddy MS, Mandel ID. Nature of salivary pellicle in microbial adherence: Role of salivary mucins. In: Mergenhagen SE, Rosan B (eds). Molecular Basis of Oral Microbial Adhesion. Washington DC: American Society of Microbiology 1985; 125–130.

93. Azen E, Prakobphol A, Fisher SJ. PRB3 null mutations result in the absence of the proline-rich glycoprotein G1 and abolish Fusobacterium nucleatum interactions with saliva in vitro. Infect Immun 1993; 61:4434–4439.

94. Kousvelari E, Tabak LA. Genetic regulation of salivary proteins in rodents. Crit Rev Oral Biol Med 1991; 2:139–151.

95. Baum BJ, Dai Y, Hiramatsu Y, Horn VJ, Ambudkar IS. Signalling mechanisms that regulate saliva formation. Crit Rev Oral Biol Med 1993; 4:379–384.

96. Reynolds EC, Johnson IH. Effect of milk on caries incidence and bacterial composition of dental plaque in the rat. Arch Oral Biol 1981; 26:927–933.

97. Vacca-Smith AM, Vanwuyckhuyse BC, Tabak LA, Bowen WH. The effect of milk and casein proteins on the adherence of Streptococcus mutans to saliva-coated hydroxyapatite. Arch Oral Biol 1994; 39:1063–1069.

98. Nesser J-R, Golliard M, Woltz A, Rouvet M, Dillmann M-L, Guggenheim B. In vitro modulation of oral bacterial adhesion to saliva-coated

hydroxyapatite beads by milk casein derivatives. Oral Microbiol Immunol 1994; 9:193–201.

99. Cox SD, Lassiter MO, Taylor KG, Doyle RJ. Fluoride inhibits the glucan-binding lectin of *Streptococcus sobrinus*. FEMS Microbiol Lett 1994; 123:331–334.

100. Wu Q, Wang Q, Taylor KG, Doyle RJ. Subinhibitory concentrations of antibiotics affect cell surface properties of *Streptococcus sobrinus*. J Bacteriol 1995; 177:1399–1401.

101. Tagg JR, Russell C. Bacteriocin production by *Streptococcus salivarius* strain P. Can J Microbiol 1981; 27:918–923.

102. Tompkins GR, Tagg JR. The ecology of bacteriocin-producing strains of *Streptococcus salivarius*. Microbiol Ecol Health Dis 1989; 2:19–28.

103. Ross KF, Ronson CW, Tagg JR. Isolation and characterization of the lantibiotic salivaricin A and its structural gene *salA* from *Streptococcus salivarius* 20P3. Appl Environ Microbiol 1993; 59:2014–2021.

104. Hillman JD, Dzuback AL, Andrews SW. Colonization of the human oral cavity by a *Streptococcus mutans* mutant producing increasing bacteriocin. J Dent Res 1987; 66:1092–1094.

105. Novak J, Caufield PW, Miller EJ. Isolation and biochemical characterization of a novel lantibiotic mutacin from *Streptococcus mutans*. J Bacteriol 1994; 176:4316–4320.

106. Morency H, Trahan L, Lavoie MC. Preliminary grouping of mutacins. Can J Microbiol 1995; 41:826–831.

107. van der Hoeven JS, Schaeken MJM. Streptococci and actinomyces inhibit regrowth of *Streptococcus mutans*. Caries Res 1995; 29:159–162.

108. Hillman JD, Socransky SS. Replacement therapy for the prevention of dental disease. Adv Dent Res 1987; 1:119–125.

109. Smith DJ, Taubman MA, Holmberg CR, Eastcott J, King WF, Ali-Salaam P. Antigenicity and immunogenicity of a synthetic peptide derived from a glucan-binding domain of mutans streptococcal glycosyltransferase. Infect Immun 1993; 61:2899–2905.

110. Frandsen EVD, Pedrazzoli V, Kilian M. Ecology of the viridans streptococci in the oral cavity and pharynx. Oral Microbiol Immunol 1991; 6:129–133.

111. Liljemark WF, Gibbons RJ. Proportional distribution and relative adherence of *Streptococcus miteor* [*"mitis"*] on various surfaces of the human oral cavity. Infect Immun 1972; 6:852–859.

112. Carlsson J. Presence of various types of non-haemolytic streptococci in dental plaque and other sites of the oral cavity. Odontol Rev 1967; 18:55–74.

113. Gibbons RJ, Kapsimalis B, Socransky SS. The source of salivary bacteria. Arch Oral Biol 1964; 9:101–103.

114. Krasse B. The proportional distribution of *Strep-*

tococcus salivarius* and other streptococci in various parts of the mouth. Odont Rev 1954; 5:203–211.

115. Carlsson J, Grahnen H, Jonsson G, Wikner S. Establishment of *Streptococcus sanguis* in the mouth of infants. Arch Oral Biol 1970; 15:1143–1148.

116. Li Y, Caufield PW. The fidelity of initial acquisition of mutans streptococci by infants from their mothers. J Dent Res 1995; 74:681–685.

117. Caufield PW, Cutter GR, Dasanayake AP. Initial acquisition of mutans streptococci by infants: evidence for a discrete window of infectivity. J Dent Res 1993; 72:37–45.

118. Sissons CH, Wong L, Cutress TW. Patterns and rates of growth of microcosm dental plaque biofilms. Oral Microbiol Immunol 1995; 10:160–167.

119. Yodzis P. Competition, mortality and community structure. In: Diamond J, Case TJ (eds). Community Ecology. New York: Harper & Row, 1986; 480–491.

120. Brecx M, Theilade J, Attstrom R. An ultrastructural quantitative study of the significance of microbial multiplication during early plaque growth. J Periodontol Res 1983; 18:177–186.

121. Li YH, Bowden GH. Characteristics of accumulation of oral gram-positive bacteria on mucin-conditioned glass surfaces in a model system. Oral Microbiol Immunol 1994; 9:1–11.

122. Loesche WJ. Role of *Streptococcus mutans* in human dental decay. Microbiol Rev 1986; 50:353–380.

123. Van Houte J, Lopman J, Kent R. The predominant cultivable flora of sound and carious human root surfaces. J Dent Res 1994; 73:1727–1734.

124. Schupbach P, Osterwalder V, Guggenheim B. Human root caries—microbiota in plaque covering sound, carious, and arrested carious root surfaces. Caries Res 1995; 29:382–395.

125. Beighton D, Lynch E. Comparison of selected microflora of plaque and underlying carious dentine associated with primary root caries lesions. Caries Res 1995; 29:154–158.

126. Switalski LM, Butcher WG, Caufield PC, Lantz MS. Collagen mediates adhesion of *Streptococcus mutans* to human dentin. Infect Immun 1993; 61:4119–4125.

127. Switalski LM, Butcher WG. An in vitro model for adhesion of bacteria to human tooth root surfaces. Arch Oral Biol 1994; 39:155–161.

128. Harrington DJ, Russell RR. Identification and characterization of two extracellular proteases of *Streptococcus mutans*. FEMS Microbiol Lett 1994; 121:237–241.

129. Stephan RM. Intra-oral hydrogen-ion concentrations associated with dental caries activity. J Dent Res 1944; 23:257–266.

130. Macrina FL, Dertzbaugh MT, Halula MC, Krah ER, Jones KR. Genetic approaches to the study

of oral microflora: a review. Crit Rev Oral Biol Med 1990; 1:207–227.

131. Kuramitsu HK. Virulence factors of mutans streptococci: role of molecular genetics. Crit Rev Oral Biol Med 1993; 4:159–176.

132. Van Houte J. The role of micro-organisms in caries etiology. J Dent Res 1994; 73:672–681.

133. LeBlanc DJ. The role of sucrose metabolism in the cariogenicity of the mutans streptococci. In: Miller VL, Kasper JB, Portnoy DA, Isberg RR (eds). Molecular Genetics of Bacterial Pathogenesis. Washington DC: American Society of Microbiology, 1994; 465–477.

134. Russell RRB. The application of molecular genetics to the microbiology of dental caries [invited mini-review]. Caries Res 1994; 28:69–82.

135. Yamamoto Y, Sato Y, Takahashi-Abbe S, Abbe K, Yamada T, Kizaki H. Cloning and sequence analysis of the *pfl* gene encoding pyruvate formate-lyase from *Streptococcus mutans*. Infect Immun 1996; 64:385–391.

136. Kleinberg I, Jenkins GN. The pH of dental plaques in the different areas of the mouth before and after meals and their relationship to the pH and rate of flow of resting saliva. Arch Oral Biol 1964; 9:493–516.

137. Dashper SG, Riley PF, Reynolds EC. Characterization of glutamine transport in *Streptococcus mutans*. Oral Microbiol Immunol 1995; 10:183–187.

138. Kleinberg I. Effect of urea concentration on human plaque pH in situ. Arch Oral Biol 1967; 12:1475–1484.

139. Chen Y-YM, Clancy KA, Burne RA. *Streptococcus salivarius* urease: genetic and biochemical characterization and expression in a dental plaque streptococcus. Infect Immun 1996; 64:585–592.

140. Bowden GH, Ellwood DC, Hamilton IR. Microbiol ecology of the oral cavity. In: Alexander M (ed). Advances in Microbial Ecology. New York: Plenum Press, 1979; 135–217.

141. Bradshaw DJ, McKee AS, Marsh PD. Effects of carbohydrate pulses and pH on population shifts within oral microbial communities. J Dent Res 1989; 68:1298–1302.

142. Kleinberg I, Chatterjee R, Denepitiya L. Effects of saliva and dietary eating habits on the pH and demineralisation-remineralisation potential of dental plaque. In: Leach SA, Edgar WM (eds). Proceedings, Demineralisation and Remineralisation of the Teeth. Washington DC: IRL Press, 1982; 25–50.

143. Zero DT, van Houte J, Russo J. The intra-oral effect on enamel demineralization of extracellular matrix material synthesized from sucrose by *Streptococcus mutans*. J Dent Res 1986; 65:918–923.

144. Clarkson BH, Krell D, Wefel JS, Crall J, Feagin FF. In vitro caries-like lesion production by *Streptococcus mutans* and *Actinomyces viscosus*

145. Wennerholm K, Birkhed D, Emilson CG. Effects of sugar restriction on *Streptococcus mutans* and *Streptococcus sobrinus* in saliva and dental plaque. Caries Res 1995; 29:54–61.

146. Alaluusa S, Nyström M, Grönroos L, Peck L. Caries-related microbiological findings in a group of teenagers and the parents. Caries Res 1989; 23:49–54.

147. Granath L, Cleaton-Jones P, Fatti LP, Grossman ES. Salivary lactobacilli explain dental caries better than salivary mutans in 4–5-year-old children. Scand J Dent Res 1994; 102:319–323.

148. Roeters FJM, van der Hoeven JS, Burgersdijk RCW, Schaeken MJM. Lactobacilli, mutans streptococci and dental caries: a longitudinal study in 2-year-old children up to the age of 5 years. Caries Res 1995; 29:272–279

149. Sigurjons H, Magnusdottir MO, Holbrook WP. Cariogenic bacteria in a longitudinal study of approximal caries. Caries Res 1995; 29:42–45.

150. Banas JA, Russell RRB, Ferretti JJ. Sequence analysis of the gene for the glucan-binding protein of *Streptococcus mutans* Ingbritt. Infect Immun 1990; 58:667–673.

151. Qian H, Dao ML. Inactivation of the *Streptococcus mutans* wall-associated protein A gene [*wapA*] results in a decrease in sucrose-dependent adherence and aggregation. Infect Immun 1993; 61:5021–5028.

151a. Harrington DJ, Russell RR. Multiple changes in cell wall antigens of isogenic mutants of *Streptococcus mutans*. J Bacteriol 1993; 175:5925–5933.

152. Slee AM, Tanzer JM. Sucrose transport by *Streptococcus mutans*: evidence for multiple transport systems. Biochim Biophys Acta 1982; 692:415–424.

153. Vadeboncoeur C, Bourgeau G, Mayrand D, Trahan L. Control of sugar utilization in the oral bacteria *Streptococcus salivarius* and *Streptococcus sanguis* by the phosphoenolpyruvate: glucose phosphotransferase system. Arch Oral Biol 1983; 28:123–131.

154. Jacobson GR, Lodge J, Poy F. Carbohydrate uptake in the oral pathogen *Streptococcus mutans*: mechanisms and regulation by protein phosphorylation. Biochimie 1989; 71:997–1004.

155. Poy F, Jacobson GR. Evidence that a low-affinity sucrose phosphotransferase activity in *Streptococcus mutans* GS-5 is a high-affinity trehalose uptake system. Infect Immun 1990; 58:1479–1480.

156. Ferretti JJ, Tao L, Aduse-Opoku J, Russell RRB. A sugar binding protein-dependent transport system in *Streptococcus mutans*. Proceedings of the International Lancefield Streptococcal Conference, 1991, Sienna, Italy.

157. Russell RRB, Aduse-Opoku J, Sutcliffe IC, Tao

L, Ferretti JJ. A binding protein-dependent transport system in *Streptococcus mutans* responsible for multiple sugar metabolism. J Biol Chem 1992; 267:4631–4637.

158. Cvitkovitch DG, Boyd DA, Thevenot T, Hamilton IR. Glucose transport by a mutant of *Streptococcus mutans* unable to transport sugars via the phosphoenolpyurvate phosphotransferase system. J Bacteriol 1995; 177:2251–2258.

159. Tao L, Sutcliffe IL, Russell RRB, Ferretti JJ. Cloning and expression of the multiple sugar metabolism (*msm*) operon of *Streptococcus mutans* in heterologous streptococcal hosts. Infect Immun 1993; 61:1121–1125.

160. Tao L, Sutcliffe IL, Russell RRB, Ferretti JJ. Transport of sugars, including sucrose, by the *msm* transport system of *Streptococcus mutans*. J Dent Res 1993; 72:1386–1390.

161. Cvitkovitch DG, Boyd DA, Hamilton IR. Regulation of sugar transport via the multiple sugar metabolism operon of *Streptococcus mutans* by the phosphoenolpyruvate phosphotransferase system. J Bacteriol 1995; 177:5704–5706.

162. Simpson CL, Russell RRB. Identification of a homolog of CcpA catabolite repressor protein in *Streptococcus mutans*. Infect Immun 1998; 66:2085–2092.

162a. Slee AM, Tanzer JM. Phosphoenolpyruvate-dependent sucrose phosphotransferase activity in five serotypes of *Streptococcus mutans*. Infect Immun 1979; 26:783–786.

163. St. Martin EJ, Wittenberger CL. Characterization of a phosphoenolpyruvate-dependent sucrose phosphotransferase system in *Streptococcus mutans*. Infect Immun 1979; 24:865–868.

164. Sato Y, Poy F, Jacobson GR, Kuramitsu HK. Characterization and sequence analysis of the *scrA* gene encoding enzyme II^scr of the *Streptococcus mutans* phosphoenolpyruvate-dependent sucrose phosphotransferase system. J Bacteriol 1989; 171:263–271.

165. Vadeboncoeur C. Structure and properties of the phosphoenolpyruvate: glucose phosphotransferase system of oral streptococci. Can J Microbiol 1984; 30:495–502.

166. Thevenot T, Brochu D, Vadeboncoeur, Hamilton IR. Regulation of ATP-dependent P-[ser]-HPr formation in *Streptococcus mutans* and *Streptococcus salivarius*. J Bacteriol 1995; 177:2751–2759.

167. St. Martin EJ, Wittenberger CL. Regulation and function of sucrose-6-phosphate hydrolase in *Streptococcus mutans*. Infect. Immun 1979; 26:487–491.

168. Hayakawa M, Aoki H, Kuramitsu HK. Isolation and characterization of the sucrose-6-phosphate hydrolase gene from *Streptococcus mutans*. Infect Immun 1986; 53:582–586.

169. Lunsford RD, Macrina FL. Molecular cloning and characterization of *scrB*, the structural gene for *Streptococcus mutans* phosphoenolpyruvate-

170. Sato Y, Kuramitsu HK. Sequence analysis of the *Streptococcus mutans scrB* gene. Infect Immun 1988; 56:1956–1960.

171. Dashper SG, Reynolds EC. Lactic acid excretion by *Streptococcus mutans*. Microbiology 1996; 142(part 1):33–39.

172. Ellwood DC, Hamilton IR. Properties of *Streptococcus mutans* Ingbritt growing on limiting sucrose in a chemostat: repression of the phosphoenolpyruvate phosphotransferase transport system. Infect Immun 1982; 36:576–581.

173. McLaughlin RE, Ferretti JJ. Multiple sugar metabolism [*msm*] gene cluster of *Streptococcus mutans* is transcribed as a single operon. FEMS Microbiol Lett 1996; 140:261–264.

174. Sutcliffe IC, Tao L, Ferretti JJ, Russell RR. MsmE, a lipoprotein involved in sugar transport in *Streptococcus mutans*. J Bacteriol 1993; 175:1853–1855.

175. Aduse-Opoku J, Tao L, Ferretti JJ, Russell RRB. Biochemical and genetic analysis of *Streptococcus mutans* α-galactosidase. J Gen Microbiol 1991; 137:2271–2272.

176. Russell RRB, Mukasa H, Shimamura A, Ferretti JJ. *Streptococcus mutans gtfA* gene specifies sucrose phosphorylase. Infect Immun 1988; 56:2763–2765.

177. Russell RRB, Ferretti JJ. Nucleotide sequence of the dextran glucosidase [*dexB*] gene of *Streptococcus mutans*. J Gen Microbiol 1990; 136:803–810.

178. Iwami Y, Hata S, Schachtele CF, Yamada T. Simultaneous monitoring of intracellular pH and proton excretion during glycolysis by *Streptococcus mutans* and *Streptococcus sanguis*—effect of low pH and fluoride. Oral Microbiol Immunol 1995; 10:355–359.

179. Hamilton IR. Effects of changing environment on sugar transport and metabolism by oral bacteria. In: Reizer J, Peterkofsky A (eds). Sugar Transport and Metabolism in Gram Positive Bacteria. Chichester: Ellis Horwood, 1987; 94–133.

180. Yang YB, Germaine GR. Effect of lysozyme on glucose fermentation, cytoplasmic pH, and intracellular potassium concentration in *Streptococcus mutans* 10449. Infect Immun 1991; 59:638–644.

181. Marquis RE. Antimicrobial actions of fluoride for oral bacteria. Can J Microbiol 1995; 41:955–964.

182. Munro C, Michalek SM, Macrina FL. Cariogenicity of *Streptococcus mutans* V403 glucosyltransferase and fructosyltransferase mutants constructed by allelic exchange. Infect Immun 1991; 59:2316–2323.

183. Burne RA, Chen YM, Wexler DW, Kuramitsu HK, Bowen WH. Cariogenicity of *Streptococ-*

cus mutans strains with defects in fructan metabolism assessed in a program-fed specific pathogen-free rat model. J Dent Res 1996; 75:1572–1577.

184. Ceska M, Granath K, Norman B, Guggenheim B. Structural and enzymatic studies on glucans synthesized with glucosyltransferases of some strains of oral streptococci. Acta Chem Scand 1972; 6:2223–2230.

185. Freedman M, Birkhed D, Granath K. Analysis of glucans from cariogenic and mutant *Streptococcus mutans*. Infect Immun 1978; 21:17–27.

186. Trautner K, Birkhed D, Svensson S. Structure of extracellular glucans synthesized by *Streptococcus mutans* of serotypes a–e in vitro. Caries Res 1982; 16:81–89.

187. Scheie AA, Eggen KH, Rølla G. Glucosyltransferase in human in vivo formed pellicle and in whole saliva. Scand J Dent Res 1986; 95:212–215.

188. Rølla G, Ciardi JE, Eggen K, Bowen WH, Afseth J. Free glucosyl- and fructosyltransferase in human saliva and adsorption of these enzymes to teeth in vivo. In: Doyle RJ, Ciardi JE (eds). Glucosyltransferases, Glucans, Sucrose and Dental Caries. Special supplement, Chemical Senses. Washington DC: IRL Press, 1983; 21–30.

189. Hanada N, Kuramitsu HK. Isolation and characterization of the *Streptococcus mutans gtfc* gene, coding for synthesis of soluble and insoluble glucans. Infect Immun 1988; 56:1999–2005.

190. Hanada N, Kuramitsu HK. Isolation and characterization of the *Streptococcus mutans gtfd* gene, coding for primer-dependent soluble glucan synthesis. Infect Immun 1989; 57:2079–2085.

191. Aoki H, Shiroza T, Hayakawa M, Sato S, Kuramitsu HK. Cloning of *Streptococcus mutans* glucosyltransferase gene coding for insoluble glucan synthesis. Infect Immun 1986; 53:587–594.

192. Kopec LK, Vacca-Smith AM, Bowen WH. Structural aspects of glucans formed in solution and on the surface of hydroxyapatite. Glycobiology 1997; 7:929–934.

193. Vacca-Smith AM, Venkitaraman AR, Quivey RG Jr, Bowen WH. Interactions of streptococcal glucosyltransferases with α-amylase and starch on the surface of saliva-coated hydroxyapatite. Arch Oral Biol 1996; 41:291–298.

194. Schilling KM, Bowen WH. Glucans synthesized in situ in experimental pellicle functions as specific binding sites for *Streptococcus mutans*. Infect Immun 1992; 60:284–295.

195. Russell RRB. Glucan-binding proteins of *Streptococcus mutans* serotype c. J Gen Microbiol 1979; 112:197–201.

196. Yamashita Y, Bowen WH, Burne RA, Kuramitsu HK. Role of the *Streptococcus mutans gtf* genes in caries induction in the specific pathogen-free rat model. Infect Immun 1993; 61:3811–3817.

197. Bowden GHW, Li YH. Nutritional influences on biofilm development. Adv Dent Res 1997; 11:81–89.

198. Carlsson J. Bacterial metabolism in dental biofilms. Adv Dent Res 1997; 11:75–80.

199. Germaine GR, Tellefson LM. Effect of endogenous phosphoenolpyruvate potential on fluoride inhibition of glucose uptake by *Streptococcus mutans*. Infect Immun 1986; 51:119–124.

200. Bender GR, Sutton SVW, Marquis RE. Acid tolerance, proton permiabilities, and membrane ATPase of oral streptococci. Infect Immun 1986; 53:331–338.

201. Hamilton IR, Buckley ND. Adaptation of *Streptococcus mutans* to acid tolerance. Oral Microbiol Immunol 1991; 6:65–71.

202. Sturr MG, Marquis RE. Comparative acid tolerances and inhibitor sensitivities of isolated F-ATPases of oral lactic acid bacteria. Appl Environ Microbiol 1992; 58:2287–2291.

203. Quivey RG Jr, Faustoferri RC, Clancy KA, Marquis RE. Acid adaptation in *Streptococcus mutans* UA159 alleviates sensitization to environmental stress due to RecA deficiency. FEMS Microbiol Lett 1995; 126:257–262.

204. Henderson B, Wilson M. Commensal communism and the oral cavity. J Dent Res 1998; 77:1674–1683.

204a. Bayston K, Tomlinson M, Cohen J. In-vitro stimulation of TNF-alpha from human whole blood by cell-free supernatants of gram-positive bacteria. Cytokine 1992; 4:397–402.

205. Bancsi MJ, Veltrop MH, Bertina RM, Thompson J. Role of phagocytosis in activation of the coagulation system in *Streptococcus sanguis* endocarditis. Infect Immun 1996; 64:5166–5170.

206. Soto A, McWhinney PH, Kibbler CC, Cohen J. Cytokine release and mitogenic activity in the viridans streptococcal shock syndrome. Cytokine 1998; 10:370–376.

207. Orlicek SL, Branum KC, English BK, McCordic R, Shenep JL, Patrick CC. Viridans streptococcal isolates from patients with septic shock induce tumor necrosis factor-alpha production by murine macrophages. J Lab Clin Med 1997; 130:515–519.

208. English BK, Patrick CC, Orlicek SL, McCordic R, Shenep JL. Lipoteichoic acid from viridans streptococci induces the production of tumor necrosis factor and nitric oxide by murine macrophages. J Infect Dis 1996; 174:1348–1351.

209. Vernier A, Diab M, Soell M, Haan-Archipoff G, Beretz A, Wachsmann D, Klein JP. Cytokine production by human epithelial and endothelial cells following exposure to oral viridans streptococci involves lectin interactions between bacteria and cell surface receptors. Infect. Immun 1996; 64:3016–3022.

210. Soto A, Evans TJ, Cohen J. Proinflammatory cytokine production by human peripheral blood mononuclear cells stimulated with cell-free su-

pernatants of viridans streptococci. Cytokine 1996; 8:300–304.

211. Le Roy D, Morand P, Lengacher S, Celio M, Grau GE, Glauser MP, Heumann D. *Streptococcus mitis* cell walls and lipopolysaccharide induce lethality in D-galactosamine-sensitized mice by a tumor necrosis factor-dependent pathway. Infect Immun 1996; 64:1846–1849.

212. Mossad SB, Longworth DL, Goormastic M, Serkey JM, Keys TF, Bolwell BJ. Early infectious complications in autologous bone marrow transplantation: a review of 219 patients. Bone Marrow Transplant 1996; 18:265–271.

213. Engel A, Kern P, Kern WV. Levels of cytokines and cytokine inhibitors in the neutropenic patient with alpha-hemolytic streptococcus shock syndrome. Clin Infect Dis 1996; 23:785–789.

214. Murakata H, Harabuchi Y, Kukuminato Y, Yokoyama Y, Kataura A. Cytokine production by tonsils lymphocytes stimulated with alpha-streptococci in patients with pustulosis palmaris et plantaris. Acta Otolaryngol Suppl (Stockh) 1996; 523:201–203.

215. Takada H, Kawabata Y, Tamura M, Matsushita K, Igarashi H, Ohkuni H, Todome Y, Uchiyama T, Kotani S. Cytokine induction by extracellular products of oral viridans group streptococci. Infect Immun 1993; 61:5152–5260.

216. Matsushita K, Fujimaki W, Kato H, Uchiyama T, Igarashi H, Ohkuni H, Nagaoka S, Kawagoe M, Kotani S, Takada H. Immunopathological activities of extracellular products of *Streptococcus mitis*, particularly a superantigenic fraction. Infect Immun 1995; 63:785–793.

217. Matsushita K, Sugiyama A, Uchiyama T, Igarashi H, Ohkuni H, Nagaoka S, Kotani S, Takada H. Induction of lymphocytes cytotoxic to oral epithelial cells by *Streptococcus mitis* superantigen. J Dent Res 1996; 75:927–934.

218. Lareau DE, Herzberg MC, Nelson RD. Human neutrophil migration under agarose to bacteria associated with the development of gingivitis. J Periodontol 1984; 55:540–549.

219. Durack DT. Prevention of infective endocarditis. New Engl J Med 1995; 332:38–44.

220. Roberts GJ, Holzel HS, Sury MR, Simmons NA, Gardner P, Longhurst P. Dental bacteremia in children. Pediatr Cardiol 1997; 18:24–27.

221. Daly C, Mitchell D, Grossberg D, Highfield J, Stewart D. Bacteraemia caused by periodontal probing. Aust Dent J 1997; 42:77–80.

222. Heimdahl A, Hall G, Hedberg M, Sandberg H, Soder PO, Tuner K, Nord CE. Detection and quantitation by lysis-filtration of bacteremia after different oral surgical procedures. J Clin Microbiol 1990; 28:2205–2209.

223. Soldado L, Esteban F, Delgado-Rodriguez M, Solanellas J, Florez C, Martin E. Bacteraemia during tonsillectomy: a study of the factors involved and clinical implications. Clin Otolaryngol 1998; 23:63–66.

224. Fujimori I, Kikushima K, Hisamatsu K, Nozawa I, Goto R, Murakami Y. Interaction between oral alpha-streptococci and group A streptococci in patients with tonsillitis. Ann Otol Rhinol Laryngol 1997; 106(7 Pt 1):571–574.

225. Lundberg C, Lonnroth J, Nord CE. Identification of attached bacteria in the nasopharynx of the child. Infection 1982; 10:58–62.

226. Mogi A, Nishi JI, Yoshinaga M, Harada H, Narahara S, Kawakami K, Maruyama I. Increased prevalence of penicillin-resistant viridans group streptococci in Japanese children with upper respiratory infection treated by beta-lactam agents and in those with oncohematologic diseases. Pediatr Infect Dis J 1997; 16:1140–1144.

227. Erickson PR, and Herzberg MC. Emergence of antibiotic resistant *Streptococcus sanguis* in dental plaque of children after treatment for otitis media. Pediatr Dent 1999; in press.

228. Guiot HF, Corel LJ, Vossen JM. Prevalence of penicillin-resistant viridans streptococci in healthy children and in patients with malignant haematological disorders. Eur J Clin Microbiol Infect Dis 1994; 13:645–650.

229. Marrie TJ. Bacteremic community-acquired pneumonia due to viridans group streptococci. Clin Invest Med 1993; 16:38–44.

230. Koorevaar CT, Scherpenzeel PG, Neijens HJ, Derksen-Lubsen G, Dzoljic-Danilovic G, de Groot R. Childhood meningitis caused by enterococci and viridans streptococci. Infection 1992; 20:118–121.

231. Devaux Y, Archimbaud E, Guyotat D, Plotton C, Maupas J, Fleurette J, Fiere D. Streptococcal bacteremia in neutropenic adult patients. Nouv Rev Fr Hematol 1992; 34:191–195.

232. Steiner M, Villablanca J, Kersey J, Ramsay N, Haake R, Ferrieri P, Weisdorf D. Viridans streptococcal shock in bone marrow transplantation patients. Am J Hematol 1993; 42:354–358.

233. Leibovici L, Drucker M, Konigsberger H, Samra Z, Harrari S, Ashkenazi S, Pitlik SD. Septic shock in bacteremic patients: risk factors, features and prognosis. Scand J Infect Dis 1997; 29:71–75.

234. Jacobs JA, Schouten HC, Stobberingh EE, Soeters PB. Viridans streptococci isolated from the bloodstream. Relevance of species identification. Diagn Microbiol Infect Dis 1995; 22:267–273.

235. Casariego E, Rodriguez A, Corredoira JC, Alonso P, Coira A, Bal M, Lopez MJ, Varela J. Prospective study of *Streptococcus milleri* bacteremia. Eur J Clin Microbiol Infect Dis 1996; 15:194–200.

236. Bochud PY, Calandra T, Francioli P. Bacteremia due to viridans streptococci in neutropenic patients: a review. Am J Med 1994; 97:256–264.

237. Richard P, Amador Del Valle G, Moreau P, Milpied N, Felice MP, Daeschler T, Hrousseau JL, Richet H. Viridans streptococcal bacter-

aemia in patients with neutropenia. Lancet 1995; 345:1607–1609.

238. Bilgrami S, Feingold JM, Dorsky D, Edwards RL, Clive J, Tutschka PJ. Streptococcus viridans bacteremia following autologous peripheral blood stem cell transplantation. Bone Marrow Transplant 1998; 21:591–595.

239. Pfaller MA, Jones RN, Marshall SA, Edmond MB, Wenzel RP. Nosocomial streptococcal blood stream infections in the SCOPE Program: species occurrence and antimicrobial resistance. The SCOPE Hospital Study Group. Diagn Microbiol Infect Dis 1997; 29:259–263.

240. Herzberg MC. Platelet-streptococcal interactions in endocarditis. Crit Rev Oral Biol Med 1996; 7:222–236.

240a. Kern WV, Engel A, Schieffer S, Prummer O, Kern P. Circulating tumor necrosis factor alpha (TNF), soluble TNF receptors, and interleukin-6 in human subacute bacterial endocarditis. Infect Immun 1993; 61:5413–5416.

241. Iga K, Hori K, Matsumura T, Tomonaga G, Gen H, Tamamura T. Native valve infective endocarditis in adults: analysis of 32 consecutive cases over a ten-year period from 1980 to 1989. Jpn Circ J 1991; 55:437–442.

242. Rohmann S, Erbel R, Darius H, Gorge G, Makowski T, Zotz R, Mohr-Kahaly S, Nixdorff U, Drexler M, Meyer J. Prediction of rapid versus prolonged healing of infective endocarditis by monitoring vegetation size. J Am Soc Echocardiogr 1991; 4:465–474.

243. Douglas CW, Heath J, Hampton KK, Preston FE. Identity of viridans streptococci isolated from cases of infective endocarditis. J Med Microbiol 1993; 39:179–182.

244. Benn M, Hagelskjaer LH, Tvede M. Infective endocarditis, 1984 through 1993: a clinical and microbiological survey. J Intern Med 1997; 242:15–22.

245. Paterson DL, Dominguez EA, Chang FY, Snydman DR, Singh N. Infective endocarditis in solid organ transplant recipients. Clin Infect Dis 1998; 26:689–694.

246. Bouvet A. Human endocarditis due to nutritionally variant streptococci: Streptococcus adjacens and Streptococcus defectivus. Eur Heart J 1995; 16 Suppl B:24–27.

247. Overholser CD, Moreillon P, Glauser MP. Experimental endocarditis following dental extractions in rats with periodontitis. J Oral Maxillofac Surg 1988; 46:857–861.

248. Overholser CD, Moreillon P, Glauser MP. Experimental bacterial endocarditis in rats with periodontitis. J Infect Dis 1988; 155:107–112.

249. Erickson PR, Herzberg MC. Altered expression of the platelet aggregation-associated protein from Streptococcus sanguis after growth in the presence of collagen. Infect Immun 1995; 63:1084–1088.

250. Summer P, Gleyzal C, Guerret S, Etienne J, Gri-

maus J-A. Induction of a putative laminin-binding protein of Streptococcus gordonii in human infective endocarditis. Infect Immun 1992; 60:360–365.

251. Herzberg MC, Meyer MW, Kiliç A, Tao L. Host-pathogen interactions in bacterial endocarditis: streptococcal virulence in the host. Adv Dent Res 1997; 11:69–74.

251a. Kiliç AO, Herzberg, MC, Meyer MW, Zhao X, Tao L. Streptococcal reporter gene-fusion vector for identification of in vivo-expressed genes. Plasmid 1999; in press.

252. Burnie JP, Brooks W, Donohoe M, Hodgetts S, al-Ghamdi A, Matthews RC. Defining antibody targets in Streptococcus oralis infection. Infect Immun 1996; 64:1600–1608.

253. Ryd M, Schennings T, Flock M, Heimdahl A, Flock JI. Streptococcus mutans major adhesion surface protein, P1 (I/II), does not contribute to attachment to valvular vegetations or to the development of endocarditis in a rat model. Arch Oral Biol 1996; 41:999–1002.

254. Burnette-Curley D, Wells V, Viscount H, Munro CL, Fenno JC, Fives-Taylor P, Macrina F. FimA, a major virulence factor associated with Streptococcus parasanguis endocarditis. Infect Immun 1995; 63:4669–4674.

255. Jenkinson HF. Cell surface protein receptors in oral streptococci. FEMS Microbiol Lett 1994; 121:133–140.

256. Viscount HB, Munro CL, Burnette-Curley D, Peterson DL, Macrina FL. Immunization with FimA protects against Streptococcus parasanguis endocarditis in rats. Infect Immun 1997; 65:994–1002.

257. Kessler CM, Nussbaum E, Tuazon CU. In vitro correlation of platelet aggregation with occurrence of disseminated intravascular coagulation and subacute bacterial endocarditis. J Lab Clin Med 1987; 109:647–652.

258. Manning JE, Hume EB, Hunter N, Knox KW. An appraisal of virulence factors associated with streptococcal endocarditis. J Med Microbiol 1994; 40:110–114.

259. Herzberg MC, Brintzenhofe KL, Clawson CC. Aggregation of human platelets and adhesion of Streptococcus sanguis. Infect Immun 1983; 39:1457–1469.

260. Sullam PM, Valone FH, Mills J. Mechanisms of platelet aggregation by viridans group streptococci. Infect Immun 1987; 55:1743–1750.

261. Douglas CWI, Brown PR, Preston FE. Platelet aggregation by oral streptococci. FEMS Microbial Lett 1990; 60:63–67.

262. Manning JE, Geyelin AJ, Ansmits LM, Oakey HJ, Knox KW. A comparative study of the aggregation of human, rat and rabbit platelets by members of the Streptococcus-Sanguis group. J Med Microbiol 1994; 41:10–13.

263. Erickson PR, Herzberg MC. A collagen-like immunodeterminant on the surface of Streptococ-

cus sanguis induces platelet aggregation. J Immunol 1987; 138:3360–3366.

264. Erickson PR, Herzberg MC. Purification and partial characterization of a 65-kDa platelet aggregation-associated protein antigen from the surface of *Streptococcus sanguis*. J Biol Chem 1990; 265:14080–14087.

265. Erickson PR, Herzberg MC. The *Streptococcus sanguis* platelet aggregation-associated protein: identification and characterization of the minimal platelet-interactive domain. J Biol Chem 1993; 268:1646–1649.

266. Herzberg MC, MacFarlane GD, Gong K, Armstrong NN, Witt AR, Erickson PR, Meyer MW. Platelet interactivity phenotype of *Streptococcus sanguis* influences the course of experimental endocarditis. Infect Immun 1992; 60:4809–4818.

267. Meyer MW, Witt AR, Krishnan LK, Yokota M, Roszkowski MJ, Rudney JD, Herzberg MO. Therapeutic advantage of recombinant human tissue plasminogen activator in endocarditis: evidence from experimental rabbits. Thromb Haemost 1995; 73:680–682.

268. Ford I, Douglas CWI, Preston FE, Lawless A, Hampton KK. Mechanisms of platelet aggregation by *Streptococcus sanguis*, a causative organism in infective endocarditis. Br J Haematol 1993; 84:95–100.

269. Sullam PM, Jarvis GA, Valone FH. Role of immunoglobulin G in platelet aggregation by viridans group streptococci. Infect Immun 1988; 56:2907–2911.

270. Sullam PM, Frank U, Yeaman MR, Tauber MA, Bayer AS, Chambers HF. Effect of thrombocytopenia on the early course of streptococcal endocarditis. J Infect Dis 1993; 168:910–914.

271. Wu T, Yeaman MR, Bayer AS. In vitro resistance to platelet microbicidal protein correlates with endocarditis source among bacteremic staphylococcal and streptococcal isolates. Antimicrob Agents Chemother 1994; 38:729–732.

272. Dankert J, VanderWerff J, Saat SAJ, Joldersma W, Klein D, Hess J. Involvement of bactericidal factors from thrombin-stimulated platelets in clearance of adherent viridans streptococci in experimental infective endocarditis. Infect Immun 1995; 63:663–671.

273. Gong K, Wen DY, Ouyang T, Rao AT, Herzberg MC. Platelet receptors for the *Streptococcus sanguis* adhesin and aggregation-associated antigens and distinguished by anti-idiotypical monoclonal antibodies. Infect Immun 1995; 63:3628–3633.

274. Gong K, Ouyang T, Herzberg MC. A streptococcal adhesion system for salivary pellicle and platelets. Infect Immun 1998; 66:5388–5392.

275. Martino R, Manteiga R, Sanchez I, Brunet S, Sureda A, Badell I, Argiles B, Subira M, Bordes R, Domingo-Albos A. Viridans streptococcal

shock syndrome during bone marrow transplantation. Acta Haematol 1995; 94:69–73.

276. Elting LS, Rubenstein EB, Rolston KV, Bodey GP. Outcomes of bacteremia in patients with cancer and neutropenia: observations from two decades of epidemiological and clinical trials. Clin Infect Dis 1997; 247–259.

277. Herzberg MC, Meyer MW. Effects of oral flora on platelets: possible consequences in cardiovascular disease. J Periodontol 1996; 67(Suppl): 1138–1142.

278. Herzberg MC, Meyer MW. Dental plaque, platelets and cardiovascular diseases. Ann Periodontol 1998; 3:151–160.

279. Meyer MW, Gong K, Herzberg MC. *Streptococcus sanguis*–induced platelet clotting in rabbits and hemodynamic and cardiopulmonary consequences. Infect Immun 1998; 66:5906–5914.

280. Beck J, Garcia R, Heiss G, Vokonas PS, Offenbacher S. Periodontal disease and cardiovascular disease. J Periodontol 1996; 67(Suppl):1123–1137.

281. DeStefano F, Anda RF, Kahn HS, Williamson DF, Russell CM. Dental disease and risk of coronary heart disease and mortality. BMJ 1993; 306:688–691.

282. Mattila KJ, Nieminen MS, Valtonen VV, Rasi VP, Kesaniemi YA, Syrjala SL, Jungell PS, Isoluoma M, Hietaniemi, Jokinen MJ. Association between dental health and myocardial infarction. BMJ 1989; 298:779–782.

283. Syrjanen J, Peltola J, Valtonen V, Iivanainen M, Kaste M, Huttunen JK. Dental infections in association with cerebral infarction in young and middle-aged men. J Intern Med 1989; 225:179–184.

284. Grau AJ, Buggle F, Ziegler C, Schwarz W, Meuser J, Tasman AJ, Buhler A, Benesch C, Becher H, Hacke W. Association between acute cerebrovascular ischemia and chronic and recurrent infection. Stroke 1997; 28:1724–1729.

284a. Matilla KJ, Valtonen VV, Nieminen MS, Asikainen S. Role of infection as a risk factor for atherosclerosis, myocardial infarction, and stroke. Clin Infect Dis 1998; 26:719–734.

285. Ogawa SK, Yurberg ER, Hatcher VB, Levitt MA, Lowy FD. Bacterial adherence to human endothelial cells in vitro. Infect Immun 1985; 50:218–224.

286. Tart RC, van de Rijn I. Analysis of *Streptococcus defectivus* and endocarditis-associated streptococci to extracellular matrix. Infect Immun 1991; 59:857–862.

287. Drake TA, Pang M. Effects of interleukin-1, lipopolysaccharide, and streptococci on procoagulant activity of cultured human cardiac valve endothelial and stromal cells. Infect Immun 1989; 57:507–512.

288. Vercellotti GM, Lussenhop D, Peterson PK, Furcht LT, McCarthy JB, Jacob HS, Moldow

CF. Bacterial adherence to fibronectin and endothelial cells: a possible mechanism for bacterial tissue tropism. J Lab Clin Med 1984; 103:34–43.

289. Smith DJ, Anderson JM, King WF, van Houte J, Taubman MA. Oral streptococcal colonization of infants. Oral Microbiol Immunol 1993; 8:1–4.

290. Koch RJ, Brodsky L. Effect of specific bacteria on lymphocyte proliferation in diseased and nondiseased tonsils. Laryngoscope 1993; 103: 1020–1026.

291. Bernstein JM, Reddy MS, Scannapieco FA, Faden HS, Ballow M. The microbial ecology and immunology of the adenoid: implications for otitis media. Ann N Y Acad Sci 1997; 830:19–31.

292. Curtis N, Levin M. Kawasaki disease thirty years on. Curr Opin Pediatr 1998; 10:24–33.

293. Nakamura Y, Yanagawa H, Ojima T, Kawasaki T, Kato H. Cardiac sequelae of Kawasaki disease among recurrent cases. Arch Dis Child 1998; 78:163–165.

294. Ohkuni H, Todome Y, Mizuse M, Ohtani N, Suzuki H, Igarashi H, Hashimoto Y, Ezaki T, Hrada K, Imada Y, Ohkawa S, Kotani S. Biologically active extracellular products of oral viridans streptococci and the aetiology of Kawasaki disease. J Med Microbiol 1993; 39:352–362.

295. Abe Y, Nakano S, Aita K, Sagishima M. Streptococcal and staphylococcal superantigen-induced lymphocytic arteritis in a local type experimental mode: comparison with acute vasculitis in the Arthus reaction. J Lab Clin Med 1998; 131:93–102.

296. Leung DY, Meissner C, Fulton D, Schlievert PM. The potential role of bacterial superantigens in the pathogenesis of Kawasaki syndrome. J Clin Immunol 1995; 15:11S–17S.

297. Costalonga M, Powdrill JM, Herzberg MC, Schlievert PM. Pyrogenic exotoxins and the pathogenesis of Streptococcus sanguis endocarditis [abstract]. J Dent Res 1994; 73:426.

298. Jason J, Gregg L, Han A, Hu A, Inge KL, Eick A, Tham I, Campbell R. Immunoregulatory changes in Kawasaki disease. Clin Immunol Immunopathol 1997; 84:296–306.

299. Choi IH, Chwae YJ, Shim WS, Kim DS, Kwon DH, Kim JD, Kim SJ. Clonal expansion of CD8+ T cells in Kawasaki disease. J Immunol 1997; 159:481–486.

300. Rowley AH, Eckerley CA, Jack HM, Shulman ST, Baker SC. IgA plasma cells in vascular tissue of patients with Kawasaki syndrome. J Immunol 1997; 159:5946–5955.

301. Falcini F, Trapani S, Turchini S, Farsi A, Ermini M, Keser G, Khamashta MA, Hughes GR. Immunological findings in Kawasaki disease: an evaluation in a cohort of Italian children. Clin Exp Rheumatol 1997; 15:685–689.

302. Kaklamani VG, Vaiopoulos G, Kaklamanis PG. Behçet's disease. Semin Arthritis Rheum 1998; 27:197–217.

303. Gurler A, Boyvat A, Tursen U. Clinical manifestation of Behçet's disease: an analysis of 2147 patients. Yonsei Med J 1997; 38:423–427.

304. Lenk N, Ozet G, Alli N, Coban O, Erbasi S. Protein C and protein S activities in Behçet's disease as risk factors of thrombosis. Int J Dermatol 1998; 37:124–125.

305. Isogai E, Isogai H, Yokota K, Hayashi S, Funii N, Oguma K, Yoshikawa K, Sasamoto Y, Kotake S, Ohno S. Platelet aggregation induced by uncommon serotypes of Streptococcus sanguis isolated from patients with Behçet's disease. Arch Oral Biol 1991; 26:425–429.

306. Yokota K, Hayashi S, Araki Y, Isogai E, Kotake S, Yoshikawa K, Fujhii N, Hirai Y, Oguma K. Characterization of Streptococcus sanguis isolated form patients with Behçet's disease. Microbiol Immunol 1995; 39:729–732.

306a. Narikawa S, Suzuki Y, Takahashi M, Furukawa A, Sakane T, Mizushima Y, Streptococcus oralis previously identified as uncommon 'Streptococcus sanguis' in Behçet's disease. Arch Oral Biol 1995; 40:685–690.

307. Yokota K, Oguma K. IgA protease produced by Streptococcus sanguis and antibody production against IgA protease in patients with Behçet's disease. Microbiol Immunol 1997; 41:925–931.

308. Yokota K, Hayashi S, Fujii N, Yoshikawa K, Kotake S, Isogai E, Ohno S, Araki Y, Oguma K. Antibody response to oral streptococci in Behçet's disease. Microbiol Immunol 1992; 36:815–822.

309. Hirohata S, Oka H, Mizushima Y. Streptococcal-related antigens stimulate production of IL-6 and interferon-gamma by T cells from patients with Behçet's disease. Cell Immunol 1992; 140:410–419.

310. Yoshikawa K, Kotake S, Kubota T, Kimura K, Isogai E, Fujii N. Cloning and sequencing of the BES-1 gene encoding the immunogenic antigen of Streptococcus sanguis KTH-1 isolated from patients with Behçet's disease. Zentralbl Bakteriol 1998; 287:449–460.

311. Lehner T. The role of heat shock protein, microbial and autoimmune agents in the aetiology of Behçet's disease. Int Rev Immunol 1997; 14:21–32.

312. Stanford MR, Kasp E, Whiston R, Hasan A, Todryk S, Shinnick T, Mizushima Y, Dumonde DC, van der Zee R, Lehner T. Heat shock protein peptides reactive in patients with Behçet's disease are uveitogenic in Lewis rats. Clin Exp Immunol 1994; 97:226–231.

313. Direskeneli H, Hasan A, Shinnick T, Mizushima R, van der Zee R, Fortune F, Stanford MR, Lehner T. Recognition of B-cell epitopes of the 65 kDa HSP in Behçet's disease. Scand J Immunol 1996; 43:464–471.

314. Hasan A, Fortune F, Wilson A, Warr K, Shinnick T, Mizushima Y, van der Zee R, Stanford MR, Sanderson J, Lehner T. Role of gamma

delta T cells in pathogenesis and diagnosis of Behçet's disease. Lancet 1996; 347:789–794.

315. Liu P, Cleary PP, Herzberg MC. Complete sequence and analysis of hsp65 gene homologue of *Streptococcus sanguis*. 1999;submitted.

316. Mochizuki M, Morita E, Yamamoto S, Yamana S. Characteristics of T cell lines established from skin lesions of Behçet's disease. J Dermatol Sci 1997; 15:9–15.

317. Lehner T, Lavery E, Smith R, van der Zee R, Mizushima Y, Shinnick T. Association between the 65-kilodalton heat shock protein, *Streptococcus sanguis*, and the corresponding antibodies in Behçet's syndrome. Infect Immun 1991; 59:1434–1441.

318. Cunningham MW, Swerlick RA. Polyspecificity of anti streptococcal murine monoclonal antibodies and their implications in autoimmunity. J Exp Med. 1986; 164:998–1012.

319. Cunningham MW, McCormick JM, Fenderson PG, Ho MK, Beachey EH, Dale JB. Human and murine antibodies cross-reactive with streptococcal M protein recognize the sequence GLN-LYS-SER-LYS-GLN in M protein. J Immunol 1989; 143:2677–2683.

320. Quinn A, Ward K, Fischetti VA, Hemric M, Cunningham MW. Immunological relationship between the class I epitope of streptococcal M protein and myosin. Infect Immun 1998; 66:4418–4424.

321. Lehner T, Ma JK, Kelly CG. A mechanism of passive immunization with monoclonal antibodies to a 185,000 M(r) streptococcal antigen. Adv Exp Med Biol 1992; 327:151–163.

322. Taubman MA, Holmberg CJ, Smith DJ. Immunization of rats with synthetic peptide constructs from the glucan-binding or catalytic region of mutans streptococcal glucosyltransferase protects against dental caries. Infect Immun 1995; 63:3088–3093.

323. Smith DJ, Akita H, King WF, Taubman MA. Purification and antigenicity of a novel glucan-binding protein of *Streptococcus mutans*. Infect Immun 1994; 62:2545–2552.

324. Ma JK, Hiatt A, Hein M, Vine ND, Wang F, Stabila P, van Dolleweerd C, Mostov K, Lehner T. Generation and assembly of secretory antibodies in plants. Science 1995; 268:716–719.

325. Ma JK, Hikmat BY, Wycoff K, Vine ND, Chargelegue D, Yu L, Hein MB, Lehner T. Characterization of a recombinant plant monoclonal secretory antibody and preventive immunotherapy in humans. Nat Med 1998; 4:601–606.

326. Kelly CG, Todryk S, Kendal HL, Munro GH, Lehner T. T-cell, adhesion, and B-cell epitopes of the cell surface *Streptococcus mutans* protein antigen I/II. Infect Immun 1995; 63:3649–3658.

327. Todryk SM, Kelly CG, Munro GH, Lehner T. Induction of immune responses to functional

determinants of a cell surface streptococcal antigen. Immunology 1996; 87:55–63.

328. Russell MW, Moldoveanu Z, White PL, Sibert GJ, Mestecky J, Michalek SM. Salivary, nasal, genital, and systemic antibody responses in monkeys immunized intranasally with a bacterial protein antigen and the cholera toxin B subunit. Infect Immun 1996; 64:1272–1283.

329. Hajishengallis G, Michalek SM, Russell MW. Persistence of serum and salivary antibody responses after oral immunization with a bacterial protein antigen genetically linked to the A2/B subunits of cholera toxin. Infect Immun 1996; 64:665–667.

330. Harokopakis E, Hajishengallis G, Greenway TE, Russell MW, Michalek SM. Mucosal immunogenicity of a recombinant *Salmonella typhimurium*–cloned heterologous antigen in the absence or presence of coexpressed cholera toxin A2 and B subunits. Infect Immun 1997; 65:1445–1454.

331. Todryk SM, Kelly CG, Lehner T. Effect of route immunisation and adjuvant on T and B cell epitope recognition with a streptococcal antigen. Vaccine 1998; 16:174–180.

332. Hajishengallis G, Russell MW, Michalek SM. Comparison of an adherence domain and a structural region of *Streptococcus mutans* antigen I/II in protective immunity against dental caries in rats after intranasal immunization. Infect Immun 1998; 66:1740–1743.

333. Smith DJ, van Houte J, Kent R, Taubman MA. Effect of antibody in gingival crevicular fluid on early colonization of exposed root surfaces by mutans streptococci. Oral Microbiol Immunol 1994; 9:65–69.

334. Smith DJ, Taubman MA, King WF, Eida S, Powell JR, Eastcott J. Immunological characteristics of a synthetic peptide associated with a catalytic domain of mutans streptococcal glucosyltransferase. Infect Immun 1994; 62:5470–5476.

335. Smith DJ, Taubman MA. Experimental immunization of rats with a *Streptococcus mutans* 59-kilodalton glucan-binding protein protects against dental caries. Infect Immun 1996; 64:3069–3073.

336. Smith DJ, Shoushtari B, Heschel RL, King WF, Taubman MA. Immunogenicity and protective immunity induced by synthetic peptides associated with a catalytic subdomain of mutans group streptococcal glucosyltransferase. Infect Immun 1997; 65:4424–4430.

337. Bowen WH. Vaccine against dental caries—a personal view. J Dent Res 1996; 75:1530–1533.

338. Russell MW, Bergmeier LA, Zanders ED, Lehner T. Protein antigens of *Streptococcus mutans*: purification and properties of a double antigen and its protease-resistant component. Infect Immun 1980; 28:486–493.

339. Koga T, Okahashi N, Takahashi I, Kanamoto T,

Asakawa H, Iwaki M. Surface hydrophobicity, adherence, and aggregation of cell surface protein antigen mutants of *Streptococcus mutans* serotype c. Infect Immun 1990; 58:289–296.

340. Russell RRB. Wall-associated protein antigens of *Streptococcus mutans*. J Gen Microbiol 1979; 114:109–114.

341. Lehner T, Russell MW, Caldwell J, Smith R. Immunization with purified protein antigens from *Streptococcus mutans* against dental caries in rhesus monkeys. Infect Immun 1981; 34:407–415.

342. Forester H, Hunter N, Knox KW. Characteristics of a high molecular weight extracellular protein of *Streptococcus mutans*. J Gen Microbiol 1983; 129:2779–2788.

343. Kelly C, Evans P, Bergmeier L, Lee SF, Progulske-Fox A, Harris AC, Aitken A, Bleiweis AS, Lehner T. Sequence analysis of the cloned streptococcal cell surface antigen I/II. FEBS Lett 1989; 258:127–132.

344. Ackermans F, Klein JP, Ogier J, Bazin H, Cormont F, Frank RM. Purification and characterization of a saliva-interacting cell wall protein from *Streptococcus mutans* serotype f by using monoclonal antibody immunoaffinity chromatography. Biochem J 1985; 228:211–217.

345. Ogier JA, Schöller M, Lepoivre Y, Pini A, Sommer P, Klein J-P. Complete nucleotide sequence of the *sr* gene from *Streptococcus mutans* OMZ175. FEMS Microbiol Lett 1990; 68:223–228.

346. Okahashi N, Sasakawa C, Yoshikawa M, Hamada S, Koga T. Cloning of a surface protein antigen gene from serotype c *Streptococcus mutans*. Mol Microbiol 1989; 3:221–228.

347. Hughes M, MacHardy SM, Sheppard AJ, Woods NC. Evidence for an immunological relationship between *Streptococcus mutans* and human cardiac tissue. Infect Immun 1980; 27:576–588.

348. Holt LG, Abiko Y, Saito S, Smorawinska M, Hansen JB, Curtiss R. *Streptococcus mutans* genes that code for extracellular proteins in *Escherichia coli* K-12. Infect Immun 1982; 38:127–156.

349. Takahashi I, Okahashi N, Sasakawa D, Yoshikawa M, Hamada S, Koga T. Homology between surface protein antigen genes of *Streptococcus sobrinus* and *Streptococcus mutans*. FEBS Lett 1989; 249:383–388.

350. Okahashi N, Koga T, Hamada S. Purification and immunochemical properties of a protein antigen from serotype c *Streptococcus mutans*. Microbiol Immunol 1986; 30:35–47.

351. Demuth DR, Davis CA, Corner AM, Lamont RJ, Laboy PS, Malamud D. Cloning and expression of a *Streptococcus sanguis* surface antigen that interacts with a human salivary agglutinin. Infect Immun 1988; 56:2484–2490.

352. Brady LJ, Piacentini, Crowley PJ, Bleiweis AS.

Identification of monoclonal antibody binding domains within antigen P1 of *Streptococcus mutans* and cross-reactivity with related surface antigens of oral streptococci. Infect Immun 1991; 59:4425–4435.

353. Jenkinson HF. Adherence, coaggregation, and hydrophobicity of *Streptococcus gordonii* associated with expression of cell surface proteins. Infect Immun 1992; 60:1225–1228.

354. Fives-Taylor PM, Macrina FL, Pritchard TJ, Peene SS. Expression of *Streptococcus sanguis* antigens in *Escherichia coli*: cloning of a structural gene for adhesion fimbriae. Infect Immun 1987; 55:123–128.

355. Fenno JC, LeBlanc DL, Fives-Taylor P. Nucleotide sequence analysis of a type 1 fimbrial gene of *Streptococcus sanguis* FW213. Infect Immun 1989; 57:3527–3533.

356. Sampson JS, O'Connor, Stinson AR, Tharpe JA, Russell H. Cloning and nucleotide sequence analysis of *psaA*, the *Streptococcus pneumoniae* gene encoding a 37-kilodalton protein homologous to previously reported *Streptococcus* sp. adhesins. Infect Immun 1994; 62:319–324.

357. Morris EJ, Ganeshkumar N, Song M, McBride BC. Identification and preliminary characterization of a *Streptococcus sanguis* fibrillar glycoprotein. J Bacteriol 1987; 169:164–171.

358. Liljemark WF, Bloomquist CG. Isolation of a protein-containing cell surface component from *Streptococcus sanguis* which affects its adherence to saliva-coated hydroxyapatite. Infect Immun 1981; 34:428–434.

359. Wu H, Mintz KP, Ladha M, Fives-Taylor PM, Isolation and characterization of a Fap1, a fimbriae-associated adhesin of *Streptococcus parasanguis* FW213. Mol Microbiol 1998; 28:487–500.

360. Lamont RJ, Rosan B, Baker CT, Nelson GM. Characterization of an adhesin antigen of *Streptococcus sanguis* G9B. Infect Immun 1988; 56:2417–2423.

361. Lamont RJ, Rosan B, Murphy GM, Baker CT. *Streptococcus sanguis* surface antigens and their interactions with saliva. Infect Immun 1988; 56:64–70.

362. Rosan B, Baker CT, Nelson GM, Berman R, Lamont RJ, Demuth DR. Cloning and expression of an adhesin antigen of *Streptococcus sanguis* G9B in *Escherichia coli*. J Gen Microbiol 1989; 135:531–538.

363. Rogers JD, Haase EM, Brown AE, Douglas CW, Gwynn JP, Scannapieco FA. Identification and analysis of a gene (*abpA*) encoding a major amylase-binding protein in *Streptococcus gordonii*. Microbiology 1998; 144:1223–1233.

364. Frithz E, Heden LO, Lindahl G. Extensive sequence homology between IgA receptor and M proteins in *Streptococcus pyogenes*. Mol Microbiol 1989; 3:1111–1119.

365. Tokuda M, Okahashi N, Takahashi I, Nakai M,

Nagaska S, Kawagoe M, Koga T. Complete nucleotide sequence of the gene for a surface protein antigen of *Streptococcus sobrinus*. Infect Immun 1991; 59:3309–3312.

366. Kronvall G. A surface component in group A, C, and G streptococci with non-immune reactivity for immunoglobulin G. J Immunol 1973; 111:1401–1406.

367. Bjorck L, Krnovall G. Purification and some properties of a streptococcal protein G, a novel IgG binding reagent. J Immunol 1984; 133:969–974.

368. Murray PA, Levine MJ, Tabak LA, Reddy MS. Specificity of salivary-bacterial interactions. II. Evidence for a lactin on *Streptococcus sanguis* with a specificity for a NeuAc(α)2,3Gal(β)1,3GalNAc sequence. Biochem Biophys Res Commun 1982; 106:390–396.

Protection Against Group A Streptococcal Infection

VINCENT A. FISCHETTI

Group A streptococci (*Streptococcus pyogenes*) are human pathogens responsible for a wide range of diseases, the most common of which are nasopharyngeal infections and impetigo. More than 25 million cases of group A streptococcal infections occur each year in the United States at a cost of over $1 billion to public, in addition to losses in productivity at work and school. In recent years, an increase in streptococcal toxic shock and invasive infections (particularly necrotizing fasciitis) has been reported with certain strains of group A streptococci, resulting in rapid fatalities in up to 30% of patients [1–3]. Initially, most of the reported invasive disease was caused by serotypes 1 and 3 [4]; however, more recently, other serotypes have been isolated from such cases, notably serotypes 5, 6, and 28R [5]. Since there have been no reports of penicillin resistance in group A streptococci, streptococcal-related diseases can be successfully treated with this antibiotic, although resistance to erythromycin, the second drug of choice for these bacteria, is beginning to be observed [6]. Prior to treatment, group A streptococcal infections are usually associated with fever, significant discomfort, and generalized lethargy. If left untreated, about 3% of individuals with streptococcal pharyngitis develop rheumatic fever and rheumatic heart disease. Whereas outbreaks of rheumatic fever in the United States are usually sporadic and infre-

quent, affecting only local areas of the country [7], in developing countries as many as 1% of school-age children are estimated to have rheumatic heart disease [8]. Because of this and the concern that penicillin-resistant strains may appear, there is a strong impetus to develop a safe and effective vaccine against group A streptococcal pharyngitis.

It has been known for decades that rheumatic fever patients have serum immunoglobulin G (IgG) to human smooth muscle tissue at levels 3–4 times that found in normal serum. While these antibodies have been found also to react with streptococcal cell-wall [9,10], membrane [11–13], and M protein N-terminal determinants [14–16], their role, if any, in the pathogenesis of rheumatic fever has not yet been proven. The fact that rheumatic fever and further cardiac damage occurs around the time of the streptococcal infection, and not between infections when cross-reactive antibodies are still elevated [12], argues against the direct involvement of these antibodies in the disease process. Despite this, and until proven otherwise, it is important to minimize the induction of cross-reactive antibodies in streptococcal vaccine preparations.

Though more prevalent during winter months, at any given time up to 30% of asymptomatic humans carry group A streptococci in their pharynx. Except under unusual circumstances [17] and for one serotype [18], there is no animal reservoir for these organisms. Thus, the eradication of, or significant reduction in, the carriage of group A streptococci in the human pharynx would have a profound effect on dissemination of this organism in the population and on the initiation of streptococcal disease [19,20]. Even in the case of highly invasive strains of streptococci, there is no evidence that they have their origins in sources other than the pharynx.

It is clear from studies carried out over 50 years ago by Lancefield [21] that the M protein is a prime candidate for a vaccine to protect against streptococcal infection. Since that time, however, we have learned that protection incurred by serum IgG to the M molecule is type specific and antibodies directed to limited portions of the type-specific region may induce protection against only a limited number of strains within an M type. More recent studies have revealed that broad protection against streptococcal infection may be achieved by the induction of a local secretory response to exposed conserved sequences found within the M molecule. This approach prevents streptococcal colonization of the upper respiratory mucosa in a mouse model. This chapter will concentrate on the progress to date toward the development of a vaccine to protect against streptococcal nasopharyngeal infection.

M PROTEIN STRUCTURE AND FUNCTION

Protective immunity from group A streptococcal infection is achieved through antibodies directed against the M protein [22,23], a major virulence factor present on the surface of all clinical isolates. M protein is a coiled-coil fibrillar protein composed of three major segments of tandem repeat sequences that extend nearly sixty nm from the surface of the streptococcal cell wall (Fig. 19.1; [22]). The A- and B-repeats located within the N-terminal half are antigenically variable among the more than 100 known streptococcal types with the N-terminal nonrepetitive region and A-repeats exhibiting hypervariability. The more C-terminal C-repeats, the majority of which are surface exposed, contain epitopes that are highly conserved among

the identified M proteins [24]. Because of its antigenically variable N-terminal region, the M protein provides the basis for the Lancefield serological typing scheme for group A streptococci [22].

The M protein is considered the major virulence determinant because of its ability to pre-

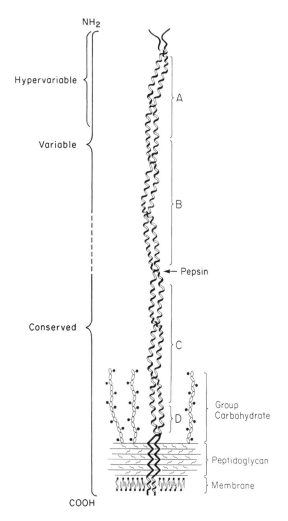

Figure 19.1 Proposed model of the M protein from M6 strain D471 [49,50]. The coiled-coil rod region extends about 60 nm from cell wall with a short nonhelical domain at the NH$_2$-terminus. The proline\ glycine-rich region of the molecule is found within the peptidoglycan [83]. The membrane anchor segment extends through the cell membrane with the charged tail extending into the cytoplasm. Data suggest that the membrane anchor may be cleaved shortly after synthesis [83]. The A-, B-, and C-repeat regions are indicated along with those segments containing conserved, variable, and hypervariable epitopes among heterologous M serotypes.

vent phagocytosis when present on the streptococcal surface; by this definition all clinical isolates express M protein. This function may be attributed in part to the specific binding of complement factor H to both the conserved C-repeat domain [25] and the fibrinogen bound to the B-repeats [26], preventing the deposition of C3b on the streptococcal surface. When the streptococcus contacts serum, the factor H bound to the M molecule inhibits or reverses the formation of C3b,Bb complexes and helps to convert C3b to its inactive form (iC3b) on the bacterial surface, preventing C3b-dependant phagocytosis. Studies have shown that antibodies directed to the B- and C-repeat regions of the M protein are unable to promote phagocytosis [27]. This may be the result of the ability of factor H to also control the binding of C3b to the Fc receptors on these antibodies, resulting in inefficient phagocytosis [28]. Antibodies directed to the hypervariable N-terminal region are opsonic, perhaps because they cannot be controlled by the factor H bound to the B- and C-repeat regions. Thus it appears that the streptococcus has devised a method to protect its conserved region from being used against itself by binding factor H to regulate the potentially opsonic antibodies that bind to these regions.

TYPE-SPECIFIC PROTECTION

The M protein has been a prime vaccine candidate to prevent group A streptococcal infections since Lancefield showed clearly that M protein–specific human and animal antibodies have the capacity to opsonize streptococci in preparation for phagocytic clearance [29]. In general, serum IgG directed to the hypervariable NH$_2$-terminal portion of M protein leads to complement fixation and opsonophagocytosis of only the homologous streptococcal serotype by polymorphonuclear leukocytes [21,27]. Even antibodies directed to whole group A streptococci will only allow phagocytosis of strains of the same M type in a phagocytic assay, suggesting that, besides the M protein, no other streptococcal antigen is able to induce antibodies to override the antiphagocytic property of the M protein. Fox's 1974 [30] reviewed of early attempts at M protein vaccine development indicates that un-

til the mid-1970s, few human trials had been realized. This is partially based on problems with hypersensitivity reactions found with the acid-extracted M protein preparations of the time [30] and the fact that only type-specific protection was observed. In addition, repeated attempts to separate heterologous protein contaminants from type-specific determinants proved unsuccessful. Except for one investigation [31], all streptococcal vaccine development since the early 1970s was based on animal studies in which analyses of the immune response to M protein preparations were performed with and without adjuvants [32–38] and in combination with other antigens [35].

In 1979 Beachey et al. [31] used pepsin-extracted M24 protein (pep M24, the N-terminal half of the native M24 molecule; see Fig. 19.1) to immunize human volunteers. Unlike earlier acid-extracted products, this highly purified fragment was found to be free of non–type-specific reactivity [30] and did not induce delayed-type hypersensitivity tests in the skin of the 37 adult volunteers. Immunization with alum-precipitated pep M24 protein led to the development of type-specific opsonic antibodies in 10 of 12 volunteers, none of whom developed heart-reactive antibodies as determined by immunofluorescence. These studies clearly indicated that M protein vaccines free of sensitizing antigens could be produced, but further emphasized the type specificity of the immune response.

Using these studies as a starting point, Beachey and co-workers began to develop a type specific–based vaccine strategy to protect against streptococcal disease. It was soon learned that the complete PepM24 fragment was not necessary, but peptides representing the first 20 or so N-terminal amino acids of the M24 protein also evoked type-specific opsonic antibodies to M24 streptococci [39]. Experiments with synthetic peptides of the N-terminus of M1, M5, M6, and M19 proteins resulted in the same conclusions [40–45]. When a hybrid peptide was chemically synthesized, representing the N-terminal sequence of both the M24 and M5 proteins, and injected into animals with complete Freund's adjuvant, opsonic antibodies to both M5 and M24 streptococci were produced [42]. Opsonic antibodies to three M proteins were obtained when the N-terminal sequences of three M protein sequences (M5–M6–M24) were synthesized in tandem and injected into rabbits [46]. In a recent study, Dale et al. [47] used recombinant technology to prepare a tandem array of the N-terminal sequence of four serotypes (M24–M5–M6–M19). When the recombinant tetravalent fusion protein was purified and used to immunize rabbits, antibodies were raised against all four M proteins with substantial variation in both the ELISA titer and opsonic activity to the four respective streptococcal types. These studies were subsequently repeated using an octavalent construct [48]; however, in these studies, opsonic antibodies were produced against six of the eight serotypes used in the vaccine construct. As in the other studies using N-terminal sequences as a vaccine, none of the rabbits developed tissue cross-reactive antibodies as measured by immunofluorescence of cardiac tissue. These studies confirm and extend the earlier experiments of Beachey and colleagues and show that such an approach may be useful for the prevention of infection by specific streptococcal serotypes.

An important factor to consider in the development of a type-specific, epitope-based vaccine is the potential of the streptococcus to generate new M serotypes by changing the amino-terminal portion of the M protein. For example, in the type 6 M protein of strain D471, type-specific opsonizing antibodies are directed against epitopes located both at the amino-terminal end (residues 1 through 21) and within the A-repeat block [27], which begins at amino acid 27 and continues to residue 96 in the 441 amino acid M6 molecule [49,50]. High-frequency, intragenic recombinational events within the A-repeat block [51] can lead to a significant loss in the opsonizing ability of monospecific antibodies directed to this region [45]. For instance, an opsonic antibody generated to the D471 parental strain showed some or no opsonizing activity to size-variant derivatives of this strain or other M6 streptococci isolated from patients (Table 19.1). In addition, Cleary et al. [52] showed that sequence variation also occurs within the non-repeating N-terminal end of the M protein sequence from strains of the same serotype and that these changes ultimately affect the binding of opsonic antibodies. More recently, Penney et

Table 19.1 Opsonization and Phagocytosis of Size-Variant M6 Strains

M6 Strains	Inoculum	CFU after 3 h Rotation with	
		No antibody	MAb3B8
D471[a]	35	2091	3
d113[b]	49	1982	30
d112	33	1628	1422
D894[c]	27	2224	941
MO-1015	38	2166	1154
MO-1018	43	2156	1270

[a]Strain D471 is the parental strain from which the opsonic MAb3B8 was prepared.

[b]d113 and d112 are M protein–size mutants that were derived from strain D471 [51].

[c]D894, MO-1015, and MO-1018 are M6 strains in the Rockefeller collection that have M proteins differing in size from D471.

al. [53] showed a significant degree of sequence variation within the N-terminal hypervariable region of several strains identified serologically as M1. These findings strongly indicate that opsonic antibodies induced by M protein N-terminal sequences from a given vaccine strain may prove to be ineffective against other strains of the same serotype. Therefore, a type-specific vaccine necessary to protect against a streptococcal infection would require a multivalent antigen corresponding to stable immunodeterminants on serotypes that together account for most of the nasopharyngeal isolates prevalent within the population at a given time. This region has not yet been identified.

MUCOSAL VACCINE FOR NON-TYPE-SPECIFIC PROTECTION

At its peak incidence, 50% of children between the ages of 5 and 7 years suffer from streptococcal infection each year (Fig. 19.2). Furthermore, the siblings of a child with a streptococcal pharyngitis are 5 times more likely to acquire the organism than one of the parents. This decreased occurrence of streptococcal pharyngitis in adults might be explained by a nonspecific, age-related host factor resulting in a decreased susceptibility to streptococci. Alternatively, protective antibodies directed to antigens common to a large number of group A streptococcal serotypes might arise as a consequence of mul-

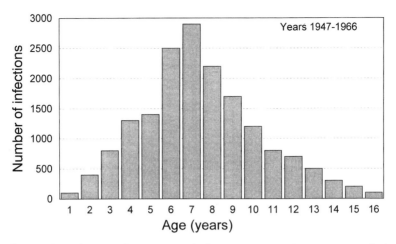

Figure 19.2 The number of cases of streptococcal pharyngitis in Rochester New York during the years 1947–1966. Because there are more children in day care now than in 1947–1966, the curve would likely be shifted to the left with a peak at ages 5–7 years. (Adapted from Breese and Hall [112], with permission.)

tiple infections or exposures experienced during childhood resulting in an elevated response to conserved M protein epitopes. This latter hypothesis is partly supported by our earlier studies on the immune response to the M protein where it was found that the B-repeat domain (see Fig. 19.1) was clearly immunodominant [36]. When rabbits were immunized with the whole M protein molecule, the first detectable antibodies were directed against the B-repeat region, which rose steadily with time. It was only after repeated M protein immunization that antibodies were produced against the hypervariable A- and conserved C-repeat regions.

Unlike antibodies to the N-terminal region, it became clear that antibodies directed to the exposed C-repeat region were not opsonic [54]. Because of this, experiments were performed to explore whether mucosal antibodies to this conserved region of M protein could play a role in protection from infection. Taking advantage of the pepsin site in the center of the M molecule (separating the variable and conserved regions; Fig. 19.1), the recombinant M6 protein was cleaved and the N- and C-terminal fragments were separated by SDS-PAGE and Western blotted. When the blots were reacted with different adult human sera, all adults tested had antibodies to the C-terminal conserved region, whereas, as expected, only sera that were opsonic for the M6 organisms reacted with the N-terminal variable region (Fig. 19.3; [38,55,56]). Simi-

lar studies performed with M protein isolated from five different common serotypes (M3, M5, M6, M24, M29) show that sera from 10 of 17 adults tested did not have N-terminal-specific

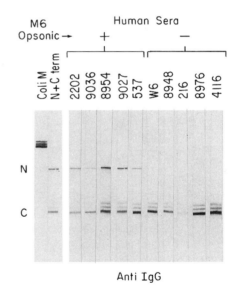

Figure 19.3 Western blot of a pepsin digest of recombinant M6 protein (ColiM) reacted with human serum. After digestion of the M protein with pepsin, the N- and C-terminal fragments (N + C term) were separated by Western blot and cut into strips, and each strip was reacted with different human sera diluted 1:500. Sera from individuals that had opsonic or did not have opsonic antibodies to the M6 streptococci were tested. Control strips (left) were reacted with monoclonal antibodies to the N- and C-terminal fragments.

antibodies to these M types (Table 19.2), while only two sera reacted with two serotypes and the remaining five sera reacted with only one serotype. However, all sera tested reacted to the C-terminal fragment of the M molecule. Similar results were seen when salivary IgA from adults and children were tested in ELISA against the N- and C-terminal halves of the M6 molecule (V.A. Fischetti, unpublished data). This provides further evidence that the relative resistance of adults to streptococcal pharyngitis is clearly not due to the presence of type-specific antibodies to multiple types but may be due to the presence of antibodies to conserved determinants.

From these findings we reasoned that an immune response to the conserved region of the M molecule might afford protection by inducing a mucosal response to prevent streptococcal colonization and ultimate infection. In view of the evidence that the conserved C-repeat epitopes of the M molecule are immunologically ex-

posed on the streptococcal surface [24], it should be possible to generate mucosal antibodies that are reactive to most streptococcal types using only a few distinct conserved-region antigens for immunization.

PASSIVE PROTECTION

Secretory IgA (sIgA) is able to protect mucosal surfaces from infection by pathogenic microorganisms [57] despite the fact that its effector functions differ from those of serum-derived immunoglobulins [58]. When streptococci are administered intranasally to mice, they are able to cause death by first colonizing and then invading the mucosal barrier resulting in dissemination of the organism to systemic sites. Using this model we first examined whether sIgA, delivered directly to the mucosa, plays a role in protecting against streptococcal infection. Live

Table 19.2 Reactivity of Human Sera to Type-Specific and Conserved Regions of the M Protein Molecule by Western Blot

	Reactivity to[a]						
		N-Terminal Half (Type-Specific) M Types					C-Terminal Half (Conserved)
Human Sera	None	29	24	6	5	3	All Types Tested
M6 opsonic							
8954				+[b]			+
9043				+			+
226			+	+			+
537				+			+
M6 not opsonic							
108	+						+
213	+						+
130						+	+
1331	+						+
8976	+						+
1337	+						+
8980	+						+
9016	+						+
8990	+						+
8939	+						+
8940	+						+
9035			+				+
1395			±[c]	±			+

[a]M protein was extracted from streptococci with pepsin at pH 5.8 [116] (N-terminal) and the bacteria washed and the remaining C-terminal half extracted with phage lysin [117]. The extracts were run on Western blots and reacted with the various human sera diluted 1:500. Controls include type-specific antibody to identify the N-terminal half and monoclonal antibody 10B6 [24] to locate the C-terminal fragment for each serotype (not shown).

[b]Positive reaction after 30 min incubation with substrate.

[c]Trace reaction after 30 min incubation with substrate.

streptococci were mixed with affinity-purified M protein–specific sIgA or IgG antibodies and administered intranasally to the animals [37]. The results clearly showed that the anti–M protein sIgA protected the mice against streptococcal infection and death, whereas the opsonic serum IgG administered in the same way had no effect, indicating that sIgA can protect at the mucosa, and may preclude the need for opsonic IgG in preventing streptococcal infection. These studies were also among the first to compare purified, antigen-specific sIgA and serum IgG for passive protection at a mucosal site.

In another laboratory, passive protection against streptococcal pharyngeal colonization was also shown by oral administration of purified lipoteichoic acid (LTA) but not deacylated LTA prior to oral challenge in mice [59]. The addition of anti-LTA by the same route also protected mice from oral streptococcal challenge. While several in vitro studies have shown the importance of M protein [60–62] and LTA [63] in streptococcal adherence, these in vivo studies together with those presented above suggest that both M protein and LTA may play a key role in the colonization of the mouse pharyngeal mucosa. However, it is uncertain whether this is also true in humans.

ACTIVE IMMUNIZATION WITH CONSERVED REGION PEPTIDES

To determine whether a local mucosal response directed to the conserved exposed epitopes of M protein can influence the course of mucosal colonization by group A streptococci, peptides corresponding to these regions were used as immunogens in a mouse model [38,56]. Overlapping synthetic peptides of the conserved region of the M6 protein were covalently linked to the mucosal adjuvant cholera toxin B (CTB) subunit and administered intranasally to the mice in three weekly doses. Thirty days later, animals were challenged intranasally with live streptococci (either homologous M6 or heterologous M14) and pharyngeal colonization by the challenge organism was monitored for 10–15 days. Mice immunized with the peptide–CTB complex showed a significant reduction in colonization with either the M6 or M14 streptococci

compared to mice receiving CTB alone (Fig. 19.4; [38,56]). Thus, despite the fact that conserved region peptides were unable to evoke an opsonic antibody response [27], these peptides have the capacity to induce a local immune response capable of influencing the colonization of group A streptococci at the nasopharyngeal mucosa in this model system. These findings were the first to demonstrate protection against a heterologous serotype of group A streptococci with a vaccine consisting of the widely shared C-repeat region of the M6 protein. These findings were confirmed independently through use of different streptococcal serotypes as the immunizing and challenge strains [64]. In another study, Pruksakorn et al. [65], used different criteria for streptococcal opsonization than those previously published [66], and found that when a peptide derived from the conserved region of the M protein was injected in mice, it induced antibodies capable of opsonizing type 5 streptococci and streptococci isolated from Aboriginal and Thai rheumatic fever patients. These findings are in sharp contrast with those of Jones and Fischetti [27], who showed that antibodies to the conserved region of M protein are not opsonic. However, since the peptide reported by Pruksakorn et al. [65] is similar to one of the peptides used by Bessen and Fischetti [38,56] in their mucosal protection studies (see above), the induction of serum IgG during mucosal immu-

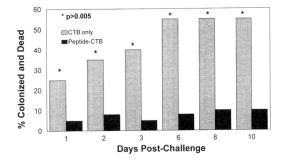

Figure 19.4 The extent of colonization of mice challenged with group A streptococci after oral immunization with M protein conserved region M6 peptides linked to cholera toxin B (CTB). Orally immunized mice were swabbed each day after challenge with M14 streptococci and plated on blood plates to determine the extent of colonization compared to that of mice vaccinated with CTB only. Plates showing group A streptococci were scored as positive.

nization may offer added protection against streptococcal infection.

Vaccinia Virus as a Vector

To further verify the validity of using the M protein–conserved region as a streptococcal vaccine, experiments were repeated in a vaccinia virus vector system. In these studies, the gene coding for the complete conserved region of the M6 molecule (from the pepsin site to the C-terminus) was cloned and expressed in vaccinia virus, producing the recombinant VV::M6 virus [67,68]. Tissue culture cells infected with this virus were found to produce the conserved region of the M6 molecule. Animals immunized intranasally with only a single dose of recombinant virus were significantly protected from heterologous streptococcal challenge compared to animals immunized with wild-type virus (Fig. 19.5). When the extent of colonization was examined in those animals immunized with wild-type or the VV::M6 recombinant, the VV::M6–immunized animals showed a marked reduction in overall colonization (Fig. 19.6), indicating that mucosal immunization reduced the bacterial load on the mucosa in these animals. Animals immunized intradermally with the VV::M6 virus and challenged intranasally showed no protection.

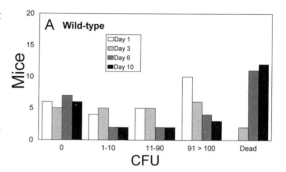

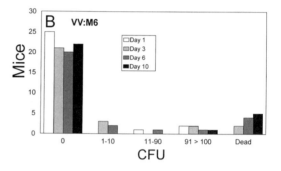

Figure 19.6 The number of colony-forming units (CFU) of M14 streptococci isolated from mice vaccinated with wild-type (*A*) or recombinant (*B*) vaccinia virus after challenge with M14 streptococci. Mice were vaccinated and swabbed as described in Figure 19.5 and the number of CFU found on the blood plates were counted. The number of mice that died after challenge are also indicated.

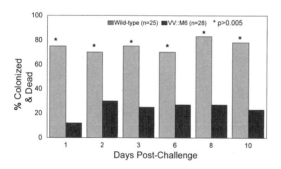

Figure 19.5 The extent of colonization of mice challenged with group A streptococci after oral immunization with recombinant vaccinia virus containing the gene for the whole conserved region of the M6 protein. Orally immunized mice were swabbed each day after challenge with M14 streptococci and plated on blood plates to determine the extent of colonization compared to that of mice vaccinated with wild-type vaccinia only. Plates showing group A streptococci were scored as positive.

The approaches described above prove that induction of a local immune response is critical for protection against streptococcal colonization and that the protection is not dependant upon an opsonic response. However, in the event that the streptococcus is successful in penetrating the mucosa and establishing an infection, only then would type-specific antibodies be necessary to eradicate the organism. This idea may explain why adults sporadically develop a streptococcal pharyngitis. The success of these strategies not only forms the basis of a broadly protective vaccine for the prevention of streptococcal pharyngitis but may offer insight into the development of other vaccines. For instance, a vaccine candidate previously shown to be ineffective by the parenteral route may prove to be successful by simply changing the site of immunization. Furthermore, these results emphasize the fact that in some cases, antigens need to be presented to the immune system in a specific fashion to ultimately induce a protective response.

GRAM-POSITIVE COMMENSALS AS VACCINE VECTORS: A MODEL SYSTEM

Although the CTB-linked peptide and vaccinia systems are successful for protection against streptococcal infection, they are not ideal. The CTB system requires large quantities of purified peptide and a linkage protocol that allows no more that two peptides per CTB molecule to enable the proper binding of CTB to GM_1 ganglioside [38]. Though possible to achieve, these requirements make this type of vaccine relatively expensive to produce, even if recombinant technology is used to prepare the fusion molecules [69]. Given the fact that such a vaccine would ultimately be administered in developing countries, the cost would likely be prohibitive. The vaccinia virus vector, on the other hand, is inexpensive but unlikely to gain U.S. Food and Drug Administration (FDA) approval, since oral/intranasal administration is required for effectiveness. Because of these limitations, we set out to develop a mucosal vaccine delivery system that was safe, effective, and inexpensive.

While several nonliving systems of delivering antigen to mucosal sites have been developed [56,70–72], live vectors may afford a better and more natural response without the need to reimmunize to gain higher response titers. In most instances, live antigen delivery vectors are derived from bacteria (usually gram-negative) [73,74] or viruses [75–78] that are normally considered mammalian pathogens, perhaps because our better understanding of these organisms has made genetic manipulations easier. Usually these organisms have been extensively engineered to reduce their pathogenicity yet maintain certain invasive qualities (e.g., to invade the M cells of the gut mucosa) to induce a mucosal immune response [73,76]. To circumvent some of the safety and environmental issues inherent in the wide-scale dissemination of engineered pathogens, we developed nonpathogenic gram-positive bacteria as vaccine vectors [79]. In this system, foreign antigens are displayed on the surface of gram-positive human commensal organisms that colonize the niche invaded by the pathogen (oral, intestinal, and vaginal). Colonization generates both an enhanced local IgA response to the foreign antigen and systemic IgG and T cell responses. Unlike many other live bacterial systems, where the foreign antigen is either retained in the cytoplasm, translocated to the periplasm, or in some cases secreted, the gram-positive vector anchors the foreign antigen to the cell for surface display [79]. Since the cell wall peptidoglycan of the gram-positive cell is a natural adjuvant, an enhanced response is obtained when the engineered organisms are processed by the host for antibody induction.

Our ability to accomplish this is based on the discovery that surface molecules from gram-positive bacteria that anchor via their C-termini (of which more than 70 have now been sequenced) have a highly conserved C-terminal region that is responsible for cell attachment [80–82]. Up to six charged amino acids are located at the C-terminus adjacent to a segment of 15–20 predominantly hydrophobic amino acids sufficient to span the cytoplasmic membrane of the cell. This amino acid arrangement likely functions as a stop sequence for these molecules [83].

Immediately N-terminal to the hydrophobic domain is a hexapeptide with the consensus sequence LPXTGX that is nearly 100% conserved among the more than 70 surface proteins of this class (Fig. 19.7; [80]). Limited substitutions are seen predominantly in positions 3 and 6 of the hexapeptide, whereas positions 1 and 2 are 100% conserved, and amino acids 4 and 5 exhibit few substitutions (Fig. 19.7). This conservation also extends to the DNA level [80], further emphasizing the importance of this region within these molecules. Exceptions to this rule include surface molecules on gram-positive bacteria that are anchored through an N-terminal acylation (for review see ref. [84]) and a few that bind to the cell surface through ionic interactions [85]. The maintenance of the conserved LPXTGX hexapeptide throughout various gram-positive species, together with the high homology seen within the hydrophobic and charged regions, indicates that the mechanism of anchoring these molecules within the bacterial cell is highly conserved.

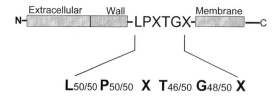

Figure 19.7 C-terminal anchor motif found in surface proteins from gram-positive bacteria. The LPXTGX anchor motif was examined from 50 surface proteins. The number of occurrences of each amino acid in the motif was scored.

Wide Range in Surface Protein Structure

Sequence and conformational analysis of many of the naturally occurring surface proteins from gram-positive bacteria reveal that their surface-exposed domains are quite diverse in both size and conformation [82,86]. To date, except for the alpha-helical coiled-coil structure established for the streptococcal M6 protein [87], and crystal and NMR structure on small segments of protein A [88,89] and protein G [90–92], respectively, there is little physicochemical information on the other surface proteins [93]. However, current data are consistent with the idea that the anchoring process is capable of managing proteins with a wide assortment of molecular attributes.

Foreign Proteins Expressed on the Surface of Gram-Positive Bacteria

The importance of the C-terminal region in the attachment process was demonstrated using the protein A from *Staphylococcus aureus* as a model system [81,94]. Surface proteins in gram-positive bacteria (which could number more than 20 in a single organism) are synthesized and exported at the septum, where new cell wall is also being produced and translocated to the surface [22,95]. Thus, the C-terminal hydrophobic domain and charged tail function to control the export and anchoring process by acting as a temporary stop to position the LPXTGX motif precisely at the outer surface of the cytoplasmic membrane. This sequence motif, which is an enzymatic recognition sequence, is cleaved, resulting in attachment of the surface-exposed segment of the protein to a cellular substrate [81]. This is supported by studies indicating that the C-terminal hydrophobic domain and charged tail are missing from the streptococcal surface M protein extracted from the cell wall [81,83].

Since the anchor region is highly conserved among a wide variety of surface molecules within several different gram-positive species, could it be fused to a foreign antigen and used to deliver the resulting fusion protein to the surface of a gram-positive bacterium, ultimately anchoring it to the cell? To answer this, the streptococcal M protein was employed in a model system (Fig. 19.8).

Using this strategy, Pozzi et al. [79,96] delivered a fusion protein to the surface of the gram-positive human oral commensal *Streptococcus gordonii*. The approach utilized knowledge of the location of the surface-exposed and wall-associated regions of the fibrillar M protein [24,83]. Thus, by deleting the surface-exposed segment of the M molecule (Fig. 19.8) and replacing it in frame with the gene for a foreign protein (Fig. 19.9) (i.e., the E7 protein from human papillomavirus, consisting of 294 base pairs [79]), it was found that, when expressed in a new gram-positive host (i.e., *Streptococcus gordonii*), the fusion molecule was presented on the cell surface and tightly anchored. Using this same strategy, a variety of protein antigens ranging from a few hundred to over 700 amino acids have been successfully expressed on the surface of *Streptococcus gordonii* ([79,97–99]; V. Fischetti, unpublished data).

To be certain that expression of the recombinant molecule would be stable for many bacterial generations, the recipient *Streptococcus gordonii* was engineered such that the recombinant gene would be expressed from the chromosome controlled by an efficient resident promotor (Fig. 19.10; [79,96]). This strategy is one of a few in which the gene in question is chromosomally expressed. In contrast, most other reported live vaccine vector systems regulate genes from high-expression plasmids. Translocation of the recombinant molecule to the surface is assured by inclusion of the signal sequence and a short segment of the N-terminal region of the carrier M protein (see Figs. 19.9 and 19.10).

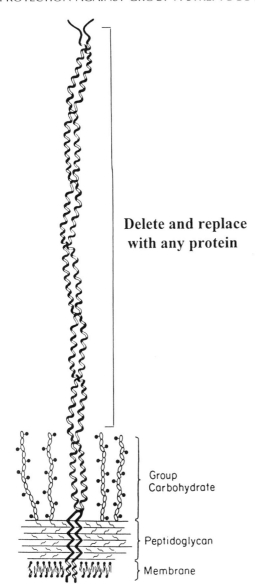

**Delete and replace
with any protein**

Figure 19.8 Schematic representation of the M protein molecule on the streptococcal surface. The segment of the M protein gene coding for the surface-exposed segment was removed and replaced with the gene for a variety of protein molecules [79,98,113].

IMMUNE RESPONSE TO SURFACE-EXPOSED FUSION PROTEINS

While the studies of Pozzi et al. [79] showed the feasibility of expressing a wide range of foreign proteins on the surface of gram-positive bacteria, an important question remained: would this

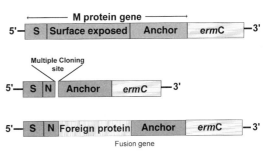

Figure 19.9 Construction of gene fusions with the M protein gene. The M protein gene fusions are constructed in *E. coli* adjacent to an *ermC* antibiotic marker. The sequence coding for the surface-exposed region of the M molecule is deleted and replaced with a multiple cloning site [98]. A heterologous gene (foreign protein) may then be inserted in frame within the M protein gene. The "anchor" region represents the region from the surface of the cell wall to the C-terminal end.

mode of delivery induce an immune response, particularly a mucosal response, in animals colonized by the recombinant organism? To answer this question and to further verify the ability to deliver a wide range of proteins to the bacterial

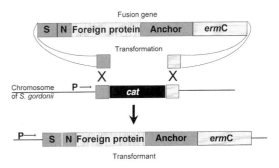

Figure 19.10 Chromosomal integration of the fusion protein gene in *Streptococcus gordonii*. The recombinant plasmid (Fig. 19.9) is used to transform recipient *Streptococcus gordonii* engineered such that a promoterless *cat* gene is flanked by two DNA fragments that are also present in the recombinant plasmid. This *cat* construct is located downstream from a strong chromosomal promoter (P). The recombinant plasmid is naturally linearized during transformation [114,115] and the recognition of the flanking homologous segments allow for the integration of the fusion gene together with the erythromycin resistance gene (*ermC*) into the chromosome of recipient *Streptococcus gordonii*. Recombinant *Streptococcus gordonii* are selected for erythromycin resistance (conferred by *ermC*) and the loss of chloramphenicol resistance (conferred by *cat*).

cell surface with this approach, Medaglini et al. elected to express a 204 amino acid protein allergen from the white-faced hornet (Ag5.2) [100] on the surface of *Streptococcus gordonii*, using essentially the same methods described above (see Figs. 19.9 and 19.10; [79,98]).

The fusion protein consisted of the 204 amino acids of Ag5.2 inserted between the N-terminal and anchor regions of the M6 protein, after deleting a 179 amino acid segment of the surface-exposed region of the M6 molecule. Immunofluorescence analysis of whole cells and Western blots of wall extracts confirmed the presence of the recombinant molecule on the bacterial cell surface. The immunogenicity of the M6::Ag5.2 fusion protein expressed on the surface of the recombinant *Streptococcus gordonii* strain DM100 was assessed in mice [98]. Animals were inoculated orally and intranasally with a single dose (about 10^9 colony-forming units [CFU]) of either live recombinant DM100 or wild-type *Streptococcus gordonii* strains. Both were capable of stably colonizing the oropharyngeal mucosa of mice for 10–12 weeks as detected by weekly oropharyngeal swabs. All recombinant organisms isolated from mice colonized during the 12 weeks still expressed Ag5.2 on the cell surface at levels comparable to those of the inoculated organisms. In mice colonized with recombinant DM100, Ag5.2-specific serum IgG was first observed 4 weeks after colonization and peaked at week 5, and titers were maintained for the duration of the experiment (12 weeks) (Fig. 19.11). Systemic

immunization with recombinant strain DM100 in complete Freund's adjuvant induced serum IgG titers comparable to those of oral immunization, but as expected, did not result in significant levels of secretory IgA (Figure 19.11). Ag5.2-specific salivary IgA was also produced in these animals during the course of the experiment, accounting for nearly 2.5% of the total IgA in the saliva (Fig. 19.12A). Colonized animals were sacrificed after 12 weeks, and Ag5.2-specific IgA and total IgA levels in lung and intestinal washes were determined in relation to total IgA in these fluids (Fig. 19.12B,C). Animals colonized with the recombinant DM100 exhibited significant increases of Ag5.2-specific IgA in lung washes compared to specific IgA found in intestinal washes, indicating a local induction of the response. Mice immunized with killed recombinant organisms expressing surface Ag5.2 showed no immune response to the antigen in any compartment tested, indicating that colonization was required for the observed responses. Furthermore, a direct correlation was found between the amount of IgA antibody produced and the length of time the animals were colonized.

Though still early in its development, the gram-positive commensal seems promising as a versatile live vector for vaccine delivery. Since the system induces not only a mucosal but a systemic immune response, it may be a more natural way of generating a protective response to a pathogen than systemic delivery alone. Although the animal studies indicate that this ap-

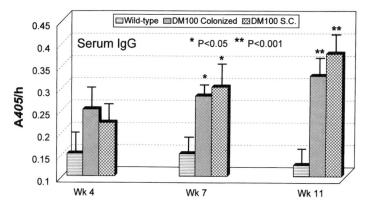

Figure 19.11 ELISA assay of Ag5.2-specific serum IgG from mice colonized with either wild-type or recombinant *Streptococcus gordonii* or immunized subcutaneously (S.C.) with DM100 in adjuvant at day 0.

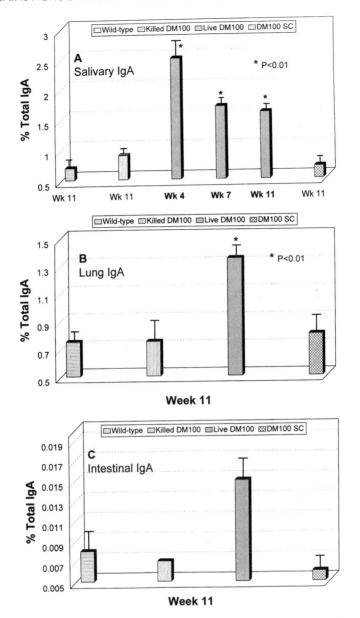

Figure 19.12 ELISA assay of Ag5.2-specific IgA from saliva (*A*), lung lavage (*B*), and intestinal lavage (*C*) from mice colonized with wild-type or recombinant (DM100) *Streptococcus gordonii* or immunized subcutaneously (S.C.) with DM100 in adjuvant at day 0. Saliva from DM100-colonized animals was taken at weeks 4, 7, and 11 while the lungs and intestines were sampled at week 11.

proach is feasible, human studies must be performed to determine if the same responses can be achieved. Early studies show that when reintroduced into the human oral cavity, *Streptococcus gordonii* is capable of persisting for over 2 years [101], therefore, it remains to be seen if the recombinant will perform similarly and in-

duce an immune response to the fusion protein expressed on its surface. Because an immune response is in fact generated to commensal flora [102] even in humans [103]; V. Fischetti, unpublished data], yet it is not a clearing response, it may be expected that the same would occur with the newly introduced recombinant strain.

NEW-GENERATION STREPTOCOCCAL VACCINE DELIVERED BY *STREPTOCOCCUS GORDONII*

Since the use of a commensal bacteria as a vaccine delivery vehicle is a safe, effective, and inexpensive way to induce a mucosal response, a recombinant *Streptococcus gordonii* was prepared that contained the C-terminal half of the M protein with the exposed conserved region of the molecule. This segment was similar to that used successfully in the vaccinia virus experiments (see above; [67,68]). *Streptococcus gordonii* expressing this segment of the M protein on its surface was used to successfully colonize all of the 10 rabbits immunized for up to 12 weeks. During this time, the animals raised a salivary IgA (Fig. 19.13) and serum IgG (Fig. 19.14) response to the intact M protein. The amount of M protein–specific sIgA was up to 5% of the total IgA in the saliva of these animals. Using the conserved region of the M molecule as a mucosal vaccine, preliminary experiments have shown that the IgA and IgG induced by this method do not cross-react with human heart tissue as determined by immunofluorescence assay [13]. Studies are in progress to determine the protective effects of this delivery system in the mouse model described above.

If proven to be successful, the commensal delivery system would be ideal for developing countries. A live vector would be easy to administer and probably would not require additional doses. Also, since gram-positive bacteria

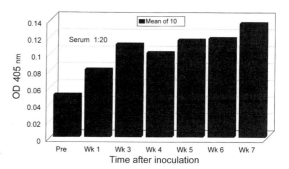

Figure 19.14 M protein–specific serum IgG in rabbits colonized with *Streptococcus gordonii* expressing the conserved region on the cell surface. Blood samples were taken at weekly intervals and tested in ELISA against the M protein.

are stable for long periods in the lyophilized state, a cold chain would not be required. Earlier studies showed that when reintroduced into the human oral cavity, *Streptococcus gordonii* is capable of persisting for over 2 years, and is transmitted to other members of the family [101]. For a developing country this factor could be ideal since rarely is the entire population immunized. However, it remains to be seen if the recombinant will induce a protective immune response in humans to the M protein fragment expressed on its surface.

NON–M PROTEIN APPROACHES FOR PROTECTION AGAINST STREPTOCOCCAL INFECTION

In recent years, other approaches have been presented that may be an alternative to using M protein as a vaccine candidate [104]. Cleary and coworkers have identified a group A streptococcal protease that specifically cleaves the human serum chemotaxin C5a, preventing its binding to polymorphonuclear neutrophils [105,106]. This cleavage has been shown to reduce the influx of inflammatory cells at the site of a streptococcal infection [107]. Capitalizing on this finding, this group demonstrated that intranasal delivery of a defective form of the streptococcal C5a peptidase molecule to mice showed promise in protecting against heterologous M serotypes [108]. In these studies, immunized animals cleared the challenge streptococci from the throat more rapidly than control animals.

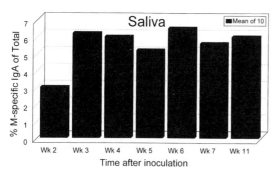

Figure 19.13 M protein–specific salivary IgA in rabbits colonized with *Streptococcus gordonii* expressing the conserved region on the cell surface. Salivary samples were taken after pylocarpine induction and tested in ELISA against the M protein.

Using a different approach, Musser and colleagues have worked on a group A streptococcal cysteine protease known as streptococcal pyrogenic exotoxin B (SpeB). The gene for this protein is found in virtually all strains of group A streptococci, and in most cases its product is secreted from these organisms. Since cysteine proteases have been implicated in bacterial pathogenicity, it was shown that a protease-negative SpeB mutant lost nearly all of its ability to cause death in mice when compared to wild-type organisms [109]. It was shown that passive immunization of mice with rabbit IgG to cysteine protease exhibited a longer time to death than control animals [110]. Active immunization with cysteine protease gave the same result. Thus, while this vaccine approach prolonged life, it did not prevent death.

The group-specific antigen for group A streptococci is N-acetyl-glucosamine, a polysaccharide component of the streptococcal cell wall. Because most people infected by streptococci will develop anti-N-acetyl-glucosamine antibodies, Zabriskie and colleagues examined whether these antibodies have any effect on protecting against streptococcal infection. Using a modified in vitro phagocytic assay and a very low inoculum, they found that anti-carbohydrate antibodies were phagocytic. A comparison of human and rabbit opsonic sera showed that only high titers of anti-N-acetyl-glucosamine–specific antibodies were effective in opsonization and phagocytosis of streptococci [111].

SUMMARY AND CONCLUSIONS

It would be naive to believe that a streptococcal infection is not a highly complex process, and perhaps no one single approach will control or prevent all aspects of infection by these organisms. While we may be able to prevent infection by using a mucosal approach, these types of vaccines are usually not 100% protective and organisms introduced at high doses may break through, resulting in sporadic infections. This scenario is akin to how we believe most adults naturally become more resistant to streptococcal infections. One of the benefits of a successful mucosal vaccination scheme would be the reduction of streptococcal colonization in general,

thus reducing the total number of these pathogens in the population. Since the main reservoir for group A streptococci responsible for most streptococcal-related illnesses is the human nasopharynx, a reduction in the carriage of these organisms by only 30% would have a profound impact on the dissemination of streptococci in the environment and thus produce a significant reduction in streptococcal disease in general.

REFERENCES

1. Stevens DL, Tanner MH, Winship J, Swarts R, Ries KM, Schlievert PM, Kaplan EL. Severe group A streptococcal infections associated with a toxic shock-like syndrome and scarlet fever toxin A. N Engl J Med 1989; 321:1–7.
2. Stevens DL. Invasive group A streptococcus infections. Clin Infect Dis 1992; 14:2–13.
3. Musser JM, Hauser AR, Kim MH, Schlievert PM, Nelson K. *Streptococcus pyogenes* causing toxic-shock-like syndrome and other invasive diseases: clonal diversity and pyrogenic exotoxin expression. Proc Natl Acad Sci USA 1991; 88:2668–2672.
4. Stevens DL. Streptococcal toxic-shock syndrome: spectrum of disease, pathogenesis, and new concepts in treatment. Emerg Infect Dis 1995; 1:69–78.
5. Invasive group A streptococcal infections: first report of enhanced surveillance. Commun Dis Rep CDR Rev 1995; 5(10):1.
6. Seppala H, Nissenen A, Jarvinen H, Huovinen S, Henriksson T, Herva E, Holm SE, Jahkola M, Katila M-L, Klaukka T, Kontiainen S, Liimatainen S, Oinonen S, Passi-Metsomaa L, Huovinen P. Resistance to erythromycin in group A streptococci. N Engl J Med 1992; 30:292–297.
7. Veasy LG, Wiedmeier SE, Orsmond GS, Ruttenberg HD, Boucek MM, Roth SJ, Tait VF. Resurgence of acute rheumatic fever in the intermountain area of the United States. N Engl J Med 1987; 316:421–427.
8. Dodu SRA, Bothig S. Rheumatic fever and rheumatic heart disease in developing countries. World Health Forum 1989; 10:203–212.
9. Kaplan MH. Immunologic relations of streptococcal and tissue antigens. I. Properties of an antigen in certain strains of group A streptococci exhibiting an immunologic cross reaction with human heart tissue. J Immunol 1963; 90:595–606.
10. Kaplan MH, Meyeserian M. An immunological cross-reaction between group A streptococcal cells and human heart tissue. Lancet 1962; 1:706.

11. Zabriskie JB, Freimer EH. An immunological relationship between the group A streptococcus and mammalian muscle. J Exp Med 1966; 124:661.

12. van de Rijn I, Zabriskie JB, McCarty M. Group A streptococcal antigens cross-reactive with myocardium. Purification of heart-reactive antibody and isolation and characterization of the streptococcal antigen. J Exp Med 1977; 146:579.

13. Zabriskie JB, Hsu KC, Seegal BC. Heart-reactive antibody associated with rheumatic fever: characterization and diagnostic significance. Clin Exp Immunol 1970; 7:147.

14. Dale JB, Ofek I, Beachey EH. Heterogeneity of type-specific and cross-reactive antigenic determinants within a single M protein of group A streptococci. J Exp Med 1980; 151:1026–1038.

15. Dale JB, Beachey EH. Epitopes of streptococcal M proteins shared with cardiac myosin. J Exp Med 1985; 162:583–591.

16. Dale JB, Beachey EH. Multiple, heart-cross-reactive epitopes of streptococcal M proteins. J Exp Med 1985; 161:113–122.

17. Copperman SM. Household pets as reservoirs of persistent or recurrent streptococcal sore throats in children. NY State J Med 1982; 82;1685–1687.

18. Hook EW, Wagner RR, Lancefield RC. An epizootic in Swiss mice caused by a group A streptococcus, newly designated type 50. Am J Hyg 1960; 72:111–119.

19. Anonymous. Acute rheumatic fever at a Navy training center—San Diego, California. MMWR Morb Mortal Wkly Rep 1988; 37:101–104.

20. Anonymous. Acute rheumatic fever among Army trainees—Fort Leonard Wood, Missouri, 1987–1988. MMWR Morb Mortal Wkly Rep 1988; 37:519–522.

21. Lancefield RC. Current knowledge of the type specific M antigens of group A streptococci. J Immunol 1962; 89:307–313.

22. Fischetti VA. Streptococcal M protein: molecular design and biological behavior. Clin Microbiol Rev 1989; 2:285–314.

23. Bessen D, Fischetti VA. Vaccination against Streptococcus pyogenes infection. In: Levine MM, Wood G (eds). New Generation Vaccines. New York: Marcel Dekker, 1988; 599–609.

24. Jones KF, Manjula BN, Johnston KH, Hollingshead SK, Scott JR, Fischetti VA. Location of variable and conserved epitopes among the multiple serotypes of streptococcal M protein. J Exp Med 1985; 161:623–628.

25. Fischetti VA, Horstmann RD, Pancholi V. Location of the complement factor H binding site on streptococcal M6 protein. Infect Immun 1995; 63:149–153.

26. Horstmann RK, Sievertsen HJ, Leippe M, Fischetti VA. Role of fibrinogen in complement inhibition by streptococcal M protein. Infect Immun 1992; 60:5036–5041.

27. Jones KF, Fischetti VA. The importance of the location of antibody binding on the M6 protein for opsonization and phagocytosis of group A M6 streptococci. J Exp Med 1988; 167:1114–1123.

28. Ehlenberger AG, Nussenzweig V. Role of C3b and C3d receptors in phagocytosis. J Exp Med 1977; 145:357–371.

29. Lancefield RC. The antigenic complex of Streptococcus hemolyticus. I. Demonstration of a type-specific substance in extracts of Streptococcus hemolyticus. J Exp Med 1928; 47:91–103.

30. Fox EN. M proteins of group A streptococci. Bacteriol Rev 1974; 38:57–86.

31. Beachey EH, Stollerman GH, Johnson RH, Ofek I, Bisno AL. Human immune response to immunization with a structurally defined polypeptide fragment of streptococcal M protein. J Exp Med 1979; 150:862–877.

32. Wittner MK, Fox EN. Homologous and heterologous protection of mice with group A streptococcal M protein vaccines. Infect Immun 1977; 15:104–108.

33. Jolivet M, Audibert F, Beachey EH, Tartar A, Gras-Masse H, Chedid L. Epitope specific immunity elicited by a synthetic streptococcal antigen without carrier or adjuvant. Biochem Biophys Res Commun 1983; 117:359–366.

34. Beachey EH. Type-specific opsonic antibodies evoked with a synthetic peptide of streptococcal M protein conjugated to polylysine without adjuvant. Infect Immun 1986; 51:362–364.

35. Chedid L, Jolivet M, Audibert F, Przewlocki G, Beachey EH, Gras-Masse H, Tartar A. Antibody responses elicited by a polyvalent vaccine containing synthetic diphtheric, streptococcal, and hepatitis peptides coupled to the same carrier. Biochem Biophys Res Commun 1983; 117:908–915.

36. Fischetti VA, Windels M. Mapping the immunodeterminants of the complete streptococcal M6 protein molecule: identification of an immunodominant region. J Immunol 1988; 141:3592–3599.

37. Bessen D, Fischetti VA. Passive acquired mucosal immunity to group A streptococci by secretory immunoglobulin A. J Exp Med 1988; 167:1945–1950.

38. Bessen D, Fischetti VA. Influence of intranasal immunization with synthetic peptides corresponding to conserved epitopes of M protein on mucosal colonization by group A streptococci. Infect Immun 1988; 56:2666–2672.

39. Beachey EH, Seyer JM, Dale JB, Simpson WA, Kang AH. Type-specific protective immunity evoked by synthetic peptide of Streptococcus pyogenes M protein. Nature 1981; 292:457–459.

40. Beachey EH, Tartar A, Seyer JM, Chedid L. Epitope-specific protective immunogenicity of chemically synthesised 13-, 18-, and 23-residue peptide fragments of streptococcal M protein. Proc Natl Acad Sci USA 1984; 81:2203–2207.

41. Beachey EH, Seyer JM. Protective and nonprotective epitopes of chemically synthesized peptides of the NH2-terminal region of type 6 streptococcal M protein. J Immunol 1986; 136:2287–2292.

42. Beachey EH, Gras-Masse H, Tarter A, Jolivet M, Audibert F, Chedid L, Seyer JM. Opsonic antibodies evoked by hybrid peptide copies of types 5 and 24 streptococcal M proteins synthesized in tandem. J Exp Med 1986; 163:1451–1458.

43. Sargent SJ, Beachey EH, Corbett CE, Dale JB. Sequence of protective epitopes of streptococcal M proteins shared with cardiac sarcolemmal membranes. J Immunol 1987; 139:1285–1290.

44. Bronze MS, Beachey EH, Dale JB. Protective and heart-cross-reactive epitopes located within the N-terminus of type 19 streptococcal M protein. J Exp Med 1988; 167:1849–1859.

45. Jones KF, Hollingshead SK, Scott JR, Fischetti VA. Spontaneous M6 protein size mutants of group A streptococci display variation in antigenic and opsonogenic epitopes. Proc Natl Acad Sci USA 1988; 85:8271–8275.

46. Beachey EH, Seyer JM, Dale JB. Protective immunogenicity and T lymphocyte specificity of a trivalent hybrid peptide containing NH2-terminal sequences of types 5, 6, and 24 proteins synthesized in tandem. J Exp Med 1987; 166:647–656.

47. Dale JB, Chiang EY, Lederer JW. Recombinant tetravalent group A streptococcal M protein vaccine. J Immunol 1993; 151:2188–2194.

48. Dale JB, Simmons M, Chiang EC, Chiang EY. Recombinant, octavalent group A streptoccal M protein vaccine. Vaccine 1996; 14:944–948.

49. Hollingshead SK, Fischetti VA, Scott JR. Complete nucleotide sequence of type 6 M protein of the group A streptococcus: repetitive structure and membrane anchor. J Biol Chem 1986; 261:1677–1686.

50. Fischetti VA, Parry DAD, Trus BL, Hollingshead SK, Scott JR, Manjula BN. Conformational characteristics of the complete sequence of group A streptococcal M6 protein. Proteins: Struct Func Genet 1988; 3:60–69.

51. Fischetti VA, Jones KF, Scott JR. Size variation of the M protein in group A streptococci. J Exp Med 1985; 161:1384–1401.

52. Harbaugh MP, Podbielski A, Hugl S, Cleary PP. Nuceotide substitutions and small-scale insertion produce size and antigenic variation in group A streptococcal M1 protein. Mol Microbiol 1993; 8:981–991.

53. Penney TJ, Martin DR, Williams LC, de Malmanche SA, Bergquist PL. A single *emm* gene-specific oligonucleotide probe does not recognize all members of the *Streptococcus pyogenes* M type 1. FEMS Microbiol Lett 1995; 130:145–150.

54. Macrina FL, Evans RP, Tobian JA, Hartley DL, Clewell DB, Jones KR. Novel shuttle plasmid vehicles for *Escherichia-Streptococcus* transgeneric cloning. Gene 1983; 25:145–150.

55. Bessen D, Fischetti VA. Role of nonopsonic antibody in protection against group A streptococcal infection. In: Lasky L (ed). Technological Advances in Vaccine Development. New York: Alan R. Liss, 1988; 493–501.

56. Bessen D, Fischetti VA. Synthetic peptide vaccine against mucosal colonization by group A streptococci. I. Protection against a heterologous M serotype with shared C repeat region epitopes. J Immunol 1990; 145:1251–1256.

57. Kiyono H, Bienenstock J, McGhee J, Ernst PB. The mucosal immune system: features of inductive and effector sites to consider in mucosal immunization and vaccine development. Reg Immunol 1992; 4:54–62.

58. McGhee JR, Fujihashi K, Xu-Amano J, Jackson RJ, Elson CO, Beagley KW, Kiyono H. New perspectives in mucosal immunity with emphasis on vaccine development. Semin Hematol 1993; 30(4):3–15.

59. Dale JB, Baird RW, Courtney HS, Hasty DL, Bronze MS. Passive protection of mice against group A streptococcal pharyngeal infection by lipoteichoic acid. J Infect Dis 1994; 169:319–323.

60. Tylewska SK, Fischetti VA, Gibbons RJ. Binding selectivity of *Streptococcus pyogenes* and M protein to epithelial cells differs from that of lipoteichoic acid. Curr Microbiol 1988; 16:209–216.

61. Alkan M, Ofek I, Beachey EH. Adherence of pharyngeal and skin strains of group A streptococci to human skin and oral epithelial cells. Infect Immun 1977; 18:555–557.

62. Caparon MG, Stephens DS, Olsen A, Scott JR. Role of M protein in adherence of group A streptococci. Infect Immun 1991; 59:1811–1817.

63. Beachey EH, Ofek I. Epithelial cell binding of group A streptococci by lipoteichoic acid on fimbriae denuded of M protein. J Exp Med 1976; 143:759–771.

64. Bronze MS, McKinsey DS, Beachey EH, Dale JB. Protective immunity evoked by locally administered group A streptococcal vaccines in mice. J Immunol 1988; 141:2767–2770.

65. Pruksakorn S, Currie B, Brandt E, Martin D, Galbraith A, Phornphutkul C, Hunsakunachal S, Manmontri A, Good MF. Towards a vaccine for rheumatic fever: identification of a conserved target epitope on M protein of group A streptococci. Lancet 1994; 344:639–642.

66. Lancefield RC. Persistence of type specific antibodies in man following infection with group A streptococci. J Exp Med 1959; 110:271–292.

67. Hruby DE, Hodges WM, Wilson EM, Franke CA, Fischetti VA. Expression of streptococcal M protein in mammalian cells. Proc Natl Acad Sci USA 1988; 85:5714–5717.

68. Fischetti VA, Hodges WM, Hruby DE. Protection against streptococcal pharyngeal colonization with a vaccinia:M protein recombinant. Science 1989; 244:1487–1490.

69. Dertzbaugh MT, Peterson DL, Macrina FL. Cholera toxin B-subunit gene fusion: structural and functional analysis of the chimeric protein. Infect Immun 1990; 58:70–79.

70. McKenzie SJ, Halsey JF. Cholera toxin B subunit as a carrier protein to stimulate a mucosal immune response. J Immunol 1984; 133:1818–1824.

71. Challacombe SJ, Rahman D, Jeffery H, Davis SS, O'Hagan DT. Enhanced secretory IgA and systemic IgG antibody responses after oral immunization with biodegradable microparticles containing antigen. Immunology 1992; 76:164–168.

72. Eldridge JH, Staas JK, Meulbroek JA, McGhee JR, Tice TR, Gilley RM. Biodegradable microspheres as a vaccine delivery system. Mol Immunol 1991; 28:287–294.

73. Tacket CO, Hone DM, Curtiss R III, Kelly SM, Losonsky G, Guers L, Harris AM, Edelman R, Levine MM. Comparison of the safety and immunogenicity of *delta-aroC delta-aroD* and *delta-cya delta-crp Salmonella typhi* strains in adult volunteers. Infect Immun 1992; 60:536–541.

74. Stover CK, de la Cruz VF, Fuerst TR, Burlein JE, Benson LA, Bennett LT, Bansal GP, Young JF, Lee MH, Hatfull GF, Snapper SB, Barletta RG, Jacobs WR Jr, Bloom BR. New use of BCG for recombinant vaccines. Nature 1991; 351:456–460.

75. Moss B. Vaccinia virus: a tool for research and vaccine development. Science 1991; 252:1662–1667.

76. Tartaglia J, Perkus ME, Taylor J, Norton EK, Adonnet J-C, Cox WI, Davis SW, van der Hoeven J, Meignier B, Riviere M, Languet B, Paoletti E. NYVAC: a highly attenuated strain of vaccinia virus. Virology 1992; 188:217–232.

77. Cadoz M, Strady A, Meignier B, Taylor J, Tartaglia J, Paoletti E, Plotkin S. Immunisation with canarypox virus expressing rabies glycoprotein. Lancet 1992; 339:1429–1431.

78. Tartaglia J, Paoletti E. Live recombinant viral vaccines. In: van Regenmorterl MHV, Neurath AR (eds). Immunochemistry of Viruses, II. New York: Elsevier Science, 1990; 125–151.

79. Pozzi G, Contorni M, Oggioni MR, Manganelli R, Tommasino M, Cavalieri F, Fischetti VA. Delivery and expression of a heterologous antigen on the surface of streptococci. Infect Immun 1992; 60:1902–1907.

80. Fischetti VA, Pancholi V, Schneewind O. Conservation of a hexapeptide sequence in the anchor region of surface proteins of gram-positive cocci. Mol Microbiol 1990; 4:1603–1605.

81. Schneewind O, Model P, Fischetti VA. Sorting of protein A to the staphylococcal cell wall. Cell 1992; 70:267–281.

82. Fischetti VA, Pancholi V, Schneewind O. Common characteristics of the surface proteins from gram-positive cocci. In: Dunney GM, Cleary PP, McKay LL (eds). Genetics and Molecular Biology of Streptococci, Lactococci, and Enterococci. Washington, DC: American Society of Microbiology 1991; 290–294.

83. Pancholi V, Fischetti VA. Isolation and characterization of the cell-associated region of group A streptococcal M6 protein. J Bacteriol 1988; 170:2618–2624.

84. Sutcliffe IC, Russell RRB. Lipoproteins of gram-positive bacteria. J Bacteriol 1995; 177:1123–1128.

85. Yother J, Briles DE. Structural properties and evolutionary relationships of PspA, a surface protein of *Streptococcus pneumoniae*, as revealed by sequence analysis. J Bacteriol 1992; 174:601–609.

86. Fischetti VA, Pancholi V, Sellers P, Schmidt J, Landau G, Xu X, Schneewind O. Streptococcal M protein: a common structural motif used by gram-positive bacteria for biologically active surface molecules. In: Korhonen TK, Hovi T, Makela PH (eds). Molecular Recognition in Host-Parasite Interactions. New York: Plenum Press, 1992; 31–38.

87. Phillips GN, Flicker PF, Cohen C, Manjula BN, Fischetti VA. Streptococcal M protein: alpha-helical coiled-coil structure and arrangement on the cell surface. Proc Natl Acad Sci USA 1981; 78:4689–4693.

88. Deisenhofer J, Jones TA, Huber R, Sjodahl J, Sjoquist J. Crystallization, crystal structure analysis and atomic model of the complex formed by a human Fc fragment and fragment B of protein A from *Staphylococcus aureus*. Hoppe-Seylers Z Physiol Chem 1978; 359:975–985.

89. Gouda H, Torigoe H, Saito A, Sato M, Arata Y, Shimada I. Three-dimensional solution structure of the B domain of staphylococcal protein A: comparisons of the solution and crystal structures. Biochemistry 1992; 31:9665–9672.

90. Barchi JJ Jr, Grasberger B, Gronenborn AM, Clore GM. Investigation of the backbone dynamics of the IgG-binding domain of streptococcal protein G by heteronuclear two-dimensional ^{1}H-^{15}N nuclear magnetic resonance spectroscopy. Protein Sci 1994; 3:15–21.

91. Lian L-Y, Derrick JP, Sutcliffe MJ, Yang JC, Roberts GCK. Determination of the solution structures of domains II and III of protein G from streptococcus by ^{1}H nuclear magnetic resonance. J Mol Biol 1992; 228:1219–1234.

92. Boutillion C, Wintjens R, Lippens G, Drobecq H, Tartar A. Synthesis, three-dimensional structure, and specific ^{15}N-labelling of the strepto-

coccal protein G B1-domain. Eur J Biochem 1995; 231:166–180.

93. Gronenborn AM, Filpula DR, Essig NZ, Achari A, Whitlow M, Wingfield PT, Clore GM. A novel, highly stable fold of the immunoglobulin binding domain of streptococcal protein G. Science 1991; 253:657–661.

94. Schneewind O, Mihaylova-Petkov D, Model P. Cell wall sorting signals in surface proteins of gram-positive bacteria. EMBO J 1993; 12:4803–4811.

95. Cole RM, Hahn JJ. Cell wall replication in *Streptococcus pyogenes*. Science 1962; 135:722–724.

96. Pozzi G, Oggioni MR, Manganelli R, Fischetti VA. Expression of M6 protein gene of *Streptococcus pyogenes* in *Streptococcus gordonii* after chromosomal integration and transcriptional fusion. Res Microbiol 1992; 143:449–457.

97. Pozzi G, Oggioni MR, Manganelli R, Medaglini D, Fischetti VA, Fenoglio D, Valle MT, Kunkl A, Manca F. Human T-helper cell recognition of an immunodominant epitome of HIV-1 gp120 expressed on the surface of *Streptococcus gordonii*. Vaccine 1994; 12:1071–1077.

98. Medaglini D, Pozzi G, King TP, Fischetti VA. Mucosal and systemic immune responses to a recombinant protein expressed on the surface of the oral commensal bacterium *Streptococcus gordonii* after oral colonization. Proc Natl Acad Sci USA 1995; 92:6868–6872.

99. Piard J-C, Hautefort I, Fischetti VA, Ehrlich SD, Fons M, Gruss A. Cell wall anchoring of the *Streptococcus pyogenes* M6 protein in various lactic acid bacteria. J Bacteriol 1997; 179:3068–3072.

100. King TP, Kochoumian L, Lam T. Immunochemical observations of antigen 5, a major venom allergen of hornets, yellow jackets and wasps. Mol Immunol 1987; 24:857–864.

101. Svanberg M, Westergren G. Persistence and spread of the orally implanted bacterium *Streptococcus sanguis* between persons. Arch Oral Biol 1986; 31:1–4.

102. Shroff KE, Meslin K, Cebra JJ. Commensal enteric bacteria engender a self-limiting humoral mucosal immune response while permanently colonizing the gut. Infect Immun 1995; 63:3904–3913.

103. Dougan G. The molecular basis for the virulence of bacterial pathogens: implications for oral vaccine development. Microbiology 1994; 140:215–224.

104. Dale JB, Cleary PP, Fischetti VA, Musser JM, Zabriskie JB. Group A and group B streptococcal vaccine development. A round table presentation. Adv Exp Med Biol 1997; 418:863–868.

105. Chen CC, Cleary PP. Cloning and expression of the streptococcal C5a petidase gene in *Es-*

cherichia coli: linkage to the type 12 M protein gene. Infect Immun 1989; 57:1740–1745.

106. Cleary PP, Prahbu U, Dale JB, Wexler DE, Handley J. Streptococcal C5a peptidase is a highly specific endopeptidase. Infect Immun 1992; 60:5219–5223.

107. Ji Y, McLandsborough L, Kondagunta A, Cleary PP. C5a peptidase alters clearance and trafficking of group A streptococci by infected mice. Infect Immun 1996; 64:503–510.

108. Ji Y, Carlson B, Kondagunta A, Cleary PP. Intranasal immunization with C5a peptidase prevents nasopharyngeal colonization of mice by the group A streptococcus. Infect Immun 1997; 65:2080–2087.

109. Lukomski S, Burns EH Jr, Wyde PR, Podbielski A, Rurangirwa J, Moore-Poveda DK, Musser JM. Genetic inactivation of an extracellular cysteine protease (SpeB) expressed by *Streptococcus pyogenes* decreases resistance to phagocytosis and dissemination to organs. Infect Immun 1998; 66:771–776.

110. Kapur V, Maffei JT, Greer RS, Li LL, Adams GJ, Musser JM. Vaccination with streptococcal extracellular cysteine protease (interleukin-1 beta convertase) protects mice against challenge with heterologous group A streptococci. Microbiol Pathog 1994; 16:443–450.

111. Salvadori LG, Blake MS, McCarty M, Tai JY, Zabriskie JB. Group A streptococcus-liposome ELISA antibody titers to group A polysaccharide and opsonophagocytic capability to the antibodies. J Infect Dis 1995; 171:593–600.

112. Breese BB, Hall CB. Beta Hemolytic Streptococcal Diseases. Boston: Houghton Mifflin, 1978; p 34–64.

113. Pozzi G, Oggioni MR, Manganelli R, Fischetti VA. Expression of M6 protein gene of *Streptococcus pyogenes* in *Streptococcus gordonii* after chromosonal integration and transcriptional fusion. Res Microbiol 1992; 143:449–457.

114. Lacks S. Uptake of curcular deoxyribonucleic acid and mechanism of deoxyribonucleic acid transport in genetic transformation of *Streptococcus pneumoniae*. J Bacteriol 1979; 138:404.

115. Saunders CW, Guild WR. Pathway of plasmid transformation in pneumococcus: open circular molecules and linear molecules are active. J Bacteriol 1981; 146:517.

116. Manjula BN, Fischetti VA. Studies on group A streptococcal M proteins: purification of type 5 M-protein and comparison of its amino terminal sequence with two immunologically unrelated M-protein molecules. J Immunol 1980; 124:261–267.

117. Fischetti VA, Gotschlich EC, Bernheimer AW. Purification and physical properties of group C streptococcal phage-associated lysin. J Exp Med 1971; 133:1105–1117.

20

Multivalent Group A Streptococcal Vaccines

JAMES B. DALE

There are several different strategies being used to develop group A streptococcal M protein–based vaccines. The previous chapter outlined current efforts to incorporate common, protective M protein epitopes into vaccines that would prevent colonization of mucosal surfaces and thus interrupt infection at the earliest steps. Another approach, which is the subject of this chapter, is to incorporate type-specific, M protein epitopes into multivalent vaccines that are designed to evoke serum bactericidal antibodies as well as mucosal IgA. The success of this strategy will depend on our ability to overcome several significant obstacles, including the identification and exclusion of tissue–cross-reactive M protein epitopes and the development of complex, multivalent constructs that retain their immunogenicity and evoke opsonic antibodies against multiple different serotypes of group A streptococci.

Early attempts to develop group A streptococcal vaccines were based on the observation that bactericidal antibodies were directed against the M protein [1] and that these antibodies could persist for as long as 30 years following natural infection [2]. Because of the documented causal relationship between streptococcal pharyngitis and acute rheumatic fever, it was clear that immunization with whole, killed organisms carried an unacceptable risk of this immunological complication. Thus, some of the earliest subunit vaccines were M proteins ex-

tracted from viable streptococci and purified to varying degrees. These early preparations were not well tolerated by human subjects because they were contaminated with streptococcal extracellular toxins. The toxicity limited the total amount of protein that could be administered and sufficiently immunogenic doses of M protein could not be achieved.

The problem of toxicity of M protein preparations was largely overcome by Beachey and colleagues, who determined that dilute solutions of pepsin released significant amounts of M protein from the surface of the organism while leaving the cell wall relatively intact [3]. The M protein from type 24 streptococci extracted with pepsin (pep M24) was purified to homogeneity using standard procedures and was shown to be immunogenic in laboratory animals [4]. The purified pepsin-extracted fragment of type 24 M protein was well tolerated in human volunteers in doses sufficient to evoke bactericidal antibodies [5].

For the first time it was conceivable that M proteins extracted from multiple serotypes of streptococci could be mixed together to form multivalent vaccines and administered to humans without the fear of toxic reactions. We next turned our attention to type 5 streptococci, a highly prevalent, rheumatogenic serotype. Initial experiments in laboratory animals revealed that pep M5 was immunogenic and evoked not only bactericidal antibodies but also antibodies that cross-reacted with human myocardium [6]. This finding was not totally unexpected, but these studies showed conclusively for the first time that autoimmune epitopes were contained within the covalent structure of type 5 M protein itself. Although there is no direct evidence that M proteins are involved in the immunopathogenesis of rheumatic fever or rheumatic carditis, the presence of tissue–cross-reactive epitopes in M proteins raised the theoretical possibility that M proteins themselves may trigger rheumatic fever, one of the very diseases the vaccines are supposed to prevent. This observation led to a series of studies to identify the structures of M proteins that contained protective and tissue–cross-reactive epitopes, in hopes of separating the two functional activities so that vaccines could be developed that were free of autoimmune epitopes.

IDENTIFICATION OF OPSONIC EPITOPES OF M PROTEINS

Early studies had shown that the pepsin-derived fragment of type 5 M protein evoked opsonic antibodies as well as heart–cross-reactive antibodies [6,7]. Some of the heart–cross-reactive antibodies also reacted with heterologous M proteins, including types 6, 18, and 19, indicating the presence of shared autoimmune epitopes. Structural analyses confirmed that the amino-terminal regions of M proteins were hypervariable and could account for type-specific immune responses [8–11]. Thus, we reasoned that the amino-terminal structures of M proteins, which were known to be oriented on the outermost surface of the organism [12], would be most likely to evoke type-specific, opsonic antibodies.

To demonstrate directly that opsonic M protein epitopes could be separated from autoimmune epitopes, we synthesized a peptide copying the amino-terminal 20 amino acids of M5 [13]. SM5(1–20) failed to react with affinity-purified pep M5 heart-reactive antibodies [13]. Rabbits immunized with SM5(1–20) coupled to tetanus toxoid developed high titers of antibodies against pep M5 that opsonized type 5 streptococci [13]. Most importantly, none of the immune sera cross-reacted with human myocardium. Thus, we had direct evidence that the opsonic and tissue–

cross-reactive epitopes of type 5 M protein were located within different covalent structures. Additional studies using synthetic peptides copying amino-terminal regions of type 6 [14] and type 24 [15] M proteins also revealed the presence of type-specific opsonic epitopes that were not tissue cross-reactive.

However, previous studies have also shown that under certain conditions, amino-terminal peptides of M proteins may elicit opsonic as well as tissue-cross-reactive antibodies. For example, a synthetic peptide of type 1 M protein, SM1(1–19)(23–26)C, that was inadvertently synthesized with a deletion of residues 20–22 evoked polyclonal antibodies that were opsonic but that also cross-reacted with vimentin [16] and monoclonal antibodies that cross-reacted with an antigen in both kidney and heart [17]. Although the tissue–cross-reactive antibodies were inhibited by the correct peptide, SM1 (1–26)C, and the native pep M1 [16,17], none of the cross-reactive antibodies was ever evoked by the peptide copying the native sequence. Similar results were obtained with a synthetic peptide of type 19 M protein [18], whose structure was based on the sequence of the pepsin-extracted M19 protein determined by Edman degradation. The SM19 peptide evoked opsonic and heart–cross-reactive antibodies in rabbits [18]. Although the heart–cross-reactive antibodies were inhibited by the native M19 protein, indicating the presence of the autoimmune epitopes, we later determined after deducing the M19 protein sequence from the gene sequence [19] that SM19(1–24) contained three incorrect amino acids. Later studies showed that the correct peptide, SM19(1–35)C, evoked only protective antibodies and not tissue–cross-reactive antibodies [19]. Thus, our conclusions that these M proteins contain autoimmune epitopes within their amino-terminal regions were correct, but the antibodies were only evoked by peptides with incorrect sequences. The autoimmune epitopes do not appear to be immunogenic when the native primary structures are used as immunogens. However, these findings underscore the need to assess vaccine constructs for their ability to evoke tissue–cross-reactive antibodies because of potential changes in immunogenicity created by making hybrid proteins (see below).

LOCALIZATION OF TISSUE–CROSS-REACTIVE EPITOPES OF M PROTEINS

M proteins evoke antibodies that cross-react with a variety of human tissues and antigens within those tissues [6,7,16,20–28]. Many of the antibodies cross-react with other alpha-helical proteins such as tropomyosin, myosin, and vimentin [16,20,25,29]. In earlier studies to determine the location of tissue–cross-reactive epitopes of M proteins, we focused on type 5 M protein. Manjula and colleagues had determined the entire covalent structure of the pep M5 molecule [9]. We synthesized a series of overlapping peptides that copied the pep M5 fragment and used the peptides to either inhibit or evoke tissue–cross-reactive antibodies. The myosin–cross-reactive antibodies evoked by pep M5 in rabbits were almost totally inhibited by peptide 84–116 of pep M5 (Fig. 20.1; [21]). This peptide spans the region between the A- and B-repeats of M5 and includes the degenerate A6 repeat. Murine and human myosin–cross-reactive antibodies reacted with an epitope in peptide 183–189, which is located in the region between the B- and C-repeats of the intact M5 molecule [25]. Additional sarcolemmal membrane cross-reactive epitopes were localized to peptide 164–197 (Fig. 20.1; [22]). Several epitopes of M5 that evoked antibodies that cross-reacted with articular cartilage and synovium were identified within the B-repeats and the region spanning the A- and B-repeats of M5 [27]. The brain–cross-reactive epitopes of M6 that were shared with other M proteins were localized to the B-repeat region of the molecule (Fig. 20.1; [28]). Many of the tissue–cross-reactive epitopes are shared among types 5, 6, 18, and 19 M proteins [7,20,27,28]. Primary structural data revealed that all of these M proteins contain similar sequences within their B-repeats [8–10,30], which is most likely the location of the shared heart–, brain–, and joint–cross-reactive epitopes.

RATIONALE FOR VACCINES CONTAINING AMINO-TERMINAL M PROTEIN FRAGMENTS

The above discussion summarizes the data that now serve as the basis for our current strategies for M protein vaccine design. Because M proteins contain protective (opsonic) as well as tissue–cross-reactive epitopes, it has been necessary to identify peptide fragments that contain only opsonic epitopes that may be included in multivalent vaccines. The data indicate that amino-terminal regions of M proteins contain epitopes that evoke antibodies with the greatest bactericidal activity [13–15,31,32] and are least likely to evoke tissue–cross-reactive antibodies. Most of the tissue–cross-reactive epitopes have been localized to the B-repeats, the A–B flanking regions, or the B–C flanking regions, which are all some distance from the type-specific, amino-terminal epitopes (Fig. 20.1). Therefore, our current approach is to incorporate limited amino-terminal fragments of multiple M proteins into multivalent vaccine constructs, either as hybrid proteins or individual peptides linked in tandem to unrelated carrier proteins that could be mixed to form multivalent vaccines.

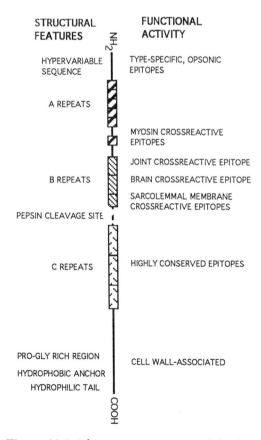

Figure 20.1 Schematic representation of the functional and structural regions of type 5 streptococcal M protein.

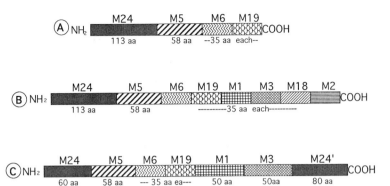

Figure 20.2 Schematic representation of the tetravalent *(A)*, octavalent *(B)*, and hexavalent *(C)* M protein–based vaccines.

The following sections will summarize our data resulting from these different approaches to M protein vaccine development.

RECOMBINANT, MULTIVALENT M PROTEIN VACCINES

We have used recombinant techniques to produce complex hybrid proteins containing N-terminal peptides of M proteins from different serotypes of GrAS [19,30,33]. We first constructed a tetravalent gene that encoded defined N-terminal fragments of M24, M5, M6, and M19 (Fig. 20.2A; [19]). Polymerase chain reaction (PCR) primers were synthesized to amplify specific 5′ sequences of each *emm* gene, and each primer was extended to contain a unique restriction enzyme site used to ligate the individual PCR products in tandem. The tetravalent gene contained 113 codons of *emm*24, 58 codons of *emm*5, and 35 each from *emm*6 and *emm*19.

Rabbits immunized with the recombinant tetravalent protein developed significant antibody levels against all four serotypes of purified native M proteins (Fig. 20.3). On the whole, the

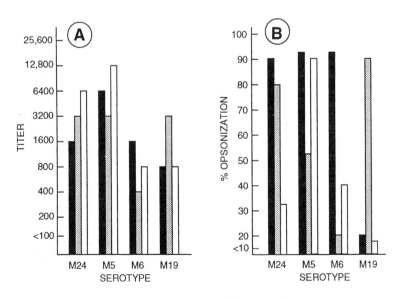

Figure 20.3 Immune responses in rabbits immunized with the tetravalent M protein vaccine. ELISA titers against the pep M proteins *(A)* and percent opsonization of each different serotype of group A streptococci *(B)* obtained using immune serum from each of three rabbits (represented by the different bars) are shown. Data adapted from Dale et al. [19].

antisera had higher titers of antibodies against pep M24 and pep M5 than against M6 and M19. The immune sera also contained opsonic antibodies against all four serotypes of group A streptococci, indicating that the antibodies were, in most cases, directed against protective M protein epitopes (Fig. 20.3). None of the antisera cross-reacted with human heart tissue. These data indicated that the tetravalent protein evoked opsonic antibodies against all four serotypes of group A streptococci, but not all rabbits responded equally to all subunits of the vaccine. The M19 fragment, located in the C-terminal position, was least immunogenic. This may have been related to an unfavorable conformation of the peptide in this position. Alternatively, this end of the protein may be susceptible to proteolytic cleavage so that the M19 fragment becomes haptenic and nonimmunogenic after injection. Rather than reconfigure the tetravalent gene to answer these questions, we chose to extend the gene to include four additional M protein fragments.

An octavalent gene [30] was constructed using the same approach outlined above for the tetravalent gene (Fig. 20.2B). The additional fragments encoded 35 amino acids each from M1, M3, M18, and M2. The purified octavalent protein evoked significant levels of antibodies in rabbits against each of the pep M proteins represented in the hybrid molecule (Fig. 20.4). The octavalent protein also evoked opsonic antibodies against six of the eight serotypes of streptococci (Fig. 20.4). None of the antisera cross-reacted with human tissues. The antisera raised against the octavalent protein did not opsonize type 18 or type 2 streptococci, despite the presence of significant levels of antibodies against the respective M proteins. These studies demonstrated the feasibility of evoking broadly protective immune responses against multiple serotypes of group A streptococci using complex hybrid M proteins. Of interest was the finding that the M19 fragment, which was converted to an internal location in the octavalent protein, was highly immunogenic and evoked opsonic antibodies in all three immunized rabbits (Fig. 20.4). As with the tetravalent protein, the octavalent vaccine failed to evoke opsonic antibodies against the M proteins represented by the peptide fragments in the C-terminal locations.

In order to enhance the protective immunogenicity of each M protein fragment, we constructed another hybrid gene encoding N-terminal peptides of six different M proteins [33]. We reasoned that the C-terminal fragments may be preferentially susceptible to proteolysis after injection, effectively converting them into haptenic peptides that failed to evoke sufficient

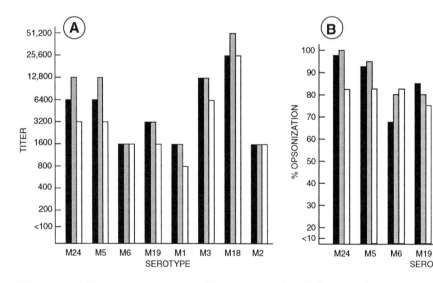

Figure 20.4 Immune responses in rabbits immunized with the octavalent M protein vaccine. ELISA titers against the pep M proteins (A) and percent opsonization of each different serotype of group A streptococci (B) using immune serum from each of three rabbits (represented by the different bars) are shown. Data adapted from Dale et al. [30].

levels of opsonic antibodies. To circumvent this problem, we reiterated the N-terminal M24 fragment on the C-terminal end of the hexavalent protein to serve as a "sacrificial" peptide (Fig. 20.2C). The hexavalent gene was ligated into an expression vector containing a polyhistidine N-terminal peptide to facilitate purification from extracts of *E. coli* [33]. Rabbits were immunized with 100 μg of the hexavalent protein adsorbed to alum at 0, 4, and 8 weeks. All of the animals developed significant antibody levels against the vaccine after the first injection and booster responses after the subsequent injections (Fig. 20.5).

One of our major goals was to design a multivalent, hybrid protein that retained the immunogenic properties of each M protein subunit. ELISAs were performed on sera obtained from the three rabbits immunized with the hexavalent vaccine in alum (Fig. 20.6). In each case the ELISA antigen was the purified pepsin-extracted M protein. Thus, the assay measured only the antibodies evoked by the hexavalent protein that react with the native M protein and

not the antibodies that may be specific for the joining segments or for conformations that are not present in the native M proteins. The hexavalent protein evoked significant levels of antibodies against each M protein represented in the vaccine construct (Fig. 20.6). Importantly, none of the antisera contained antibodies that cross-reacted with human heart, brain, or kidney tissue, as determined by indirect immunofluorescence assays (data not shown). Sera from all three rabbits contained opsonic antibodies against each serotype of group A streptococci represented in the vaccine (Fig. 20.6). Taken together, the results indicate that the individual components of the hexavalent vaccine retain the conformation and immunogenicity necessary to elicit antibodies that react with the native M proteins on the surface of each respective serotype of group A streptococci.

In order to show directly the protective efficacy of opsonic antibodies evoked by the hexavalent vaccine, mice were immunized with the vaccine adsorbed to alum and then challenged with two of the serotypes represented in the vaccine. Female outbred white Swiss mice were immunized intramuscularly with four 25-μg doses of the vaccine at 3-week intervals. Serum was obtained prior to the first injection and at 8 and 15 weeks. Serum antibody determinations were performed by ELISA using a single 1:200 dilution and the native pep M proteins. Most of the animals developed significant levels of antibodies against each M protein represented in the vaccine 15 weeks after the first injection (Fig. 20.7). Challenge experiments were performed on the 20 immunized mice and 20 control, unimmunized mice (Table 20.1). The challenge strains were types 24 and 19, with the reasoning that the M24 peptide was the largest fragment in the hexavalent protein and was reiterated and the M19 fragment is one of two that are only 35 amino acids long. Two groups of ten mice each received an inoculum that approximated the LD_{70}–LD_{100} for each serotype, which was 2×10^4 colony-forming units (CFU). The mice that were immunized with the hexavalent vaccine and challenged with type 24 streptococci were significantly protected from death compared to the control group ($P = .0001$). The mice challenged with type 19 streptococci were protected by vaccination, but the level was not statistically

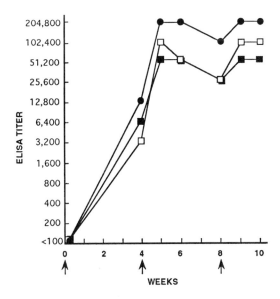

Figure 20.5 Immune responses in rabbits immunized with the hexavalent M protein vaccine adsorbed to alum. Three rabbits, represented by the symbols, received 100 μg doses of the vaccine at the times indicated by the arrows. ELISA titers were determined on serum obtained at the times indicated using the hexavalent protein as the solid-phase antigen. Data adapted from Dale [33].

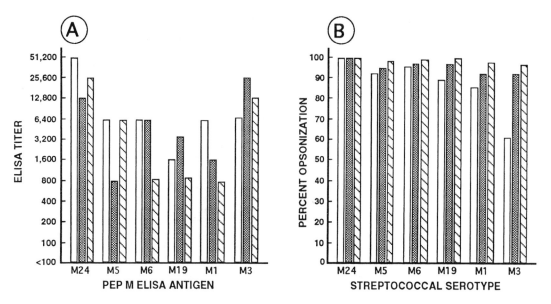

Figure 20.6 Immune responses in rabbits immunized with the hexavalent M protein vaccine in alum. ELISA titers against the pep M proteins *(A)* and percent opsonization of each different serotype of group A streptococci *(B)* using immune serum from each of three rabbits (represented by the different bars) are shown. Data adapted from Dale [33].

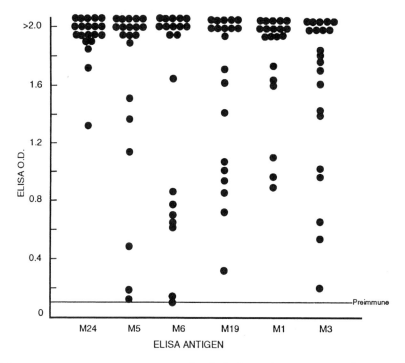

Figure 20.7 Immune responses in mice immunized with the hexavalent vaccine on alum. ELISAs were performed using serum that was obtained 15 weeks after the first injection. Serum obtained from each of 20 mice was diluted 1:200 prior to performing the assay. The solid-phase ELISA antigens were the native pep M proteins.

Table 20.1 Protective Immunogenicity of Hexavalent Vaccine in Mice Challenged Intraperitoneally with Virulent Type 24 and Type 19 Streptococci

	Dead/Survivors (% survival)		
Group	Type 24	Type 19	Total
Immunized mice	0/10 (100)	4/6 (60)	4/16 (80) $P = .0002^a$
Control mice	9/1 (10)	7/3 (30)	16/4 (20)

$^a P$ value was calculated using the Fisher exact test.

significant ($P = .15$). When the survival of the entire immunized group of mice was analyzed (Table 20.1), the level of protection was highly significant ($P = .0002$).

MUCOSAL DELIVERY OF RECOMBINANT M PROTEIN VACCINES

The recombinant hybrid proteins described above were designed to evoke opsonic antibodies following parenteral injection. Another approach is to develop M protein vaccines that may be delivered via mucosal routes to evoke secretory antibodies as well as serum opsonic antibodies. In initial experiments, we constructed a hybrid gene that encoded the entire B subunit of *E. coli* labile toxin (LT-B) linked to 15 amino-terminal amino acids of type 5 M protein (Fig. 20.8; [34]). In this construct, LT-B serves as a carrier for the haptenic peptide and also as a mucosal adjuvant. In order to maintain the antigenicity of the M5 fragment, a seven-residue proline-glycine-rich linker was inserted between the LT-B and M5 components. The purified hybrid protein retained the ganglioside-binding activity of LT-B [34], which is thought to enhance its immunomodulating potential when delivered mucosally. Therefore, we immunized groups of mice intranasally with 30 mg LT-B-M5 or LT-B. Mice that were immunized with LT-B-M5 developed significant levels of serum anti-

bodies against SM5(1–15) and LT-B as determined by ELISA (data not shown). Many of the mice immunized with LT-B-M5 also developed salivary immunoglobulin A (IgA) against the M5 peptide and LT-B. The presence of serum antibodies after intranasal immunization suggested that the animals may be protected against systemic challenge infections with group A streptococci. Therefore, we challenged both groups with 10^6 virulent type 5 streptococci intraperitoneally, which is a stringent assay for bactericidal antibodies. Of 18 mice immunized with LT-B-M5, only 2 died of infection (Table 20.2). Of 20 mice immunized with LT-B, 15 died after intraperitoneal challenge infection ($P < .001$, Fisher's exact test).

These studies showed for the first time that serum opsonic antibodies could be evoked after intranasal immunization with an M protein fragment. We have since extended this observation and have constructed a fusion protein containing LT-B linked to the tetravalent M protein described above (Fig. 20.9). Mice immunized intranasally with the purified LT-B-tetravalent protein developed significant levels of serum antibodies against pep M24, pep M5, and pep M6, but not pep M19 (Fig. 20.10A). Most importantly, the mice also developed opsonic antibodies against type 24, 5, and 6 streptococci (Fig. 20.10B). As discussed above, the finding that the M19 component is not immunogenic may be re-

Table 20.2 Survival of Mice Immunized Intranasally with LT-B-M5 Following Intraperitoneal Challenge Infections with Type 5 Streptococci^a

Immunization	Survived/Challenged	Survival (%)
LT-B-M5	16/18 ($P < .001$)	89
LT-B	5/20	25

^{a}Data adapted from Dale and Chiang [34].

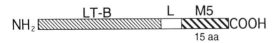

Figure 20.8 Schematic representation of the recombinant fusion protein LT-B-M5. The seven-residue proline-glycine-rich linker is indicated by L.

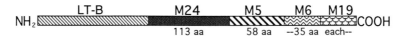

Figure 20.9 Schematic representation of the recombinant fusion protein LT-B-tetravalent M protein.

lated to its carboxy-terminal location within the hybrid protein. Despite this disappointment, the ability to evoke serum opsonic antibodies against three of the four M protein fragments after intranasal immunization suggests that this approach may be feasible. Mucosal delivery of M protein fragments has the advantage of evoking mucosal IgA, which may block adherence and colonization, and serum opsonic antibodies, which prevent infection at the level of the mucosa and in deeper tissues.

CONCLUSIONS AND FUTURE STUDIES

The data presented in this chapter indicate the feasibility of developing multivalent M protein vaccines designed to evoke serum opsonic antibodies. The major problems associated with this approach center on the complexity of the vaccine constructs. Epidemiologic data suggest that not all serotypes of group A streptococci have the ability to trigger acute rheumatic fever [35].

In addition, most serious life-threatening group A streptococcal infections in this country are caused by a limited number of serotypes [36]. In a recent survey of over 1100 group A streptococcal isolates collected in the United States, serotypes 1, 3, and 18 were more frequently isolated from patients with serious invasive infections and types 3 and 18 were more frequently recovered from patients with rheumatic fever, compared to control isolates from uncomplicated cases of pharyngitis [36]. The serotypes most commonly associated with uncomplicated infections were types 1, 2, 4, and 12. Assuming 100% serotype-specific efficacy, the octavalent vaccine described above would prevent 77% of the infections causing rheumatic fever, 52% of those that cause severe infections, and 40% of uncomplicated infections [36]. By adding types 4, 12, 22, and 28, thereby increasing the number of serotypes represented in the vaccine to 12, immunization could potentially prevent 84% of infections causing rheumatic fever, 73% of those that cause serious infections, and 69% of uncomplicated infections [36].

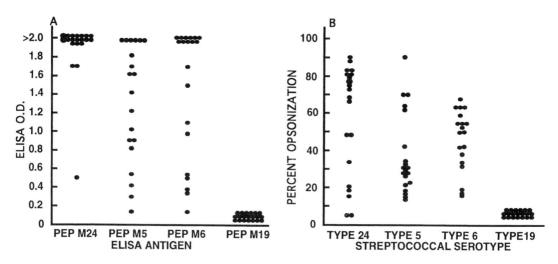

Figure 20.10 Serum immune responses of mice immunized intranasally with LT-B-tetravalent M protein. ELISA optical densities (A) were obtained using a 1:100 dilution of immune serum. Opsonization assays (B) were performed using undiluted serum. Preimmune sera resulted in ELISA O.D.s of <0.1 and opsonization levels of <10%.

These predictions of efficacy are based on several assumptions, the first of which is that each strain of streptococci within a given serotype expresses an M protein with similar or identical type-specific epitopes. The actual impact of strain variation of M protein structures on vaccine efficacy cannot adequately be predicted at the present time because sequences of multiple *emm* genes have only been determined for a few serotypes. Studies by Musser et al. have shown that the 5′ region of the *emm*1 gene may vary considerably among strains collected from various locations in the world [37]. In addition, variations in amino-terminal sequences of the type 1 M protein may influence opsonization of strains within the same serotype [38]. On the other hand, the sequences of three M5 proteins have previously been determined [9,10]; unpublished results, J. B. Dale). Two of the strains expressed M proteins that were identical through the first 40 amino acids and the other differed by only two amino acids. These minor structural differences were shown to have no impact on bactericidal activity [39]. The potential for structural variation within M proteins of the same serotype suggests that future studies should be designed to assess the functional significance of the different M protein structures. If certain strains that appear to be epidemiologically important are not opsonized by vaccine antisera, the *emm* genes will need to be sequenced so that additions to the multivalent vaccines can be made.

Another important determinant of serotype-specific M protein vaccine efficacy is the proportion of strains within a population that is nontypeable. If *emm* gene mutations lead to new M types, it is likely that these new serotypes will not be opsonized by antisera evoked by small amino-terminal fragments of M proteins from known serotypes. The prevalence of nontypeable strains appears to vary depending on location. For example, in the survey by Johnson et al., only 19% of the strains recovered from patients with uncomplicated infections were nontypeable, 26% from cases of severe infection were nontypeable, and none of the isolates from rheumatic fever cases were nontypeable [36]. On the other hand, in a similar study in Thailand, only 20% of the isolates of group A streptococci were typeable [40]. Similarly, a signifi-

cant proportion of streptococci isolated in Australia are nontypeable [41]. Recent studies have begun to answer the question of how many new serotypes may be represented in the nontypeable collection from a given geographic area [42]. A significant percentage of the strains associated with rheumatic fever in Northern Australia appear to belong to the M5 family of M proteins [41]. Future studies may show that the number of distinct serotypes represented by the nontypeable organisms is limited. Therefore, vaccine efficacy may be improved significantly by including these M protein structures in multivalent vaccines.

Although future studies in the laboratory will address questions related to strain variation of M proteins and the absolute number of distinct serotypes within the nontypeable strains, ultimate determinations of efficacy will depend on large-scale clinical trials and prospective surveillance. Long-term efficacy may also rely on ongoing epidemiologic studies to identify serotypes not represented in multivalent vaccines that may enter the immunized population under the influence of vaccine-induced, type-specific antibodies. It may be necessary to reformulate vaccine constructs periodically to represent serotypes that become prevalent or cause serious disease in the future. Although there remain some important issues related to the potential efficacy of streptococcal M protein vaccines, the approaches outlined in this chapter may lead to safe and effective vaccines that will prevent a significant proportion of these infections. The most effective vaccines may be combinations that include multivalent, type-specific M protein epitopes and conserved epitopes that evoke broadly protective immune responses [42,43]. Such vaccines are not likely to prevent all group A streptococcal disease, but careful attention to the design of multivalent vaccines, possibly combined with broadly protective M protein epitopes, may have significant impact on the overall incidence of group A streptococcal infections.

These studies were supported by research funds from the Department of Veterans Affairs and from the U.S. Public Health Service, NIH grant AI-10085. The author thanks Edna Chiang for expert technical assistance and Drs. Harry Courtney and David Hasty for their critical review of the manuscript.

REFERENCES

1. Lancefield RC. Current knowledge of the type specific M antigens of group A streptococci. J Immunol 1962; 89:307–313.
2. Lancefield RC. Persistence of type-specific antibodies in man following infection with group A streptococci. J Exp Med 1959; 110:271–282.
3. Beachey EH, Campbell GL, Ofek I. Peptic digestion of streptococcal M protein. II. Extraction of M antigen from group A streptococci with pepsin. Infect Immun 1974; 9:891–896.
4. Beachey EH, Seyer JM, Kang AH. Repeating covalent structure of streptococcal M protein. Proc Natl Acad Sci USA 1978; 75:3163–3167.
5. Beachey EH, Stollerman GH, Johnson RH, Ofek I, Bisno AL. Human immune response to immunization with a structurally defined polypeptide fragment of streptococcal M protein. J Exp Med 1979; 150:862–877.
6. Dale JB, Beachey EH. Protective antigenic determinant of streptococcal M protein shared with sarcolemmal membrane protein of human heart. J Exp Med 1982; 156:1165–1176.
7. Dale JB, Beachey EH. Multiple heart-cross-reactive epitopes of streptococcal M proteins. J Exp Med 1985; 161:113–122.
8. Hollingshead SK, Fischetti VA, Scott JR. Complete nucleotide sequence of type 6 M protein of the group A streptococcus. Repetitive structure and membrane anchor. J Biol Chem 1986; 261:1677–1686.
9. Manjula BN, Seetharma-Acharya A, Mische SM, Fairwell T, Fischetti VA. The complete amino acid sequence of a biologically active 197-residue fragment of M protein isolated from type 5 group A streptococci. J Biol Chem 1984; 259:3686–3693.
10. Miller L, Gray L, Beachey EH, Kehoe M. Antigenic variation among group A streptococcal M proteins: nucleotide sequence of the serotype 5 M protein gene and its relationship with genes encoding types 1, 6 and 24 M proteins. J Biol Chem 1988; 263:5668–5673.
11. Mouw AR, Beachey EH, Burdett V. Molecular evolution of streptococcal M protein: cloning and nucleotide sequence of the type 24 M protein gene and relation to other genes of *Streptococcus pyogenes*. J Bacteriol 1988; 170:676–684.
12. Phillips GN, Flicker PF, Cohen C, Manjula BN, Fischetti VA. Streptococcal M protein: alpha-helical coiled-coil structure and arrangement on the cell surface. Proc Natl Acad Sci USA 1981; 78:4689–4693.
13. Dale JB, Seyer JM, Beachey EH. Type-specific immunogenicity of a chemically synthesized peptide fragment of type 5 streptococcal M protein. J Exp Med 1983; 158:1727–1732.
14. Beachey EH, Seyer JM. Protective and nonprotective epitopes of chemically synthesized peptides of the NH_2-terminal region of type 6 streptococcal M protein. J Immunol 1986; 136:2287–2292.
15. Beachey EH, Bronze MS, Dale JB, Kraus W, Poirier TP, Sargent SJ. Protective and autoimmune epitopes of streptococcal M protein vaccine. Vaccine 1988; 6:192–196.
16. Kraus W, Ohyama K, Snyder DS, Beachey EH. Autoimmune sequence of streptococcal M protein shared with the intermediate filament protein, vimentin. J Exp Med 1989; 169:481–492.
17. Kraus W, Dale JB, Beachey EH. Identification of an epitope of type 1 streptococcal M protein that is shared with a 43-kD protein of human myocardium and renal glomeruli. J Immunol 1990; 145:4089–4093.
18. Bronze MS, Beachey EH, Dale JB. Protective and heart-crossreactive epitopes located within the NH_2-terminus of type 19 streptococcal M protein. J Exp Med 1988; 167:1849–1859.
19. Dale JB, Chiang EY, Lederer JW. Recombinant tetravalent group A streptococcal M protein vaccine. J Immunol 1993; 151:2188–2194.
20. Dale JB, Beachey EH. Epitopes of streptococcal M proteins shared with cardiac myosin. J Exp Med 1985; 162:583–591.
21. Dale JB, Beachey EH. Sequence of myosin-crossreactive epitopes of streptococcal M protein. J Exp Med 1986; 164:1785–1790.
22. Sargent SJ, Beachey EH, Corbett CE, Dale JB. Sequence of protective epitopes of streptococcal M proteins shared with cardiac sarcolemmal membranes. J Immunol 1987; 139:1285–1290.
23. Cunningham MW, Russell SM. Study of heart-reactive antibody in antisera and hybridoma culture fluids against group A streptococci. Infect Immun 1983; 42:531–538.
24. Cunningham MW, Swerlick RA. Polyspecificity of antistreptococcal murine monoclonal antibodies and their implications in autoimmunity. J Exp Med 1986; 164:988–1012.
25. Cuningham MW, McCormack JM, Fenderson PG, Ho MK, Beachey EH, Dale JB. Human and murine antibodies cross-reactive with streptococcal M protein and myosin recognize the sequence GLN-LYS-SER-LYS-GLN in M protein. J Immunol 1989; 143:2677.
26. Krisher K, Cunningham MW. Myosin: a link between streptococci and heart. Science 1985; 227:413–415.
27. Baird RW, Bronze MS, Kraus W, Hill HR, Veasey LG, Dale JB. Epitopes of group A streptococcal M protein shared with antigens of articular cartilage and synovium. J Immunol 1991; 146:3132–3137.
28. Bronze MS, Dale JB. Epitopes of streptococcal M proteins that evoke antibodies that cross-react with human brain. J Immunol 1993; 151:2820–2828.
29. Fischetti VA. Streptococcal M protein: molecular design and biological behavior. Clin Microbiol Rev 1989; 2:285.

30. Dale JB, Simmons M, Chiang EC, Chiang EY. Recombinant, octavalent group A streptococcal M protein vaccine. Vaccine 1996; 14:944–948.

31. Beachey EH, Seyer JM, Dale JB. Protective immunogenicity and T lymphocyte specificity of a trivalent hybrid peptide containing NH2-terminal sequences of types 5, 6 and 24 M proteins synthesized in tandem. J Exp Med 1987; 166:647–656.

32. Jones KF, Fischetti VA. The importance of the location of antibody binding on the M6 protein for opsonization and phagocytosis of group A M6 streptococci. J Exp Med 1988; 167:1114–1123.

33. Dale JB. Multivalent group A streptococcal vaccine designed to optimize the immunogenicity of six tandem M protein fragments. Vaccine 1999; 17:193–200.

34. Dale JB, Chiang EC. Intranasal immunization with recombinant group a streptococcal M protein fragment fused to the B subunit of *Escherichia coli* labile toxin protects mice against systemic challenge infections. J Infect Dis 1995; 171:1038–1041.

35. Bisno AL. The concept of rheumatogenic and nonrheumatogenic group A streptococci. In: Reed SE, Zabriskie JB (eds). Streptococcal Diseases and the Immune Response. New York: Academic Press, 1980; 789–803.

36. Johnson DR, Stevens DL, Kaplan EL. Epidemiologic analysis of group A streptococcal serotypes associated with severe systemic infections, rheumatic fever, or uncomplicated pharyngitis. J Infect Dis 1992; 166:374.

37. Musser JM, Kapur V, Szeto J, Pan X, Swanson DS, Martin DR. Genetic diversity and relationships among Streptococcus pyogenes strains expressing serotype M1 protein: recent intercontinental spread of a subclone causing epidoes of invasive disease. Infect Immun 1995; 63:994.

38. Harbaugh MP, Podbielski A, Hugh S, Cleary PP. Nucleotide substitution and small-scale insertion produce size and antigenic variation in group A streptococcal M1 protein. Mol Microbiol 1993; 8:981.

39. Dale JB, Beachey EH. Localization of protective epitopes of the amino terminus of type 5 streptococcal M protein. J Exp Med 1986; 163:1191–1202.

40. Kaplan EL, Johnson DR. Nanthapisud P, Sirilertpomrana S, Chumdermpadetsuk S. A comparison of group A streptococcal serotypes isolated from the upper respiratory tract in the USA and Thailand: implications. Bull World Health Organ 1992; 70:433.

41. Hartas J, Goodfellow AM, Currie BS, Sriprakash KS. Characterization of group A streptococcal isolates from tropical Australia with high prevalence of rheumatic fever: probing for signature sequences to identify members of the family of serotype 5. Microb Pathog 1995; 18:345–354.

42. Bronze MS, Courtney HS, Dale JB. Epitopes of group A streptococcal M protein that evoke cross-protective local immune responses. J Immunol 1992; 148:888–893.

43. Bessen D, Fischetti VA. Influence of intranasal immunization with synthetic peptides corresponding to conserved epitopes of M protein on mucosal colonization by group A streptococci. Infect Immun 1988; 56:2666–2672.

21

Group B Streptococcal Vaccines

MICHAEL R. WESSELS
DENNIS L. KASPER

With the virtual eradication of serious *Hemophilus influenzae* disease following the introduction of effective polysaccharide–protein conjugate vaccines, group B streptococcus (GBS) has become the most common cause of fatal bacterial infection among infants and young children in the United States and other developed countries. The attack rate for invasive neonatal GBS infection is estimated at 1 to 2 cases per 1000 live births, or approximately 8000 cases annually in the United States. Group B streptococcus is one of the few major bacterial infections of childhood for which no vaccine is commercially available. Yet, evidence is accumulating that GBS infection is a vaccine-preventable disease. In light of recent progress in GBS vaccine development, it appears that the technology is now available to produce an immunogenic and broadly protective vaccine to prevent neonatal and maternal GBS infections. A similar number of serious GBS infections is estimated to occur among nonpregnant adults, primarily those with diabetes, cancer, and other chronic illnesses. Whether a vaccine may be useful to prevent GBS infections among particular high-risk groups in the nonpregnant adult population remains to be determined.

IMMUNITY TO GROUP B STREPTOCOCCUS

The GBS, like other gram-positive organisms, are resistant to direct complement-mediated lysis in serum. Therefore, immune defense against GBS, particularly after the organisms gain access to the bloodstream, depends upon effective ingestion and killing by phagocytic leukocytes. Evidence from in vitro assays of phagocytosis and from in vivo studies in experimental animals has demonstrated an essential role for serum complement in opsonophagocytosis of GBS and in host defense in vivo. Heat-inactivation of human sera containing GBS antibodies abrogated the ability of these sera to opsonize type III GBS for killing by blood leukocytes, indicating that complement was required for effective antibody-mediated opsonophagocytosis [1]. The same conclusion was supported by studies showing that an immunoglobulin M (IgM) monoclonal antibody to type III GBS capsular polysaccharide failed to protect rats from GBS challenge if the animals were first depleted of C3 by treatment with cobra venom factor [2]. Edwards and coworkers showed that the sialic acid–rich capsule of type III GBS inhibited activation of the alternative complement pathway, whereas organisms from which sialic acid was removed by treatment with neuraminidase activated the alternative pathway, resulting in deposition of opsonically active C3 on the bacterial surface. These observations were supported by subsequent studies showing that alternative pathway–mediated deposition of C3 on type III GBS was inversely related to the amount of capsular polysaccharide on the bacterial surface—large amounts of C3 were bound to poorly encapsulated strains, whereas highly encapsulated strains bound little [3]. Studies of genetically manipulated strains of type III GBS demonstrated a striking reduction in animal virulence of mutants expressing either no capsule or capsule lacking sialic acid [4–7]. These results confirmed that capsular sialic acid not only regulated complement activation in vitro but was critical to virulence of the organisms in experimental infection.

Although the GBS type III capsular polysaccharide inhibits alternative pathway complement activation, this inhibition can be overcome by specific antibodies. Human sera containing antibodies to the type III capsular polysaccharide effectively opsonize type III GBS for killing by human blood leukocytes and protect mice against lethal GBS infection [8,9]. The relevance of these observations for human immunity was supported by the finding that infants with type III GBS sepsis had low or undetectable levels of type III polysaccharide–specific antibodies [10,11]. Taken together, this body of experimental and epidemiologic evidence strongly suggests that, in the setting of an immunocompetent host, antibodies to the GBS capsular polysaccharide confer protective immunity.

RATIONALE FOR A GROUP B STREPTOCOCCAL VACCINE

Development of a vaccine to prevent GBS infection is an appealing approach for several reasons. The first is the abundance of experimental and clinical evidence that specific antibodies are protective. Second, a target population at high risk of infection is well defined: pregnant women and their newborn infants. Third, because maternal IgG crosses the placenta during the third trimester of pregnancy, a maternal GBS vaccine given before or during pregnancy could confer immunity to peripartum maternal infection as well as passive immunity to the newborn during the period of highest risk for neonatal infection. Finally, although intrapartum chemoprophylaxis of high-risk GBS carriers has been shown to reduce the risk of infant infection, large-scale implementation of a chemoprophylaxis program has been hampered by uncertainty over the best screening and prophylaxis

methods as well as concern about overuse of antibiotics with resultant allergic reactions and the potential for selection of resistant flora. Two strategies for selective intrapartum chemoprophylaxis have been proposed by the Centers for Disease Control and Prevention and endorsed by the American College of Obstetrics and Gynecology and the American Academy of Pediatrics; however, chemoprophylaxis is viewed as an interim measure to reduce the incidence of early-onset GBS disease, rather than a final solution [12]. A cost-benefit analysis comparing various chemoprophylaxis strategies with a hypothetical maternal vaccine concluded that a moderately immunogenic vaccine could save more lives at lower cost than any of the proposed chemoprophylaxis regimes [13].

CANDIDATE GROUP B STREPTOCOCCAL ANTIGENS: GROUP B CARBOHYDRATE

Rebecca Lancefield's studies in the 1930s to classify beta-hemolytic streptococci identified an acid-extractable antigen that reacted with antisera raised to formalin-killed GBS organisms. This group B antigen was later shown to be a complex carbohydrate associated with the cell wall of all GBS strains. The group B carbohydrate is composed of rhamnose as the predominant sugar, as well as N-acetylglucosamine, galactose, and glucitol. It extends from the cell wall in a tetra-antennary array with immunodominant $\alpha(1 \rightarrow 2)$linked rhamnose trisaccharides at the terminus of each saccharide chain [14,15]. Because the group B carbohydrate is common to all strains of GBS, it is an appealing candidate antigen for a vaccine. However, Lancefield found that antisera raised in rabbits against whole GBS organisms protected mice only against challenge with GBS of the same capsular type, leading her to conclude that antibodies to the capsular polysaccharide were protective, whereas those to the common group B antigen were not [16]. The potential utility of group B antigen in a vaccine was raised again in studies by Raff and co-workers, who found that human IgM monoclonal antibodies to group B antigen had opsonic and animal-protective activity against multiple GBS serotypes [17,18].

The antibodies were protective in neonatal rats only in high doses and lost activity upon class-switching from IgM to IgG1. Marques et al. studied the functional activities of antibodies elicited in rabbits by a group B carbohydrate–protein conjugate vaccine. Although high levels of IgG class antibodies were elicited by the conjugate, the antibodies had minimal opsonic power in vitro or protective activity in a neonatal mouse infection model [19]. Taken together, these studies suggest that the group B carbohydrate will not be useful as a vaccine component.

CAPSULAR POLYSACCHARIDES

Immunochemistry

In addition to the group B antigen, Lancefield found that strains of GBS could be serotyped into subgroups based on antigenic differences in a type-specific carbohydrate antigen, distinct from the common group B antigen. The type-specific antigen has since been shown to represent a capsular polysaccharide located exterior to the cell wall (Fig. 21.1). More than 90%, and perhaps all, isolates of GBS associated with human infection express one of nine identified capsular polysaccharides, although many isolates of GBS from animal sources do not. Each of the identified capsular polysaccharides has been purified and the covalent repeating structure determined [20–27]. Each is a high molecular weight (MW) linear polymer made up of oligosaccharide repeating units. Although the sugar composition of the capsular polysaccharides is very similar, the precise arrangement of the component sugars varies, accounting for their antigenic distinctness (Fig. 21.2). Cross-reactions have been described for antibodies to the Ia or Ib polysaccharides, the two polysaccharides with the highest degree of structural relatedness [28,29]. A common feature of all the identified GBS capsular polysaccharides is the presence of short side chains with terminal residues of N-acetylneuraminic acid, or sialic acid.

Capsular types Ia, Ib, II, III, and V are the predominant serotypes associated with human colonization and disease [30–33]. Type III has been the single most common serotype in inva-

sive neonatal disease, although types Ia and V have also become relatively common in recent years. The antigenic properties of the type III polysaccharide have been studied in considerable detail. An early observation was that sialic acid residues of the type III polysaccharide were an important part of the epitope recognized by protective antibodies: in human sera, the concentration of antibodies directed to the native (sialylated) polysaccharide correlated with immunity to GBS infection, whereas the concentration of antibodies to the desialylated polysaccharide did not [8]. Desialylated type III polysaccharide gave a reaction of partial identity with the sialylated (native) polysaccharide in immunodiffusion reactions against GBS antiserum, indicating that the desialylated polysaccharide did not contain the complete native epitope [34]. An equivalent loss of antigenicity could be achieved by reduction of carboxyl groups of the sialic acid residues, rather than removal of sialic acid. Nuclear magnetic resonance (NMR) studies suggested that desialylation or reduction of the type III polysaccharide resulted in a change in the torsion angle of the side chain with respect to the backbone of the polysaccharide [35]. In other words, the charged sialic acid residues played an important role in controlling the conformation of the polysaccharide epitope recognized by protective antibodies. Interestingly, oxidation of the polysaccharide, a modification that removed carbons 8 and/or 9 from sialic acid, but left intact the carboxyl group, had no effect on antigenicity or conformation, as reflected in the NMR spectrum [35].

These immunologic and physicochemical studies established that sialic acid was a critical part of the epitope of the GBS type III polysaccharide. Although sialic acid was essential to the immunodeterminant, neither sialic acid itself nor sialylated oligosaccharides competed with the type III polysaccharide for binding to capsule-specific antibodies. Further insight into the nature of the type III polysaccharide epitope came from studies examining binding of polysaccharide-specific antibodies to oligosaccharides derived from the type III polysaccharide—in this context, the term "oligosaccharide" is used to denote any saccharides of smaller molecular size than the native polysaccharide. Oligosaccharides consisting of one or more pen-

Surface antigens

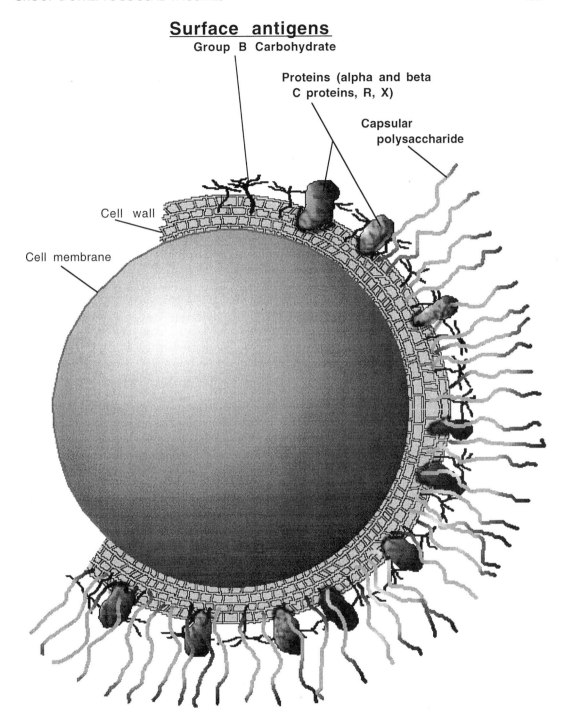

Figure 21.1 Schematic representation of surface antigens of group B Streptococcus that have been considered candidates for vaccine development (illustration courtesy of Tom DiCesare).

tasaccharide repeating units were derived from the type III polysaccharide by enzymatic digestion using an endo-β-galactosidase that cleaves the backbone of the polysaccharide once per repeating unit [22,36]. Binding studies using derivative oligosaccharides of various chain lengths showed that the overall affinity of antigen–antibody binding increased dramatically as the sac-

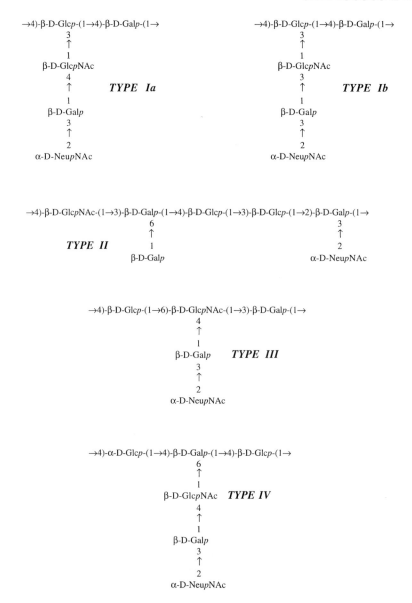

Figure 21.2 Repeating unit structures of group B streptococcal capsular polysaccharides [20–27].

charide size increased up to a molecular size of at least 100,000 [36]. This unexpected result was interpreted to mean that type III polysaccharide–specific antibodies recognize a conformational epitope that is optimally expressed only in high MW forms of the antigen. Since the repeating unit structure of the type III polysaccharide is very similar to the oligosaccharide component of certain mammalian glycoproteins, it may be that polysaccharide antibodies specific for a molecular size–dependent conformational

epitope are selected by a self-tolerance mechanism. In any case, antibodies to the type III polysaccharide from rabbit or human sources show minimal or no reaction with simple oligosaccharides such as those represented on eukaryotic cells or serum glycoproteins [36,37].

Capsular Polysaccharide Vaccines

Purified capsular polysaccharides of GBS types Ia, II, and III have been tested as immunogens

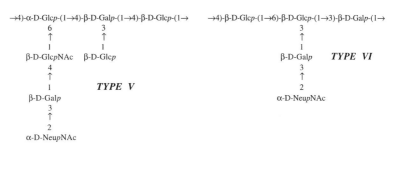

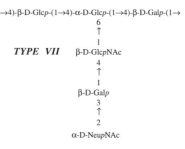

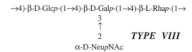

Figure 21.2 (continued).

in animals and human subjects. The immunogenicity in previously nonimmune humans varied from 40% for type Ia to 88% for type II [38–41]. Most subjects have low or undetectable levels of antibodies to GBS polysaccharides; virtually all subjects with pre-existing antibody responded to vaccination with an increase in specific antibody, whereas the responses among previously nonimmune subjects were much more variable. Baker et al. vaccinated a group of women with type III polysaccharide during the third trimester of pregnancy. The response rate was 63%, and the antibody levels in the infants, all of whom were healthy, were closely correlated to maternal levels [42]. This study demonstrated that maternal IgG antibodies were transported across the placenta, supporting the feasibility of maternal vaccination to prevent neonatal GBS infection, if immunogenicity of the vaccine could be improved.

POLYSACCHARIDE–PROTEIN CONJUGATE VACCINES

Group B Streptococcal Type III Polysaccharide–Protein Conjugate Vaccines

A major advance in GBS vaccine development occurred in 1990 with the publication of three reports describing experimental vaccines constructed by the covalent coupling of the type III GBS polysaccharide or a derivative oligosaccharide to a carrier protein [43–45]. Polysaccharides, in general, are considered T-independent antigens, a class of molecules that is less predictable in eliciting a brisk IgG class antibody response than T-dependent antigens such as most proteins. The general approach of conjugating a polysaccharide or oligosaccharide to a carrier protein is one that has been used to improve the immunogenicity of several bacterial polysaccharides, the most notable example being the type b capsular polysaccharide of *H. influenzae* [46]. Presumably, by recruiting T cell help, these semi-synthetic conjugate vaccines may enhance the antibody response to the polysaccharide component in several ways, including the ability to elicit a response in young infants, an increased amount of specific antibody with a predominance of IgG class antibodies, and an anamnestic or memory response to booster vaccinations.

Lagergard et al. prepared a GBS type III polysaccharide–protein conjugate by activating the polysaccharide with cyanogen bromide, then using adipic acid dihydrazide as a bifunctional spacer to link the activated polysaccharide to tetanus toxoid [43]. The polysaccharide–protein conjugate was more effective than polysaccharide alone in eliciting a polysaccharide-specific antibody response in mice. Furthermore, antibodies elicited by the conjugate were predominantly of the IgG isotype, while those elicited by polysaccharide alone were exclusively IgM.

Wessels et al. used a different approach to synthesize a GBS type III polysaccharide–protein conjugate [44]. To introduce sites for protein coupling, the GBS type III polysaccharide was chemically modified by controlled oxidation with sodium meta-periodate resulting in cleavage, between carbons 8 and 9, of approximately 25% of the sialic acid residues, and the introduction of an aldehyde group on carbon 8 of the modified residues. The newly created aldehyde functions served as sites for direct coupling to amino groups on tetanus toxoid in a reductive amination reaction in the presence of sodium cyanoborohydride (Fig. 21.3). A polysaccharide–protein conjugate of this design has a theoretical advantage over conjugates synthesized by random-site coupling methods such as cyanogen bromide activation: in contrast to random-site coupling methods, controlled periodate oxidation modifies the polysaccharide in a very specific and predictable way that is readily verifiable by GC-MS analysis. As a result, the nature of the polysaccharide–protein linkage is well defined and lot-to-lot variation in conjugate structure can be minimized. This general conjugate design, coupling a carrier protein to a partially oxidized polysaccharide by reductive amination, has proved to be of general utility in the development of GBS polysaccharide–protein conjugate vaccines (see below).

The type III polysaccharide–tetanus toxoid conjugate (III-TT) developed using this technology was first tested for immunogenicity in rabbits. This conjugate elicited type III polysaccharide–specific IgG class antibodies after a single dose with further increases after boosters [44]. Rabbits vaccinated with uncoupled type III GBS polysaccharide had no response. The antibodies evoked in rabbits were shown to opsonize type III GBS for killing by human peripheral blood leukocytes in an in vitro assay and protected mice against lethal challenge with type III GBS. These results provide evidence that the III-TT vaccine could elicit polysaccharide-specific antibodies that are opsonically active in vitro and that have protective activity in vivo.

Evidence from certain model systems has suggested that oligosaccharides or short-chain polysaccharides may be superior to a full-length polysaccharide as a component of a conjugate vaccine [47]. A lower MW carbohydrate hapten linked to a protein may result in closer proximity of B cell epitopes on the carbohydrate moiety to T cell epitopes on the protein and enhance T cell help. Oligosaccharide–protein conjugates based on the type III GBS polysaccharide were synthesized and tested by Paoletti et al. [45,48]. The oligosaccharides or short-chain polysaccharides were derived from GBS type III polysaccharide by partial enzymatic digestion with endo-β-galactosidase, as described above. Saccharides of three different molecular sizes were purified by gel filtration chromatography and coupled separately to tetanus toxoid to create conjugates of large (Mr ~27,000), medium (Mr ~14,500), and small (Mr ~7,000) molecule-size saccharides. These conjugates were constructed not by oxidation of sialic acid residues but by single-site coupling of the reducing end of the saccharide chain to a synthetic spacer molecule that was then coupled to tetanus toxoid in a second reductive amination reaction. All three oligosaccharide–TT conjugates were immunogenic in rabbits. Analysis of opsonic antibodies elicited by the vaccines demonstrated a higher proportion of IgG class antibodies in response to the short-chain conjugate with relatively more IgM for the long-chain conjugate. Antibodies evoked by the long-chain conjugate, however, exhibited a

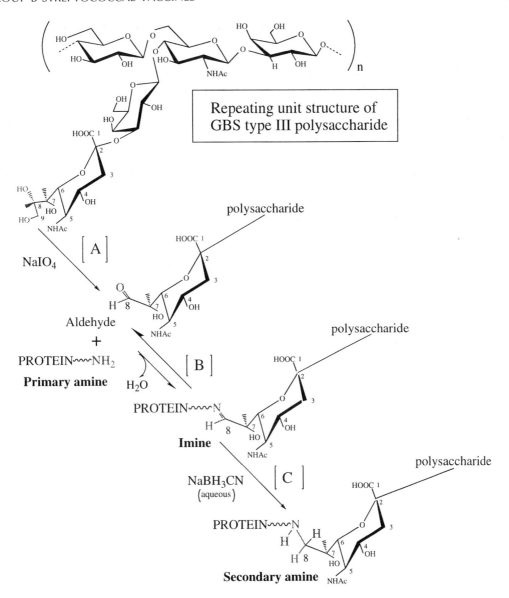

Figure 21.3 Reaction sequence in synthesis of group B streptococcal type III polysaccharide–tetanus toxoid conjugate vaccine. (*A*) Oxidation with sodium periodate cleaves carbon 9 from sialic acid and creates an aldehyde group on carbon 8; (*B*) the aldehyde on the modified sialic acid residue reacts with a primary amino group on the carrier protein to form an unstable imine bond; (*C*) reduction by sodium cyanoborohydride converts the imine to a secondary amine, resulting in a stable covalent bond between polysaccharide and protein. (From Kasper et al. [79], with permission.)

greater relative binding affinity for high MW type III polysaccharide relative to lower MW oligosaccharides. The intermediate size conjugate was the best immunogen with respect to eliciting protective antibodies, perhaps because it represents a size optimum of the opposing trends of T cell dependence (better with smaller saccharides) and expression of the polysaccharide's conformational epitope (better with large saccharides).

The GBS type III–TT polysaccharide–protein conjugate was more immunogenic than any of the type III oligosaccharide–protein conjugates. The III-TT conjugate may be a better immunogen because it binds the polysaccharide to the carrier protein at multiple sites, presumably creating a complex lattice of several polysaccharide and protein molecules, in contrast to the single-site attachment of the oligosaccharide conjugates. Both the approximation of multiple polysaccharide and protein epitopes as well as the formation of a higher MW complex may enhance immunogenicity. For these reasons, as well as relative technical simplicity, multi-site coupling via oxidized sialic acid residues is the approach that has been utilized for further GBS polysaccharide–protein conjugate vaccine development.

Polysaccharide–Protein Conjugate Vaccines for other Group B Streptococcal Serotypes

Because all the known GBS capsular polysaccharides have side chains with terminal residues of sialic acid, all are amenable to the same chemical modification used to create the III-TT conjugate. Using essentially the same technology, a GBS type Ia polysaccharide–tetanus toxoid conjugate (Ia-TT) was synthesized [49]. The Ia-TT vaccine utilized a GBS type Ia polysaccharide in which 10% of the sialic acid residues were modified by periodate oxidation. Antibodies elicited in rabbits by the Ia-TT vaccine were shown to bind not only to type Ia polysaccharide but also to the structurally related type Ib polysaccharide, albeit at 100-fold lower affinity. Despite the lower binding affinity for Ib polysaccharide, antibodies elicited by Ia-TT were shown to opsonize both type Ia and type Ib GBS for phagocytic killing in vitro and to confer protective immunity to both serotypes in a mouse maternal immunization/neonatal challenge model.

Group B streptococcal polysaccharide–tetanus toxoid conjugate vaccines of the same basic design have also been synthesized for serotypes Ib, II, and V [50–52]. All have been immunogenic in rabbits, eliciting predominantly IgG class antibodies that are opsonically active in vitro against organisms of homologous capsular type and are protective in vivo. To test the potential efficacy of a multivalent conjugate vaccine, two such combination conjugate vaccines were tested in the mouse maternal vaccination/neonatal challenge model [50]. Adult female mice received one dose

of vaccine before and a second dose after breeding. Their pups were challenged within 36 h of delivery with a lethal dose of type Ia, Ib, II, or III GBS. Pups born to dams vaccinated with a tetravalent vaccine were protected against challenge with each of the four vaccine serotypes, whereas control litters born to dams receiving a tetravalent polysaccharide vaccine or tetanus toxoid were not (Fig. 21.4). Interestingly, although rabbit antiserum to Ia-TT had shown functional activity against Ib GBS, a trivalent (Ia-TT, II-TT, III-TT) vaccine failed to protect against Ib challenge, presumably reflecting the lower binding affinity of Ia-TT-elicited antibodies for Ib polysaccharide [50]. These studies supported the possibility of maternal vaccination with a multivalent conjugate vaccine to protect neonates against multiple serotypes of GBS.

PROTEIN ANTIGENS

X and R Proteins

Several antigenically distinct proteins are variably expressed on the surface of GBS. Protein X is commonly present on bovine mastitis isolates of GBS, but is found rarely on human clinical isolates [53–55]. A protein designated R (for resistance to trypsin) was first described on certain strains of group A streptococci. An antigenically related protein (or proteins) was later discovered on some strains of streptococci in several other Lancefield groups, including group B. Some investigators have distinguished serologically several species of R proteins [56]. Flores and Ferrieri found R proteins on 37% of GBS clinical isolates, with the majority being of the R4 type [57]. Antiserum raised to R protein had protective activity in mice challenged with R protein–bearing type II GBS, suggesting a potential role for R proteins in immunity [58]. However, the same antiserum failed to protect against challenge with R protein–bearing type III GBS.

C Proteins

The GBS proteins that have received the most attention as potential vaccine components are the C proteins, formerly known as Ibc proteins

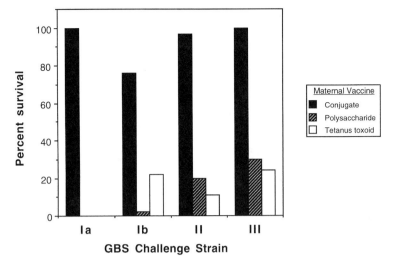

Figure 21.4 Protective efficacy of a tetravalent group B streptococcal polysaccharide–tetanus toxoid conjugate vaccine in a mouse maternal vaccination/neonatal challenge model. The graph shows survival of neonatal mice challenged with a lethal dose of type Ia, Ib, II, or III group B streptococci. These mice were born to dams vaccinated previously with a tetravalent conjugate vaccine containing type Ia, Ib, II, and III polysaccharides coupled to tetanus toxoid (conjugate), or with a tetravalent polysaccharide vaccine containing type Ia, Ib, II, and III polysaccharides (polysaccharide), or with tetanus toxoid. Maternal vaccination with the tetravalent conjugate vaccine protected pups against challenge with all four vaccine serotypes, but vaccination with the uncoupled polysaccharides or with tetanus toxoid alone did not. (From Paoletti et al. [50], with permission.)

[29,59]. Two distinct C proteins, alpha and beta, each encoded by a separate gene, are expressed singly or together in approximately 60% of GBS strains isolated from human sources [60,61]. Two other varieties of C proteins, gamma and delta, have been described, but not characterized extensively [62]. Both the alpha and beta C proteins have been cloned and expressed in *E. coli* [63,64]. Antibodies raised in rabbits to the recombinant proteins were shown to be opsonic and to protect mice against lethal challenge with GBS strains expressing the immunizing protein [64].

While both the alpha and beta C proteins can elicit protective immunity, the proteins differ in several interesting ways. The alpha c protein is resistant to trypsin, while the beta C protein is susceptible to trypsin digestion [59]. By PAGE and Western blot analysis, the beta C protein occurs as a single polypeptide of approximately 130 kDa, while the alpha C protein exhibits a distinctive ladder pattern, consisting of several regularly spaced protein bands [65–67]. Analysis of alpha C protein extracts from various GBS strains has shown, as well, that the apparent molecular size of the largest alpha C protein band

may vary from 62.5 to 167 kDa, depending on the strain examined [68]. The ladder pattern and variability in maximum size of the alpha protein are related to the presence within the alpha C protein gene of a series of identical repeated sequences, each consisting of 246 nucleotides (Fig. 21.5; [69]). Madoff and co-workers have shown that in at least two instances the alpha C protein expressed by a GBS isolate from an infant was smaller in size than the otherwise identical GBS isolate colonizing the infant's mother [70]. This observation suggests that the size of the alpha C protein expressed by a particular strain may change, presumably through recombination/deletion events involving the repeated sequences. Since truncated forms of the alpha C protein may not be recognized by antibodies to the full-length protein, such variations might be a mechanism through which the organism evades a protective immune response. These considerations raise a cautionary note in developing a vaccine based on the alpha C protein.

Because the C proteins are present on many GBS strains of various capsular types (with the notable exception of type III), they are appealing candidates for use as a carrier protein in a

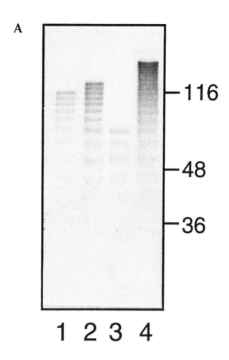

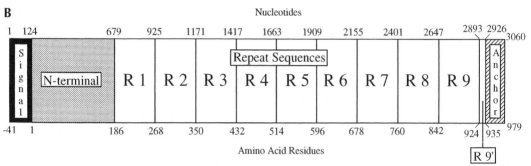

Figure 21.5 The alpha C protein and its structural gene. (*A*) Western immunoblot showing the characteristic "ladder" pattern of protein bands recognized by an alpha C protein–specific monoclonal antibody in protein extracts from four different alpha C protein–bearing strains of group B streptococcus. Molecular weight standards are indicated in kilodaltons on the right side of the figure. Both the ladder pattern and the variation among strains in molecular size of the largest protein band result from the presence within the protein of a variable number of tandem repeats, each consisting of 82 amino acids (photograph courtesy of L.C. Madoff). (*B*) Schematic diagram of the structure of the alpha C protein gene (*bca*). The gene consists of a signal sequence, unique amino terminal domain (N-terminal), a variable number of identical tandem repeats (R1–R9), and a short carboxy-terminal domain including a typical cell wall anchor consensus motif (anchor). (From Michel et al. [69], with permission.)

GBS polysaccharide–protein conjugate vaccine. Such a conjugate was synthesized by Madoff et al., using the beta C protein as a carrier and coupling to it the type III polysaccharide by the method described above for preparation of GBS polysaccharide–tetanus toxoid conjugates [71]. The III-beta conjugate elicited in rabbits antibodies to both components of the vaccine, and the antiserum was opsonically active against both type III and beta C protein–bearing strains. Pups born to vaccinated female mice were protected against lethal challenge with either type III or type Ia/c (beta C protein–expressing) organisms. A limitation to the potential utility of the beta C protein as a vaccine component is the limited number of disease isolates expressing this protein (approximately 10%). Another potential concern is the capacity of the beta C protein to bind human IgA [72]. The consequences of IgA binding are not known, but it has been suggested to represent a virulence mechanism for the organism. Variants of the beta C protein have been described that lack IgA-binding activity, suggesting it might be possible to utilize a naturally occurring variant or genetically engineered form of the antigen to circumvent this issue [73]. Also, binding of human serum IgA to the beta C protein was markedly reduced after coupling the protein to the type III GBS polysaccharide [71].

Other Group B Streptococcal Surface Proteins

A protein antigenically distinct from the alpha and beta C proteins has been identified in a high proportion of type III GBS, although it appears to be uncommon on non–type III isolates. The protein, designated Rib by Stalhammer-Carlemalm et al., exhibited a ladder pattern on Western blot, similar to the alpha C protein [74]. In addition, like the alpha C proteins, protein Rib is resistant to trypsin. Comparison of the nucleotide sequence of the gene encoding Rib with that of the alpha C protein gene revealed substantial similarity in predicted amino acid sequence and overall protein structure, although the two proteins are not immunologically cross-reactive. Like the alpha C protein, the Rib protein contains identical tandem repeat elements that share 47% amino acid residue identity with the repeat sequences of the alpha C protein [75]. Antibodies to protein Rib protected mice against lethal challenge with Rib-bearing GBS strains, suggesting the protein may be a candidate for vaccine development. Protein Rib may be identical or closely related to the R4 protein described earlier. It is not clear, however, why earlier mouse-protection studies failed to demonstrate activity of R4 antiserum against R4-bearing type III GBS if R4 and Rib are the same protein [58].

Lachenauer and Madoff purified a trypsin-resistant, surface protein from type V GBS that exhibited a ladder-like pattern on SDS-PAGE and Western immunoblots, similar to that of the alpha C protein and protein Rib [76]. The protein, which was detected on 61% of type V strains, was cross-reactive with antibodies to alpha C protein, and had a nearly identical N-terminal amino acid sequence to that of alpha. Antibodies to the type V protein had protective activity in a neonatal mouse model of GBS infection. The similarities between the alpha C protein, Rib, and the type V protein suggest that they may be members of a family of GBS surface proteins with similar structure and function. Antibodies to all three of these proteins have been shown to have protective activity; however, the usefulness as candidate vaccine antigens may be mitigated by the potential for variation in antigenic structure mediated by deletion of their repeat elements, as noted above for the alpha C protein.

HUMAN TESTING OF POLYSACCHARIDE-PROTEIN CONJUGATE VACCINES

The first GBS polysaccharide–protein conjugate vaccine to be tested in human subjects was a III-TT conjugate. The vaccine was prepared by coupling partially oxidized type III polysaccharide to tetanus toxoid by reductive amination, as described above. In phase I and phase II testing of the vaccine, women from 18 to 40 years of age were vaccinated with a single intramuscular (i.m.) injection of III-TT vaccine at one of three doses. The vaccine was well tolerated with minimal side effects. Evaluation of antibody responses at 8 weeks after vaccination demonstrated a ≥4-fold rise in polysaccharide-specific IgG levels in 90% of III-TT recipients, compared to 50% of recipients of uncoupled polysaccharide [77]. The vaccine-induced antibodies were predominantly of the IgG2 subclass. They were opsonic for type III GBS in an in vitro assay of opsonophagocytic killing by human blood leukocytes and had protective activity in a passive maternal immunization/neonatal challenge model in mice. Antibodies evoked by III-TT had similar affinity for type III GBS polysaccharide and similar specificity for the polysaccharide chain length–dependent conformational epitope as those evoked by uncoupled polysaccharide.

Polysaccharide–protein conjugate vaccines for human use have also been prepared for serotypes

Ia, Ib, II, and V. Each of the four polysaccharides has been coupled to tetanus toxoid and the type V polysaccharide has been coupled to CRM197, a nontoxic derivative of diphtheria toxin. Results of initial phase I and II testing suggest that these GBS polysaccharide–protein conjugate vaccines, like III-TT, are safe and highly immunogenic [78–80].

DIRECTIONS FOR FUTURE RESEARCH

Extensive testing in animals and results of phase I and II trials in humans suggest that a multivalent polysaccharide–protein conjugate vaccine will provide a safe and efficacious means to elicit protective antibodies in women and, by placental transfer, in their newborn infants. However, many basic questions about the optimal design and implementation of such a vaccine remain unanswered. One important issue is the choice of serotypes covered by such a vaccine. According to data gathered in the United States over the past decade, serotypes Ia, Ib, II, III, and V account for at least 95% of invasive GBS disease, both in neonates and adults. The relative prevalence of particular serotypes today has changed somewhat since several hospital-based surveys in the 1970s; in particular, serotype V, which accounted for <5%–10% of disease isolates in the 1970s, now represents the third-most common serotype among neonatal disease isolates. Shifts in the serotype distribution of GBS in the future may dictate reformulation of a multivalent vaccine.

Choice of a carrier protein is another aspect of vaccine design that may require modification. Tetanus toxoid is an appealing carrier for several reasons: it is acceptable for use during pregnancy, pre-existing immunity in most subjects may enhance T cell help in the immune response to the polysaccharide component, and prototype GBS polysaccharide–tetanus toxoid conjugates have already been synthesized and tested. However, as the number of GBS polysaccharide–protein conjugates increases in a multivalent vaccine, the total dose of tetanus toxoid may become high enough to increase side effects or to suppress the immune response. Alternative carriers for some or all of the component polysaccharides might be an unrelated protein (such

as diphtheria toxoid) or a GBS protein, such as the alpha or beta C proteins. A GBS protein would have the additional theoretical advantage of eliciting antibodies against an additional GBS antigen, resulting in broader protective efficacy and, perhaps, increased opsonic activity against strains bearing both polysaccharide and protein antigens.

It remains to be determined how such a vaccine should be used clinically. The primary target population is child-bearing women. Various approaches have been suggested to reach this population group, including administration of a GBS vaccine as part of a vaccine package to be given to adolescent or pre-adolescent girls, or as part of an initial or early visit for routine gynecologic care. An appealing alternative strategy is target the vaccine specifically to pregnant women. The kinetics of the human antibody response to III-TT suggest that maximum antibody levels are achieved within 2 weeks of vaccination, so the vaccine could be given as late as the third trimester and still produce protective levels in the fetus before delivery. The target population is well defined and more likely to seek medical care than nonpregnant healthy women. Finally, since the duration of the antibody response is not yet defined, vaccination during pregnancy would ensure adequate antibody levels at delivery. It remains to be determined whether booster vaccinations would be required for subsequent pregnancies, and at what intervals.

It is likely, although unproven, that a GBS vaccine also would provide a significant level of protection to pregnant women against GBS bacteremia, chorioamnionitis, and postpartum endometritis. Whether such a vaccine could protect nonpregnant adults with diabetes mellitus, cancer, or other chronic illnesses against invasive GBS infections is not known. Further research is needed to define the factors that govern susceptibility to GBS infection among adults, and the potential utility of a vaccine in these populations.

We thank all the investigators who have contributed to the work summarized in this chapter. We are especially indebted to Harold Jennings, Carol Baker, Lawrence Paoletti, and Lawrence Madoff for their contributions to group B streptococcal vaccine research and for insightful discussions that helped us to formulate this chapter. Research reviewed in this chapter was supported in part by NIH grants AI23339, AI28040, and AI30628 and by NIH contract AI25152.

REFERENCES

1. Edwards MS, Nicholson-Weller A, Baker CJ, Kasper DL. The role of specific antibody in alternative pathway-mediated opsonophagocytosis of type III, group B *Streptococcus*. J Exp Med 1980; 151:1275–1287.

2. Shigeoka AO, Pincus SH, Rote NS, Hill HR. Protective efficacy of hybridoma type specific antibody against experimental infection with group B *Streptococcus*. J Infect Dis 1984; 149:363–372.

3. Marques MB, Kasper DL, Pangburn MK, Wessels MR. Prevention of C3 deposition is a virulence mechanism of type III group B *Streptococcus* capsular polysaccharide. Infect Immun 1992; 60:3986–3993.

4. Rubens CE, Wessels MR, Heggen LM, Kasper DL. Transposon mutagenesis of group B streptococcal type III capsular polysaccharide: correlation of capsule expression with virulence. Proc Natl Acad Sci USA 1987; 84:7208–7212.

5. Rubens CE, Heggen LM, Haft RF, Wessels MR. Identification of *cpsD*, a gene essential for type III capsule expression in group B streptococci. Mol Microbiol 1993; 8:843–855.

6. Wessels MR, Rubens CE, Benedi V-J, Kasper DL. Definition of a bacterial virulence factor: sialylation of the group B streptococcal capsule. Proc Natl Acad Sci USA 1989; 86:8983–8987.

7. Wessels MR, Haft RF, Heggen LM, Rubens CE. Identification of a genetic locus essential for capsule sialylation in type III group B streptococci. Infect Immun 1992; 60:392–400.

8. Kasper DL, Baker CJ, Baltimore RS, Crabb JH, Schiffman G, Jennings HJ. Immunodeterminant specificity of human immunity to type III group B *Streptococcus*. J Exp Med 1979; 149:327–339.

9. Baltimore RS, Baker CJ, Kasper DL. Antibody to group B *Streptococcus* type III in human sera measured by a mouse protection test. Infect Immun 1981; 32:56–61.

10. Baker CJ, Kasper DL. Correlation of maternal antibody deficiency with susceptibility to neonatal group B streptococcal infection. N Engl J Med 1976; 294:753–756.

11. Baker CJ, Edwards MS, Kasper DL. Role of antibody to native type III polysaccharide of group B *Streptococcus* in infant infection. Pediatrics 1981; 68:544–549.

12. CDC. Prevention of perinatal group B streptococcal disease: a public health perspective. MMWR Morb Mortal Wkly Rep 1996; 45 (RR-7):1–25.

13. Mohle-Boetani JC, Schuchat A, Plikaytis BD, Smith JD, Broome CV. Comparison of prevention strategies for neonatal group B streptococcal

14. Michon F, Brisson JR, Dell A, Kasper DL, Jennings HJ. Multiantennary group-specific polysaccharide of group B *Streptococcus*. Biochemistry 1988; 27:5341–5351.

15. Michon F, Chalifour R, Feldman R, Wessels M, Kasper DL, Gamian A, Pozsgay V, Jennings HJ. The α-L-(12)-trirhamnopyranoside epitope on the group-specific polysaccharide of group B streptococci. Infect Immun 1991; 59:1690–1696.

16. Lancefield RC. Antigens of group B streptococci in relation to mouse-protective antibodies and immunity. In: Robbins J, et al (eds). New Approaches for Inducing Natural Immunity to Pyogenic Organisms. Bethesda, MD: NIH, 1975; 145–151.

17. Raff HV, Siscoe PJ, Wolff EA, Maloney G, Shuford W. Human monoclonal antibodies to group B streptococcus. J Exp Med 1988; 168:905–917.

18. Raff HV, Bradley C, Brady W, Donaldson K, Lipsich L, Maloney G, Shuford W, Walls M, Ward P, Wolff E, Harris LJ. Comparison of functional activities between IgG1 and IgM class-switched human monoclonal antibodies reactive with group B streptococci or Escherichia coli K1. J Infect Dis 1991; 163:346–354.

19. Marques MB, Kasper DL, Shroff A, Michon F, Jennings HJ, Wessels MR. Functional activity of antibodies to the group B polysaccharide of group B streptococci elicited by a polysaccharide-protein conjugate vaccine. Infect Immun 1994; 62:1593–1599.

20. Jennings HJ, Katzenellenbogen E, Lugowski C, Kasper DL. Structure of the native polysaccharide antigens of type Ia and type Ib group B *Streptococcus*. Biochemistry 1983; 22:1258–1263.

21. Jennings HJ, Rosell K-G, Katzenellenbogen E, Kasper DL. Structural determination of the capsular polysaccharide antigen of type II group B streptococcus. J Biol Chem 1983; 258:1793–1798.

22. Wessels MR, Pozsgay V, Kasper DL, Jennings HJ. Structure and immunochemistry of an oligosaccharide repeating unit of the capsular polysaccharide of type III group B *Streptococcus*. J Biol Chem 1987; 262:8262–8267.

23. DiFabio JL, Michon F, Brisson J-R, Jennings HJ, Wessels MR, Benedí V-J, Kasper DL. Structure of the capsular polysaccharide antigen of type IV group B *Streptococcus*. Can J Chem 1989; 67:877–882.

24. Wessels MR, DiFabio JL, Benedi V-J, Kasper DL, Michon F, Brisson J-R, Jelinkova J, Jennings HJ. Structural determination and immunochemical characterization of the type V group B *Streptococcus* capsular polysaccharide. J Biol Chem 1991; 266:6714–6719.

25. Kogan G, Uhrin D, Brisson J-R, Paoletti LC, Kasper DL, von Hunolstein C, Orefici G, Jennings HJ. Structure of the type VI group B *Streptococcus* capsular polysaccharide determined by

high resolution NMR spectroscopy. J Carbohydr Chem 1994; 13:1071–1078.

26. Kogan G, Brisson J-R, Kasper DL, von Hunolstein C, Orefici G, Jennings HJ. Structure of the novel type VII group B *Streptococcus* capsular polysaccharide by high resolution NMR spectroscopy. Carbohydr Res 1995; 277:1–9.

27. Kogan G, Uhrin D, Brisson J-R, Paoletti LC, Blodgett AE, Kasper DL, Jennings HJ. Structural and immunochemical characterization of the type VIII group B *Streptococcus* capsular polysaccharide. J. Biol. Chem. 1996; 271:8786–8790.

28. Schifferle RE, Jennings HJ, Wessels MR, Katzenellenbogen E, Roy R, Kasper DL. Immunochemical analysis of the types Ia and Ib group B streptococcal polysaccharides. J Immunol 1985; 135:4164–4170.

29. Lancefield RC, McCarty M, Everly WN. Multiple mouse-protective antibodies directed against group B streptococci. Special reference to antibodies effective against protein antigens. J Exp Med 1975; 142:165–179.

30. Dillon HC Jr, Khare S, Gray BM. Group B streptococcal carriage and disease: a 6-year prospective study. J Pediatr 1987; 110:31–36.

31. Wenger JD, Hightower AW, Facklam RR, Gaventa S, Broome CV. Bacterial meningitis in the United States, 1986: Report of a multistate surveillance study. J Infect Dis 1990; 162:1316–1323.

32. Blumberg HM, Stephens DS, Modansky M, Erwin M, Elliott J, Facklam RR, Schuchat A, Baughman W, Farley MM. Invasive group B streptococcal disease: the emergence of serotype V. J Infect Dis 1996; 173:365–373.

33. Harrison LH, Elliott JA, Dwyer DM, et al. Serotype distribution of invasive group B streptococcal isolates in Maryland: implications for vaccine development. J. Infect. Dis. 1998; 177: 998–1002.

34. Jennings HJ, Rosell K-G, Kasper DL. Structural determination and serology of the native polysaccharide antigen of type-III group B streptococcus. Can J Biochem 1980; 58:112–120.

35. Jennings HJ, Lugowski C, Kasper DL. Conformational aspects critical to the immunospecificity of the type III group B streptococcal polysaccharide. Biochemistry 1981; 20:4511–4518.

36. Wessels MR, Munoz A, Kasper DL. A model of high-affinity antibody binding to type III group B Streptococcus capsular polysaccharide. Proc Natl Acad Sci USA 1987; 84:9170–9174.

37. Hayrinen J, Pelkonen S, Finne J. Structural similarity of the type-specific group B streptococcal polysaccharides and the carbohydrate units of tissue glycoproteins: evaluation of possible cross-reactivity. Vaccine 1989; 7:217–224.

38. Baker CJ, Edwards MS, Kasper DL. Immunogenicity of polysaccharides from type III, group B *Streptococcus*. J Clin Invest 1978; 61:1107–1110.

39. Kasper L, Baker CJ, Galdes B, Katzenellenbogen E, Jennings HJ. Immunochemical analysis and immunogenicity of the type II group B streptococcal capsular polysaccharide. J Clin Invest 1983; 72:260–269.

40. Eisenstein TK, De Cueninck BJ, Resavy D, Shockman GD, Carey RB, Swenson RM. Quantitative determination in human sera of vaccine-induced antibody to type-specific polysaccharides of group B streptococci using an enzyme-linked immunosorbent assay. J Infect Dis 1983; 147:847–856.

41. Baker CJ, Kasper DL. Group B streptococcal vaccines. Rev Infect Dis 1985; 7:458–467.

42. Baker CJ, Rench MA, Edwards MS, Carpenter RJ, Hays BM, Kasper DL. Immunization of pregnant women with a polysaccharide vaccine of group B *Streptococcus*. N Engl J Med 1988; 319:1180–1185.

43. Lagergard T, Shiloach J, Robbins JB, Schneerson R. Synthesis and immunological properties of conjugates composed of group B streptococcus type III capsular polysaccharide covalently bound to tetanus toxoid. Infect Immun 1990; 58:687–694.

44. Wessels MR, Paoletti LC, Kasper DL, DiFabio JL, Michon F, Holme K, Jennings HJ. Immunogenicity in animals of a polysaccharide–protein conjugate vaccine against type III group B *Streptococcus*. J Clin Invest 1990; 86:1428–1433.

45. Paoletti LC, Kasper DL, Michon F, DiFabio JL, Holme K, Jennings HJ. An oligosaccharide-tetanus toxoid conjugate vaccine against type III group B *Streptococcus*. J Biol Chem 1990; 265:18278–18283.

46. Dick WE Jr, Beurret M. Glycoconjugates of bacterial carbohydrate antigens. In: Cruse JM, Lewis RE Jr (eds.) Conjugate Vaccines, Vol. 10. Basel: Karger, 1989; 48–114.

47. Seppala I, Makela O. Antigenicity of dextran-protein conjugates in mice. Effect of molecular weight of the carbohydrate and comparison of two modes of coupling. J Immunol 1989; 143:1259–1264.

48. Paoletti LC, Kasper DL, Michon F, DiFabio JL, Jennings HJ, Tosteson TD, Wessels MR. Effects of chain length on the immunogenicity in rabbits of group B *Streptococcus* type III oligosaccharide-tetanus toxoid conjugates. J Clin Invest. 1992; 89:203–209.

49. Wessels MR, Paoletti LC, Rodewald AK, Michon F, DiFabio J, Jennings HJ, Kasper DL. Stimulation of protective antibodies against type Ia and Ib group B streptococci by a type Ia polysaccharide-tetanus toxoid conjugate vaccine. Infect Immun 1993; 61:4760–4766.

50. Paoletti LC, Wessels MR, Rodewald AK, Shroff AA, Jennings HJ, Kasper DL. Neonatal mouse protection against infection with multiple group B streptococcal serotypes by maternal immunization with a tetravalent GBS polysaccharide-

tetanus toxoid conjugate vaccine. Infect Immun 1994; 62:3236–3243.

51. Paoletti LC, Wessels MR, Michon F, DiFabio J, Jennings HJ, Kasper DL. Group B *Streptococcus* type II polysaccharide-tetanus toxoid conjugate vaccine. Infect Immun 1992; 60:4009–4014.

52. Wessels MR, Paoletti LC, Pinel J, Kasper DL. Immunogenicity and protective activity in animals of a group B *Streptococcus* type V polysaccharide-tetanus toxoid conjugate vaccine. J Infect Dis 1995; 171:879–884.

53. Jensen NE. Distribution of serotypes of group B streptococci in herds and cows within an area of Denmark. Acta Vet Scand 1980; 21:354–366.

54. Parisibu FH, Lammler C, Blobel H. Serotyping of bovine and human group B streptococci by co-agglutination. IRCS Med Sci 1985; 13:24–25.

55. Wilkinson HW. Group B streptococcal infection in humans. Annu Rev Microbiol 1978; 32:41–57.

56. Wilkinson HW. Comparison of streptococcal R antigens. Appl Microbiol 1972; 24:669–670.

57. Flores A, Ferrieri P. Molecular species of R-protein antigens produced by clinical isolates of group B streptococci. J Clin Microbiol 1989; 27:1050–1054.

58. Linden V. Mouse-protective effect of rabbit anti-R-protein antibodies against group B streptococci type II carrying R-protein. Acta Pathol Microbiol Immunol Scand 1983; 91:145–151.

59. Wilkinson HW, Eagon RG. Type-specific antigens of group B type Ic streptococci. Infect Immun 1971; 4:596–604.

60. Bevanger L, Maeland JA. Complete and incomplete Ibc protein fraction in group B streptococci. Acta Pathol Microbiol Scand Sect B 1979; 87:51–54.

61. Johnson DR, Ferrieri P. Group B streptococcal Ibc protein antigen: distribution of two determinants in wild-type strains of common serotypes. J Clin Microbiol 1984; 19:506–510.

62. Brady LJ, Daphtary UD, Ayoub EM, Boyle MD. Two novel antigens associated with group B streptococci identified by a rapid two-stage radioimmunoassay. J Infect Dis 1988; 158:965–972.

63. Cleat PH, Timmis KN. Cloning and expression in *Escherichia coli* of the Ibc protein genes of group B streptococci: binding of human immunoglobulin A to the beta antigen. Infect Immun 1987; 55:1151–1155.

64. Michel JL, Madoff LC, Kling DE, Kasper DL, Ausubel FM. Cloned alpha and beta c-protein antigens of group B streptococci elicit protective immunity. Infect Immun 1991; 59:2023–2028.

65. Russell-Jones GJ, Gotschlich EC. Identification of protein antigens of group B streptococci, with special reference to the Ibc antigens. J Exp Med 1984; 160:1476–1484.

66. Madoff LC, Michel JL, Gong EW, Rodewald AK, Kasper DL. Protection of neonatal mice from group B streptococcal infection by maternal immunization with beta C protein. Infect Immun 1992; 60:4989–4994.

67. Madoff LC, Michel JL, Kasper DL. A monoclonal antibody identifies a protective c-protein alpha-antigen epitope in group B streptococci. Infect Immun 1991; 59:204–210.

68. Madoff LC, Hori S, Michel JL, Baker CJ, Kasper DL. Phenotypic diversity in the alpha C protein of group B *Streptococcus*. Infect Immun 1991; 59:2638–2644.

69. Michel JL, Madoff LC, Olson K, Kling DE, Kasper DL, Ausubel FM. Large, identical, tandem repeating units in the C protein alpha antigen gene, *bca*, of group B streptococci. Proc Natl Acad Sci USA 1992; 89:10060–10064.

70. Madoff LC, Michel JL, Gong EW, Kling DE, Kasper DL. Group B streptococci escape host immunity by deletion of tandem repeat elements of the alpha C protein. Proc Natl Acad Sci USA 1996; 93:4131–4136.

71. Madoff LC, Paoletti LC, Tai JY, Kasper DL. Maternal immunization of mice with group B streptococcal type III polysaccharide-beta C protein conjugate elicits protective antibody to multiple serotypes. J Clin Invest 1994; 94:286–292.

72. Russell-Jones GJ, Gotschlich EC, Blake MS. A surface receptor specific for human IgA on group B streptococci possessing the Ibc protein antigen. J Exp Med 1984; 160:1467–1475.

73. Brady LJ, Boyle MD. Identification of non-immunoglobulin A-Fc-binding forms and low-molecular-weight secreted forms of the group B streptococcal beta antigen. Infect Immun 1989; 57:1573–1581.

74. Stalhammer-Carlemalm M, Stenberg L, Lindahl G. Protein Rib: a novel group B streptococcal cell surface protein that confers protective immunity and is expressed by most strains causing invasive infections. J Exp Med 1993; 177:1593–1603.

75. Wastfelt M, Stalhammar-Carlemalm M, Delisse AM, Cabezon T, Lindahl G. Identification of a family of streptococcal surface proteins with extremely repetitive structure. J Biol Chem 1996; 271:18892–18897.

76. Lachenauer CS, Madoff LC. A protective surface protein from type V group B streptococci shares N-terminal sequence homology with the alpha C protein. Infect Immun 1996; 64:4255–4260.

77. Kasper DL, Paoletti LC, Wessels MR, Guttormsen H-K, Carey VJ, Jennings HJ, Baker CJ. Immune response to type III group B streptococcal polysaccharide-tetanus toxoid conjugate vaccine. J Clin Invest 1996; 98:2308–2314.

78. Paoletti LC, Baker CJ, Kasper DL. Neonatal group B streptococcal disease: progress towards a multivalent maternal vaccine. Abstr. P16, p. 43. *Abstr. First Annual Conference on Vaccine Research.* National Foundation for Infectious Diseases, Washington, D.C.

79. Kasper DL, Paoletti LC, Madoff LC, Michel JL, Wessels MR, Jennings HJ. Glycoconjugate vac-

cines for the prevention of group B streptococcal infections. In: Norrby E, Brown F, Chanock RM, Ginsberg HS (eds.) Vaccines 94: Modern Approaches to New Vaccines Including Prevention of AIDS. Cold Spring Harbor, NY: Cold Spring Harbor Laboratory Press, 1994; 113–117.

80. Baker CJ, Paoletti LC, Wessels MR, Guttormsen HK, Rench MA, Hickman ME, Kasper DL. Safety and immunogenicity of capsular polysaccharide-tetanus toxoid conjugate vaccines for group B streptococcal types Ia and Ib. J Infect Dis 1999; 179:142–150.

22

Vaccine Strategies for *Streptococcus pneumoniae*

DAVID E. BRILES
EDWIN SWIATLO
KATHRYN EDWARDS

Streptococcus pneumoniae is one of the most important and ubiquitous bacterial pathogens of humans. It is the most common cause of community-acquired pneumonia and meningitis in all ages greater than 6 months and is the most frequently isolated pathogen from children with acute otitis media [1–8]. Although difficult to assess, the pneumococcus is thought to be the most common cause of serious respiratory tract infections in children in developing countries [9–11] and is a frequent cause of invasive infection in human immunodeficiency virus (HIV)–infected persons and those with sickle cell disease [12–15]. The polysaccharide capsule of pneumococcus was the first described virulence factor [16] and is still generally thought to make the greatest contribution to pathogenesis of infection (for reviews see refs. 17–21].

Even before the description of the polysaccharide capsule, attempts were made to prevent pneumococcal infection with vaccine preparations consisting simply of heat-killed organisms. In the first two decades of the twentieth century whole-cell vaccines were administered to high-risk populations with an apparent reduction of disease incidence [22]. These vaccination regimens were designed primarily to curtail ongoing outbreaks of pneumonia and the nature of these trials made firm conclusions regarding vaccine

efficacy difficult to extract. During this time animal protection studies defined serotypes 1 and 2 and passive transfer of type-specific antibodies was shown to be protective [23,24]. From these studies anticapsular horse antisera were developed at the Rockefeller Institute and were used successfully to treat pneumococcal infection in the pre-antibiotic era [22].

It was not long after the initiation of whole-cell vaccines and antiserum therapy that the targets of protective antibody were elucidated. Recovery from pneumococcal infection was found to be associated with the appearance of antibodies directed to the polysaccharide capsule [25] and humans injected with capsule-derived polysaccharide developed type-specific antibodies [26]. While antiserum therapy continued until the development of effective antimicrobial chemotherapy, subsequent pneumococcal vaccines focused on the polysaccharide capsule.

Purified capsular polysaccharide was first used as a vaccine in the 1930s to abrogate pneumonia epidemics [27,28] and polyvalent vaccines were used in military recruits throughout World War II [29]. These early formulations were effective in preventing bacteremic pneumococcal pneumonia caused by serotypes included in the vaccines. In the latter part of the 1940s, two pneumococcal vaccines were introduced commercially in the United States, but by this time antimicrobial agents were widely available and the perceived impact of pneumococcal infection was greatly diminished. The two vaccines were quickly withdrawn from the market for lack of demand.

Despite the use of effective antibiotics, the mortality related to pneumococcal infection was still excessively high [30]. It was not until 30 years after the first commercial pneumococcal vaccine were introduced that renewed interest in prevention of pneumococcal disease led to well-controlled clinical vaccine trials. In South Africa and New Guinea the efficacy of a multivalent pneumococcal polysaccharide vaccine was demonstrated in healthy adults [31–33]. On the basis of these trials, a 14-valent polysaccharide vaccine was licensed in the United States in 1977. This was expanded in 1983 to contain 23 capsule types and this formulation is the one currently used in the United States. Depending on the reference population, this vaccine contains serotypes responsible for 80%–90% of invasive pneumococcal infections (Table 22.1; [34,35]).

Following the introduction of the pneumococcal vaccine, clinical trials continued with mixed results. The polysaccharide vaccine has had a demonstrated impact on the incidence of invasive pneumococcal infection in adults, however, a significant number of clinical studies have failed to show efficacy similar to that originally seen in South Africa and New Guinea [33,36–41]. Although the minimum amount of anticapsular antibody necessary for protection is unknown, certain adult high-risk groups, such as the elderly and persons infected with HIV, have antibody responses less than those in normal control groups when measured by in vitro assays [42–50]. For included serotypes the vaccine is generally considered to be approximately 60% effective for prevention of invasive infection in immunocompetent adults [51].

Soon after capsular polysaccharide was described as an important protective antigen of pneumococci, it was found that infants respond poorly to these antigens [52]. Children less than 2 years of age respond poorly, or not at all, to T cell–independent antigens such as polysaccharides [53]. This has hindered preventive strategies in one of the largest groups at risk for pneumococcal infection. The present polyvalent vaccine is not recommended for children less than 2 years of age. A recently described strat-

Table 22.1 Distribution of *Streptococcus pneumoniae* Serotypes Responsible for Approximately 90% of Invasive Infections in Humans in the United States

Serotypes in Current 23-Valent Vaccine	Children <2 years		Adults	
	Serotype	% of Total	Serotype	% of Total
1	14	27.8	14	14.7
2	6B	13.4	6A,B	11.7
3	19F	11.8	4	9.4
4	18C	7.2	19F	7.7
5	23F	6.7	18C	7.5
6B	4	5.8	9V	5.4
7F	9V	5.8	3	4.5
8	19A	3.9	7F	3.5
9N, 9V	6A	3.3	8	3.5
10A	3	1.6	19A	3.3
11A	7F	1.4	1	3.2
12F	9N	0.9	9N	2.4
14	1	0.8	12F	2.2
15B	22F	0.8	22F	1.9
17F			15B,C	1.0
18C			5	0.8
19A, 19F			13	0.8
20			16	0.8
22F			20	0.8
23F				
33F				

Data derived from Butler et al. [35] and Robbins et al. [153].

egy to enhance humoral immune responses to T-independent antigens using CD40 antibodies suggests that polysaccharide antigens may yet be useful in this population [54]. Overall, most populations at risk for invasive pneumococcal disease have a low or inadequate antibody response to polysaccharide antigens.

CONJUGATE VACCINES

A major advancement in the development of effective polysaccharide vaccines has been the conjugation of polysaccharide antigens to carrier proteins, thus enabling T-independent antigens such as polysaccharides to elicit Th2-type cytokine responses. B cells stimulated by cytokines of a Th2-like pattern have significant memory responses and antibody secretion can be boosted with repeated immunization. An example of a successful conjugate vaccine is the one currently licensed for *Haemophilus influenzae* serotype b (Hib). As for the pneumococcus, Hib has a polysaccharide capsule that is a prominent virulence factor and is a target of protective antibodies during natural infection. This carbohydrate antigen is also poorly immunogenic in high-risk groups, specifically, children less than 12 months of age. Conjugation of Hib capsular polysaccharide to diphtheria toxoid, tetanus toxoid, or meningococcal outer membrane protein complex results in a vigorous antibody response to the polysaccharide and prevents invasive Hib infections in infants [55–59]. Interestingly, the Hib conjugate vaccine has also been shown to elicit

a secretory IgA response when given intramuscularly and reduces nasopharyngeal carriage [60,61].

Pneumococcal conjugate vaccines have been developed in a manner similar to that for Hib. Conjugates of capsular polysaccharide with diphtheria toxoid, tetanus toxoid, and meningococcal outer membrane proteins have been shown to be both safe and immunogenic in healthy adult volunteers [62–64]. These studies confirm that conjugates can readily induce 8- to 20-fold increase in specific anti-capsule antibodies compared to preimmune sera. In contrast, purified polysaccharide was able to elicit only two- to sixfold increases in antibody over preimmune levels. Recent trials have shown that pneumococcal polysaccharide–protein conjugates are safe and immunogenic in infants as young as 2 months of age [65–68] and concomitant administration with Hib vaccine may boost the response to *Haemophilus* polysaccharide [69]. Additionally, immunization with a conjugate vaccine may reduce pneumococcal carriage in children in a manner similar to that seen for *Haemophilus* and the Hib vaccine [70]. Pneumococcal conjugates using tetanus or diphtheria toxoids have been shown to induce a secretory immune response in adults [71]. Phase II/III clinical trials are in progress in the U.S. to evaluate the efficacy of pneumococcal conjugate vaccines (Table 22.2).

Despite the proven success of the Hib conjugate vaccine and the initial promising results from pneumococcal conjugate vaccine trials, a polysaccharide-based pneumococcal vaccine is

Table 22.2 Conjugate Pneumococcal Vaccine Trials

Organizing Group	Protein Carrier	Included Capsular Serotypes in Vaccine	Status of Trials
Pasteur-Merieux/ Connaught	Tetanus toxoid Diphtheria toxoid	6, 14, 19, 23 (proposed to add 3, 4, 9, and 18)	Phase I/II
Lederle-Praxis	CRM_{197} (diphtheria toxoid)	6, 14, 18, 19, 23 (Proposed to add 4 and 9 for U.S. and 1 and 5 for developing countries)	Phase III
Merck	OMP- meningococcus B	4, 6, 9, 14, 18, 19, 23	Phase I/II
University of Rochester	CRM_{197} Tetanus toxoid	6, 14, 19, 23	Phase I
National Institute of Child Health and Human Development	Tetanus toxoid	6, 12	Phase I

From National Institute of Allergy and Infectious Diseases, 1994.

inherently problematic. The number of type-specific polysaccharides that can be included in a conjugate vaccine may be limited by the suppression of epitope antigenicity with excessive quantities of protein carrier [72,73]. Even if conjugate vaccines could be extended to include all of the 23 serotypes currently included in the polysaccharide vaccine, this would miss at least 10% of invasive serotypes. Although pediatric pneumococcal infections are more limited in number of predominant capsular types, it would not be realistic to expect 100% coverage by conjugate vaccines. The prevalent capsular serotypes in adults and children vary among countries, moreover, the epidemiology of invasive pneumococcal serotypes could potentially shift over time to nonvaccine types. Conjugation of polysaccharide to protein is a complex and variably efficient process that increases the cost per dose of vaccine. Additionally, persons infected with HIV may have poor immune responses to even conjugate vaccines. In one study of pentavalent pneumococcal conjugate vaccine, HIV-infected persons, regardless of immunologic status reflected in CD4 cell count, responded to polysaccharide vaccine better than conjugate for serotypes 14 and 19F. Only one serotype (18C) was more immunogenic as a conjugate in subjects with less than 200 CD4 cells [42]. Protein-conjugated vaccines in healthy older adults have shown mixed results when total type-specific immunoglobulins are measured, however, the qualitative differences of antibody subclasses may be clinically relevant [74,75]. For these reasons, alternatives to pneumococcal capsule have been studied that would circumvent the deficiencies of polysaccharide immunogens.

POTENTIAL OF NONCAPSULAR PNEUMOCOCCAL ANTIGENS AS IMMUNOGENS

Evidence that noncapsular antigens of pneumococci are able to protect against infection was first acquired in animal models soon after the description of capsule [76]. Immediately following this study, many poorly characterized noncapsular components of pneumococcus were described as effective protection-eliciting antigens [77–81]. However, it was not until 1981 that the

first noncapsule pneumococcal antigen that could induce protective antibodies was identified as phosphocholine (see below). Since that time, a number of additional virulence factors have been identified and in some cases, tested as protective antigens.

Protein antigens can induce a vigorous immune response in infants and other high-risk groups that do not respond optimally to polysaccharides. Antibody levels to protein antigens can be boosted by repeated immunization with a subsequent rapid anamnestic response. Generally, there is little or no serologic diversity among proteins, even across capsular types, and they can be produced relatively inexpensively on a large scale as recombinant DNA products. Several protein virulence factors of pneumococcus have been identified that can induce protective immune responses in animal models.

Pneumococcal Surface Protein A

This surface-exposed protein was originally identified in a study using hybridoma fusions to search for protective antigens of pneumococci [82]. Prior to the work describing pneumococcal surface protein A (PspA), a species-specific, serologically variable pneumococcal protein(s) had been demonstrated and designated M protein [83]. Although not possible to prove, it may be that this early work described some serotypes of PspA [84]. PspA has been shown to inhibit clearance of pneumococci from blood and monoclonal antibodies to PspA can protect passively immunized mice against virulent pneumococci [85,86]. Systemic immunization of mice with purified native or recombinant PspA can protect mice against infection with multiple capsule types of virulent pneumococci [87–89]. Mucosal immunization with PspA has also been shown to protect against invasive disease as well as nasopharyngeal carriage in animal models [90].

The deduced amino acid sequence of PspA from strain Rx1 has been derived from the nucleotide sequence of the cloned gene [91,92]. The N-terminal half of the protein is an alpha-helical coiled-coil structure, which suggests that PspA exists as a dimer. The protective epitopes of PspA have been mapped to this N-terminal, alpha-helical region of the protein [88,89,93].

Adjacent to this is a proline-rich region thought to span the cell wall in a manner similar to that of other bacterial surface proteins. At the C-terminus of PspA are 10 repeats of 20 uncharged amino acids each, followed by a unique 17 amino acid sequence at the terminus that lacks a typical membrane-spanning region and has unknown function. The attachment of PspA to the cell surface involves a unique interaction between the C-terminal repeats and choline in the pneumococcal lipoteichoic acid [94] (Fig. 22.1).

Unlike other protein antigens studied in pneumococci, PspA is serologically variable [95] and immunization with a single serotype will probably not provide optimal protection against all invasive strains. Variation in the N-terminus is responsible for the serologic variability, however, this domain has been mapped and there are protective epitopes conserved across serotypes of PspA [93]. These conserved epitopes may permit immunization with a few select peptides or a single-fusion polypeptide containing PspA epitopes found on all, or nearly all, clinically important strains.

Pneumolysin

Pneumolysin is a thiol-activated toxin expressed by all strains of pneumococcus and is an important virulence factor [96–98]. This toxin has been shown to activate complement by directly binding the Fc portion of immunoglobulin G (IgG)

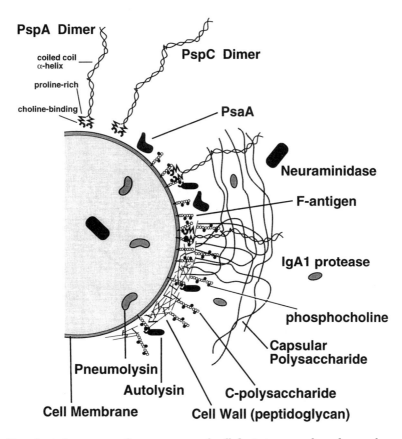

Figure 22.1 Hypothetical structure of a pneumococcal cell depicting capsule and several noncapsular antigens. F-antigen (lipoteichoic acid) and C-polysaccharide (teichoic acid) are identical except for the presence of fatty acids that allow F-antigen to insert into the plasma membrane. Neuraminidase is thought to be a secreted protein, however, pneumolysin is a cytoplasmic protein that is released upon lysis of the pneumococcal cell. PspA is shown extending from the cell surface and is to scale with relation to the cell wall and capsule. PsaA is shown at the cell surface but its exact relation to other surface components is unknown. Not shown are CbpA, SpsA, and other choline-binding proteins.

[99] and also has a distinct functional domain that binds cholesterol in cell membranes, resulting in cytolysis [100]. Both of these activities are important during the pathogenesis of pneumococcal pneumonia [101]. Purified pneumolysin is toxic to pulmonary epithelial and endothelial cells in vitro [102,103] and alone is able to reproduce all histopathologic changes characteristic of pneumococcal pneumonia in a rat model [104]. In a mouse model, pneumolysin-deficient mutants of pneumococci cause a chronic low-grade bacteremia rather than rapidly fatal sepsis [98]. Recent comprehensive reviews provide an overview of the role of pneumolysin in the pathogenesis of pneumococcal infection [20,105].

Antibodies to pneumolysin have been detected in adults recovering from acute pneumococcal pneumonia [106] and in upper airway secretions of children with acute otitis media caused by pneumococcus [107]. Adults infected with HIV may be at increased risk for invasive pneumococcal infection if levels of naturally occurring pneumolysin antibodies are low [108]. Appearance of secretory IgA (sIgA) against pneumolysin in middle ear fluid of children as young as 6 months with otitis media attests to the potent antigenicity of this protein [109]. These studies showed that many children had detectable anti-pneumolysin antibodies in their upper respiratory secretions even before the onset of symptomatic infection. This suggests that carriage of pneumococci in the upper airways may be able to induce an immune response to pneumolysin. The type or magnitude of immune response to pneumolysin in the middle ear that protects against clinical disease is still unsettled.

Studies in mice suggest that pre-existing antibodies to pneumolysin can protect from otherwise fatal septicemia. Initially, mice were immunized with native [110] or genetically obtained pneumolysin toxoids [111] and protected from infection with capsular type 2 pneumococci. The protective capacity of pneumolysin toxoid has subsequently been demonstrated for nine serotypes and has also been shown to protect mice when challenged by the intranasal route [112]. This study showed marked differences in the ability of pneumolysin to protect against different capsular types and, although all strains of pneumococcus express pneumolysin, there are significant differences in quantity produced among strains, at least in vitro, that may affect pneumococcal virulence. If these differences occur in vivo, this may explain, in part, the variable effectiveness of pneumolysin in eliciting protection to different capsular types.

An additional utility of pneumolysin may be as the protein component of a conjugated polysaccharide vaccine. Conjugates of pneumolysin with polysaccharide from capsule types 18C and 19F were able to induce high titers of protective antibodies in mice. Antibodies were detected to both the protein and polysaccharide moieties of the vaccine and large increases in antibody were produced by two booster injections [111,113]. Other pneumococcal proteins have not yet been studied as carriers in conjugate vaccines but inclusion of protein virulence factors is an attractive technique to broaden the target of inducible protective antibodies.

Neuraminidase

Pneumococcus produces two distinct enzymes with the ability to remove terminal N-acetyl-neuraminic acid residues from glycoproteins and gangliosides [114,115]. By screening a small number of strains, it appears that all pneumococci contain genes for both enzymes. At least one of these contains a C-terminal LPXTGX amino acid motif with an adjacent hydrophobic domain characteristic of many proteins anchored to the cell wall in gram-positive organisms [116]. The neuraminidase enzyme NanA elicits a brisk antibody response; however, it offers little protection as a single antigen in a mouse model [117]. In mice challenged intranasally with a virulent type 2 pneumococcus, immunization with formaldehyde-denatured neuraminidase plus pneumolysin added little protection compared to immunization with pneumolysin alone. The second neuraminidase enzyme encoded by nanB has little amino acid homology to NanA [118] but has not been studied as a protective antigen. Although not an effective antigen when used alone for protection against sepsis, neuraminidase antibodies may have a role in attenuating carriage, pneumonia, or invasion.

Autolysin

Lysis of the pneumococcal cell has been postulated to be important in the pathogenesis of pneumococcal infection. This may result from release of cytoplasmic contents, including pneumolysin, and release of highly pro-inflammatory cell-wall breakdown products [119,120]. A cell wall–associated amidase of pneumococcus, autolysin, and a highly homologous phage-encoded amidase can hydrolyze N-acetylmuramic acid–alanine in the cell-wall peptidoglycan and cause cell lysis [121,122]. Autolysin has been shown to contribute to virulence [97,123,124] but its ability to induce a protective immune response appears limited. Mice immunized with autolysin, pneumolysin, or autolysin plus pneumolysin are all protected against challenge with wild-type pneumococci [125]. Autolysin in combination with pneumolysin, however, is no more protective than pneumolysin alone and immunization with autolysin alone does not protect against challenge with mutant pneumococci unable to produce pneumolysin.

These findings imply that the main effect of autolysin on virulence is to release pneumolysin from the cytoplasm by autolysis and, indeed, mutations in either pneumolysin or autolysin have similar effects on virulence when tested by intraperitoneal (i.p.) infection [125]. In contrast to immunization results, autolysin-negative mutants are significantly less virulent than pneumolysin mutants as demonstrated by intranasal infection of mice [124]. It is possible that autolysin releases factor(s) other than pneumolysin or that autolysin itself is involved in interactions at the mucosal surface. Autolysin alleles have been shown to vary at the nucleotide level among clinical isolates [126] and the resultant variability in amino acid sequence may have implications for the immunogenicity and vaccine development of autolysin.

Pneumococcal Surface Adhesin A

A pneumococcal protein with nucleotide sequence homology to other streptococcal adhesins has been cloned [127,128] and functional studies suggest that it has a role in virulence and host-cell adhesion. Pneumococcal surface adhesin A (PsaA) has been shown to induce anti-bodies that protect against intravenous (i.v.) infection with type 3 pneumococci in mice [129]. Further studies will confirm the function of PsaA and the extent of protection induced by this protein.

OTHER POTENTIALLY IMMUNOGENIC PNEUMOCOCCAL PROTEINS

There are many other pneumococcal components that have been described but their potential as immunogens has not been fully investigated. Serine protease activity has been described in pneumococcus, however, its role in pathogenesis remains unknown [130]. A hyaluronidase gene has been cloned and sequenced [131] and this should facilitate studies into the role of this enzyme in pathogenesis. Pneumococci have specific enzymes that are able to inactivate components of the humoral immune response. Specific hydrolysis of human IgA by a pneumococcal protease has been demonstrated [132] and may facilitate carriage of pneumococci in the nasopharynx. Likewise, a surface protein of pneumococcus, SpsA, has been shown to specifically bind the secretory component of sIgA [133]. Inactivation of this important mucosal defense mechanism could certainly be important in establishing colonization of the upper airways by pneumococci. If these two IgA-inactivating proteins can be delivered as effective antigens to the mucosal immune system, a resultant immune response may potentially reduce the number of pneumococci in the nasopharynx during the carrier state. One obvious obstacle to such a strategy is that induced immune responses will be largely sIgA, a host defense for which pneumococci have apparently acquired quite capable mechanisms for avoiding. Complement activation is critical for effective clearance of pneumococci in nonimmune hosts and C3 degradation has been ascribed to a pneumococcal cell-associated enzyme [134]. Immune response to this protein has implications for protection against invasive disease as well as carriage.

Three heat shock proteins (HSPs) from pneumococcus have been described and monoclonal antibodies to one of them have been obtained [135]. It is known that HSPs are immunodominant antigens of intracellular bacterial pathogens but they are poorly understood for extracellular gram-positive organisms. The role of HSPs in pneumococcal virulence and immunity awaits further clarification.

A number of choline-binding proteins are known to exist in pneumococci and are likely surface-exposed molecules that represent potential immunogens. One of these molecules, CbpA, has been shown to be involved in adhesion to host cells and can induce a protective immune response in a mouse model [136]. Choline-binding proteins such as PspA, CbpA, and others as yet uncharacterized are rapidly gaining significant attention as protein-based pneumococcal vaccine candidates.

C-POLYSACCHARIDE

The first noncapsule antigen of pneumococcus that was well characterized was phosphocholine (PC), present on C-polysaccharide and F-antigen (teichoic and lipoteichoic acid, respectively) [137]. The original studies showing the protective capacity of anti-PC antibodies against virulent type 3 pneumococci in mice have since been extended to demonstrate protection against several capsular types [138,139]. Levels of naturally occurring anti-PC antibodies in mice can be boosted by immunization with PC with concomitant keyhole limpet hemocyanin [140].

Antibodies directed against PC in mice consist of idiotypes utilizing three different heavy chains. One of these idiotypes, T15, has been shown to be far superior to others in its capacity to protect against pneumococcal infection [141,142]. Immunization of mice with nonviable pneumococci results in protective T15 antibodies directed against PC. Subsequent booster immunizations with PC–protein conjugates selects for B cell clones that secrete non-T15 antibodies that are much less protective. In contrast, immunization of *Xid* mice with either nonviable pneumococci or PC–protein conjugates does not result in protective anti-PC antibodies. *Xid* mice lack Lyb-3 and (5) B cell markers and are genetically unable to respond to polysaccharide antigens. These mice also have a minimal amount of naturally occurring antibody to PC. Against this background, promising results were described in a study of immunization of *Xid* mice with the PC analog *p*-nitrophenyl-6-(O-phosphocholine) hydroxyhexanoate. This antigen was

able to elicit protective antibodies that were not of the T15 idiotype [143]. This hapten is able to select B cell clones that secrete protective antibody by a mechanism other than boosting the intrinsic anti-PC response.

Despite these encouraging results, it is known that anti-PC antibodies are less protective than anti-capsule antibodies on a weight basis [144,145], and, in fact, some studies suggest that antibodies to C-polysaccharide may not be protective in humans [146,147]. There is evidence for other protective epitopes on C-polysaccharide [148] and the usefulness of teichoic acid antigens as vaccine candidates remains controversial. It is not known, however, what conditions are necessary to induce the most highly protective antibody to PC in humans. If methods can be devised to stimulate protective anti-PC antibodies in humans then this antigen may be a promising pneumococcal vaccine alone or as a component of a multi-antigen vaccine protocol.

MUCOSAL IMMUNITY AND CARRIAGE OF PNEUMOCOCCI

From experience with Hib conjugate vaccine and the first pneumococcal conjugate vaccines, it is becoming evident that systemic immunization can induce a mucosal immune response sufficient to eliminate carriage in the upper airways. Although the mechanism of this response is not proven, one possibility is that bacterial polysaccharides in the gastrointestinal tract share cross-reactive epitopes with capsules of organisms that inhabit the nasopharynx [149]. This cross-reactivity may prime gut- and mucosa-associated lymphoid tissue and thus facilitate an enhanced generalized mucosal response after systemic immunization. Preliminary work suggests that induction of mucosal immunity by systemic immunization can reduce carriage of pneumococci in mice [150]. It remains to be seen if polysaccharide–protein conjugates can reduce carriage of pneumococci in a manner similar to the reduction in Hib carriage as a result of the conjugate vaccine.

Elimination of carriage is a desirable goal for pathogens that can be carried asymptomatically in the upper airways. Pneumococci are spread person-to-person by respiratory droplets and in this way are disseminated in human populations. Interruption of transmission would greatly decrease exposure of nonimmune hosts to new serotypes and decrease the incidence of invasive disease in this group. An effective mucosal vaccine that eliminates carriage of pneumococci would reduce the overall infection rate even in those who are not immunized or who have a suboptimal response to vaccination. Also, mucosal immune response to pneumococcal proteins and polysaccharides appears at an early age in response to natural exposure [107,109] and immunization via mucosal surfaces may elicit immunity at an earlier age than would otherwise be possible. An animal model of pneumococcal carriage has recently been established [151] and early results suggest that oral or intranasal immunization with PspA or polysaccharide–tetanus toxoid conjugate can prevent nasopharyngeal carriage in mice [90,152]. Immunization by mucosal routes would be easily administered and a protective immune response induced directly at mucosal surfaces may be the most effective method to reduce the incidence of pneumococcal infection in humans. Further studies with pneumococcal noncapsular antigens hold the potential to ultimately define the optimal methods to prevent pneumococcal carriage, as well as the morbidity and mortality of invasive infection.

SUMMARY

Streptococcus pneumoniae continues to be one of the most widespread and important human pathogens. The current preventive strategy is immunization of high-risk groups with a 23-valent polysaccharide vaccine based on the most common capsular serotypes. Some common capsule serotypes included in the vaccine are poorly immunogenic in children less than 2 years of age, the elderly, and those with advanced HIV infection. These groups represent a significant percentage of patients at risk for invasive pneumococcal infection. Alternative strategies to polysaccharide antigens are proteins or protein conjugate–based vaccines. Conjugates have proven successful for other encapsulated organisms and may potentially be effective in preventing pneumococcal infection. However, the

expense and logistical difficulties of using conjugates to protect against such a large number of pneumococcal serotypes is considerable. A number of protein virulence factors of pneumococci have been described and a few of these have been studied for their ability to induce a protective immune response in animal models. If any noncapsular antigens are found to be effective human vaccines, it could greatly reduce the cost and complexity of the production of a pneumococcal vaccine and make immunization available to more people throughout the world.

REFERENCES

1. Bohte R, van Furth R, van den Broek PJ. Aetiology of community-acquired pneumonia: a prospective study among adults requiring admission to hospital. Thorax 1995; 50:543–547.
2. Bradley JS, Kaplan SL, Klugman KP, Leggiadro RJ. Consensus: management of infections in children caused by *Streptococcus pneumoniae* with decreased susceptibility to penicillin. Pediatr Infect Dis J 1995; 14:1037–1041.
3. Cherian T, Steinhoff MC, Harrison LH, Rohn D, McDougal LK, Dick J. A cluster of invasive pneumococcal disease in young children in child care. JAMA 1994; 271:695–697.
4. Davidson M, Parkinson AJ, Bulkow LR, Fitzgerald MA, Peters HV, Parks DJ. The epidemiology of invasive pneumococcal disease in Alaska, 1986–1990—ethnic differences and opportunities for prevention. J Infect Dis 1994; 170:368–376.
5. Fiebach N, Beckett W. Prevention of respiratory infections in adults: influenza and pneumococcal vaccines. Arch Intern Med 1994; 154:2545–2557.
6. Johnston RB Jr. Pathogenesis of pneumococcal pneumonia. Rev Infect Dis 1991; 13(Suppl 6):S509–S517.
7. Takala AK, Jero J, Kela E, Ronnberg PR, Koskenniemi E, Eskola J. Risk factors for primary invasive pneumococcal disease among children in Finland. JAMA 1995; 273:859–864.
8. Kornelisse RF, Westerbeek ML, Spoor AB, van der Heijde B, Spanjaard L, Neijens HJ, de Groot R. Pneumococcal meningitis in children: prognostic indicators and outcome. Clin Infect Dis 1995; 21:1390–1397.
9. Sniadack DH, Schwartz B, Lipman H, Bogaerts J, Butler JC, Dagan R, Echaniz-Aviles G, Lloyd-Evans N, Fenoll A, Girgis NI, Henrichsen J, Klugman K, Lehmann D, Takala AK, Vandepitte J, Gove S, Breiman RF. Potential interventions for the prevention of childhood pneumonia: geographic and temporal differences in

serotype and serogroup distribution of sterile site pneumococcal isolates from children—implications for vaccine strategies. Pediatr Infect Dis J 1995; 14:503–510.

10. Steinhoff MC. Developing and deploying pneumococcal and haemophilus vaccines. Lancet 1993; 342:630–631.

11. Shann F. Etiology of severe pneumonia in children in developing countries. Pediatr Infect Dis J 1986; 5:247–252.

12. Janoff EN, Breiman RF, Daley CL, Hopewell PC. Pneumococcal disease during HIV infection: epidemiologic, clinical, and immunologic perspectives. Ann Intern Med 1992; 117:314–324.

13. Wong WY, Overturf GD, Powars DR. Infection caused by *Streptococcus pneumoniae* in children with sickle cell disease: epidemiology, immunologic mechanisms, prophylaxis, and vaccination. Clin Infect Dis 1992; 14:1124–1136.

14. Mao C, Harper M, McIntosh K, Reddington C, Cohen J, Bachur R, Caldwell B, Hsu HW. Invasive pneumococcal infections in human immunodeficiency virus–infected children. J Infect Dis 1996; 173:870–876.

15. John AB, Ramlal A, Jackson H, Maude GH, Sharma AW, Serjeant GR. Prevention of pneumococcal infection in children with homozygous sickle cell disease. BMJ 1984; 288:1567–1570.

16. Avery OT, Dubos R. The protective action of a specific enzyme against type III pneumococcus infection in mice. J Exp Med 1931; 54:73–85.

17. Boulnois GJ. Pneumococcal proteins and the pathogenesis of disease caused by *Streptococcus pneumoniae*. J Gen Microbiol 1992; 138:249–259.

18. Gillespie SH. Aspects of pneumococcal infection including bacterial virulence, host response and vaccination. J Med Microbiol 1989; 28:237–248.

19. Lee C-J, Banks SD, Li JP. Virulence, immunity, and vaccine related to *Streptococcus pneumoniae*. Crit Rev Microbiol 1991; 18:89–114.

20. Paton JC, Andrew PW, Boulnois GJ, Mitchell TJ. Molecular analysis of the pathogenicity of *Streptococcus pneumoniae*: the role of pneumococcal proteins. Annu Rev Microbiol 1993; 47:89–115.

21. Watson DA, Musher DM, Verhoef J. Pneumococcal virulence factors and host immune responses to them. Eur J Clin Microbiol Infect Dis 1995; 14:479–490.

22. White B. The Biology of the Pneumococcus. New York: The Commonwealth Fund, 1938.

23. Heffron R. Pneumonia: With Special Reference to Pneumococcus Lobar Pneumonia. Cambridge, MA: Harvard University Press, 1939.

24. Avery OT, Goebel WF. Chemoimmunological studies of the soluble specific substance of pneumococcus. 1. The isolation and properties of the acetyl polysaccharide of pneumococcus type I. J Exp Med 1933; 58:731 755.

25. Heidelberger M, Avery OT. The soluble specific substance of the pneumococcus. J Exp Med 1923; 38:73–79.

26. Francis T Jr, Tillett WS. The development of antibodies following the intradermal injection of type-specific polysaccharide. J Exp Med 1930; 52:573–581.

27. Smillie WG, Wornock GH, White HJ. A study of a type 1 pneumococcus epidemic at the State Hospital at Worcester, Mass. Am J Publ Health 1938; 28:293–302.

28. Felton LD. Studies on the immunizing substances of pneumococcus. II. Separation of the organism into acid soluble and acid insoluble fractions. J Immunol 1934; 27:379–393.

29. McLeod CM, Hodges RG, Heidelberger M, Bernhard WG. Prevention of pneumococcal pneumonia by immunization with specific capsular polysaccharides. J Exp Med 1945; 82:445–455.

30. Austrian R, Gold J. Pneumococcal bacteremia with special reference to bacteremic pneumococcal pneumonia. Ann Intern Med 1964; 60:759–776.

31. Austrian R, Douglas RM, Schiffman G, Coetzee AN, Koornhof HJ, Hayden-Smith S, Reid RW. Prevention of pneumococcal pneumonia by vaccination. Trans Assoc Am Phys 1976; 89:184–189.

32. Riley ID, Andrews M, Howard R, Tarr PI, Pfeiffer M, Challands P, Jennison G, Douglas RM. Immunisation with a polyvalent pneumococcal vaccine: reduction of adult respiratory mortality in a New Guinea highlands community. Lancet 1977; 1:1338–1341.

33. Smit P, Oberholzer D, Hatden-Smith S, Koornhof HJ, Hilleman MR. Protective efficacy of pneumococcal polysacharide vaccines. JAMA 1977; 238:2613–2616.

34. Jorgensen JH, Howell AW, Maher LA, Facklam RR. Serotypes of respiratory isolates of *Streptococcus pneumoniae* compared with the capsular types included in the current pneumococcal vaccine. J Infect Dis 1991; 163:644–646.

35. Butler JC, Breiman RF, Lipman HB, Hofmann J, Facklam RR. Serotype distribution of *Streptococcus pneumoniae* infections among preschool children in the United States, 1978–1994: implications for the development of a conjugate vaccine. J Infect Dis 1995; 171:885– 889.

36. McMahon BJ, Parkinson AJ, Bulkow L, Davidson M, Wainwright K, Wolfe P, Schiffman GS. Immunogenecity of the 23-valent pneumococcal polysaccharide vaccine in Alaska native chronic alcoholics compared with nonalcoholic native and non-native controls. Am J Med 1993; 95:589–594.

37. Shapiro ED, Berg AT, Austrian R, Schroeder D, Parcells V, Margolis A, Adair RK, Clemens JD.

The protective efficacy of polyvalent pneumococcal polysaccharide vaccine. N Eng J Med 1991; 325:1453–1460.

38. Forrester HL, Jahnigen DW, LaForce FM. Inefficacy of pneumococcal vaccine in a high-risk population. Am J Med 1987; 83:425–430.

39. Sims RV, Steinman WC, McConville JH, King LR, Zwick WC, Schwartz JS. The clinical effectiveness of pneumococcal vaccine in the elderly. Ann Intern Med 1988; 108:653–657.

40. Bolan G, Broome CV, Facklam RR, Plikaytis BD, Fraser DW, Schlech WF. Pneumococcal vaccine efficacy in selected populations in the United States. Ann Intern Med 1986; 104:1–6.

41. Leech JA, Gervais A, Ruben FL. Efficacy of pneumococcal vaccine in severe chronic obstructive pulmonary disease. Can Med Assoc J 1987; 136:361–365.

42. Ahmed F, Steinhoff MC, Rodriguez-Barradas MC, Hamilton RG, Musher DM, Nelson KE. Effect of human immunodeficiency virus type 1 infection on the antibody response to a glycoprotein conjugate pneumococcal vaccine: results from a randomized trial. J Infect Dis 1996; 173:83–90.

43. Carson PJ, Schutt RL, Simpson ML, O'Brien J, Janoff EN. Antibody class and subclass responses to pneumococcal polysaccharides following immunization of human immunodeficiency virus–infected patients. J Infect Dis 1995; 172:340–345.

44. Hedlund JU, Kalin ME, Ortqvist AB, Henrichsen J. Antibody response to pneumococcal vaccine in middle-aged and elderly patients recently treated for pneumonia. Arch Intern Med 1994; 154:1961–1965.

45. Mascart-Lemone F, Gerard M, Libin M, Crusiaux A, Franchioly P, Lambrechts A, Goldman M, Clumek N. Differential effect of human immunodeficiency virus infection on the IgA and IgG antibody responses to pneumococcal vaccine. J Infect Dis 1995; 172:1253–1260.

46. Musher DM, Groover JE, Rowland JM, Watson DA, Struewing JB, Baughn RE, Mufson MA. Antibody to capsular polysaccharides of *Streptococcus pneumoniae*: prevalence, persistence, and response to revaccination. Clin Infect Dis 1993; 17:66–73.

47. Rao SP, Rajkumar K, Schiffman G, Desai N, Unger C, Miller ST. Anti-pneumococcal antibody levels three to seven years after first booster immunization in children with sickle cell disease, and after a second booster. J Pediatr 1995; 127:590–592.

48. Sankilampi U, Honkanen PO, Bloigu A, Herva E, Leinonen M. Antibody response to pneumococcal capsular polysaccharide vaccine in the elderly. J Infect Dis 1996; 173:387–393.

49. Rodriguez-Barradas MC, Groover JE, Lacke CE, Gump DW, Lahart CJ, Pandey JP, Musher DM. IgG antibody to pneumococcal capsular polysaccharide in human immunodeficiency virus–infected subjects: persistence of antibody in responders, revaccination in nonresponders, and relationship of immunuglobulin allotype to response. J Infect Dis 1996; 173:1347–1353.

50. Janoff EN, Fasching C, Ojoo JC, O'Brien J, Gilks CF. Responsiveness of human immunodeficiency virus type1-infected Kenyan women with or without prior pneumococcal disease to pneumococcal vaccine. J Infect Dis 1997; 175:975–978.

51. Shapiro ED, Berg AT, Austrian R, Schroeder D, Parcells V, Margolis A, Adair RK, Clemens JD. The protective efficacy of polyvalent pneumococcal polysaccharide vaccine. N Engl J Med 1991; 325:1453–1460.

52. Davies JAV. The response of infants to inoculation with type I pneumoocccus. J Immunol 1937; 33:1.

53. Borgono JM, McLean AA, Vella PP, Woodhour AF, Canepa I, Davidson WL, Hilleman MR. Vaccination and revaccination with polyvalent and pneumococcal polysaccharide vaccines in adults and infants. Proc Soc Exp Biol Med 1978; 157:148–155.

54. Dullforce P, Sutton DC, Heath AW. Enhancement of T cell–independent immune responses in vivo by CD40 antibodies. Nat Med 1998; 4:88–91.

55. Decker MD, Edwards KM, Bradley R, Palmer P. Comparative trial in infants of four conjugate *Haemophilus influenzae* type b vaccines. J Pediatr 1992; 120:184–189.

56. Granoff DM, Anderson EL, Osterholm MT, Holmes SJ, Medley F, McHugh JE, Murphy TV, Belshe RB. Differences in the immunogenicity of three *Haemophilus influenzae* type b conjugate vaccines in infants. J Pediatr 1992; 121:187–194.

57. Lepow ML, Barkin RM, Berkowitz CD, Brunell PA, James D, Meier K, Ward J, Zahradnik JM, Samuelson J, McVerry PH, Gordon LK. Safety and immunogenicity of *Haemophilus influenzae* type b polysaccharide diphtheria toxoid conjugate vaccine PRP-D in infants. J Infect Dis 1987; 156:591–596.

58. Madore DV, Johnson CL, Phipps DC, Eby R, Popejoy LA, Smith DH. Safety and immunologic response to *Haemophilus influenzae* type b oligosaccharide-CRM$_{197}$ conjugate vaccine in 1 to 6 month old infants. Pediatrics 1990; 85:331–337.

59. Park JC, Schneerson R, Reimer C, Black C, Welfare S, Bryla D, Levi L, Pavliakova D, Cramton T, Schulz D, Cadoz M, Robbins JB. Clinical and immunologic responses to *Haemophilus influenzae* type b—tetanus toxoid conjugate vaccine in infants injected at 3, 5, 7, and 18 months of age. J Pediatr 1991; 118:184–190.

60. Kauppi M, Eskola J, Kayhty H. Antibodies to

capsular polysaccharide in the saliva of children immunized with the *Haemophilus influenzae* b vaccine. Pediatr Infect Dis J 1995; 14:286–294.

61. Barbour ML, Mayon-White RT, Coles C, Crook DWM, Moxon ER. The impact of conjugate vaccine on carriage of *Haemophilus influenzae* type b. J Infect Dis 1995; 171:93–98.

62. Schneerson R, Robbins JR, Parke JC, Bell C, Schlesselman JJ, Sutton A, Wang Z, Schiffman G, Karpas A, Shiloach J. Quantitative and qualitative analyses of serum antibodies elicited in adults by *Haemophilus influenzae* type b and pneumococcus type 6A capsular polysaccharide–tetanus toxoid conjugates. Infect Immun 1986; 52:519–528.

63. Fattom A, Lue C, Szu SC, Mestecky J, Schiffman G, Bryla D, Vann WF, Watson D, Kimzey LM, Robbins JB, Schneerson R. Serum antibody response in adult volunteers elicited by injection of *Streptococcus pneumoniae* type 12F polysaccharide alone or conjugated to diphtheria toxoid. Infect Immun 1990; 58:2309–2312.

64. Anderson P, Betts R. Human adult immunogenicity of protein-coupled pneumococcal capsular antigens of serotypes prevalent in otitis media. Pediatr Infect Dis J 1989; 8:S50–S55.

65. Kayhty H, Ahman H, Ronnberg P-R, Tillikainen R, Eskola J. Pneumococcal polysaccharide-meningococcal outer membrane protein complex conjugate vaccine is immunogenic in infants and children. J Infect Dis 1995; 172:1273–1278.

66. Ahman H, Kayhty H, Tamminen P, Vuorela A, Malinoski F, Eskola J. Pentavalent pneumococcal oligosaccharide conjugate vaccine PncCRM is well tolerated and able to induce an antibody response in infants. Pediatr Infect Dis J 1996; 15:134–139.

67. Anderson EL, Kennedy DJ, Geldmacher KM, Donnelly J, Mendelman PM. Immunogenicity of heptavalent pneumococcal conjugate vaccine in infants. J Pediatr 1996; 128:649–653.

68. Ahman H, Kayhty H, Lehtonen H, Leroy O, Froeschle J, Eskola J. *Streptococcus pneumoniae* capsular polysaccharide-diphtheria toxoid conjugate vaccine is immunogenic in early infancy and able to induce immunologic memory. Pediatr Infect Dis J 1998; 17:211–216.

69. Daum RS, Hogerman D, Rennels MB, Bewley K, Malinoski F, Rothstein E, Reisinger K, Block S, Keyserling H, Steinhoff M. Infant immunization with pneumococcal CRM$_{197}$ vaccines: effect of saccharide size on immonogenicity and interactions with simultaneously administered vaccines. J Infect Dis 1997; 176:445–455.

70. Dagan R, Melamed R, Muallem M, Piglansky L, Greenberg D, Abramson O, Mendelman PM, Bohidar N, Yagupsky P. Reduction of nasopharyngeal carriage of pneumococci during the second year of life by a heptavalent conjugate pneumococcal vaccine. J Infect Dis 1996; 174:1271–1278.

71. Nieminen T, Eskola J, Kayhty H. Pneumococcal conjugate vaccination in adults: circulating antibody secreting cell response and humoral antibody responses in saliva and in serum. Vaccine 1998; 16:630–636.

72. Schutze MP, Leclerc C, Jolivet M, Audibert F, Chedid L. Carrier-induced epitopic suppression, a major issue for synthetic vaccines. J Immunol 1985; 135:2319–2322.

73. Peeters CCAM, Tenbergen-Meekes A-M, Poolman JT, Beurret M, Zegers BJM, Rijkers GT. Effect of carrier priming on immunogenicity of saccharide–protein conjugate vaccines. Infect Immun 1991; 59:3504–3510.

74. Shelly MA, Jacoby H, Riley GJ, Graves BT, Pichichero M, Treanor JJ. Comparison of pneumococcal polysaccharide and CRM 197 conjugated pneumococcal oligosaccharide vaccines in young and elderly adults. Infect Immun 1997; 65:242–247.

75. Powers DC, Anderson EL, Lottenbach K, Mink CM. Reactogenicity and immunogenicity of a protein-conjugated pneumococcal oligosaccharide vaccine in older adults. J Infect Dis 1996; 173:1014–1018.

76. Tillett WS. Active and passive immunity to pneumococcus infection induced in rabbits by immunization with R pneumococci. J Exp Med 1928; 48:791–804.

77. Day HB. Preparation of pneumococcal species antigen. J Pathol Bacteriol 1934; 38:171.

78. Dubos RJ. Immunization of experimental animals with a soluble antigen extracted from pneumococci. J Exp Med 1938; 67:799–808.

79. Felton LD. Essential immunizing antigen of pneumococci. J Bacteriol 1937; 33:335–337.

80. Harley D. Species immunity to pneumococcus. Br J Exp Pathol 1935; 16:14–20.

81. Julianella L. Reactions of rabbits to intracutaneous injections of pneumococci and their products. II. Resistance to infection. J Exp Med 1930; 52:895.

82. McDaniel LS, Scott G, Kearney JF, Briles DE. Monoclonal antibodies against protease-sensitive pneumococcal antigens can protect mice from fatal infection with *Streptococcus pneumoniae*. J Exp Med 1984; 160:386–397.

83. Austrian R, Macleod OM. A type specific protein from pneumococcus. J Exp Med 1949; 89:439–450.

84. McDaniel LS, Scott G, Widenhofer K, Carroll JM, Briles DE. Analysis of a surface protein of *Streptococcus pneumoniae* recognised by protective monoclonal antibodies. Microb Pathog 1986; 1:519–531.

85. Briles DE, Yother J, McDaniel LS. Role of pneumococcal surface protein A in the virulence of *Streptococcus pneumoniae*. Rev Infect Dis 1988; 10(Suppl. 2):S372–S374.

86. McDaniel LS, Yother J, Vijayakumar M, McGarry L, Guild WR, Briles DE. Use of inser-

tional inactivation to facilitate studies of biological properties of pneumococcal surface protein A (PspA). J Exp Med 1987; 165:381–394.

87. McDaniel LS, Sheffield JS, Delucchi PA, Briles DE. PspA, a surface protein of *Streptococcus pneumoniae*, is capable of eliciting protection against pneumococci of more than one capsular type. Infect Immun 1991; 59:222–228.

88. Talkington DF, Crimmins DL, Voellinger DC, Yother J, Briles DE. A 43-kilodalton pneumococcal surface protein, PspA: isolation, protective abilities, and structural analysis of the amino-terminal sequence. Infect Immun 1991; 59:1285–1289.

89. Briles DE, King JD, Gray MA, McDaniel LS, Swiatlo E, Benton KA. PspA, a protection-eliciting pneumococcal protein: immunogenicity of isolated native PspA in mice. Vaccine 1996; 14:858–867.

90. Wu H-Y, Nahm MH, Guo Y, Russell MW, Briles DE. Intranasal immunization of mice with PspA (pneumococcal surface protein A) can prevent intranasal carriage, pulmonary infection, and sepsis with *Streptococcus pneumoniae*. J Infect Dis 1997; 175:839–846.

91. Yother J, Handsome GL, Briles DE. Truncated forms of PspA that are secreted from *Streptococcus pneumoniae* and their use in functional studies and cloning of the *psp*A gene. J Bacteriol 1992; 174:610–618.

92. Yother J, Briles DE. Structural properties and evolutionary relationships of PspA, a surface protein of *Streptococcus pneumoniae*, as revealed by sequence analysis. J Bacteriol 1992; 174:601–609.

93. McDaniel LS, Ralph BA, D.O. M, Briles DE. Localization of protection-eliciting epitopes on PspA of *Streptococcus pneumoniae* between amino acid residues 192 and 260. Microb Pathog 1994; 17:323–337.

94. Yother J, White JM. Novel surface attachment mechanism of the *Streptococcus pneumoniae* protein PspA. J Bacteriol 1994; 176:2976–2985.

95. Crain MJ, Waltman WD, Turner JS, Yother J, Talkington DF, McDaniel LS, Gray BM, Briles DE. Pneumococcal surface protein A (PspA) is serologically highly variable and is expressed by all clinically important capsular serotypes of *Streptococcus pneumoniae*. Infect Immun 1990; 58:3293–3299.

96. Berry AM, Yother J, Briles DE, Hansman D, Paton JC. Reduced virulence of a defined pneumolysin-negative mutant of *Streptococcus pneumoniae*. Infect Immun 1989; 57:2037–2042.

97. Berry AM, Paton JC, Hansman D. Effect of insertional inactivation of the genes encoding pneumolysin and autolysin on the virulence of *Streptococcus pneumoniae* type 3. Microb Pathog 1992; 12:87–93.

98. Benton KA, Everson MP, Briles DE. A pneumolysin-negative mutant of *Streptococcus pneu-*

moniae causes chronic bacteremia rather than acute sepsis in mice. Infect Immun 1995; 63:448–455.

99. Mitchell TJ, Andrew PW, Saunders FK, Smith AN, Boulnois GJ. Complement activation and antibody binding by pneumolysin via a region of the toxin homologous to a human acute-phase protein. Mol Microbiol 1991; 5:1883–1888.

100. Johnson MK, Geoffroy C, Alouf JE. Binding of cholesterol by sulfhydryl-activated cytolysins. Infect Immun 1980; 27:97–101.

101. Rubins JB, Charboneau D, Fasching C, Berry AM, Paton JC, Alexander JE, Andrew PW, Mitchell TJ, Janoff EN. Distinct roles for pneumolysin's cytotoxic and complement activities in the pathogenesis of pneumococcal pneumonia. Am J Respir Crit Care Med 1996; 153:1339–1346.

102. Rubins JB, Duane PG, Clawson D, Charboneau D, Young J, Niewoehner DE. Toxicity of pneumolysin to pulmonary alveolar epithelial cells. Infect Immun 1993; 61:1352–1358.

103. Rubins JB, Duane PG, Charboneau D, Janoff EN. Toxicity of pneumolysin to pulmonary endothelial cells in vitro. Infect Immun 1992; 60:1740–1746.

104. Feldman C, Munro NC, Jeffrey PK, Wilson R, Mitchell TJ, Boulnois GJ, Todd HC, Andrew PW, Guerreiro D, Cole PJ, Rohde JAL. Pneumolysin induces the salient features of pneumococcal infection in the rat lung in vivo. Am J Respir Cell Mol Biol 1991; 5:416–423.

105. Boulnois GJ, Paton JC, Mitchell TJ, Andrew PW. Structure and function of pneumolysin, the multifunctional, thiol-activated toxin of *Streptococcus pneumoniae*. Mol Microbiol 1991; 5: 2611–2616.

106. Kanclerski K, Blomquist S, Granstrom M, Mollby R. Serum-antibodies to pneumolysin in patients with pneumonia. J Clin Microbiol 1988; 26:96–100.

107. Virolainen A, Jero J, Kayhty H, Karma P, Eskola J, Leinonen M. Nasopharyngeal antibodies to pneumococcal pneumolysin in children with acute otitis media. Clin Diagn Lab Immunol 1995; 2:704–707.

108. Amdahl BM, Rubins JB, Daley CL, Gilks CF, Hopewell PC, Janoff EN. Impaired immunity to pneumolysin during human immunodeficiency virus infection in the United States and Africa. Am J Respir Crit Care Med 1995; 152:2000–2004.

109. Virolainen A, Jero J, Kayhty H, Karma P, Leinonen M, Eskola J. Antibodies to pneumolysin and pneumococcal capsular polysaccharides in middle ear fluid of children with acute otitis media. Acta Otolaryngol 1995; 115:796–803.

110. Paton JC, Lock RA, Hansman DJ. Effect of immunization with pneumolysin on survival time of mice challenged with *Streptococcus pneumoniae*. Infect Immun 1983; 40:548–552.

111. Paton JC, Lock RA, Lee CJ, Li JP, Berry AM, Mitchell TJ, Andrew PW, Hansman D, Boulnois GJ. Purification and immunogenicity of genetically obtained pneumolysin toxoids and their conjugation to *Streptococcus pneumoniae* type 19F polysaccharide. Infect Immun 1991; 59: 2297–2304.

112. Alexander JE, Lock RA, Peeters CCAM, Poolman JT, Andrew PW, Mitchell TJ, Hansman D, Paton JC. Immunization of mice with pneumolysin toxoid confers a significant degree of protection against at least nine serotypes of *Streptococcus pneumoniae*. Infect Immun 1994; 62:5683–5688.

113. Kuo J, Douglas M, Ree HK, Lindberg AA. Characterization of a recombinant pneumolysin and its use as a protein carrier for pneumococcal type 18C conjugate vaccines. Infect Immun 1995; 63:2706–2713.

114. Camara M, Mitchell TJ, Andrew PW, Boulnois GJ. *Streptococcus pneumoniae* produces at least two distinct enzymes with neuraminidase activity: cloning and expression of a second neuraminidase gene in *Escherichia coli*. Infect Immun 1991; 59:2856–2858.

115. Berry AM, Paton JC, Glare EM, Hansman D, Catcheside DEA. Cloning and expression of the pneumococcal neuraminidase gene in *Escherichia coli*. Gene 1988; 71:299–305.

116. Camara M, Boulnois GJ, Andrew PW, Mitchell TJ. A neuraminidase from *Streptococcus pneumoniae* has the features of a surface protein. Infect Immun 1994; 62:3688–3695.

117. Lock RA, Paton JC, Hansman D. Comparative efficacy of pneumococcal neuraminidase and pneumolysin as immunogens protective against *Streptococcus pneumoniae*. Microb Pathog 1988; 5:461–467.

118. Berry AM, Lock RA, Paton JC. Cloning and characterization of *nan*B, a second *Streptococcus pneumoniae* neuraminidase gene, and purification of the NanB enzyme from recombinant *Escherichia coli*. J Bacteriol 1996; 178: 4854–4860.

119. Tuomanen E, Liu H, Hengstler B, Zak O, Tomasz A. The induction of meningeal inflammation by components of the pneumococcal cell wall. J Infect Dis 1985; 151:859–868.

120. Geelen S, Bhattacharyya C, Tuomanen E. The cell wall mediates pneumococcal attachment to and cytopathology in human endothelial cells. Infect Immun 1993; 61:1538–1543.

121. Romero A, Lopez R, Garcia P. Sequence of the *Streptococcus pneumoniae* bacteriophage HB-3 amidase reveals high homology with the major host autolysin. J Bacteriol 1990; 172:5064–5070.

122. Mosser JL, Tomasz A. Choline-containing teichoic acid as a structural component of pneumococcal cell wall and its role in sensitivity to lysis by an autolytic enzyme. J Biol Chem 1970; 245:287–290.

123. Diaz E, Lopez R, Garcia JL. Role of the major pneumococcal autolysin in the atypical response of a clinical isolate of *Streptococcus pneumoniae*. J Bacteriol 1992; 174:5508–5515.

124. Canvin JR, Marvin AP, Sivakumaran M, Paton JC, Boulnois GJ, Andrew PW, Mitchell TJ. The role of pneumolysin and autolysin in the pathology of pneumonia and septicemia in mice infected with a type 2 pneumococcus. J Infect Dis 1995; 172:119–123.

125. Lock RA, Hansman D, Paton JC. Comparative efficacy of autolysin and pneumolysin as immunogens protecting mice against infection by *Streptococcus pneumoniae*. Microb Pathog 1992; 12:137–143.

126. Gillespie SH, McHugh TD, Ayres H, Dickens A, Efstratiou A, Whiting GC. Allelic variation in *Streptococcus pneumoniae* autolysin (*N*-acetyl muramoyl-L-alanine amidase). Infect Immun 1997; 65:3936–3938.

127. Sampson JS, O'Connor SP, Stinson AR, Tharpe JA, Russell H. Cloning and nucleotide sequence analysis of *psa*A, the *Streptococcus pneumoniae* gene encoding a 37-kilodalton protein homologous to previously reported *Streptococcus* sp. adhesins. Infect Immun 1994; 62:319–324.

128. Berry AM, Paton JC. Sequence heterogeneity of PsaA, a 37-kilodalton putative adhesin essential for virulence of *Streptococcus pneumoniae*. Infect Immun 1996; 64:5255–5262.

129. Talkington DF, Brown BG, Tharpe JA, Koenig A, Russell H. Protection of mice against fatal pneumococcal challenge by immunization with pneumococcal surface adhesin A (PsaA). Microb Pathog 1996; 21:17–22.

130. Courtney HS. Degradation of connective tissue proteins by serine proteases from *Streptococcus pneumoniae*. Biochem Biophys Res Commun 1991; 175:1023–1028.

131. Berry AM, Lock RA, Thomas SM, Rajan DP, Hansman D, Paton JC. Cloning and nucleotide sequence of the *Streptococcus pneumoniae* hyaluronidase gene and purification of the enzyme from recombinant *Escherichia coli*. Infect Immun 1994; 62:1101–1108.

132. Mulks MH, Kornfeld SJ, Plaut AG. Specific proteolysis of human IgA by *Streptococcus pneumoniae* and *Haemophilus influenzae*. J Infect Dis 1980; 141:450–456.

133. Hammerschmidt S, Talay SR, Brandtzaeg P, Chhatwal GS. SpsA, a novel pneumococcal surface protein with specific binding to secretory immunoglobulin A and secretory component. Mol Microbiol 1997; 25:1113–1124.

134. Angel CS, Ruzek M, Hostetter MK. Degradation of C3 by *Streptococcus pneumoniae*. J Infect Dis 1994; 170:600–608.

135. Hamel J, Martin D, Brodeur BR. Heat shock response and heat shock protein antigens of *Streptococcus pneumoniae*. In: American Society for Microbiology General Meeting, New Orleans,

LA. Washington, DC: American Society for Microbiology, 1996; Abstract no. B-270.

136. Rosenow C, Ryan P, Weiser JN, Johnson S, Fontan P, Ortqvist A, Masure HR. Contribution of novel choline-binding proteins to adherence, colonization and immunogenicity of *Streptococcus pneumoniae*. Mol Microbiol 1997; 25:819–829.

137. Briles DE, Nahm M, Schroer K, Davie J, Baker P, Kearney J, Barletta R. Antiphosphocholine antibodies found in normal mouse serum are protective against intravenous infection with type 3 *Streptococcus pneumoniae*. J Exp Med 1981; 153:694–705.

138. Szu SC, Clarke S, Robbins JB. Protection against pneumococcal infection in mice conferred by phosphocholine-binding antibodies: specificity of the phosphocholine binding and relation to several types. Infect Immun 1983; 39:993–999.

139. Briles DE, Forman C, Crain MC. Mouse antibody to phosphocholine can protect mice from infection with mouse-virulent human isolates of *Streptococcus pneumoniae*. Infect Immun 1992; 60:1957–1962.

140. Wallick S, Claflin L, Briles DE. Resistance to *Streptococcus pneumoniae* is induced by phosphocholine-protein conjugate. J Immunol 1983; 130:2871–2875.

141. Briles DE, Forman C, Hudak S, Claflin JL. The effects of idiotype on the ability of IgG1 antiphosphorylcholine antibodies to protect mice from fatal infection with *Streptococcus pneumoniae*. Eur J Immunol 1984; 14:1027–1030.

142. Briles DE, Forman C, Hudak S, Claflin JL. Anti-PC antibodies of the T15 idiotype are optimally protective against *Streptococcus pneumoniae*. J Exp Med 1982; 156:1177–1185.

143. Kenny JJ, Guelde G, Fisher RT, Longo DL. Induction of phosphocholine-specific antibodies in X-linked immune deficient mice: in vivo protection against a *Streptococcus pneumoniae* challenge. Int Immunol 1993; 6:561–568.

144. Briles DE, Claflin JL, Schroer K, Forman C. Mouse IgG3 antibodies are highly protective against infection with *Streptococcus pneumoniae*. Nature 1981; 294:88–90.

145. McDaniel LS, Benjamin Jr, WH, Forman C, Briles DE. Blood clearance by anti-phosphocholine antibodies as a mechanism of protection in experimental pneumococcal bacteremia. J Immunol 1984; 133:3308–3312.

146. Musher DM, Watson DA, Baughn RE. Does naturally acquired IgG antibody to cell wall polysaccharide protect human subjects against pneumococcal infection? J Infect Dis 1990; 161:736–740.

147. Nielsen SV, Skov Sorensen UB, Henrichsen J. Antibodies against pneumococcal C-polysaccharide are not protective. Microb Pathog 1993; 14:299–305.

148. McDaniel LS, Waltman WD, Gray B, Briles DE. A protective monoclonal antibody that reacts with a novel antigen of pneumococcal teichoic acid. Microb Pathog 1987; 3:249–260.

149. Brandtzaeg P. Humoral immune response patterns of human mucosae: induction and relation to respiratory tract infections. J Infect Dis 1992; 165(Suppl 1):S167–S176.

150. Briles DE, Tart RC, Wu H-Y, Ralph BA, Russell MW, McDaniel LS. Systemic and mucosal protective immunity to pneumococcal surface protein A. Ann NY Acad Sci 1996; 797: 118–126.

151. Wu H-Y, Virolainen A, Mathews B, King J, Russell MW, Briles DE. Establishment of a *Streptococcus pneumoniae* nasopharyngeal colonization model in adult mice. Microb Pathog 1997; 23:127–137.

152. Yamamoto M, McDaniel LS, Kawabata K, Briles DE, Jackson RJ, McGhee JR, Kiyono H. Oral immunization with PspA elicits protective humoral immunity against *Streptococcus pneumoniae* infection. Infect Immun 1997; 65: 640–644.

153. Robbins JB, Austrian R, Lee C-J, Rastogi SC, Schiffman G, Henrichsen J, Makela PH, Broome CV, Facklam RR, Tiesjema RH, Parke Jr, JC. Considerations for formulating the second-generation pneumococcal capsular polysaccharide vaccine with emphasis on cross-reactive types within groups. J Infect Dis 1983; 148:1136–1159.

Index